CLINICAL PHARMACOLOGY
AND THERAPEUTICS FOR THE
VETERINARY TECHNICIAN

CLINICAL PHARMACOLOGY AND THERAPEUTICS FOR THE VETERINARY TECHNICIAN

THIRD EDITION

ROBERT L. BILL, DVM, PhD

Veterinary Physiology and Pharmacology
School of Veterinary Medicine
Purdue University
West Lafayette, Indiana

With 55 illustrations

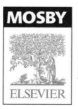

MOSBY

ELSEVIER

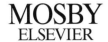

11830 Westline Industrial Drive
St. Louis, Missouri 63146

Notice

Knowledge and best practice in pharmacology are constantly changing. As new research and experience broaden our knowledge, changes in practice, treatment, and drug therapy may become necessary or appropriate. Readers are advised to check the most current information provided (i) on procedures featured or (ii) by the manufacturer of each product to be administered, to verify the recommended dose of the practitioner, relying on his or her own experience and knowledge of the patient, to make diagnoses, to determine dosages and the best treatment for each individual patient, and to take all appropriate safety precautions. To the fullest extent of the law, neither the publisher nor the author assumes any liability for any injury and/or damage to persons or property arising out or related to any use of the material contained in this book.

The Publisher

Previous editions copyrighted 1997, 1993

Library of Congress Cataloging-in-Publication Data
Bill, Robert.
    Clinical pharmacology and therapeutics for the veterinary technician / Robert L. Bill. -- 3rd ed.
        p. ; cm.
    Rev. ed. of: Pharmacology for veterinary technicians. 2nd ed. 1997.
    Includes bibliographical references and index.
    ISBN-13: 978-0-323-01113-6   ISBN-10: 0-323-01113-6
    1. Veterinary pharmacology. I. Bill, Robert. Pharmacology for veterinary technicians. II. Title.
    [DNLM: 1. Veterinary Drugs--pharmacology. 2. Veterinary Drugs--therapeutic use. 3. Animal
    Technicians. SF 917 B596c 2006]
    SF915.B55 2006
    636.089'51--dc22   2006044857

ISBN-13: 978-0-323-01113-6
ISBN-10: 0-323-01113-6

Publishing Director: Linda L. Duncan
Publisher: Penny Rudolph
Managing Editor: Teri Merchant
Publishing Services Manager: Pat Joiner
Project Manager: David Stein
Design Director: Amy Buxton

Printed in the United States of America

Last digit is the print number: 9 8 7 6 5 4 3 2

To all veterinary technology students, past, present, and future.

Preface

THE CHANGING ROLE OF VETERINARY TECHNICIANS

The expectations for today's veterinary technician in terms of the technician's level of performance, degree of medical understanding, and ability to make independent decisions are different than for the technician we educated 10 or 15 years ago. When the profession began, the primary role of the veterinary technician was to be an extension of the veterinarian's hands, and therefore the technician was used primarily for completing manual procedures and tasks.

Today, with the increasing sophistication of veterinary care, contemporary veterinary practice has shifted toward utilizing the veterinary technician not only to complete nursing/surgical techniques quickly and efficiently, but also to work more independently to assess and monitor patient status, to implement therapeutic protocols, and to obtain or perform needed diagnostic procedures. Today's well-utilized veterinary technician often works on a team with the veterinarian and the veterinary assistants and depends heavily on medical knowledge, problem-solving skills, management skills, and decision making skills to carry out his or her responsibilities. Thus today's veterinary technician must *know and think* as well as "do."

A greater understanding of the medicine and science behind the diagnostics, therapeutics, and surgical interventions used in veterinary medicine is essential for today's veterinary technician to effectively assess his or her patient's current status, anticipate the patient's immediate medical and nursing needs, know what the veterinarian is likely to need next, and be one step ahead of the progression of the patient's condition. Knowledge of clinical pharmacology and therapeutics helps the veterinary technician function in this manner.

The breadth and depth of information in clinical pharmacology and therapeutics at the veterinary technician level have increased as the sophistication of veterinary medicine has advanced. When the first edition of this veterinary technician pharmacology text was published in 1993, it was the only one of its kind. Today there are many texts on pharmacology and therapeutics targeted towards veterinary technicians, as well as regular features in the veterinary technician journals that present current information on drugs and therapeutic agents. Originally titled *Pharmacology for Veterinary Technicians*, this edition has been appropriately re-titled to reflect the need for *understanding* the clinical applications of these drugs.

Like its predecessors, this edition provides understandable explanations of the "how" and "why" behind drugs, their actions, their mechanisms, and their problems. In this third edition, all drug groups have been updated to reflect changes in both the therapeutic agents themselves and the medical philosophies that determine how these drugs are used in different species. New to this edition are several case studies that illustrate how the information presented in the text translates to "real world" examples. Also new to this edition are the self-assessment test questions at the end of the chapters that provide an excellent review of pharmacology and therapeutic knowledge for certification examinations. A convenient answer key for all of the questions is included to assist in the reader's review of the content and for self-testing.

Instructors will find the "systems" organization of the chapters easy to follow and to modify as needed to fit their own curriculum or program emphasis. The questions at the back of the chapters can readily be modified to create an examination for the classroom while still providing the students with a review of the content in each chapter. Supplemental instructional materials that follow the outline of the textbook are also available from the author.

My ultimate goal with this text is to help improve veterinary care, animal health, and patient well-being by helping veterinary technicians understand how and why drugs work the way they do. By using this text to understand how drugs can be safely used and how potential problems can be avoided, a veterinary technician will be able to provide better care for his or her patients, as well as to help educate the owners who love these patients.

"As veterinary professionals, our education is not for our benefit, but for the benefit of the patients we serve."

Pete Bill

Contents

4 DRUGS AFFECTING THE GASTROINTESTINAL TRACT, 93

5 DRUGS AFFECTING THE CARDIOVASCULAR SYSTEM, 123

6 DRUGS AFFECTING THE RESPIRATORY SYSTEM, 157

7 DRUGS AFFECTING THE ENDOCRINE SYSTEM, 175

8 DRUGS AFFECTING THE NERVOUS SYSTEM: ANALGESICS, ANESTHETICS, AND STIMULANTS, 203

9 DRUGS AFFECTING THE NERVOUS SYSTEM: ANTICONVULSANTS AND BEHAVIOR-MODIFYING DRUGS, 233

12 ANTIPARASITICS, 305

13 ANTIINFLAMMATORY DRUGS, 343

Chapter 1

Introduction to Veterinary Pharmacology and Therapeutic Applications

key terms

active ingredient
adverse drug reaction
ampule
caplets
chemical name
contraindication
controlled substance
depot drug
dosage
dosage form
dosage regimen
dose
drug package insert
elixir
emulsion
enteric-coated tablet

extract
extra-label use
formulary
gel caps
generic equivalent
generic name
indication
inert ingredient
injectable dosage form
liniment
lotion
molded tablets
multidose vial
nonproprietary name
off-label use
ointment

paste
precaution
proprietary name
repository form
side effect
single-dose vial
solution
suspension
sustained-release
    formulation
syrup
tincture
topical application
trade name
troche
warning

After studying this chapter, the veterinary technician should be able to:

1. Describe why a veterinary technician needs to know information about drugs

2. Explain what the different types of drug names are

3. Recognize the characteristics of different solid and liquid dosage formulations

4. Identify several different sources of drug information

5. Explain the significance of the terminology used in drug references to describe drugs

6. List and describe the criteria for acceptable extra-label use of drugs

7. Know how to report adverse drug reactions

ROLE AND RESPONSIBILITIES OF TODAY'S VETERINARY TECHNICIAN AND TECHNOLOGIST

"Today's veterinary technician is a professional, and as such, has the responsibility to understand the reasons and the expected outcomes for the treatments they perform. Today's veterinary technician is more than a skilled set of hands. Today's veterinary technician must know how to critically evaluate, problem solve, think, and adapt to their patient's needs."

Pete Bill, DVM, PhD during a panel presentation on the topic of veterinary technician and paraprofessional utilization at the American Association of Colleges of Veterinary Medicine meeting, Washington, DC, April 2, 2001.

Veterinary medicine as a whole continues to become more sophisticated in all aspects of diagnostics, understanding of disease, surgery, and therapeutics. Accordingly, veterinary technicians today must be much more sophisticated in their understanding of veterinary medicine than they were 10 years ago. Although technicians are still legally prohibited from making diagnoses, performing surgeries, rendering prognoses, and prescribing treatments, today's veterinary technician must understand why the diagnosis was made, why the surgery was performed, why the prognosis was rendered, and why the treatment was prescribed.

In the area of clinical pharmacology and therapeutics, veterinary technicians can no longer simply know the names of medications or by which route drugs are administered; they must understand the "why" of clinical pharmacology and therapeutics behind the medications. As veterinary medicine continues to evolve, the veterinary technician will increasingly be the professional team member who monitors anesthesia induction and recovery, checks the status of hospitalized animals on medications, administers treatments under the veterinarian's directions, and interacts with clients on advising or fielding questions related to medications. In that capacity, the veterinary technician may be the first person to identify that an in-house patient is showing signs of anaphylactic reaction (a type of allergic reaction) to the medication being prescribed. The veterinary technician may be the one who detects during a client telephone conversation that the pet is showing early signs of digoxin (a common cardiovascular medication) toxicity. Veterinary technicians may find themselves in situations in which they are expected to explain issues pertaining to drug residues in livestock and how that affects human health and safety in the food society eats. But veterinary technicians cannot function fully in this role on the professional veterinary team unless they understand the decisions leading to selection of the treatments, the underlying physiology of the drug's mechanisms of action, and the means by which the *side effects* or adverse reactions manifest themselves as clinical signs. Today's veterinary technician has to *know* as well as *do*.

The goal of this text is to help students become familiar with the "why" of clinical pharmacology and therapeutics used in veterinary medicine.

ALL DRUGS ARE POISONS

Every drug is potentially a poison. The way a drug is administered often makes the difference between its ability to save life and its ability to take life away. For example, small amounts of poisonous arsenic-type compounds are used to safely treat heartworms in dogs. Drugs that might otherwise devastate an animal's (or person's) bone marrow can be successfully used with the appropriate *dose* to kill deadly cancer cells. A drug that is perfectly safe to administer by injection into the muscle could cause a severe reaction if injected intravenously. The drug acetaminophen (Tylenol), which is safe in human beings and tolerated in dogs, can easily kill a cat. The amount and method of administration of a medication can potentially determine whether a drug cures or kills.

All members of the veterinary team, which includes the veterinary technician, must guard against complacency when administering common medications to patients. Using particular medications over and over again can lead to forgetting that the next animal could potentially have a violent, allergic reaction to it, or that improper administration could damage an animal's kidneys, liver, or other vital body system.

Drugs are not "silver bullets" to be dispensed in a "cookbook" manner. A certain disease is not always treated the same way with the same drug. Each animal is different; because the normal physiology of an animal is altered by disease, each animal may require an adjustment of *dosage* or kind of medication on the basis of breed, sex, disease state, and various preexisting conditions. Any dosages listed for a medication are an estimation of the amount of drug that should work on most of the population of animals. But some animals will not fall into this ideal range. Therefore the state of the animal and the characteristics of the drug should be considered each time a medication is administered. Veterinary professionals have a responsibility to be vigilant about correctly calculating doses, adhering to a proper dose schedule, consistently using the appropriate method or route of administration of the medication, and being aware and observant for possible side effects or adverse reactions.

TERMINOLOGY USED IN DESCRIBING THERAPEUTIC AGENTS

DRUG NAMES

Drugs are generally referred to by three different names (Figure 1-1). The *chemical name*, such as D(-)-α-amino-p-hydroxybenzyl-penicillin trihydrate, describes the chemical composition of a drug (in this case, amoxicillin) and is used by chemists and pharmacologists but is of little practical use for the veterinary professional. The *nonproprietary name*, also called the *generic name*, is a more concise name given to the specific chemical compound. Examples of nonproprietary names include aspirin, acetaminophen, and amoxicillin. The nonproprietary names are usually listed as the *active ingredient* on drug labels and can be found on the drug labels from many different drug manufacturers. In contrast, the *proprietary name*, or *trade name*, is a unique name a manufacturer gives its particular brand of a drug. Examples of proprietary or trade names include Tylenol, Lasix, Valium, and Amoxi-Tabs. Because trade names are proper nouns, they are capitalized. The names are followed by the marks ® or ™ to signify that the trade name is a registered trademark and cannot be legally used by other manufacturers. Because

CHEMICAL NAME	NONPROPRIETARY NAME	PROPRIETARY/TRADE NAME
D(-)-α-amino-p-hydroxybenzyl-penicillin trihydrate	amoxicillin	Amoxi-Drop® Biomox® Robamox-V®
[(3-phenoxyphenyl) methyl cis-trans-3-(2,2-dichloroethenyl)-2,2-dimethylcyclopropanecarboxylate)]	permethrin insecticide	Atroban® Defend® Flysect®
dl 2-(o-chlorophenyl)-2-(methylamino) cyclohexanone hydrochloride	ketamine hydrochloride	Ketaset® Vetalar®

Figure 1-1 Drug chemical, generic, and trade names.

many drug manufacturers produce similar products with the same active ingredient as their competitors, a generic drug may be sold under multiple trade names. For example, the antibiotic amoxicillin is manufactured by several different companies, each of which uses its own trade name: Amoxi-Drop (Pfizer, Inc., New York, NY), Robamox-V (Fort Dodge, Overland Park, Kan.), Biomox (Virbac, Peakhurst, NSW, Australia).

When a drug company develops, patents, and completes the extensive testing required to obtain Food and Drug Administration (FDA) approval to sell a new drug, the company has the exclusive rights to manufacture this drug for a number of years. During that time, no other drug manufacturer can produce the same drug. This theoretically allows the drug company time to sell enough of the new drug to recover the costs of the research, development, and testing required to bring the drug to market.

After a number of years the exclusive rights to manufacture the drug expire, and other companies are then permitted to produce the drug. Drugs produced by companies other than the original developer are called *generic equivalent* drugs because they have properties equivalent to those of the original compound. Generic equivalents are usually sold at a much lower price than the original manufacturer's product because the generic manufacturer did not have to underwrite development of the original drug.

As a general rule, generic drugs are equivalent drugs and are as effective as the original patented compound. On occasion, however, differences in the manufacturing process produce minor fluctuations in the physical characteristics of the generic drug's tablet or capsule composition. Because of these minor differences between the original tablet form and the generic drug tablet form, and because many of these drugs are developed for use in human beings, differences in effectiveness of the drug may occur in the veterinary patient. For example, one *dosage form* may be formulated into a tablet that uses a different binder to hold the tablet's shape. However, different binders may affect the rate at which the tablet dissolves. Human beings have a relatively long intestinal tract, so small differences in time required for dissolving may not be significant. However, in the dog or cat, which has a shorter intestinal tract, the longer time to dissolve results in less of the drug being in a form that can be absorbed. Hence the difference in the physical composition of the dosage form could result in variable effectiveness of the drug from different manufacturers even though the amount of active ingredient is identical.

DOSE VERSUS DOSAGE

The terms "dose" and "dosage" seem to be used interchangeably in medicine. Technically, a dose is the amount of drug that is administered at one time to the patient. Thus 1 mL or 2 tablets are considered doses for an animal. Dosage

CLINICAL APPLICATION
Switching Medicines Produces Seizures

A 10-pound, 7-year-old, FS (female spay) miniature poodle (Jackie) presented with a history of increased seizure activity. The dog had been diagnosed with idiopathic epilepsy 2 years previously. Idiopathic means "cause unknown"; idiopathic epilepsy is a common default diagnosis for recurrent seizure activity. Jackie had been placed on phenobarbital, a common anticonvulsant medication used to control seizures, at a dose of 15 mg every 12 hours. Jackie's veterinarian drew blood every 6 months from Jackie to determine the concentration of phenobarbital in the blood (plasma) and to verify that the dose given was achieving concentrations in the blood sufficient to control seizures. The plasma concentrations of phenobarbital were always within acceptable concentrations. Jackie did well for 16 months but then started to show signs of seizure activity again. The veterinarian checked another plasma concentration of phenobarbital and found it significantly lower than the previously checked concentrations. The veterinarian increased the dose to 30 mg every 12 hours, based on the new plasma concentrations. Doubling the dose kept Jackie's seizures well under control for 4 months. Then Jackie's owners reported that Jackie was acting more sedated and lethargic and would occasionally be ataxic (wobble a bit in the hind end). The veterinarian examined Jackie and took another plasma concentration of phenobarbital. To his surprise, the plasma concentration of phenobarbital was significantly higher than previous concentrations and sufficiently high enough to produce signs of sedation and ataxia. He ordered Jackie's owners to skip a dose of phenobarbital (to allow concentrations to drop lower) and reduce the dose to the original 15 mg every 12 hours. The sedation and ataxia resolved by the next day. A recheck of plasma concentrations revealed drug levels had returned to the normal, acceptable range. What had happened?

Careful questioning of Jackie's owners and review of inventory records of the veterinary hospital revealed that the increase in seizure activity occurred 2 weeks after Jackie's owners had picked up a new refill of phenobarbital tablets from the hospital. The onset of sedation 4 months later had occurred 2 days after Jackie's owners had picked up another refill. Examination of inventory records revealed that the hospital had switched from one generic phenobarbital drug to another manufacturer because the second generic was cheaper. The second generic was likely dispensed to Jackie's owners at the refill that occurred just before the return of the seizure activity. The plasma concentrations at that time confirmed that less drug was present in the body despite Jackie's owners' strict adherence to the dose schedule. Adjustment of the dose of the second generic temporarily solved the problem. However, when the hospital inventory of the second generic ran out, the hospital ordered more of the first generic that it had always carried. The first generic was then dispensed to Jackie's owners and, when dosed at the higher adjusted dose, caused the sedation and ataxia associated with phenobarbital overdose. Confirmation of higher phenobarbital concentrations was verified, indicating more of the drug was entering the body. The only explanation was the generic drug's form. The first generic drug was apparently better absorbed by Jackie than the second, even though both tablets contained the identical amount of phenobarbital.

What should be learned from this situation: For animals on long-term treatments such as seizure control, thyroid supplementation, or long-term chronic disease, selecting the correct generic is not as important as consistently providing the same generic drug. Switching brands based on whatever is the most inexpensive at the time may invite problems. For many animals switching does not cause a clinically apparent change; however, many more do show some significant variability between generic brands, as Jackie did.

refers to the general amount that any animal or patient should be given over time. Dosage might also be applied to a general description of how a drug is to be administered. For example, 10 mg/kg or 1 mL/lb are dosages. "Apply to bandages as directed by a veterinarian" would also be an example of a dosage. If the dosage of 10 mg/kg is used for a 5-kg dog, the dose would be 50 mg.

Dosages are often referred to as *dosage regimens*. An example of a dosage regimen would be "give 2 mg/kg every 8 hours for 10 days." In this dosage regimen, there are 8 hours between each dose. If the animal gains weight, the dose would increase, but the dosage would not because it was based on the amount of drug per kilogram of body weight.

Although these definitions seem fairly easy to understand, the terms dose and dosage are often used in ways that seem synonymous. The important thing is for the veterinary professional to be aware of the differences and definitions for these two terms and how to safely follow the dosage regimen to calculate an accurate dose properly.

DOSAGE FORMS

A drug's dosage form is the description of its physical appearance or type. Tablets, capsules, *solutions*, and *liniments* are types of dosage forms. The description of the dosage form often indicates the method by which the drug is administered. Solid dosage forms for delivering the drug include tablets or *caplets*, which are powdered drugs compressed into disks or capsule-shaped tablets. Tablet dosage forms exist in many variations other than the standard white pill. For example, *molded tablets* are soft, chewable tablets in which the powdered drug is mixed with lactose, sucrose, or dextrose and a flavoring to encourage the patient to chew the tablet. Examples of molded tablets include chewable vitamins and chewable heartworm preventive. Often tablets intended for swallowing without chewing are coated with a glossy, sugar compound used

to disguise the taste of the medication, make administration of the tablet easier (coated tablets slide more readily), or identify the tablet concentration (e.g., the 400-mg tablet might be green and the 200-mg tablet red). The tablet coating may serve other functions. For example, *enteric-coated tablets* have a special covering over the powdered drug that protects the drug from the harsh acidic environment of the stomach and prevents dissolution of the tablet until it enters the more alkaline environment of the small intestine.

Tablets or caplets can come in special *sustained-release formulations*. These oral dosage forms are designed to release only small amounts of drug into the intestinal lumen over an extended period. In human beings, this allows the drug to be absorbed over a longer period, thereby reducing the number of times the drug must be administered each day. Unfortunately, many oral sustained-release medications developed for use in human beings fail to work as planned in veterinary patients because the intestinal tract transit time for dogs and cats is quicker. Thus a sustained-release tablet may not release all the medication before it passes beyond the area of absorption in the intestinal tract. Sustained-release and enteric-coated tablets or caplets should not be broken into halves or sections. Breaking an enteric-coated tablet would allow the drug within the tablet to be exposed to the damaging acidic stomach environment. Breaking a sustained-release tablet ruins the sustained-release nature of the formulation, which depends on uniform dissolution of the tablet from the outside surface inward.

Gel caps (formerly, and sometimes still, called capsules) are powdered drugs placed in a gelatin capsule. The gelatin becomes soft and readily dissolves in the stomach, releasing the powdered drug. *Troches*, or lozenges, are powdered drugs incorporated into a hard, candy-like tablet. These dosage forms are intended to be held in the mouth and slowly dissolved, releasing small amounts of drug as they dissolve (e.g., cough tablets and throat lozenges). Because veterinary patients are unlikely to cooperate and hold lozenges in their mouths long enough to dissolve, this dosage form is not used in veterinary medicine.

Unlike orally administered drugs, suppositories are dosage forms designed to be placed in the rectum, where they dissolve and release the drug to be absorbed across the membranes of the intestinal wall. This route of administration is used in animals or people who cannot tolerate ingesting drugs by mouth (e.g., in cases of persistent vomiting).

Liquid forms of drugs are usually called solutions or *suspensions*. A drug solution is a drug completely dissolved in a liquid vehicle that does not settle out, or precipitate, if left standing. In contrast, a suspension contains drug particles that are suspended, but not dissolved, in the liquid vehicle. Suspended drug particles usually settle to the bottom of an undisturbed container, requiring the veterinary technician to shake the container to ensure that the drug is evenly resuspended in the liquid and provides accurate drug dosing.

Suspensions and solutions can be further classified into different types based on the liquid in which the drug is suspended or dissolved. For example, an *emulsion* is a suspension in which the drug is mixed with a liquid fat or an oil. *Syrups*, such as cough syrups, are solutions in which the drug is dissolved in sugar water (e.g., 85% sucrose). The sugar in syrups is used to disguise the unpleasant taste of a drug and is a popular dosage form for children's medications. Unlike the sweet-tasting syrups, *elixirs* are orally administered solutions of drug dissolved in alcohol. Elixirs are used for drugs that do not readily dissolve in water; therefore they should not be diluted or mixed with water because the alcohol and water will separate into distinct layers. The strong alcohol taste usually makes administration of these drugs to veterinary patients difficult.

Tinctures are alcohol solutions meant for application to the skin (*topical application*). Tincture of iodine, for example, is iodine in an alcohol base that is dabbed on the skin as an antiseptic. Other topical dosage forms include liniments, which are drugs dissolved or suspended in an oil base and applied to the skin by rubbing, or *lotions*, which are drug suspensions or solutions that are dabbed, brushed, or dripped onto the skin without rubbing. An example of a common lotion is poison ivy lotion, which is swabbed onto the surface of the skin with a cotton ball.

Semisolid dosage forms for external use include *ointments* and creams. Ointments and creams can be either suspensions or solutions and are designed to liquefy at body temperatures. By liquefying, the ointment or cream can spread more readily across or into an area such as the ear canal. In contrast to semiliquid creams and ointments, *pastes* are semisolid, orally administered dosage forms that tend to keep their semisolid form at body temperature. Pastes are commonly packaged in large plastic syringes for administering oral deworming medications to horses, cattle, sheep, and occasionally dogs. Gels are drugs suspended in a semisolid or jelly-like form, such as toothpaste.

Injectable dosage forms are administered by a needle and syringe. Injectables are often referred to by the type of container in which they are supplied. For example, *ampules* are small, airtight glass containers; the neck of the ampule is broken to access the drug. Drugs contained within ampules are meant to be used completely at one time because the ampule cannot be resealed, and the drug contained in the ampule often does not have any additional chemicals to retard the growth of bacteria or other contaminants. Vials are glass bottles with rubber stoppers through which the drug can be withdrawn with a sterile needle. Vials may be *multidose vials*, in which multiple doses can be withdrawn over time, or *single-dose vials*, in which all the drug is used at one time. Most injectable antibiotic, anesthetic, antiinflammatory, and other commonly used drugs in veterinary medicine come in the multidose vial form. The single-dose vial is used with vaccines. The rubber stopper on multidose vials should be kept clean because reinsertion of needles through a contaminated stopper can introduce bacteria or other contaminants.

In addition to the standard injectable dosage form, repository, or depot, forms of injectable drugs are available. These drugs are formulated to prolong absorption of the drug from the site of administration and thus provide a more sustained, effective drug concentration in the body. Implants are another form of repository solid dosage forms that are injected or inserted under the skin. Once in place, the implants are designed to dissolve or release medication over an extended period (weeks to months).

Finally, a drug form may be called an *extract*, a term that describes where the drug came from. An extract is a therapeutic agent composed of specially prepared plant or animal parts rather than synthesized chemicals in a laboratory. Examples of extracts include thyroid supplements made from pig or cattle thyroid glands and pancreatic enzyme powder extract derived from prepared livestock pancreas. Although many extracts provide reasonably consistent effects from bottle to bottle, the potency of different batches may vary as a result of variation in amounts of extracted natural drug contained in the plant or animal part. Although extracts might be less expensive to purchase, they may not provide as consistent a clinical effect as a compound developed by conventional manufacturing processes.

SOURCES OF DRUG INFORMATION

Information on appropriate and safe drug use in veterinary medicine is constantly changing as new drugs are developed, new applications for old drugs are approved, and new problems with existing drugs are discovered. The veterinary professional must have access to a current drug reference guide. The most up-to-date information is usually found in the *drug package inserts*, which are included with each container of drug sent to a veterinarian. These inserts provide the essential information on the drug as required by the FDA guidelines and must be updated as new data or new information is developed and released on the drug.

Printed publications, such as this text, are generally 4 to 6 months out of date by the day they are released. Still, publications provide additional information that the drug manufacturers are not allowed to include in their drug package inserts, such as dosages or uses of the drugs common in veterinary medicine but not specifically approved by the FDA. Generally, more descriptive information can be included in the publications than can be included in the package inserts.

Good publication resources for veterinary professionals include *formularies*, which are small booklets containing common drug doses, or larger reference books, such as *Veterinary Pharmaceuticals and Biologicals, Mosby's Veterinary Drug Reference, Compendium of Veterinary Products,* and *Veterinary Drug Handbook*. Because information on pharmaceuticals changes rapidly, the veterinary technician should have the most current edition of any drug references used.

Information on most human drugs is not contained in most veterinary resources. However, the veterinary professional may need human drug information when pets accidentally ingest human medications or when needing a dosage form of a drug not available as a veterinary drug (e.g., using pediatric formulations of drugs for small veterinary patients). This information may be found in references such as *Physician's GenRx* and *Physicians' Desk Reference (PDR)*, the latter of which also has several smaller spin-off publications such as *Nonprescription Drugs* and *Ophthalmic Drugs*. Most human references are also available on CD-ROM for easy reference on a computer. Although these publications contain detailed information on thousands of drugs and their effects in human beings, they do not provide any information about effects in veterinary patients. Specific characteristics of these drugs and how they act in veterinary patients should always be obtained from current veterinary resources.

INFORMATION LISTED IN DRUG REFERENCES

The information in most drug references and package inserts conveys a large amount of data in a standard format for quick access by the veterinary professional. In drug references such as the *PDR* or *Veterinary Drug Reference*, each drug description begins with a standard heading that contains several pieces of important information (Figure 1-2).

The boldface, capital letters with the circled-R (®) indicate the registered copyrighted proprietary or trade (brand) name of the product (Nembutal®). In some cases the registered mark is replaced by a trademark symbol (™), which indicates that the name is a registered trademark owned by the company and, like the copyrighted brand name, cannot be used by other manufacturers.

The "Rx" in the heading indicates that this product is available only by prescription or on the order of a licensed veterinarian. Selling drugs with this designation as over-the-counter (OTC) drugs in grocery stores, feed stores, or discount stores is illegal.

The "C" and "II" in the drug heading in Figure 1-2 indicate that the drug is a federally *controlled substance* or schedule drug and therefore has special requirements for dispensing, prescribing, and using within a veterinary facility. The Roman numeral II indicates the general level of abuse potential for the drug and the degree of regulatory control imposed on it to prevent diversion into illicit or illegal drug sales. Categories, or schedules, of controlled substances range from a designation of C-I to C-V. The higher the Roman numeral, the less potential for abuse of the drug. Drugs classified as C-I have the highest potential for abuse; drugs classified as C-V have the least. Controlled substance regulations are discussed in greater detail in Chapter 2.

A somewhat recent addition to the drug heading by some publishers has been the phonetic spelling of the drug shown in brackets below the trade name. This is helpful for the veterinary professional when communicating the drug name to other veterinarians, veterinary technicians, physicians, or pharmacists.

The nonproprietary name (e.g., pentobarbital sodium) is printed in smaller type below the boldface name and phonetic spelling and usually includes a descriptor of the dosage form (e.g., tablets, syrup, or injectable). In this example the heading states that the drug form is for injectable use.

The "USP" designation in the nonproprietary name stands for United States Pharmacopeia. The United States Pharmacopeia is an organization that sets the standards for manufacture of drugs sold in the United States. The USP is one of the standards ensuring that drugs are produced in a manner that delivers a safe and consistent effect. The USP designation indicates that this drug has been manufactured to the standards required by the United States Pharmacopeia.

Finally, the heading may have a separate line that confers additional information about the drug. In this example, the dose form also comes in ampules and vials.

The information after the heading is broken into categories; each category contains specific information for quick access. The first category is the description, or composition statement, which describes the physical characteristics and ingredients of the drug or drug combination. This section lists the drug itself as the active ingredient and *inert ingredients* such as any preservatives, stabilizers, liquid media, or other additives that make up the dosage form. Although often overlooked, some inert ingredients can produce *adverse drug reactions* in sensitive patients.

NEMBUTAL® SODIUM SOLUTION   ℞   Ⓒ

[*nêm'–bū–tal sō'–dĭ–um*]
(pentobarbital sodium injection, USP)
Ampules – Vials

Figure 1-2 Information contained in the heading of a drug listing.

CLINICAL APPLICATION
Watch the Inert Ingredients

A practitioner called a veterinary referral hospital with a question regarding the possibility of an ear medication causing signs associated with ototoxicity (*oto*, meaning ear, and *toxic*, meaning poisonous). A young puppy was showing signs of circling (walking around in circles), head tilting to one side, and nystagmus (rapid eye movement back and forth). These signs were consistent with inflammation, disease, or damage to the inner ear, where the organs of balance are located. The practitioner knew that certain ear medications had a reputation for producing ototoxicosis, but she also knew that the otic (ear) preparation that she had prescribed did not have any of those ingredients listed on the active ingredient label. However, although the active ingredient was not associated with ototoxicity, the solvent added to the otic preparation to soften the ear wax had occasionally been reported as producing an ototoxicity exhibiting these signs. The otic medication was stopped and the puppy recovered within 12 hours.

What should be learned from this situation: Reactions to medications can come from the additives, not just the main ingredient. For example, intravenous drugs dissolved in propylene glycol appear to have a much greater potential to produce side effects if given rapidly than the same drug dissolved in water and given just as rapidly.

Therefore this section of the drug listing can be important in attempting to identify causes of an adverse drug reaction.

The *indications* section of the drug listing tells for what purposes the drug may be used. Indications are the specific, FDA-approved uses for the drug. When the FDA approves a drug for use in veterinary medicine, it is for a specific species (e.g., dog, cat, cattle), for a specific disease, and at a specific dose. Even though the drug may have other effective medical uses, the specific indications for which the drug has been tested and approved are the only ones that can be listed on the drug package insert.

Drug manufacturers continually apply to the FDA to expand the approved indications for their drugs. The motivation is that a drug with a broader range of indications is more likely to sell than a similar drug with more limited indications. For example, a drug product having an approved indication for killing fleas and ticks will be more popular, and sell more readily, than a product whose approved indication is for fleas but not ticks. Because the FDA-approved indications for drugs often change over the market life of a drug, the veterinary professional should always consult the most recent information on the product to identify the indications for which it has been approved.

As mentioned, a drug may have medically effective uses for which the drug is not FDA approved. For example, ivermectin is a broad-spectrum antiparasitic drug. It is effective against many more types of parasites than the indications on the drug listing or label indicate. However, the company is not willing to invest large sums of money to obtain FDA approval for legal label indications for use against each of these parasites. If a veterinarian prescribes ivermectin for a non-approved use, the veterinarian is using the drug as an extra-label, or off-label, medication. *Extra-label use*, or *off-label use*, means that the drug is being used in a manner other than that listed on the drug's label or listing. Extra-label use includes the use of a different dose or route of administration, use in another species, or another purpose other than that intended by the drug's manufacturer and approved by the FDA.

Extra-label use is necessary in veterinary medicine. For example, the use of human-approved drugs in animals is a generally accepted practice in veterinary medicine (e.g., phenobarbital tablets for control of epileptic seizures). Veterinary drugs approved for use in one species are also sometimes used in other species for which few drugs are approved (e.g., so called minor species such as sheep, goats, pigs, and llamas).

Because extra-label use of drugs in food animal species has the potential to introduce drug residues into human food products, some conflict exists between the need to maintain the health of livestock and the food production industry versus the need to keep drug residues out of the meat, milk, eggs, and other food products that human beings consume. The veterinary professional should be well aware of all sides of this issue. See the Clinical Application on p. 12 for more complete information on this topic.

Several sections of the drug listing are devoted to unwanted effects of the drug. A side effect or an adverse drug reaction (ADR) is any effect of the drug other than its intended beneficial effect. Side effects for a drug can range from mildly annoying to potentially fatal. The side effects for a drug are found in the *precautions*, *warnings*, and *contraindications* sections for the drug. If a drug has a history of risky side effects, the drug may have a separate section on adverse reactions.

Generally, precaution listings describe fairly rare adverse reactions or mild side effects.

TABLE **1-1** Reporting Adverse Drug Reactions

The FDA's toll-free phone number for reporting adverse drug reactions (1-888-FDA-VETS) is available from 7:00 AM to 4:00 PM EST, with next-day callback service available after hours.

The United States Pharmacopeia is an organization that establishes state-of-the-art standards for manufacturing of drugs in the United States. They also provide the Veterinary Practitioner's Reporting Program for reporting adverse reactions. Information is available at their web site (see Web Resources) or by phone at 800-4-USP-PRN or 800-487-7776).

Most drug manufacturers have technical service veterinarians to accept reports of drug reactions or discuss problems or concerns with one of their drugs. The phone numbers of selected veterinary drug manufacturers are listed with their web pages in this table.

COMPANY	PHONE	WEB SITE
AgriLaboratories	816-233-9533	www.agrilabs.com
Aspen Veterinary Resources	816-413-1444	
Bayer Animal Health	800-633-3796*	www.bayer-ah.com
Boehringer Ingelheim Vetmedica, Inc.	800-325-9167	www.bi-vetmedica.com
Butler Animal Health Supply	800-848-5983	www.AccessButler.com
DermaPet Inc.	800-755-4738	www.dermapet.com
Durvet, Inc. Animal Health Products	816-229-9101	www.durvet.com
DVM Pharmaceutical Animal Health	800-367-4902	www.DVMPharmaceuticals.com
ELANCO	800-428-4441	www.elanco.com
EVSCO Pharmaceuticals	856-697-1441	
Fort Dodge Animal Health	800-533-8536*	www.wyeth.com/divisions/fort_dodge/asp
Intervet, Inc.	800-441-8272	www.intervetusa.com
Lloyd, Inc.	712-246-4000	www.lloydinc.com
Luitpold Animal Health	631-924-4000	www.luitpoldanimalhealth.com
Merial	678-638-3000	www.merial.com
Novartis Animal Health	800-637-0281*	www.ah.novartis.com
Pfizer Inc.	800-366-5288*	www.pfizer.com/pfizer/do/mn_animal.jsp
Schering-Plough Animal Health	800-521-5767*	www.sp-animalhealth.com
Vedco, Inc.	816-238-8840	www.vedco.com/dvmonly
Vet-a-Mix	800-831-0004	www.lloydinc.com
Veterinary Products Laboratories	888-241-9545	www.vpl.com
Virbac	817-831-5030	www.virbac.com
Webster Veterinary	800-225-7911	www.webstervet.com

*Technical service veterinarian or professional service phone number.

The Food and Drug Administration (FDA) has the responsibility of ensuring the safety and effectiveness of all drugs and is charged with monitoring the safety of the food supply. This tremendous responsibility, as defined by the Federal Food, Drug, and Cosmetics Act, places the FDA in the role of watchdog over the ways veterinary drugs are used. Section 512 of the Act states that an animal drug is considered unsafe unless it has been approved and the intended use of the drug conforms to that approval. Alteration of any of the following from what is described and approved on the drug label is considered extra-label use:

- Use in a species not listed
- Use for an indication (disease or condition) not listed
- Use of a different dosage
- Use of a different frequency of administration
- Use of a different route of administration
- Deviation from labeled withdrawal time (time from last administration of the drug until the animal or the animal's products can be safely taken to market)

Because the FDA is charged with safety of the human food supply, and drug residues in meat, egg, milk, and food products are an adulteration of the food, the act is primarily directed toward the use of drugs in food animals (e.g., cattle, sheep). Veterinarians are often limited by what drugs they can use to treat food animal species because of the concern over drug residues in human food products and the tight restrictions on extra-label use.

In 1994 Congress passed the Animal Medicinal Drug Use Clarification Act (AMDUCA) which gave veterinarians the authority to use approved animal drugs in an extra-label manner. In other words, a drug approved for use in cattle for respiratory infection could be used for respiratory disease in sheep if the "health of the animal is threatened, or suffering or death may result from failure to treat." In addition, extra-label use is only valid and legal when the following criteria are met:

- No approved drug exists that is specifically labeled to treat the condition diagnosed, or the approved drug at the dosage on the label has been found by the veterinarian to be clinically ineffective in the animals to be treated.

- A careful medical diagnosis is made by the attending veterinarian within the context of a valid veterinarian-client-patient relationship (VCPR). A valid VCPR according to the American Veterinarian Medical Association Membership Directory and Resource Manual exists when the veterinarian has assumed the responsibility for making clinical judgments, the client has agreed to follow the veterinarian's instruction, the veterinarian has sufficient knowledge of the animal to make a preliminary diagnosis, and the veterinarian is readily available for follow-up evaluation in the event of an adverse reaction or treatment failure.
- Procedures are instituted to ensure that the identity of the treated animal is carefully maintained.
- A significantly extended period is assigned for drug withdrawal before marketing meat, milk, or eggs from treated animals, and steps are taken to ensure that the assigned time frames are met and that no illegal residues occur.
- The prescribed or dispensed extra-label drugs bear labeling information that is adequate to ensure the safe and proper use of the product. This would include the following:
  - Name and address of the prescribing veterinarian
  - The active ingredients
  - Animal the drug is to be used on (identification, class, or species)
  - Dosage, frequency, route of administration, and duration of therapy
  - Any cautionary statements specified by the veterinarian
  - Veterinarian's specified withdrawal/discard time for meat, milk, eggs, or food
  - Products derived from the treated animals

Veterinary professionals have an obligation to the public to support the veterinarian's and FDA's efforts to ensure that extra-label drugs are used in a safe and responsible manner. Veterinary technicians may have to explain or defend this policy or may be challenged to bend the rules "just this once." Veterinary technicians must understand both the intent of the regulations and the physiologic reasons that form the rationale behind appropriate extra-label drug use.

For example, stomach upset caused by aspirin is considered a mild side effect and is included under precautions. The veterinarian must then use clinical judgment to decide whether the benefits of the drug outweigh the potential side effect. By listing the precautions (including even mild side effects), the drug manufacturer has legally informed the veterinarian of the potential side effects or adverse reactions and placed the responsibility for administering the drug on the veterinary professional.

Warnings are more serious or frequent side effects than those found in the precautions section, such as the potential for hallucinations in an aspirin-sensitive person taking aspirin compounds. Because many of the adverse reactions in the warnings section are potentially life threatening, veterinary professionals have a moral and ethical obligation to thoroughly understand the key points of warnings and to inform the client or owner of the potential

problems that may arise. Drugs that contain warnings can still be given if the potential benefit, in the judgment of the attending veterinarian, outweighs the risk.

Contraindications are circumstances in which the drug should not be used. For example, giving penicillin to an animal or person who has severe and life-threatening allergic reactions to penicillin is contraindicated. The potential for a hypersensitivity reaction in a patient is a contraindication condition for penicillin. Failure to heed a known contraindication for a drug, with subsequent death of the veterinary patient because of administration, could constitute malpractice.

When applicable, information on a drug overdose or overdosage is also supplied in the drug inserts and drug information bulletins. Overdose can occur from a dose miscalculation or when illness changes the normal physiologic state, causing an administration of a correct dose of drug to accumulate and produce signs

CLINICAL APPLICATION
The Long Regulatory Arm of the Law

In 1997 the U.S. District Court convicted a livestock dealer for providing false information to the U.S. government and for introducing adulterated food. The United States Department of Agriculture Food Safety and Inspection Service reported more than 50 instances of animals offered for slaughter for human food that contained illegal levels of antibiotics and other drugs. Although the plea agreement resulted in tougher regulation for this livestock producer, the potential penalty for providing false information to the U.S. government is imprisonment for 5 years, a fine of $250,000, and a 3-year period of supervised release. The maximal penalty for introduction of adulterated food into interstate commerce is imprisonment for 1 year, a fine of $100,000, and a 1-year period of supervised release.[1]

A veterinarian was sentenced in U.S. District Court to 8 months in federal prison and fined $15,000 after pleading guilty to a charge that he conspired to smuggle an illegal substance into the United States. The veterinarian admitted to selling

more than $75,000 worth of clenbuterol to six customers whose children used the beta-agonist drug to improve the appearance of several show animals from 1986 to 1994. Clenbuterol has been used illegally to increase muscle mass and decrease fat deposition, giving show livestock an appearance that is an advantage in showing competition. The veterinarian was dispensing the medication to animals that he knew would be slaughtered for food, thus potentially introducing drug residues into human food sources.[2] Clenbuterol leaves a drug residue that cannot be eliminated by cooking and if eaten can potentially be dangerous. What should be learned from this situation: In these cases the veterinarian and livestock producer had been doing this illegal practice for several years and appeared to be complacent in their concern for the potential impact on the food human beings eat. Veterinary professionals can help keep this from happening by following the rules and regulations for the use of animal drugs in veterinary patients.

of overdose. Understanding how disease alters normal physiology and being aware of how a drug interacts with these alterations help the veterinary professional reduce the chances of this happening. However, if overdose occurs, this section of the drug information listing can be extremely valuable.

The information listed under dosage and administration lists the only dosage and route of administration approved by the FDA. Failure to follow the dosage and administration procedures could result in administration of insufficient or excessive medication and harm to the patient. Additionally, failure to follow dosage and administration procedures is considered an extra-label use and therefore makes the veterinary professional who orders or administers the drug potentially subject to legal action if an adverse drug reaction occurs or if regulatory statutes are violated.

REFERENCES

1. *FDA Veterinarian*, November/December xii(vi):3, 1997.
2. *JAVMA* 214(3):319, 1999.

RECOMMENDED READING

Formularies

Mosby's drug consult, St. Louis, 2004, Elsevier.
Papich MG: *Saunders Handbook of Veterinary Drugs*, ed 2, St. Louis, 2007, Saunders.
Physicians' desk reference, Montvale, NJ, 2005, Thompson Healthcare.
Plumb DC: *Veterinary drug handbook*, ed 5, Ames, IA, 2005, Blackwell.

Veterinary Drug Information

Allen DG, Pringle JK: *Handbook of veterinary drugs*, ed 2, Philadelphia, 2001, Lippincott-Raven.
Boothe D: *Small animal clinical pharmacology and therapeutics*, St. Louis, 2001, WB Saunders.

WEB RESOURCES

www.usp.org

The United States Pharmacopeia (USP) is an organization that sets standards that manufacturers must meet to sell their products in the United States. The USP home page provides links to veterinary drug information, quality standards, and the Veterinary Practitioner's Reporting (VPR) Program.

www.cvm.tamu.edu/vcpl

The site for the Veterinary Clinical Pharmacology Laboratory at Texas A&M University contains articles regarding anticonvulsant and antibiotic use that can be downloaded and printed.

www.fda.gov

The FDA's web site contains a large amount of information regarding extra-label use guidelines. Use the site's search engine to find more detailed information on a particular topic.

Self-Assessment

Fill in the following blanks with the correct item from the Key Terms list.

1. _____ liquid dose form in an alcohol solution administered orally.

2. _____ drug suspended within an oil or liquid fat.

3. _____ topically applied dose form; drug is dissolved in alcohol.

4. _____ drug made from processed animal organs (e.g., pancreas, thyroid) or plants.

5. _____ solid (powdered) dose form covered in gelatin.

6. _____ semisolid dose form that liquefies at body temperature.

7. _____ sucrose or other sugar-based liquid dose form administered orally.

8. _____ semisolid dose form that does not melt at body temperature.

9. _____ oral dosage form formulated to dissolve slowly as it moves through the gastrointestinal tract.

10. _____ drug form formulated to be protected against stomach acid.

11. _____ drug produced by companies other than the original developer.

12. _____ small, airtight glass containers containing drug; meant to be broken open to extract the drug; used only one time.

13. _____ type of drug meant to be absorbed over a prolonged period after being injected (e.g., implants).

14. _____ the ingredient of the drug formulation that includes preservatives, stabilizers, and liquid media into which the drug is dissolved or suspended.

15. _____ the term that means the *reason* or the *condition* for which the drug is to be used.

16. _____ any use of a drug in a manner other than that approved by the FDA.

17. _____ any effect of the drug other than the intended effect.

18. _____ Identify the proprietary name in the following sentence: "Cats should never be given Tylenol® or any acetaminophen product."

Indicate whether the following statements are true or false.

19. A *precaution* is a condition or situation in which a drug should not be given.

20. "10 mg/lb every 6 hours for 3 days" is an example of a dose, and "250 mg" is an example of a dosage.

21. Extra-label drugs can be legally used by veterinarians in animals intended for use as human food.

22. Suspensions must be shaken before administering; solutions do not need to be shaken.

23. Troches are commonly used with veterinary patients.

24. The ® symbol indicates that the drug is restricted to use only by a veterinarian.

25. The Animal Medicinal Drug Use Clarification Act of 1994 gave veterinarians the authority to use approved animal drugs in an extra-label manner.

APPLICATION QUESTIONS

1. You are speaking at a local high school day about the veterinary technology profession. As you are describing the education required to become a credentialed veterinary technician, one of the students raises his hand and asks, "Why do veterinary technicians have to learn about drugs? After all, they aren't going to be veterinarians!" How might you address this legitimate question?

2. The veterinarian has given a client a prescription. On the prescription is marked "generic drug can be substituted." After the veterinarian has left, the client has several questions for you: What is a generic drug? How is it different from a regular drug? Why are generic forms of drugs so much less expensive than trade name drugs? Are generic drugs as good as the better-known drugs?

3. Mrs. Jones is a well-informed client. She dutifully researches the information on medications for her pet. When she asks you "What is the reason for having an enteric coating on a tablet?" for a medication her pet is taking, what should you tell her?

4. Mr. Smith has some respiratory medication that is very similar to the medication his dog is prescribed. But his dog's medication is marked SR for "sustained release." Mr. Smith wants to know how a sustained-release tablet is different from a regular tablet. How do you respond?

5. Which liquid formulation of a drug can be safely given intravenously, as a solution, or as a suspension? Which needs to be shaken before administration?

6. If the standard injectable form of a drug is given every 12 hours, is the *repository form* more likely to be given every 6 hours or every 96 hours? Would it be the same for a *depot drug*?

7. Mr. Jones found a compound for hypothyroidism (low levels of thyroid hormone) on the Internet. It is listed as an extract. What is an extract, and how is it different from a regular drug? He notes that the extract is much less expensive than the other drug formulations. Why are extracts fairly inexpensive? Do extracts have potential problems?

8. An owner reports an unusual side effect for a drug the veterinarian prescribed. To whom should such information be reported?

9. The veterinarian makes the statement that a drug "would be indicated for disease X but contraindicated for condition Y." What does this mean?

10. Explain whether each of the following situations is considered a legitimate and legal use of an extra-label drug.

   A. The owner of a cow telephones to describe the clinical signs that the cow is showing. The veterinarian dispenses an extra-label drug for the cow that has been used to treat other cattle on adjoining farms.

   B. The veterinarian dispenses an off-label drug because it is as effective as the FDA-approved drug but half the price.

   C. After making a farm call, the veterinarian leaves a bottle of medication with a livestock producer to use on any other livestock showing similar signs, thus saving the producer the cost of multiple farm calls.

   D. The veterinarian uses an off-label drug on a producing dairy cow that he has examined and tells the dairy farmer not to send the cow to slaughter for 3 weeks because of the worry over drug residues.

   E. The veterinarian examines a goat and dispenses a medication used in calves because veterinary journals have published studies showing the drug is effective in goats.

   F. The veterinarian examines a dairy cow, determines that an off-label drug would be the best alternative to treat the condition, informs the livestock producer of the withdrawal times according to FDA guidelines, writes the information into the record, then dispenses it in a bottle with the cow's ID tag number and the drug name on it.

Chapter 2

Pharmacy Procedures, Drug Handling, and Dosage Calculations

key terms

antineoplastic agent
apothecary system
carcinogenic effect
compounding drugs
controlled substance/
  drug
cytotoxic drug
dosage range

household measurement
  system
material safety data sheet
  (MSDS)
metric system
mutagenic effect
Occupational Safety and
  Health Administration
  (OSHA)

over the counter (OTC)
percentage solution
prescription drugs
schedule drugs
teratogenic effect

objectives

*After studying
this chapter,
the veterinary
technician
should be
able to:*

1. Describe the differences between over-the-counter and prescription drugs

2. Describe the requirements for prescriptions and drug labels

3. Accurately read and write abbreviations commonly used in drug orders

4. Describe regulations and warnings regarding dispensing containers

5. Describe reasons and procedures for handling and storing drugs

6. Describe legal requirements for dispensing and storing controlled substances

7. Describe special storage and handling requirements for cytotoxic and hazardous drugs

8. Describe the issues surrounding and guidelines required for acceptable drug compounding

9. Accurately arrive at a dose given an animal's weight and a dosage

Veterinary practices, research institutions, and other areas of employment for today's veterinary technician are increasingly required to comply with regulations from the Drug Enforcement Administration (DEA), Food and Drug Administration (FDA), U.S. Department of Agriculture (USDA), and Environmental Protection Agency (EPA). Because veterinary technicians are involved in the day-to-day operation of a veterinary practice or workplace, part of the responsibility for compliance with these different regulations falls on their shoulders. Therefore all veterinary professionals must be aware of their responsibilities to store medications safely; calculate doses; and prepare, dispense, and record medications used.

PRESCRIPTION DRUGS VERSUS OVER-THE-COUNTER DRUGS

The FDA is responsible for determining whether a drug can be sold *over the counter (OTC)* or must be a prescription (Rx) drug. This decision is based on the toxicity of the drug, the method by which the drug is used, and how adequately directions for use can be written so that the layperson can clearly and consistently understand them. A drug that is considered toxic, potentially toxic if misused, or too readily misused is classified as a *prescription drug*. Only those drugs considered safe for the animal, the person administering the medication, people coming into contact with the animal, the human food chain, and the environment can be classified as OTC drugs. Some drugs can be formulated into different dose forms of different concentrations or means of administration, resulting in some dose forms marketed as OTC drugs and other forms as prescription only. For example, some deworming medications are produced in a high-concentration dose form for prescription use and a much lower concentration form for OTC sales.

Prescription drugs can only be dispensed "upon the lawful order of a licensed veterinarian." Their label must contain the phrase "Caution: Federal law restricts this drug to use by or on the order of a licensed veterinarian."

PRESCRIPTIONS AND DRUG ORDERS

The FDA has interpreted the word "prescription" to apply only to the veterinary practitioner's direction to a pharmacist or a person legally allowed by the state to fill prescription orders. Therefore the orders given by a veterinarian to a veterinary technician for a client are technically drug "orders" and not prescriptions.

Because veterinary technicians often help fill drug orders, dispense medications, and keep records, they must understand the responsibilities and limitations of their actions. Veterinary technicians cannot legally write prescriptions, but they can fill drug orders and dispense medications as instructed by veterinarians within their practice. In most states, veterinarians and technicians from one practice cannot legally fill a prescription from another practice because that would place the veterinary professional in the role of pharmacist. Still, veterinary technicians must understand the proper format of a typical prescription and the meaning of the abbreviations used in prescription writing to fill a drug order and dispense medicine properly.

A hypothetical prescription for a pharmacist is shown in Figure 2-1. For a prescription to be valid, it must contain the following items:
- Name of veterinary hospital or veterinarian, address, and telephone number
- Date on which the prescription was written
- Client's (owner's) name and address and species of animal (animal's name optional)
- Rx symbol (from the Latin, meaning *take thou of*)
- Drug name, concentration, and number of units to be dispensed

---

HOMETOWN VETERINARY ASSOCIATES
2000 West Chelsea Ave., Brookside, PA 13233
(324) 555-0214

Date: *November 22, 2001*

Patient: *Cricket*   Species: *Canine*

Owner: *Kathy Gagnier*   Phone: *555-0127*

Address: *2000 Christopher Ln,*
West Brookside, PA 13235

℞   *Amoxicillin tablets 100 mg #30 tabs*
Sig: 1 tab q8h PO PRN until gone

Robert L. Bill D.V.M.

Figure 2-1 A hypothetical prescription for a pharmacist.

- Sig (from the Latin *signa*, meaning *write* or *label*), which indicates directions for treatment of the animal
- Signature of the veterinarian
- DEA registration number if the drug is a *controlled substance*

Other items frequently found on the prescription include refill status, which shows whether the client may obtain a refill of the prescription, and internal inventory or record-keeping numbers. The FDA requires specific information to be placed on the label of the drug dispensed from a pharmacy. Regulations for medications dispensed from veterinary hospitals should theoretically follow the same regulations as from a pharmacy; however, as shown in Figure 2-2, labels from veterinary hospitals need to follow generally accepted practice guidelines, which include the following:

- Name, address, and telephone number of the veterinarian or veterinary hospital
- Name of the client and client's address
- Identification of the animal (e.g., ID tag, name)

- Drug name, concentration, and number of units dispensed
- Clear instructions for dosage, frequency, route of administration, and duration of treatment
- Cautionary statements (e.g., give on an empty stomach)
- Specified withdrawal or discard times (for food animals)

This information helps clearly communicate to the client how the medication is to be used and documents the directions given to the client or owner if a question arises about the medication's intended use.

ABBREVIATIONS USED IN DRUG ORDERS

Generally, the same abbreviations used for prescriptions sent to a pharmacy are used for filling in-house drug orders and recording treatments in the patient record. These abbreviations constitute a common form of communication in veterinary medicine; thus the veterinary technician should recognize and know how to use them appropriately. A list of the most commonly used abbreviations and their meanings is provided in Table 2-1.

These abbreviations may be capitalized or lower case and may or may not use periods after each letter. Note that some of the abbreviations used in veterinary medicine are rarely used in human medicine and are therefore not recognized by all pharmacists. For example, an abbreviation used to indicate "once a day" in veterinary medicine is "s.i.d.," whereas in human medicine the abbreviation "qd" is considered

the standard means of indicating "once daily" and s.i.d. is never used. If any doubt exists about the interpretation of the written drug order, the technician should always check with the veterinarian for verification. Taking a few moments to ask for clarification is far better than making a guess, something that could cause the animal harm if the guess is incorrect.

CONTAINERS FOR DISPENSING MEDICATION

Veterinary professionals have a moral obligation to keep medications from being misused or falling into the hands of children. In most veterinary practices today, childproof containers are commonly used to help deter children from getting into the medications. However, some veterinary practices continue to dispense medication in the less expensive paper pill "envelopes" to reduce the expenses associated with the medication. Is this method of dispensing medication in a veterinary practice illegal?

The Poison Prevention Packaging Act of 1970 enabled the FDA to require special packaging for drugs that may be dangerous to children. However, current regulations apply to drug manufacturers and pharmacists but not veterinarians. Therefore dispensing veterinary medication in pill envelopes is not illegal. However, if medication dispensed in a pill envelope is accessible to a child who ingests it, the veterinarian could theoretically be accused of negligence for placing the child at risk.

Sometimes dispensing medication in containers that are not childproof is necessary, such as for elderly clients with arthritic hands. In these circumstances veterinarians are probably justified giving these clients medications packaged in dispensing vials with lids that are not childproof. Nevertheless, veterinary professionals are morally and ethically obligated to inform clients when containers are not childproof and advise them to keep medication out of the reach of children.

TABLE **2-1** Abbreviations Commonly Used in Prescriptions

b.i.d.	twice a day
cc	cubic centimeter
disp	dispense
g (or gm)	gram
gr	grain
gtt	drop
h (or hr)	hour
IM	intramuscular
IP	intraperitoneal
IV	intravenous
L	liter
lb	pound
mg	milligram
mL (or ml)	milliliter
OD	right eye
OS	left eye
OU	both eyes
oz	ounce
PO	by mouth
prn	as needed
q	every
q4h	every 4 hours
q8h	every 8 hours
qd	every day (daily)
qh	every hour
q.i.d.	four times daily
q.o.d.	every other day
s.i.d.	once a day
SQ (or SC)	subcutaneous
stat	immediately
TBL or Tbsp	tablespoon
t.i.d.	three times daily
tsp	teaspoon

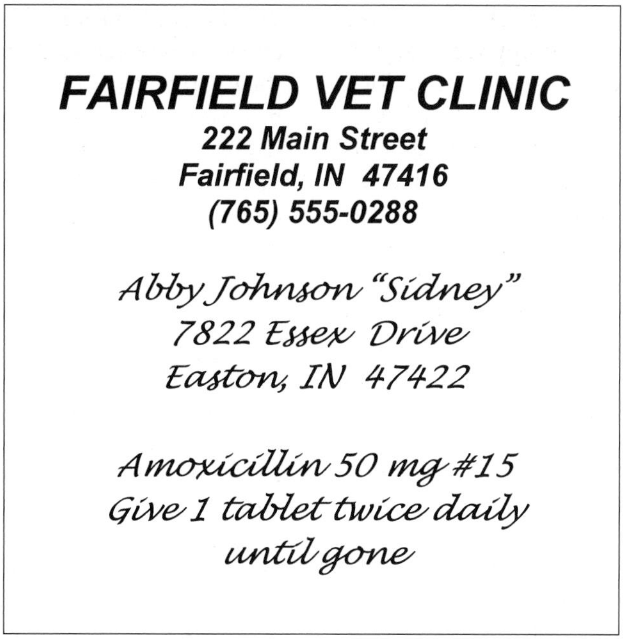

FAIRFIELD VET CLINIC
222 Main Street
Fairfield, IN 47416
(765) 555-0288

Abby Johnson "Sidney"
7822 Essex Drive
Easton, IN 47422

Amoxicillin 50 mg #15
Give 1 tablet twice daily
until gone

Figure 2-2 Labels from veterinary hospitals need to follow generally accepted practice guidelines.

STORAGE OF DRUGS IN THE VETERINARY FACILITY

Techniques for inventory control of drugs and other supplies are usually taught in conjunction with business management concepts.

However, besides the business aspects, medical and legal reasons exist for proper storage and handling of drugs. For example, drugs that are not stored in the proper temperature and light can degenerate or become inactivated, providing little or no benefit. Drugs that remain

---

CLINICAL APPLICATION
A Good Idea That Did Not Work

A veterinarian thought he was doing his clients a favor when he instructed his technician to unwrap each foil-wrapped tablet of the medication he was going to dispense. His reasoning was that he could get more of the tablets in a pill vial with a childproof safety lid, and it would be easier for his clients because they would not have to open the foil wrapping. Unfortunately, what the veterinarian failed to consider was the hygroscopic (water absorbing) nature of the dose form, which is why the manufacturer sealed each individual tablet in foil. After 2 days the tablets turned into mushy crumbles inside the pill vial. The clients returned the tablets and received replacement tablets (in their foil wrapping). The veterinarian learned, at some loss of profit to his practice, that his good intentions failed to consider the physical makeup of the medication.

What should be learned from this situation: The manufacturer knows best how to store its medications. Tampering with the environmental or physical storage properties of a medication or failing to follow the manufacturer's guidelines for storage of the drug can result in the drug becoming useless. Always read and follow the manufacturer's guidelines for storage and dispensing of medications.

CLINICAL APPLICATION
Detective Work to Solve a Diabetic's Problem

A client was having a difficult time regulating her diabetic poodle at home. The dog would repeatedly present to the veterinary hospital with blood glucose concentrations well above the normal range, indicating that either the insulin was not being administered appropriately, the insulin was not working, or the physiologic balance of the insulin and blood-glucose elevating mechanisms was off. In each case, the animal was hospitalized, the insulin regimen was evaluated, and the animal became regulated within a few days. The owner would again be shown how to administer the medication and was observed giving the insulin injection (which she did very well). Why the animal would become unregulated after a week of being at home was troubling, especially when the owner was very concerned and capable and seemed to be following every letter of the directions.

The veterinarian ruled out a physiologic problem such as insulin resistance, wherein the body is less responsive to administered insulin, or an inappropriate amount of insulin being administered based on the ability of the veterinary technician hospital staff to regulate the dog within a few days of hospitalization by using the same insulin dose that was used at home. Feeding schedules, documented by the owner in a daily diary, were closely scrutinized. The owner was very good about adhering to a tight feeding schedule and not giving snacks or treats. When the same feeding schedule was used with the prescribed dose of insulin in the veterinary hospital, the animal was consistently well regulated. What was the difference between the hospital conditions and the conditions at home that would explain this mystery?

The veterinarian wondered if a problem occurred during the transportation of the insulin home from the veterinary hospital or pharmacy. Perhaps the insulin had been left in a hot car? Was the insulin not being stored properly at home? Further questioning of the owner ruled out problems that might arise with improper storage while transporting the insulin home, and the owner seemed to be following the guidelines for proper storage of insulin.

Finally, the veterinarian had the owner bring in the bottle of insulin she had been using at home, the syringes, and the cotton balls for swabbing the injection site with alcohol and had her demonstrate exactly what she did to administer the medication. As soon as she started the procedure, the veterinarian thought he had solved the problem.

The owner was very conscientious (almost too conscientious) about following all the instructions written for her. She had been told that insulin is a suspension and would need to be shaken to resuspend it evenly in the liquid. She had indeed shaken the insulin—thoroughly, almost violently—for almost a minute. The problem is that physical disruption of the insulin molecule is possible from vigorous shaking. When she did this with each dose, she likely disrupted more and more of the insulin molecules, resulting in medication that was increasingly ineffective. The owner was gently informed that rolling the medication slowly between the hands to resuspend the drug was probably better than shaking. The owner, willing to comply with any instructions, did so. The result was a significant improvement in the ability of the owner to control the dog's diabetes at home.

What should be learned from this situation: Owners often take whatever instructions are provided to them literally. If they are told to mix a medication but are not given detailed instructions, they have no idea to what extent they should mix it, how long, or how vigorously. In the case of certain medications, shaking too vigorously can physically affect the drug. Therefore drug handling instructions, storage requirements, and any precautions for handling the drug should be clearly written, documented in sufficient detail, and if necessary demonstrated for the client to protect both the patient and the client.

on the pharmacy shelf after the listed expiration date may be less effective. In some cases, such as with tetracycline, these expired drugs may actually become unsafe. Thus responsible storage and handling of therapeutic agents are essential to facilitate safe, effective veterinary care.

ENVIRONMENTAL CONSIDERATIONS

Drugs should be stored at their optimal temperature to prevent damage. According to label specifications, temperatures for drug storage are as follows:

Cold: not exceeding 8° C (46° F)
Cool: 8° to 15° C (46° to 59° F)
Room temperature: 15° to 30° C (59° to 86° F)
Warm: 30° to 40° C (86° to 104° F)
Excessive heat: greater than 40° C (104° F)

Note that "cold" temperatures may include temperatures below freezing. Unless the package or label states "do not freeze," drugs classified as needing to be stored in cold temperatures are probably safe to freeze.

Large animal practitioners must be especially aware of environmental conditions because of the tendency to forget about drugs stored in the practice vehicle. These drugs can be subjected to wide variations in temperature, changing the physical composition of the drug. When frozen, some drugs undergo a physical change resulting in a crystalline formation that is more difficult to keep in suspension and causes pain on injection.

Drugs that are sensitive to light are usually kept in a dark amber container and have a notice on the label to not expose the drug to light. If dispensing a light-sensitive liquid drug from a larger container into a smaller dispensing container, dark amber dispensing bottles should be used.

Tablets and powders are sensitive to moisture, so their bottles usually contain silica packets designed to absorb moisture. The binders and other inert ingredients that make up tablets may be sensitive to humidity, resulting in the tablets becoming soggy. Capsules (gel caps) are especially sensitive to humidity and will stick together in a container that becomes warm or humid.

Other threats exist to medications improperly stored. Ionizing radiation can destroy some complex drug molecules, and other drugs are destroyed by physical stress such as vibrations.

Drugs that must be reconstituted before use (for example, a powder to which a liquid is added) often do not contain preservative agents to prevent bacterial growth if the container becomes contaminated after reconstitution. Reconstituted drugs may be easily contaminated by repeated insertion of needles or because the reconstituted product is often chemically unstable; therefore keeping reconstituted drugs for several days so that the contents may be completely used in several animals is inappropriate. The manufacturers of these products specify the time during which the product is considered safe and effective to use.

SPECIAL STORAGE AND HANDLING REQUIREMENTS FOR CONTROLLED SUBSTANCES

As mentioned in Chapter 1, a capital C followed by a roman numeral on a drug label indicates that the drug is considered a controlled substance or *schedule drug* (in reference to the different C levels, or "schedules"). A controlled substance is defined by law as a substance that has the potential for physical addiction, psychological addiction, and/or abuse. The Roman numeral denotes the drug's theoretic potential for abuse.

C-I: Has an extreme potential for abuse and no approved medicinal purpose in the United States; includes such drugs as heroin, LSD, and marijuana

C-II: Has a high potential for abuse and may lead to severe physical or psychological dependence; includes such drugs as opium, pentobarbital, morphine, and wild-animal restraint drugs such as etorphine hydrochloride

CLINICAL APPLICATION
The Forgotten Medication

A veterinarian posed this question on an electronic bulletin board regarding whether she handled the following situation correctly. The veterinarian works in what she described as a small tourist town with many out-of-town visitors. One night she received a call from someone, not a client, who said he had left his dog's phenobarbital tablets in the last hotel room. The caller reported that the dog was a controlled epileptic, meaning it was prone to seizures, but that the seizures were controlled by the daily administration of phenobarbital tablets. Phenobarbital tablets are classified as a controlled substance. The owner stated he had already talked with his veterinarian at home who said (correctly) that he could not prescribe medication across state lines. Being stuck without medication, the caller wanted the local veterinarian to phone in a prescription for enough phenobarbital tablets to get the dog by until they left for home. The veterinarian refused to call in a prescription for the animal but offered to see them that evening or the next morning. The client then "got snippy" and demanded to know why the veterinarian would not prescribe 10 pills. The caller was reported to have said, "If my dog has a seizure and dies, it will be your fault!"

Was the veterinarian correct in refusing to write the prescription? Absolutely. The basis of any prescription, especially controlled substance prescriptions, is a valid veterinarian/client/patient relationship. This did not exist in this case. It would be easy for someone wanting phenobarbital for abuse purposes to call with such a story, hoping it would play on the compassionate side of the veterinarian and convince him or her to phone in the prescription. If the veterinarian had complied with the dog owner's wishes, she would have been in violation of the law. Had the veterinarian given a prescription to this owner without examining the dog and this ploy turned out to be a scam to get illegal drugs, the veterinarian would also have been in serious trouble if the perpetrators had been caught.

What should be learned from this situation: Stick to the law. The veterinary profession generally attracts people who want to be veterinarians and veterinary technicians to help people and animals in need. Unfortunately, this sometimes means they are preyed on by those who would manipulate or scam them with emotional tactics for illegal or immoral purposes. Do not give in to the temptation to look the other way "just this once."

C-III: Has some potential for abuse but less than that of C-II drugs; may lead to low to moderate physical dependence or high psychological dependence; includes ultrashort-acting barbiturates, ketamine, Telazol (zolazepam and tiletamine), and drugs with limited amounts of narcotics (e.g., Tylenol plus codeine).

C-IV: Has a low potential for abuse; may lead to limited physical or psychological dependence; includes such drugs as butorphanol and diazepam (Valium)

C-V: Is subject to state and local regulation; has a low potential for abuse

Regulations for the prescribing, handling, and storing of controlled drugs are specified in the Controlled Substances Act of 1970 and enforced by the DEA. Veterinarians must have a certification number from the DEA to legally use, prescribe, or buy controlled substances from an approved manufacturer or distributor. This DEA certification number must be included on all prescriptions or any order forms for schedule (controlled) drugs. This means, for example, a veterinarian could not order or prescribe phenobarbital tablets for a dog with epilepsy unless he or she has a valid, current DEA number.

Even with a valid DEA number, veterinarians cannot prescribe schedule I (C-I) drugs, which are illegal substances such as heroin and LSD. Prescriptions for schedule II (C-II) drugs, which have a high potential for abuse, must be in written form. Many states have special forms for C-II drug prescriptions.

These prescriptions cannot be telephoned to a pharmacist except in an emergency, in which case the verbal prescription must be followed by a written order within 72 hours. Schedule II drug prescriptions may not be refilled; a new prescription must be written for each treatment period.

A controlled substance of schedule II, III, or IV rating that is dispensed from the veterinary hospital pharmacy must be packaged in a childproof container, which must include on its label the following warning: "Caution: Federal law prohibits the transfer of this drug to any person other than the [client and] patient for whom it was prescribed."

The Controlled Substances Act also gives general guidelines for how these drugs must be stored. A veterinary practice or research facility storing controlled substances must keep them in a locked storage cabinet of "substantial construction," such as a sturdy metal cabinet or heavy safe, to prevent access or removal of the storage container by unauthorized personnel. Glass-fronted cabinets, lightweight portable safes, or locked tackle boxes hidden on a closet shelf are not considered legally sufficient for storage of controlled substances. For farm-call practice vehicles, a strong locked steel toolbox bolted or chained to the vehicle itself may meet the requirements. Unfortunately the Act does not describe in specific detail what is, or is not, considered adequate compliance with the storage requirements. For example, drugs stored in a locked laboratory drawer, in a sturdy pressed fiberboard cabinet, or in a portable lock box behind a locked metal room door may or may not be considered adequate storage for schedule drugs.

The Act also requires that a log be kept of controlled substances ordered, received, dispensed, and used within the veterinary facility. Although few specifics are provided in the federal law, at a minimum retaining and recording the receipt for any controlled substances purchased is good practice, as is recording the date, purpose, and number/amount of any schedule drug dispensed or used within the veterinary facility. Note that a specific state may impose regulations in addition to these requirements. These records and logs must be maintained for 2 years. Log books with bound pages (not three-ring notebooks or spiral notebooks) that are sequentially numbered (imprinted) are advisable to provide additional documentation that the log itself has not been altered to hide the diversion (the term used for redirecting drugs for illegal purposes) of the controlled substances.

Computer logs of controlled substances can be considered legitimate record keeping if the software allows only minor editing of log entries and creates an uneditable note file of any such changes made to the record. In other words, deletion or alteration of electronic log entries must be almost impossible. Many states require hard copy (paper) documentation be kept in addition to the computer record and an auxiliary record-keeping system be established in the event that the computer documentation becomes inoperable. As with all aspects of controlled substance regulation, the state may have additional requirements for computer-kept logs for them to be considered valid documentation.

Because the veterinary technician is often the one designated for recording the in-hospital use of medications, and because improper logging of controlled substances can have serious ramifications for the veterinarian, the veterinary technician has an important responsibility to document all controlled substance transactions consistently and accurately.

Additional information on storing and handling controlled substances can be obtained from the American Veterinary Medical Association (AVMA), the local state DEA office, or most of the pharmacies at veterinary school teaching hospitals in the United States.

STORAGE AND HANDLING OF CYTOTOXIC AND HAZARDOUS DRUGS

As has been emphasized, all drugs need to be stored and handled in a way that is safe for the patient, client, and any veterinary professional or layperson treating the animal. The concern for safe handling and storage becomes even more important when *cytotoxic drugs* are being used. Cytotoxic ("cell poison") drugs are especially poisonous to mammalian cells and include *antineoplastic agents,* which are drugs used to treat cancer, and antifungal agents, which are drugs used to treat fungal infections.

At therapeutic doses, improper handling of these hazardous drugs can cause birth defects (*teratogenic* or *mutagenic effects*) in the fetus of a pregnant veterinary professional or induce cancer or preneoplastic changes *(carcinogenic effects)* in animals and human beings. Because little is known about the long-term effects of many of these drugs, the veterinary professional must handle mutagenic and carcinogenic drugs with great care.

Guidelines for safe handling of cytotoxic agents and hazardous compounds have been published. The *Occupational Safety and Health Administration (OSHA)* has developed guidelines for safe storage, use, and disposal of chemicals and drugs. The American Animal Hospital Association offers a series of videotapes on general hospital procedures, some of which relate to handling cytotoxic agents. Veterinary texts about oncology also contain guidelines and procedures for safe administration of antineoplastic agents.

The first step in protecting oneself from exposure to hazardous or cytotoxic drugs is to understand how accidental exposure can occur. Veterinary professionals may be exposed to toxic drugs during routine procedures in the following situations:

- Absorption of the drug through the skin from spillage from a syringe or drug vial or from other skin contact with the drug

- Inhalation of an aerosolized drug as the needle is withdrawn from a vial that has been pressurized by the technician injecting air into the vial to facilitate removal of the drug
- Ingestion of food contaminated with drug by aerosolization or direct contact
- Inhalation resulting from crushing or breaking of tablets and subsequent aerosolization of drug powder
- Absorption or inhalation during opening of glass ampules containing antineoplastic agents

Unfortunately, veterinarians and veterinary technicians sometimes become complacent about common sense hygiene that would make nonveterinarian professionals cringe. Veterinarian and technician lunches are commonly stored in a refrigerator next to a specimen jar containing formalin, a container with a fecal sample, or a vial of antineoplastic medication. In a busy practice, veterinary professionals often quickly eat lunch between procedures and may briefly place food on a countertop while administering medication. Practices such as these may be modeled by lay staff who have less understanding of the consequences of unhygienic practices, such as if their food encounters hazardous drugs or materials. Therefore veterinary professionals are responsible to set a model for safe practices that reduce the risk for exposure by all professional and lay staff to cytotoxic or hazardous drugs.

In addition to being aware of potential exposure situations and modeling good practice procedures and hygiene, the veterinary facility should take responsibility to educate all involved personnel on the safe handling and storage of hazardous drugs. Training may be in-house or through workshops available in many communities. Safety training should be periodically repeated to emphasize the importance of handling precautions and serve as a refresher for staff members. Regulations from OSHA may dictate what training is required based on the type of institution or facility, the types of hazardous materials staff are likely to encounter, and the type of work that is performed in the facility.

Training should include educating the staff and employees on where to find necessary information on potentially hazardous materials used within the facility. Information on all cytotoxic agents or hazardous compounds should be compiled in a readily accessible format (e.g., a notebook) in a location known to all staff members and employees. This notebook should include the following items:

- A *material safety data sheet (MSDS)* for every cytotoxic agent or hazardous compound used in the practice. The MSDS must contain guidelines for protective precautions, cleanup procedures, and first aid for accidental exposure.
- A package insert for every drug used in the practice.
- Hospital policies and descriptions of procedures for handling a cytotoxic or hazardous drug spill or an exposure and routine disposal of drugs, contaminated syringes or equipment, and empty vials (based on manufacturer's recommendations in the MSDS and package insert).

Cytotoxic drugs and hazardous compounds should be stored separately from other drugs, with particular attention paid to environmental requirements such as temperature and exposure to light. Every compound must be clearly labeled with easily read information about what the compound is, the hazards that it poses, and any additional precautionary information required or recommended by OSHA or other regulatory laws.

When cytotoxic drugs are ready to be administered, special steps must be taken to prevent contamination of the environment, the patient, and the staff administering the drug. If preparation of the drug is required before administration (e.g., mixing of dry drug and liquid diluent), it should be done just before administration of the drug to the patient to

decrease the risk of the active prepared drug being spilled or otherwise contaminating the treatment area. The veterinary professional should adhere to the following general guidelines and steps for safe preparation, administration, and disposal of toxic drugs:

1. Prepare and administer toxic drugs in a low-traffic, well-ventilated area. A ventilated hood is preferred.
2. Wear proper protective attire when preparing or administering the drug. Such attire should include the following
   - A high-efficiency filter mask (surgical masks do not protect against inhalation of aerosols)
   - Some form of gloves, either two pairs of surgical-quality latex gloves (all latex gloves are porous to some degree), commercially available heavy-weight gloves for use with cytotoxic agents, or latex gloves with large animal obstetric sleeves to protect the arms
   - A long-sleeved, nonporous gown with close-fitting cuffs over which the gloves are worn
   - Goggles to protect the eyes from aerosol exposure
3. Use syringes and intravenous lines with screw-on attachments to prevent spillage.
4. Recheck the calculated dose.
5. Confirm that the catheter is correctly placed within the vein and is still patent.
6. Place all syringes, intravenous lines, catheters, and discarded vials in sealable plastic bags immediately after use.
7. Place all items in a leak-proof, puncture-proof container designed for and labeled as hazardous waste.

Veterinary professionals should ensure that the treatment area is properly cleaned and decontaminated rather than depend on the lay staff to do so. A chemotherapy spill kit should be readily available. This kit should include a complete set of protective clothing as outlined above, absorbent pads with nonporous backing, a "sharps" container for needles and other sharp objects used, and a hazardous materials disposal bag. Because of the potential for human and animal injury with use of these drugs, the time and effort spent learning the way to safely store, prepare, administer, and dispose of these agents are well invested.

COMPOUNDING DRUGS

Originally drugs were made by mixing herbs, chemicals, extracts, and compounds together with a mortar and pestle. This process of creating a "new" drug from various ingredients is still used today in veterinary medicine and is known as compounding. Compounding is defined by the Federal Food, Drug, and Cosmetic Act as any manipulation to produce a dose form of a drug in any form other than what is approved by the FDA. Because compounding produces a "new" drug, it is considered drug manufacture and therefore, as with extra-label use, is subject to all regulations for new drugs. Compounding is not permitted by the Act even if the person performing the compounding is a veterinarian or pharmacist. However, the Center for Veterinary Medicine, the FDA division that deals with veterinary matters, "acknowledges the medical need for compounding may exist within certain areas of veterinary practice." A selected number of human pharmacies now advertise that they perform compounding for veterinarians. Examples of compounding done by pharmacies include the following:

- Formulating drugs with flavored compounds (e.g., fish, beef) so they are more readily accepted by a dog or a cat
- Formulating drugs into capsules or tablets that are no longer available as human drugs (e.g., diethylstilbestrol for urinary incontinence, cisapride for cats with megacolon)
- Formulating drugs into different forms (e.g., gels, pastes, dermal patches, rectal suppositories) to facilitate administration
- Formulating a raw chemical into a dose form for administration to animals (e.g., potassium bromide reagent used as an anticonvulsant into a syrup or elixir formulation)

Veterinary professionals often compound drugs without being aware that they are creating an unapproved drug according to the law. For example, the practice of creating "anesthetic cocktails" by combining various tranquilizers, analgesics, and anesthetic agents is an example of compounding. Other examples of compounding include diluting commercially prepared drugs with saline, another drug, or glycerol; crushing a tablet or emptying a capsule into a liquid to create a suspension or solution; and mixing two or more drugs in the same syringe.

The FDA has issued a policy on compounding titled Compounding of Drugs for Use in Animals. This document and other FDA documents can be obtained by written request from the FDA, Freedom of Information Staff (HFI-35), 5600 Fishers Lane, Rockville, MD 20857.

In addition, the Animal Medicinal Drug Use Clarification Act of 1994 (AMDUCA) provides guidelines and regulations for compounding and use of compounded medications. The guidelines for compounding can be summarized as follows:

- Compounding is considered acceptable if done by a practitioner (or a pharmacist on the prescription by a veterinarian), if the resulting product will be used within the practice, and if the benefit to the animal is much greater than the health risk to the animal or public.
- Compounding is considered unacceptable when the health risk to the general public is significant, such as from drug residues in food, regardless of potential benefit to the animal.
- Compounding a drug for use by others outside the practice is considered illegal manufacturing of a new drug.
- Compounding must be done by a veterinarian or pharmacist. Veterinarians must decide whether compounding requires the skills of a pharmacist.

- A valid relationship must exist between the veterinarian and the client and patient.
- The veterinarian or pharmacist must dispense the compound.
- No drug residue violation can occur with use of the compounded substance.
- The safety and efficacy of the compounded new drug must be consistent with current standards of pharmaceutical and pharmacologic practices.
- Appropriate patient records must be maintained.
- All compounds must be labeled with the following information: name and address of the attending veterinarian, date on which the drug was dispensed and date of expiration (expiration date not to exceed the length of prescribed treatment), medically active ingredients, identity of treated animals, directions for use, cautionary statements if applicable, withdrawal times if needed, and the condition or disease for which the compound is being used.

An interesting distinction is the difference between compounding a medication for use in the veterinary practice as opposed to compounding a product for sale or use outside the veterinary practice. Compounding different types of deworming medications for use in a veterinary professional's own practice is technically acceptable; however, the professional cannot legally sell those medications to another veterinary practice because that would constitute illegal manufacturing of a new drug. Repackaging bulk materials into smaller packages for sale would also be considered a form of compounding or drug manufacture and in violation of the Act and the guidelines set by the FDA.

Veterinary professionals must be aware of the regulations governing safe compounding of drugs in veterinary practices. Failure to comply with regulations may result in public safety issues, litigation against the veterinary professionals involved (possibly including the technician who makes up the compounded material on the order of the veterinarian), and ultimately tighter government regulation of veterinary drug use in response to public demand for safe food and water.

CALCULATING DRUG DOSES

Statistics would likely show that almost every day an animal in a veterinary hospital somewhere is receiving the wrong amount of a drug because of a miscalculated dose. In many cases the error may only result in mild or no side effects. However, if the animal dies or is injured by such a mistake, the veterinarian and the veterinary technician who miscalculated the dose would potentially be legally liable for the animal's death. Therefore good math skills and constant practice will help the veterinary professional consistently calculate the correct dose.

An explanation of how to calculate drug doses relies on a short introduction to the different measurement systems used in veterinary medicine. Different systems have historically been used to describe mass (weight), volume, and length. Today in veterinary medicine the *metric system* is the system of measurement most commonly used. However, vestiges of the *apothecary system* and the *household measurement system* are still used.

The metric system uses different prefixes to designate units of 10, 100, 1000, 1/10, and so forth. The basic metric unit of mass is the gram (e.g., kilograms, grams, milligrams), the basic metric unit of volume is the liter (e.g., kiloliters, liters, milliliters), and the basic metric unit of length is the meter (e.g., kilometers, meters, millimeters). Conversion within the metric system is much easier than within the other systems because all conversions are even multiples of 10 (e.g., 1, 10, 100, 1000). See Table 2-2 for the common prefixes of the metric system used in veterinary medicine.

The apothecary system, which is a much older system than the metric system, is not

TABLE **2-2** Common Prefixes Used in the Metric System

kilo (k)	multiplies by 1000	×10³
hecto	multiplies by 100	×10²
deka	multiplies by 10	×10
deci (d)	multiplies by 1/10	×10⁻¹
centi (c)	multiplies by 1/100	×10⁻²
milli (m)	multiplies by 1/1000	×10⁻³
micro (μ or mc)*	multiplies by 1/1,000,000	×10⁻⁶
nano (n)	multiplies by 1/1,000,000,000	×10⁻⁹

When referring to more than one metric unit (e.g., 300 kilograms), the abbreviation does not end with the letter s. So 300 kilograms would be 300 kg, not 300 kgs.
*Micro- is typically noted by the Greek letter mu. However, when "μ" is handwritten, it can look similar to a script letter m or printed letter u. Therefore mc is becoming more commonly used in handwritten dosing orders, although μ is still often seen in typewritten text.

used much in veterinary medicine, but volumes are occasionally measured as fluid ounces (fl oz) and mass measured as grains (gr). Tablet strengths of aspirin, phenobarbital, and several household antiinflammatory drugs are commonly listed in grains instead of the metric form of milligrams.

The household system, as the name implies, is based on common household units of measurement (e.g., teaspoon, tablespoon, cup, pint, gallon, pound). Oral medications are often dispensed with directions stated in household measurements (e.g., "give 1 teaspoon twice daily"). Because these three systems of measurement are still used in veterinary medicine, the veterinary professional must be able to readily convert among these systems. The common equivalent conversions used in veterinary medicine are shown in Table 2-3.

When calculating a dose for an animal, the veterinary professional will discover that several methods are advocated by different writers and different texts. They go by names such as the proportional method, dimensional analysis, the factor-label method, and the cancel-out method. Several excellent texts for human nurses and some for veterinary professionals (e.g., *Dimensional Analysis for Meds, Medical Math and Dosage Calculations for the Veterinary Professional*) explain the underlying math concepts of dosage calculation in detail and illustrate different methods for calculating drug doses.

Regardless of which method of dose calculation is used, all the methods use the same basic high-school algebra techniques to manipulate the equation to solve for X. The method used in this text is the dimensional analysis, or "cancel-out" method, so named because it uses multiplication of fractions set up so that units in the numerators (top part of the fraction) cancel out the same units in the denominators (bottom part of the fraction), leaving only the units required by the answer.

To determine a dose for a particular animal, the following elements need to be known:
- The weight of the animal
- The recommended dosage of the drug for animals of this species
- The concentration of the drug

The weight of the animal is typically expressed as units of mass (e.g., ounces, pounds, kilograms, milligrams). The dosage of the drug is usually expressed as some mass of drug per unit mass (weight) of animal. For example, a dosage may be expressed as 10 mg/kg, meaning that 10 mg of drug are administered for each kilogram of the animal's body weight. Dosages may be listed as a *dosage range*, which allows the veterinary professional to select a dosage within this range. An example of a dosage range is 1 to 3 mg/lb, meaning that a dose can be calculated for any number of milligrams between 1 and 3 for each pound of body weight.

TABLE **2-3** Equivalents Used to Convert Within or Between Metric, Apothecary, and Household Systems of Measurement

WEIGHT OR MASS		
1 kilogram (kg)	=	2.2 pounds (lb)
1 kilogram (kg)	=	1000 grams (g)
1 kilogram (kg)	=	1,000,000 milligrams (mg)
1 gram (g)	=	1000 milligrams (mg)
1 gram (g)	=	0.001 kilogram (kg)
1 milligram (mg)	=	0.001 gram (g)
1 milligram (mg)	=	1000 micrograms (µg or mcg)
1 pound (lb)	=	0.454 kilogram (kg)
1 pound (lb)	=	16 ounces (oz)
1 grain (gr)	=	64.8 milligrams (mg) (household system)
1 grain (gr)	=	60 milligrams (mg) (apothecary)
VOLUME		
1 liter (L)	=	1000 milliliters (mL)
1 liter (L)	=	10 deciliters (dL)
1 milliliter (mL)	=	1 cubic centimeter (cc)
1 milliliter (mL)	=	1000 microliters (µL or mcL)
1 tablespoon (TBL or Tbsp)	=	3 teaspoons (tsp)
1 tablespoon (TBL or Tbsp)	=	15 milliliters (mL)
1 teaspoon (tsp)	=	5 milliliters (mL)
1 gallon (gal)	=	3.786 liters (L)
1 gallon (gal)	=	4 quarts (qt)
1 gallon (gal)	=	8 pints (pt)
1 pint (pt)	=	2 cups (c)
1 pint (pt)	=	16 fluid ounces (fl oz)
1 pint (pt)	=	473 milliliters (mL)

Both the household and apothecary systems for grain to milligram conversion are still used in both human medicine and veterinary medicine.

The concentration of the drug is expressed as mass of drug per volume of liquid or mass of drug per solid dose form. For example, a multidose vial may have the concentration of drug listed as 10 mg/mL, meaning that each 1 milliliter of liquid withdrawn from the vial contains 10 mg of actual drug. Tablets, capsules, caplets, and other solid dose forms are commonly described according to the amount of drug in each dose form unit (e.g., 400-mg strength, 150-mg strength). A 400-mg strength tablet means that 400 mg of drug is delivered to the animal with each tablet.

Liquid dose form concentrations are occasionally expressed as *percentage solutions*. The percentage solution simply describes the number of grams of drug in 100 mL of liquid.

Thus a 1% solution would have 1 gram of drug in each 100 mL withdrawn. Notice that a 1% solution also equals 10 mg/mL (convert 1 gram to 1000 milligrams and divide by 100). The most common problem veterinary technician students have in converting a percentage solution concentration to the more familiar milligrams per milliliter concentration is they forget that an X percentage solution is X grams per 100 mL of liquid and not X grams/mL.

Step 1

Compare the unit of mass for the animal's weight with the unit of mass used for body weight in the drug dosage. If the animal's weight is given in the same units as the body weight in the drug dosage, step 1 can be skipped. For example, if a dog weighs 15 kg and the drug dose is listed as 2 mg/kg (2 mg of drug per kilogram of body weight), then proceed to step 2 because both the animal's body weight and the dosage body weight are expressed in the same units (kilograms). If the dosage for the 15-kg dog is listed as 2 mg/lb instead of 2 mg/kg, then the animal's weight must be converted to the same units as the body weight units in the dosage.

In this case of a 15-kg dog and a 2-mg/lb dosage, kilograms must be converted to an equivalent number of pounds by using the conversion factors listed in Table 2-3 to form a fraction by which the original unit is multiplied.

$$\text{Animal's weight} \times \frac{\overset{\text{Conversion factor}}{\text{New unit}}}{\text{Original unit}}$$

$$= \text{Equivalent weight in new units}$$

$$\text{Dog's weight } 15 \text{ kg} \times \frac{2.2 \text{ lb}}{\text{kg}} = 33\text{-lb dog}$$

Note that the conversion factor fraction is set up with the kilogram unit (body weight) located in the denominator (lower part) of the fraction so that the kilogram unit in the dog's weight can cancel it out. In the example above, the kilogram of the dog's weight in the numerator (15 kg is the same as the fraction 15 kg/1) cancels the kilogram in the denominator of the conversion factor fraction, leaving only pound as the unit to be multiplied.

$$\text{Dog's weight } 15 \cancel{\text{kg}} \times \frac{2.2 \text{ lb}}{\cancel{\text{kg}}} = 33\text{-lb dog}$$

$$\text{Dog's weight } 15 \times 2.2 \text{ lb} = 33\text{-lb dog}$$

The convenience of this method is that the equation is always set up properly when the units cancel each other out, leaving only the unit needed for the answer.

Listed below are several examples illustrating how to convert the animal's weight to an equivalent value in new units. Notice how the conversion fractions are set up to cancel out all the units except the one needed for the answer.

$$10 \cancel{\text{lb}} \text{ dog} \times \frac{1 \text{ kg}}{2.2 \cancel{\text{lb}}} = 22\text{-kg dog}$$

$$44 \cancel{\text{kg}} \text{ dog} \times \frac{2.2 \text{ lb}}{1 \cancel{\text{kg}}} = 20\text{-lb dog}$$

$$100 \cancel{\text{g}} \text{ rat} \times \frac{1 \text{ kg}}{1000 \cancel{\text{g}}} = 0.1\text{-kg rat}$$

$$2 \cancel{\text{kg}} \text{ kitten} \times \frac{1000 \text{ g}}{1 \cancel{\text{kg}}} = 2000\text{-g kitten}$$

Now that the animal's weight units have been converted to the equivalent body weight units as the dosage, step 2 calculates the actual amount of drug to be administered.

Step 2

In step 2 the animal's body weight and the drug's listed dosage or dosage range are used to calculate the actual amount of drug to be administered one time (the dose).

$$\text{Animal's weight} \times \frac{\overset{\text{Dosage}}{\text{Mass of drug}}}{\text{Body weight}}$$

$$= \text{Dose for animal}$$

The dosage is set up as a fraction, with the body weight unit in the denominator so that it will cancel out the unit of the animal's weight.

$$10 \cancel{\text{lb}} \text{ dog} \times \frac{2 \text{ mg drug}}{\cancel{\text{lb}}} = 20 \text{ mg drug}$$

$$2 \cancel{\text{kg}} \text{ cat} \times \frac{50 \text{ mg drug}}{\cancel{\text{kg}}} = 100 \text{ mg drug}$$

$$100 \cancel{\text{g}} \text{ rat} \times \frac{0.5 \text{ mg drug}}{\cancel{\text{g}}} = 50 \text{ mg drug}$$

In the event of a dosage range, any number within the range can be used. For example, if a drug has a dosage range of 2 to 4 mg/lb, any of the following would be legitimate doses:

$$10\text{-lb dog} \times \frac{2\text{ mg drug}}{\text{lb}} = 20\text{ mg drug}$$

$$10\text{-lb dog} \times \frac{3\text{ mg drug}}{\text{lb}} = 30\text{ mg drug}$$

$$10\text{-lb dog} \times \frac{4\text{ mg drug}}{\text{lb}} = 40\text{ mg drug}$$

Step 3

Step 2 defines how much drug mass to give. Step 3 determines how much of the dose form to give (e.g., how much liquid, how many tablets), which requires knowing the drug dose that needs to be given to this particular animal (from step 2) and the concentration or strength of the dose form.

$$\text{Dose (Mass)} \times \frac{\text{Volume}}{\text{Mass of drug}}$$
$$= \text{Amount of dose form to be given}$$

$$\text{Dose (Mass)} \times \frac{\text{Tablet}}{\text{Mass of drug}}$$
$$= \text{Amount of dose form to be given}$$

Although liquid concentrations of drugs are listed as drug mass per unit of volume (e.g., 50 mg/mL) or drug mass per tablet (e.g., 200 mg/tablet), to properly calculate the amount of dose form to be given the fraction must be inverted to put the tablet or volume in the numerator (top part of the fraction). By doing this, the dose mass units in the numerator and drug mass units in the denominator cancel each other out, leaving the number of tablets or volume for the answer.

For example, if the calculations in step 2 determine that a 5-lb animal needs 10 mg of drug, and given that the drug comes in a liquid concentration of 2 mg/mL, the equation would be set up as shown:

$$10\text{ mg drug} \times \frac{1\text{ mL}}{2\text{ mg}} =$$

$$10\,\cancel{\text{mg}}\text{ drug} \times \frac{1\text{ mL}}{2\,\cancel{\text{mg}}} =$$

$$10 \times \frac{1\text{ mL}}{2} = 5\text{ mL of liquid to be given}$$

For tablets, the problem is set up in a similar manner by replacing the unit of volume with the unit for the solid dose. Continuing with the example above, change the dose form to 2-mg tablet strength.

$$10\text{ mg drug} \times \frac{1\text{ tablet}}{2\text{ mg}} =$$

$$10\,\cancel{\text{mg}}\text{ drug} \times \frac{1\text{ tablet}}{2\,\cancel{\text{mg}}} =$$

$$10 \times \frac{1\text{ tablet}}{2} = 5\text{ tablets given per dose}$$

Tablets are rarely broken into anything smaller than one half; therefore rounding the calculated number of tablets needed to the nearest whole or half tablet size may be necessary.

Step 4

The client must be dispensed enough dose forms (tablets, etc.) to last several days or longer. Once the number of dose forms per dose (e.g., 5 tablets per dose) has been determined, the following equation can be used to determine the total number to be dispensed:

$$\frac{\#\text{Tablet}}{\text{Dose}} \times \frac{\#\text{Doses}}{\text{Day}} \times \#\text{Days}$$
$$= \text{Total tablets dispensed}$$

Notice how the units of "dose" and "days" cancel out, leaving the answer in tablets. If 5 tablets per dose q8h (every 8 hours, or three times daily) were given for 4 days, the equation would be set up and solved as follows:

$$\frac{5\text{ tablets}}{\text{Dose}} \times \frac{3\text{ doses}}{\text{Day}} \times 4\text{ days} =$$

$$\frac{5 \text{ tablets}}{\cancel{\text{Dose}}} \times \frac{3 \cancel{\text{ doses}}}{\text{Day}} \times 4 \text{ days} =$$

$$5 \text{ tablets} \times \frac{3}{\cancel{\text{Day}}} \times 4 \cancel{\text{ days}} =$$

$$5 \text{ tablets} \times 3 \times 4 = 60 \text{ tablets to be dispensed}$$

For liquid formulations, the tablets are replaced with units of volume. If 2 mL per dose were needed to be given twice daily (b.i.d. or q12h) for 1 week, the problem would be solved as follows:

$$\frac{2 \text{ mL}}{\text{Dose}} \times \frac{2 \text{ doses}}{\text{Day}} \times 7 \text{ days} =$$

$$\frac{2 \text{ mL}}{\cancel{\text{Dose}}} \times \frac{2 \cancel{\text{ doses}}}{\text{Day}} \times 7 \text{ days} =$$

$$2 \text{ mL} \times \frac{2}{\cancel{\text{Day}}} \times 7 \cancel{\text{ days}} =$$

$$2 \text{ mL} \times 2 \times 7 = 28 \text{ mL to be dispensed}$$

One of the most common mistakes for a veterinary technician is shown in the following example. Try to identify where the problem occurred.

$$44\text{-lb dog}$$

Dosage = 2 mg/kg t.i.d. (three times daily)

for 5 days

Tablet size = 60 mg

$$44 \text{ lb} \times \frac{\text{kg}}{2.2 \text{ lb}} = 20\text{-kg dog}$$

$$20\text{-kg dog} \times \frac{2 \text{ mg}}{\text{kg}} = 40 \text{ mg of drug per dose}$$

$$\frac{40 \text{ mg drug}}{\text{Dose}} \times \frac{3 \text{ doses}}{\text{Day}} \times 5 \text{ days}$$

$$= 600 \text{ mg total for 5 days}$$

$$600 \text{ mg} \times \frac{1 \text{ tablet}}{60 \text{ mg}} = 10 \text{ tablets}$$

This answer seems reasonable, but those 10 tablets have to be split evenly at three doses a day for 5 days or 15 doses. That means the client is going to have to give the animal two thirds of a tablet with each dose. What went wrong? The student did the calculation in the wrong order:

Step 1

$$44 \text{ lb} \times \frac{\text{kg}}{2.2 \text{ lb}} = 20\text{-kg dog}$$

Step 2

$$20\text{-kg dog} \times \frac{2 \text{ mg}}{\text{kg}} = 40 \text{ mg of drug per dose}$$

Step 4

$$\frac{40 \text{ mg drug}}{\text{Dose}} \times \frac{3 \text{ doses}}{\text{Day}} \times 5 \text{ days}$$

$$= 600 \text{ mg total for 5 days}$$

Step 3

$$600 \text{ mg} \times \frac{1 \text{ tablet}}{60 \text{ mg}} = 10 \text{ tablets}$$

Once the mass of drug is calculated (40 mg of drug per dose), the next step is to calculate how many tablets will be used per dose. Rounding the tablet to the nearest half or whole tablet takes place at this stage.

Step 1

$$44 \text{ lb} \times \frac{\text{kg}}{2.2 \text{ lb}} = 20\text{-kg dog}$$

Step 2

$$20\text{-kg dog} \times \frac{2 \text{ mg}}{\text{kg}} = 40 \text{ mg of drug per dose}$$

Step 3

$$40 \text{ mg} \times \frac{1 \text{ tablet}}{60 \text{ mg}} = 0.66 \text{ tablets}$$

Round down to

$$\frac{1}{2} \text{ tablet} \left(0.66 \text{ is closer to } 0.5 \text{ than } 1.0 \right)$$

Step 4

$$\frac{\frac{1}{2} \text{ tablet}}{\text{Dose}} \times \frac{3 \text{ doses}}{\text{Day}} \times 5 \text{ days}$$

$$= 7\frac{1}{2} \text{ tablets total for 5 days}$$

Frequent practice of dosage calculations will reduce the chances of mistakes occurring and veterinary patients receiving an inappropriate amount of medication.

RECOMMENDED READING RESOURCES

American Veterinary Medical Association: *AVMA guidelines for veterinary prescription drugs,* Schaumburg, Ill., 2005, AVMA.

Apley MD: *Current drug use regulations.* In Proceedings of the Western Veterinary Conference, Las Vegas, NV, Feb 17-20, 2003.

Boothe DM: *Optimizing antibacterial therapy for small animals using the professional flexible label.* In Proceedings of the North American Veterinary Conference, Orlando, Fla., 2000.

Boothe DM: *Small animal clinical pharmacology and therapeutics,* Philadelphia, 2001, WB Saunders.

Dickinson KL, Ogilview GK: Safe handling and administration of chemotherapeutic agents in veterinary medicine. In Bonagura JD, editor: *Kirk's current veterinary therapy XII,* Philadelphia, 1995, WB Saunders.

Kitchell BD: *How to give chemotherapeutic drugs in practice and still sleep at night.* In Proceedings of the American College of Veterinary Internal Medicine Annual Meeting, San Antonio, TX, 2002.

Lacroix CA: *Illegal drug compounding: your legal nightmare waiting to happen!* In Proceedings of the Atlantic Coast Veterinary Conference, Atlantic City, NJ, 2004.

Legendre AM: *The use of chemotherapy drugs in practice.* In Proceedings of the American College of Veterinary Internal Medicine Annual Meeting, Charlotte, NC, 2003.

Webb AI: *Legal requirements of using pharmaceuticals.* In Proceedings of the Western Veterinary Conference, Las Vegas, NV, 2004.

WEB RESOURCES

www.osha.gov

The official site of OSHA, a division of the U.S. Department of Labor, contains a large amount of information regarding OSHA standards, news, issues and events, and related resources.

www.fda.gov/search.html

This site, sponsored by the U.S. Food and Drug Administration, has a search feature that uses key words (e.g., "compounding") to locate relevant articles and documents.

www.usp.org

The United States Pharmacopeia is an organization that sets standards that manufacturers must meet to sell their products in the United States. The USP home page provides links to veterinary drug information, quality standards, and the Veterinary Practitioner's Reporting (VPR) Program.

Self-Assessment

REVIEW QUESTIONS

1. What is missing from the following prescription?

   _____

   Johnstown Veterinary Hospital, INC
   3526 E. Caroline Ave SW
   Johnstown, IA 74214-2441
   (315) 521-2151

   August 21st, 1998

   Mr. James Morrisi "Felix" (feline)

   215 Boxwood Apt. 3a, Johnstown   523-4111

   ℞ Amoxitabs #24

   SIG: 1 tablet q12h PO for 12 days

   Dr. Lucenda Morgenstine

Fill in the following blanks with the correct item from the Key Terms list.

2. _____ an abbreviation meaning the drug is available for purchase without a prescription or a veterinarian's order.

3. _____ a level of controlled substance (C-V though C-I) that cannot be prescribed by a veterinarian because it contains a substance of high abuse with no approved medical purpose.

4. _____ This term means "poisonous to cells."

5. _____ What does MSDS stand for?

6. _____   What does OSHA stand for?

7. _____   mixing two drugs together to create a "new" drug.

8. _____   type of dangerous drugs used to treat cancer.

9. _____   system of measurement that includes tablespoon, pint, gallon, and pound.

10. _____   capable of producing birth defects; often considered to be similar to the term teratogenic.

Indicate whether each of the following statements is true or false.

11. The DEA typically requires maintaining the controlled substance logs for a minimum of 5 years.

12. Adding acepromazine tranquilizer to a bottle of ketamine is not considered compounding as long as it is not sold to another practice.

13. If a drug is labeled as "store at room temperature," then keeping it in a refrigerator to keep it cool is acceptable.

14. The use of pill vial caps that are not childproof is illegal in veterinary medicine because they violate the Poison Prevention Packaging Act of 1970.

15. Schedule C-III substances have a greater potential for abuse than C-V substances.

16. Schedule C-II drug prescriptions may not be refilled; a new prescription must be written for each treatment period.

17. Generally, a three-ring notebook or spiral notebook is sufficient for maintaining a controlled substance log.

18. Make the following conversions:

2 g = _____ mg

5 mg = _____ g

14 lb = _____ kg

23 kg = _____ lb

83 kg = _____ mg

65 kg = _____ lb

0.4 kg = _____ g

0.003 lb = _____ mg

15 lb = _____ g

0.00043 kg = _____ mg

25,488 mg = _____ lb

0.0092 lb = _____ mg

25 mL = _____ L

43 cc = _____ mL

1.5 L = _____ mL

800 cc = _____ L

0.055 L = _____ mL

0.25 mL = _____ L

19. The doctor asks you to prepare a dose of ketamine sufficient to restrain a 15-lb cat. The drug formulary recommends using 15 mg/kg intravenously or intramuscularly. The concentration of ketamine in the vial is 100 mg/mL. What volume of ketamine is required for this cat?

20. The veterinarian asks you to fill a prescription for butorphanol for a coughing dog, dispensing sufficient tablets for 5 days of treatment. The dog weighs 55 lb. The recommended dose is 0.08 mg/kg. The tablets are available in 1-, 5-, and 10-mg sizes. The charge is $0.35 per tablet. How many tablets are required for a single dose? If the dosage specifies use q6h, how many tablets are required for each day of treatment? How many tablets should you dispense for the total 5 days of treatment? What is the charge for the dispensed medication?

21. The veterinarian wants to medicate a 16-lb Chihuahua, a 27-lb terrier, and a 66-lb collie. The recommended dosage is 3 to 5 mg/kg given once daily. You are to dispense enough medication to last each dog 180 days (6 months). The 50-mg tablets cost $0.03 each, the 100-mg tablets cost $0.05 each, and the 200-mg tablets cost $0.07 each. What are the minimal and maximal daily doses (in milligrams) for each dog based on the recommended dosage range? How many tablets and what size are required for each dog each day? How much does the medication for the 180 days of treatment cost for each dog?

22. What is the concentration of drug (in milligrams per milliliter) in a 10% solution? In a 43% solution?

23. How many milligrams of drug are in 0.13 L of a 7.5% solution?

APPLICATION QUESTIONS

1. A pet owner is passing through town and stops by your veterinary clinic to see whether she can pick up some "car sickness" tablets for her dog. The owner is on a cross-country car trip and has no more of the motion sickness medication that was dispensed by her veterinarian. The doctor is not in the clinic at the moment. Is it legal to dispense the medication if you first telephone the doctor to obtain permission?

2. Translate the following drug orders.

   - give 3 mg q4h PO prn
   - disp 1 bottle–give 2 gtt OU b.i.d.
   - give 2 cc IP stat
   - needs to have 3L qd

- 15 mg IV t.i.d.

- 4.5 mL of the 5 mg/mL concentration q.i.d.

3. You are the technician who orders most of the drugs for your veterinary practice. Can you legally order drugs that are listed as C-II? Can any licensed veterinarian order such drugs?

4. The veterinarian stores his controlled substances in a 1-cubic-foot metal tool box with a heavy-duty padlock. Is this adequate storage for schedule drugs? What about a wooden cabinet with a lock?

5. The veterinarian wants to clear out some old records, including some controlled substance logs that are 6 years old. Is it legal to discard these logs?

6. A fellow staff member routinely uses a surgical mask and a single pair of latex surgical gloves during preparation and administration of antineoplastic drugs. Is this adequate protection?

7. A veterinarian in another practice sees that there is a market for the "blue goo" concoction that he compounded as a teat dip to prevent mastitis. Can the doctor legally sell this product to your practice if he applies a label to each bottle stating "for use by or on the order of a licensed veterinarian"?

8. A diabetic dog is being treated in the clinic. The dog requires 3.2 units (U) of insulin in both the morning and evening. U-100 insulin has a concentration of 100 units of insulin/mL and is supplied as 10-mL vials. At the insulin dosage listed above, how many full doses (3.2 units) of insulin for this dog are contained in this vial?

9. The veterinarian asks you to dispense digoxin for a client's dog. The recommended dose is 0.22 mg/m^2, with m^2 being the number of square meters of body surface area. The dog's body surface area is 0.8 m^2. The digoxin elixir is available in a concentration of 0.15 mg/mL. To prevent overdosing, the doctor instructs you to use 60% of the calculated normal dose for this dog. How many milliliters of digoxin elixir should this dog receive for each dose?

10. You were calculating the total number of tablets to be dispensed and somehow came up with an unusable answer. The dog weighs 42 lb (19.1 kg). The dose is 10 mg/kg t.i.d. for 10 days and the tablet size is 50 mg. You calculated the dose by multiplying 19.1 kg by 10 mg/kg to get 191 mg per dose. You wanted to determine the total milligrams needed for the 10 days, so you took the 191 mg per dose and multiplied it by three doses per day (t.i.d.) to get 573 mg and then multiplied that by 10 days to get 5730 mg total for 10 days. The 5730 mg total comes out to 114.6, the 50-mg tablets that you rounded to 115 tablets to cover the 10 days. But when you attempt to determine how many tablets the owner needs to give the dog with each dose, the number of tablets per dose does not make sense. Determine how many tablets this animal would get per dose based on this calculation of total milligrams of drug needed for the 10 days and determine where the mistake in logic was made in doing this calculation.

11. A client wants to buy $10 worth of vitamins for his dog. The doctor asks you to dispense the medication but not to exceed the $10 value. The dog weighs 8 lb. The recommended dosage is 8 mg/kg given once daily. The medication is supplied as 15-mg tablets. A bottle of 1000 tablets costs $130. How many days' worth of tablets can you dispense for $10?

Pharmacokinetics and Pharmacodynamics: The Principles of How Drugs Work

key terms

absorption
acid drug
acidic pH
active secretion (renal)
active transport
aerosol administration
agonist
alkaline drug
alkaline pH
antagonist
aqueous
basic drug
basic environmental pH
biliary excretion
bioavailability
biotransformation
blood-brain barrier
Bowman's capsule
chelator
clearance
collecting ducts (kidney)
competitive, reversible
   antagonism
concentration gradient
dissolution
distal convoluted tubule
distribution
elimination
enterohepatic circulation
equilibrium
excretion
extracellular fluid
extravascular injection
facilitated diffusion
fenestrations
filtration (renal)
first-pass effect

free form of the drug
   molecules
gastric motility
glomerulus
half-life of elimination
hepatic excretion
hepatic portal system
hydrophilic
induced metabolism
intestinal motility
ion trapping
intraarterial injection
intradermal (ID) injection
intramuscular (IM) injection
intraperitoneal (IP) injection
intravenous (IV)
intravenous bolus
intravenous infusion
intrinsic activity
lipophilic
loading dose
loop of Henle
maintenance dose
maximum effective
   concentration
metabolism
metabolite
minimum effective
   concentration
noncompetitive,
   irreversible, or
   insurmountable
   antagonism
non–receptor-mediated
   drug reaction
parenteral administration
partial agonist
partial antagonist

passive diffusion
perfusion
perivascular injection
per os (PO)
phagocytosis
pharmacodynamics
pharmacokinetics
pinocytosis
pKa
plasma (serum)
   concentrations
prodrug
protein-bound drug
proximal convoluted
   tubule
reabsorption (renal)
receptor
redistribution
renal excretion
route of administration
saturated
steady state
subcutaneous (SC or SQ)
subtherapeutic
surmountable antagonism
therapeutic range/window
t-max
tolerance to drug
topically administered
   drugs
total daily dose
vasoconstriction
vasodilation
volume of distribution
   (Vd)
weak acid/base
xenobiotics

1. The factors that affect movement of drug molecules throughout the body

2. The characteristics of each route of drug administration

3. The physiologic factors that change the way drugs move through the body

4. The factors that alter the way drugs are absorbed, distributed, metabolized, and excreted

5. The interaction between drugs and receptors and how that produces cellular effects

6. How pharmacokinetics and pharmacodynamics affect every drug treatment

Pharmacokinetics is the study of how a drug moves into, through, and out of the body. *Pharmacodynamics* is the study of how the drug produces its effects on the body. This chapter explains the basics of pharmacokinetics and pharmacodynamics to provide the veterinary technician with a basic comprehension of what a drug is doing inside the body and how it is doing it.

As stated in Chapter 1, all drugs are poisons. Compounds such as strychnine, mercury, arsenic, and snake venoms were once considered useful drugs capable of curing a variety of ailments. Today, medical personnel know that these compounds, if given in sufficient quantities, can kill an animal or person. Although today's drugs are much safer, they can be just as deadly as strychnine or snake venom if given in excessive amounts or if inappropriately administered. Only proper administration determines whether a compound is beneficial or deadly.

The drug dosages listed in drug formularies or from the manufacturer will work for the majority of animals. However, the alteration of normal physiology by disease can result in the body accumulating a greater amount of a drug or responding to the drug in a way that results in harm. Therefore the veterinary professional must be familiar with how a change in the animal's physiology or body state requires alteration of drug dosages.

THERAPEUTIC RANGE

Poisons such as lead and arsenic will not produce signs of clinical toxicity if given a single time in a small quantity. In contrast, even beneficial drugs can be toxic if given in quantities that exceed the normal recommended dose. Therefore the amount of drug administered and the resulting concentration achieved in the body are quite important in determining whether a drug is beneficial or detrimental to an animal. The ideal range of drug concentrations within the body is referred to as the *therapeutic range,* or *therapeutic window.*

Administering the manufacturer's approved drug dose should achieve concentrations within the therapeutic range. If too much drug is given, an excessive accumulation of drug occurs and concentrations will exceed the top end of the normal therapeutic range. The top end of the normal therapeutic range is called the *maximum effective concentration* and represents the border between those concentrations that are beneficial and those concentrations at which signs of toxicity develop (Figure 3-1).

If insufficient drug is administered, the concentration of drug achieved within the body will be below the concentrations in the therapeutic range. The bottom end of the normal therapeutic range is the *minimum effective concentration.* At concentrations of drug below the minimum effective concentration the drug will

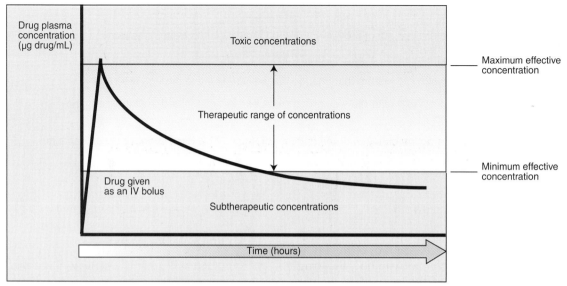

Figure 3-1 The therapeutic range of concentrations of a drug in the plasma.

not achieve its beneficial effect. These concentrations are said to be *subtherapeutic.*

If the goal of drug therapy is to maintain a drug in the body within the therapeutic range of concentration, the amount of drug entering the body must be balanced by the rate that the drug leaves the body. The proper balance allows just enough drugs to accumulate to achieve therapeutic concentrations. A simple analogy may help explain this concept. Think of the body as a bucket with a small hole in the bottom. Water poured in the bucket will leak out at a rate determined by the size of the hole. To maintain a certain water level in the bucket, the rate at which water is poured into the bucket must balance with the rate at which the water is leaking out. In this analogy, the addition of the water to the bucket is the drug dose, the leaking of the water is the *elimination* or *metabolism* of the drug, and the desired water level in the bucket is the therapeutic range for the drug.

To maintain therapeutic concentrations of a drug in an animal, the amount of the drug administered and the rate at which it is absorbed must match the rate at which it is eliminated from the body. As shown in Figure 3-2, if the hole in the bucket suddenly becomes smaller, the rate at which the water is poured into the bucket (the drug dose administered) must be decreased to prevent overflow (toxicity). The liver and kidneys are the primary organs involved in removing drugs from the body. If these organs are damaged and elimination of the drug is slowed, the drug dose (drug amount) or the frequency of administration of the drug dose must be reduced to prevent accumulation to toxic levels.

In contrast, if the hole in the bucket is made larger and the rate of water addition remains constant, the water level falls. Similarly, if the rate of drug elimination is increased, the dosage (amount and frequency of administration) must be increased to compensate and maintain concentrations within the therapeutic range.

DOSAGE REGIMEN AND ROUTES OF ADMINISTRATION

The three components of the therapeutic administration of drugs are the dose, dosage interval, and *route of administration.* Altering any

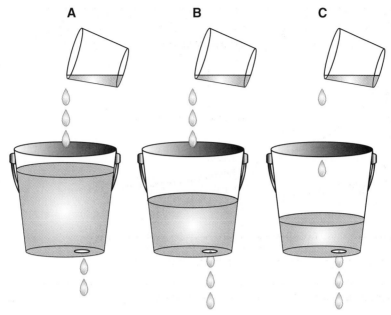

Figure 3-2 The bucket analogy for understanding the impact of pharmacokinetics on therapeutic concentrations. **A,** If the rate at which water is poured into a bucket (drug dose administered) is greater than the rate at which it is leaving (drug excreted from the body), the water level will rise. **B,** If the rate at which water is poured into a bucket is equal to the rate at which it is leaving, the water level will remain stable. **C,** If the rate at which water is poured into a bucket is less than the rate at which it is leaving, the water level will fall.

component can result in drug concentrations that are too high or too low.

DRUG DOSE

A drug's dose is the amount of drug administered at one time. Drug doses are expressed most accurately as units of mass, such as milligrams, grams, or grains, rather than the number of product units, such as tablets or capsules, or volume such as milliliters. For example, the veterinary technician should avoid writing in the patient record that an animal received "1 tablet of amoxicillin" because amoxicillin is available in tablet sizes ranging from 50 mg to 400 mg. The same is true of the statement "give 3 mL of xylazine" because 3 mL of a xylazine solution with a concentration of 20 mg/mL contains much less xylazine than 3 mL of a solution with a concentration of 100 mg/mL. Therefore the dose should be stated in units of mass unless the strength

of tablet or concentration of liquid is also mentioned (e.g., 3 mL of the 20 mg/mL xylazine).

A drug dose may be described as a *loading dose* or a *maintenance dose.* The loading dose for a drug is larger than the drug's maintenance dose and is designed to raise the drug concentration to the therapeutic range in a short time. A loading dose is administered either as a larger amount administered once or as a smaller amount (maintenance dose size) administered more frequently. Referring again to the bucket analogy, to get the water to the desired level in a dry bucket, a larger amount of water or frequent additions of smaller amounts of water must be poured in initially to accumulate to the desired level.

Once therapeutic concentrations are achieved, periodic, smaller maintenance drug doses maintain the therapeutic concentrations established by the loading dose. In the bucket analogy, once the desired water level is attained, then smaller amounts of water are added at intervals to maintain the desired level. Loading doses are used in medical situations for which achieving the beneficial therapeutic effect quickly is critical (e.g., life-threatening infections, critical conditions such as shock).

DOSAGE INTERVAL

The time between administrations of separate drug doses is referred to as the dosage interval. Dosage intervals are often expressed by Latin abbreviations such as "b.i.d." or abbreviations such as "q8h." Veterinary technicians must understand the common abbreviations shown in Table 3-1 to administer the appropriate drug amount at the proper time.

The combined amount of drug (mass) administered in a given day is referred to as the *total daily dose*. For example, a 100-mg tablet given four times daily results in a total daily dose of 400 mg. Veterinary professionals use the total daily dose to adjust the dosage interval, dose for medical reasons, or increase client compliance (the owner's willingness to administer the medication as directed). For example, the following dosage regimens provide equivalent total daily doses of 480 mg:

480 mg s.i.d. = 480 mg × 1 time a day = 480 mg
240 mg b.i.d. = 240 mg × 2 times a day = 480 mg
160 mg q8h = 160 mg × 3 times a day = 480 mg
120 mg q6h = 120 mg × 4 times a day = 480 mg
80 mg q4h = 80 mg × 6 times a day = 480 mg

If an owner is much more likely to comply with a once-daily dosage regimen (dosage interval of 24 hours) than with a dosage regimen where the drug is given three times a day, why aren't all dosage regimens once daily? Think back to the bucket analogy. As the water drains out through the bottom of the bucket and the water level falls, the level would fall much further after a longer wait to add water again than it would with a shorter wait. In this situation, a larger volume of water must be added to compensate for the longer interval between additions of water and to prevent all of the water from

TABLE **3-1** Commonly Used Dosage Regimen Abbreviations

ABBREVIATION	DOSAGE INTERVAL
s.i.d.*	Once daily
b.i.d.	Twice daily
t.i.d.	Three times daily
q.i.d.	Four times daily
q4h	Every 4 hours
q6h	Every 6 hours
q8h	Every 8 hours
q12h	Every 12 hours
qd†	Every day
q2d	Every 2 days
prn	As needed

*The abbreviation s.i.d. is not recognized outside veterinary medicine. Pharmacists and physicians that treat human beings are usually unaware of what s.i.d. means.
†If "qd" is written "q.d.", it can be easily confused with "qid" without periods, the result of which would be a 4× overdose.

draining out of the bucket during those intervals. Thus, adding the larger volume of water results in a higher level of water in the bucket than when smaller volumes were added more frequently. Even though the average amount of water in the bucket over the course of time between bucket fillings is at the desired level of water, the high and low levels of water in the bucket are significantly above and below the desired water level. In contrast, if small amounts of water are added more frequently, the average amount of water in the bucket would be the same as that with the longer interval and larger amounts of added water, but the high and low water levels would be less extreme and much closer to the desired water level.

Applying this concept to drug administration, a once-daily dosage interval results in a wider swing of concentration from high to low than a three times daily dosage interval. The concentrations resulting from the once-daily dosage interval may exceed the maximum effective concentration at the peak concentration (resulting in toxicity) and fall below the minimum effective concentration at the low end (resulting in subtherapeutic concentrations). The same amount of drug would be delivered but with less dramatic swings in drug concentrations by giving an equivalent total daily dose with a three times daily dosage interval.

ROUTES OF ADMINISTRATION

The route of administration is the means by which the drug is given and is the third component of the dosage information (dose, dosage interval, route of administration). Even if the correct dose is administered at the appropriate dosage interval, the amount of drug that reaches the target tissues in the body can be significantly altered if an inappropriate route of administration is used.

Routes of administration are identified by where the drug is placed. Drugs given by injection are said to be parenterally administered. Parenteral translates to "beside, beyond, or apart from the intestines" and refers to the space between the intestinal tract and the surface of the skin. As shown in Figure 3-3, *parenteral administration* of drugs is further divided into specific routes based on where the needle

is introduced. *Intravenous* (IV) administration means the drug is injected directly into a vein. IV injections can be given as a single, large volume at one time, called an *intravenous bolus*, or slowly injected or "dripped" into a vein over a period of several seconds, minutes, or even hours as an *intravenous infusion*. As shown in Figure 3-4 a constant-rate IV infusion results in a steady accumulation of drug concentrations in the body until the drug concentrations reach a plateau, or *steady state*, and remain there until the infusion is stopped. An IV bolus is comparable to dumping all the required water into the empty bucket at once, whereas an IV infusion is comparable to dribbling water into the bucket at a faster rate than it leaks out.

IV administration can be used to safely administer a drug that would be irritating or painful if injected into the muscle or beneath the skin. The accidental injection of an IV-administered drug outside the blood vessel is called an *extravascular injection* or *perivascular injection* because

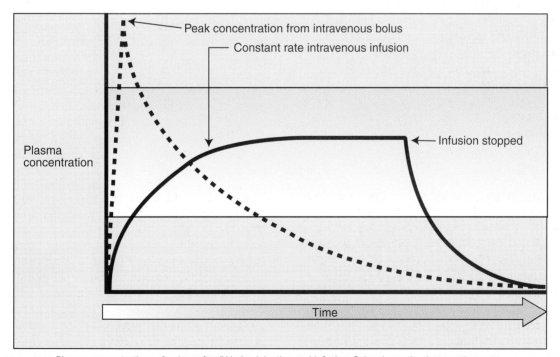

Figure 3-3 Plasma concentrations of a drug after IV bolus injection and infusion. Color shows the therapeutic range.

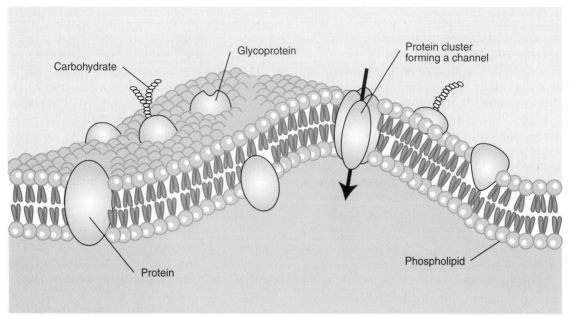

Figure 3-4 Cellular membrane structure.

it is outside (extra-) or around (peri-) the blood vessel. Some drugs injected extravascularly can cause extreme tissue inflammation and tissue necrosis (tissue death).

Although an *intraarterial injection* places the drug directly into the blood vessel, intraarterial administration of a drug produces quite different effects from the same drug given intravenously. Drugs given by the intraarterial route are injected into an artery, not a vein; thus the blood carries the injected drug away from the heart and toward a specific tissue or organ. By contrast, a drug injected intravenously is carried from the tissues toward the heart where it is diluted by the venous blood returning to the heart from the body. By the time an IV drug passes through the heart and the lungs and returns to the tissues, it has been well mixed and diluted in the blood. Unfortunately, an intraarterial injection results in the entire drug being delivered at high concentrations directly to the tissues supplied by that artery. The tissues supplied by this artery would receive drug concentrations that would far exceed the

normal therapeutic range and produce local toxicosis.

Intramuscular administration is another example of the parenteral route of administration. The prefix *intra-* means *within,* so an intramuscularly administered medication is put within the muscle. *Subcutaneous (SC or SQ)* injections are administered "beneath the skin," but not so deep as to be injected into the underlying muscle. *Intradermal (ID) injections* are administered within (intra-), not beneath, the skin with very small needles. The intradermal route is usually reserved for skin testing procedures, such as testing for tuberculosis or reaction to allergenic substances. *Intraperitoneal (IP) injections* are administered into the abdominal body cavity and are frequently used when IV or *intramuscular (IM) injections* are not practical (as in some laboratory animals) or when large volumes of solution must be administered for rapid *absorption.*

Drugs given by mouth are given *per os (PO),* meaning *"via a body opening."* Drugs that are applied to the surface of the skin such as lotions and liniments are *topically administered drugs.*

Aerosol administration, meaning "air or gas solution," indicates that the drug is administered in an inhaled mist or gas and absorbed within the lung airways.

Drugs given by each route of administration described above will be absorbed at a different speed and efficiency. In veterinary medicine the different characteristics of the route of administration provide the appropriate amount of drug to the correct part of the body. Because each route of administration can also be affected by disease in a different way, the veterinary technician must know these patterns to identify potential problems with a route of administration and take appropriate measures to compensate for any problems. These clinical challenges are further discussed below.

MOVEMENT OF DRUG MOLECULES

Part of the reason different routes of administration result in varied drug concentration curves is because of the way drug molecules move from one site to another by different mechanisms. Drug molecules move from point A to point B by four different mechanisms: *passive diffusion, facilitated diffusion, active transport,* and *pinocytosis* and *phagocytosis.*

PASSIVE DIFFUSION

The majority of drug movement through tissue fluid or membrane barriers is by passive diffusion.

Passive diffusion is the random movement of drug molecules from an area of high concentration to an area of lower concentration, or down the *concentration gradient.* For example, when a colored liquid is poured into a glass of water, the color spreads, or diffuses, to all parts of the water. Similarly, when a drug is injected in the body, it passively diffuses down the concentration gradient from the injection site to the surrounding areas of lower concentrations, eventually reaching a blood capillary and entering the systemic circulation. In this process no active cellular energy is expended by the body to direct the movement of drug molecules; hence the term passive diffusion.

The concept of diffusion of substances throughout liquid is readily grasped because it is observed in everyday life (e.g., mixing sugar in iced tea, adding milk to coffee). Diffusion is also involved in the movement of drug molecules through cell membranes. For a drug to diffuse from one side of a biologic membrane to the other, the drug must dissolve in the membrane. Cell membranes, on a molecular level, are not solid structures (Figure 3-4). The cell membranes are composed primarily of phospholipids (a molecule with phosphate groups and fatty acid components). These phospholipids give the cell membrane the characteristics of fat. Therefore, for a drug molecule to diffuse from one side of the cell membrane to the other, it must be capable of dissolving in fat or oils. In such cases, the drug molecule passes from the side of the cell membrane with a high concentration of drug molecules to the side with the lower concentration by passive diffusion and without any expenditure of cellular energy.

Whether passive diffusion occurs within a liquid or across a cellular membrane, the drug molecules continue to pass from an area of higher concentration to an area of lower concentration until the drug molecules are equally distributed. In other words, at *equilibrium* the number of molecules at point A are the same as they are at point B. In actuality, once equilibrium is reached, diffusion of the molecules does not stop. The molecules are still moving around, but no net direction of diffusion can be detected because the number of molecules moving from point A to point B is the same as the number moving from point B to point A.

FACILITATED DIFFUSION

Facilitated diffusion is a passive transport mechanism across cell membranes that involves a special "carrier molecule" located in the cellular membrane. The carrier molecule, usually a protein floating among the phospholipid molecules in the cell membrane, has a specific site to which a drug molecule can attach. When a drug molecule combines with the carrier the carrier molecule changes, allowing the drug molecule to pass through the cell membrane at that point (Figure 3-5, *A*). Thus the drug molecule does not have to dissolve in the cell membrane to pass through it. As in passive diffusion, facilitated diffusion involves no energy expended by the cell to move the drug molecules. The direction of drug movement is determined by the concentration gradient; once equilibrium is attained, the number of drug molecules crossing the membrane in either direction via the carrier is equal.

Facilitated diffusion can be thought of as functioning in the same way a revolving door allows people to move through a wall (Figure 3-5, *B*). The

people (drug molecules) provide the "push" that moves the revolving door (the carrier molecule). The building or the wall (cell and cell membrane) does not have any kind of a motor to move the revolving door and therefore does not use any electricity to make the revolving door work.

ACTIVE TRANSPORT

Active transport is a less common method for movement of drug molecules than diffusion. As with facilitated diffusion, active transport of drug molecules involves a specialized carrier molecule. However, in active transport the cell expends energy to either move the drug molecule across the cell membrane or to "reset" the carrier molecule after transport so that it can transport again. Unlike passive or facilitated diffusion, in which the direction of net drug

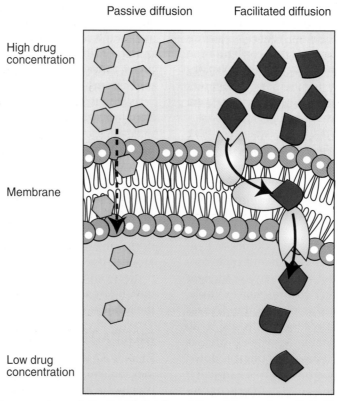

Figure 3-5 Diffusion across a membrane. **A,** Passive diffusion through the cellular membrane. **B,** Facilitated diffusion using a carrier molecule that moves the drug molecule across the membrane.

movement is determined by the concentration gradient, active transport can move drug molecules against the concentration gradient, moving drug molecules from areas of low concentration to areas of higher concentration. Thus active transport mechanisms do not stop when equilibrium is reached, but can result in a large accumulation of drug molecules within a cell or body compartment.

Whereas facilitated diffusion can be thought of as a revolving door, active transport can be thought of as a pump. A pump requires electrical energy to operate, but it can also move tremendous quantities of water from one area to another without any consideration of equilibrium between the source of the water and where it is being pumped.

PINOCYTOSIS AND PHAGOCYTOSIS

Pinocytosis and phagocytosis are forms of active transport. Both processes involve physically engulfing the drug molecule by the cell membrane. Pinocytosis (meaning *cell drinking*) involves a small invagination forming in the cell membrane that surrounds the drug molecule and brings it into the cell. Phagocytosis (meaning *cell eating*) is a process in which most or the entire cell surrounds the molecule. Both processes obviously require cellular energy, but they are relatively rare methods by which drugs are moved across membranes. The intact movement of very large molecules such as complex proteins or antibodies into cells requires this mechanism.

FACTORS THAT AFFECT RATE OF DRUG MOLECULE TRANSPORT

Different drug transport mechanisms can determine the direction of drug molecule movement and the rate at which the molecules can move from one compartment to the next or through a membrane barrier. In facilitated diffusion and active transport, in which a carrier molecule is involved to transport the drug molecule across the cell membrane, the transport mechanism can only move a limited number of drug molecules at one time. If

more drug molecules are available for transport than available carrier molecules, all the carrier molecules are continuously occupied with drug molecules and the transport system is said to be *saturated*. The rate at which drug molecules move across the membrane cannot be increased, and the transport system is said to be operating at its transportation maximum *(t-max)*. When a carrier system becomes saturated, drug molecules needing to be transported may accumulate on one side of the membrane until the carrier molecules can transport the backlog. This situation is similar to what can be seen on a crowded toll road when cars back up at the toll booths. If all the toll booths are continuously occupied, the toll booths are saturated and the processing of toll collection is operating at t-max. If cars arrive at a rate that exceeds t-max, cars will line up in front of the toll booths.

In contrast to carrier transport systems, the rate of transport of molecules by passive diffusion is not limited by the number of available carrier molecules. However, the rate at which molecules can diffuse across the membrane is related to the following:
- The concentration gradient on either side of the membrane
- The drug molecule size (with smaller molecules moving more rapidly than larger molecules)
- The *lipophilic* ("fat loving") nature of the molecule, reflecting the molecule's ability to dissolve in the phospholipids of the cell membranes
- The temperature of the cellular environment (the lower the temperature, the slower the diffusion)
- The thickness of the membrane (the thicker the membrane, the slower the diffusion)

Thus the maximal rate of drug molecule diffusion across a cellular membrane occurs when a large concentration gradient is present, the drug molecule is small and lipophilic, the temperature at the cellular membrane (and hence the random molecular movements) is increased, and the membrane is quite thin.

CLINICAL APPLICATION
Ototoxicosis and Nephrotoxicosis from Drug Accumulation

An older, intact female dog presented to a veterinary hospital with a history of lethargy, not eating, and discharge from the vulva. The veterinarian determined that the dog had a pyometra, an infection of the uterus in which a great deal of pus is produced. The veterinarian recommended surgery to remove the infected uterus and the ovaries (ovariohysterectomy). During removal of the infected uterus, the surgical site was contaminated (bacteria was introduced to the site). The veterinarian chose to use gentamicin, a potent antibiotic, to combat the infection introduced into the abdomen during surgery. Because of his concern over the potentially serious nature of the infection, he chose to give the dog a high dose on a three times daily basis.

Over the next 2 days the dog became feverish, continued to be lethargic, was not interested in eating, and seemed to have pain in the abdomen. By day 3, however, the fever started to decrease and the dog seemed more alert. To be safe, the veterinarian continued to hospitalize the animal and administer gentamicin for an additional 7 days (9 days total). On day 10 the veterinarian was going to send the dog home. A blood test and urinalysis suggested that the animal may have kidney damage or disease. The veterinarian stopped the gentamicin and hospitalized the dog for an additional 3 days on IV fluids. After that time the blood tests and urinalysis indicated that renal function had improved. The dog was sent home and recovered uneventfully.

Why did the veterinarian stop the antibiotic? Was it related to the suggested kidney damage?

In this case the veterinarian was using an antibiotic that is known to be potentially damaging to the kidney. He stopped the drug and provided supportive care for kidney injury. In this case the dog recovered.

Gentamicin and other aminoglycoside antibiotics (e.g., amikacin, neomycin, streptomycin) are potentially nephrotoxic drugs, meaning they have the ability to be poisonous to the kidney (*nephro-*, pertaining to the kidney). These drugs are nephrotoxic because they accumulate in high concentrations within the kidney cells. Gentamicin concentration within the kidney cells can be much higher than the concentration within the blood because the drug is actively transported from the blood into the kidney cells by pinocytosis. The only way for gentamicin to move back out of the kidney cell and avoid lethal concentrations is by passive diffusion from the cell back into the blood. Unless the gentamicin concentration in the blood drops low enough to create a concentration gradient for diffusion back out of the cell, gentamicin can accumulate to the point where it becomes toxic or deadly to the kidney cell. The result is a condition called nephrotoxicosis.

The cells that comprise part of the inner ear (balance and hearing function) also actively transport gentamicin into the cells. The accumulation of gentamicin or any aminoglycoside antibiotic in these cells can result in damage to the cells responsible for hearing and balance. This condition is called ototoxicosis (*oto-*, referring to the ear) and presents clinically as an animal with a reduced ability to hear, inability to stand without falling, or inability to walk without staggering or circling.

What should be learned from this situation: Active transport mechanisms of drugs can be beneficial for veterinary patients if the active transport of the drug is to the site intended. For example, active transport of an antibiotic to a site of infection is useful. However, active transport of drugs into other areas of the body may result in drug concentrations that exceed the therapeutic range and become toxic. Knowing which drugs are transported in this manner and in what tissues they accumulate allows us to take steps to prevent the local toxicity from occurring from active transport of the drug.

Pinocytosis and phagocytosis are relatively slower mechanisms for drug transport because they involve a complex series of changes in the cell membrane as the cell imbibes or ingests the drug molecules.

EFFECT OF A DRUG'S LIPOPHILIC OR HYDROPHILIC NATURE ON DRUG MOLECULE MOVEMENT

As stated previously, drugs must dissolve, or be soluble, in a membrane to move across it by passive diffusion. Biologic membranes are largely composed of phospholipids, which are fats. Therefore to move across a membrane, drug molecules must be in a lipophilic ("fat loving") form that dissolves in fat or oil. Not all molecules readily dissolve in fats. When fat or oil is mixed with water the fat or oil will separate into distinct globules that eventually come together into a layer of oil separate from water (e.g., salad dressings, gravy, grease). Molecules that do not readily dissolve in fat or oil are said to be *hydrophilic*, meaning "water loving." Technically, these molecules should be referred to as lipophobic, meaning "fat fearing"; however, a drug molecule that does not dissolve readily in fats or oils is assumed to dissolve readily in water and is therefore called hydrophilic.

Because membranes are largely phospholipids and have a lipophilic nature, drug molecules that are hydrophilic have a difficult time dissolving in and passing through the cellular membranes by passive diffusion. Hydrophilic drug molecules are dependent on carrier-mediated transport mechanisms to be transported across membranes. Conversely, lipophilic drugs do not dissolve in water readily and if introduced into an *aqueous* (water-based) medium, the lipophilic drug molecules will clump together and not readily disperse throughout the medium.

What makes a drug molecule hydrophilic or lipophilic? Hydrophilic drugs are either polarized, meaning they contain charges at the ends of the molecule, or ionized, meaning they contain a net positive or negative charge such as HCO_3^- or NH_4^+. The charged nature allows the drug molecule to dissolve more readily in water. In contrast, lipophilic drug molecules tend to be nonpolarized and nonionized molecules. When drug molecules are introduced to the body, not all the molecules may go into the hydrophilic or lipophilic form. Often a set ratio of hydrophilic molecules to lipophilic molecules is present based on characteristics of the drug molecule and the environmental conditions. For example, a drug may primarily exist in the lipophilic drug molecule form in the acidic environment of the stomach but exist primarily in a hydrophilic form in the more alkaline environment of the intestines. These changes in drug form from hydrophilic to lipophilic and vice versa change the ability of the drug overall to penetrate a drug membrane or disperse within an aqueous medium. The impact of the lipophilic and hydrophilic forms is discussed in greater detail below in terms of absorption, *distribution,* and *excretion* from the body.

PHARMACOKINETICS: ABSORPTION

Pharmacokinetics is the study (including mathematic descriptions) of how physiologic or drug characteristics affect drug movement and concentrations within the body. The pharmacokinetics of drugs is usually described in four basic steps: absorption, distribution, metabolism, and excretion (or elimination). Listed and approved drug dosages are designed to result in drug concentrations within the normal therapeutic range based on normal absorption, distribution, metabolism, and excretion (A.D.M.E.) of the drug. Each of these four pharmacokinetic steps can be altered by disease or physiologic conditions. Therefore the veterinarian and veterinary technician must recognize conditions that may potentially alter pharmacokinetics so that the drug dosage can be changed to maintain drug concentrations within the therapeutic range.

DRUG ABSORPTION AND BIOAVAILABILITY

After a drug has been ingested, injected, inhaled, or applied to the skin, it must be absorbed into the blood and travel to the body areas (target tissues) where it will have its intended effect. Absorption of a drug is defined as the movement of drug molecules from the site of administration to the systemic circulation. Generally a drug is useless unless it is absorbed. Exceptions to this are drugs designed to work only where they are applied, such as local anesthetics, topical insecticides such as flea powders, topical antibiotics, and drugs that are intended to work within the lumen of the intestine. With the exception of these locally acting medications, rapid, total absorption of the drug is desirable.

Because of characteristics of the drug's dose form, the physical characteristic of the drug molecule, and the way a drug may be given not all the drug administered may be absorbed. The degree to which an administered drug is absorbed is referred to as its *bioavailability*. If 100% of the drug administered makes it to systemic circulation, the drug is said to have a bioavailability of 100%, or 1. The letter F is sometimes used to represent bioavailability; a drug that is 100% bioavailable may be noted as F = 1. A drug that is only half absorbed may be noted as F = 0.5.

EFFECT OF ROUTE OF ADMINISTRATION ON ABSORPTION

The route of administration (e.g., PO, IM, SQ) directly affects the drug's bioavailability. The IV route of administration has no absorption phase because the administered drug is placed directly into the systemic circulation. Therefore 100% of a drug that is administered intravenously is absorbed, and these drugs have a bioavailability of 1. Drugs administered intramuscularly are usually rapidly and almost completely absorbed and therefore have a bioavailability only slightly less than drugs administered intravenously. PO and SQ administered drugs must overcome several barriers to be absorbed and therefore may have a bioavailability significantly less than 1.

The route of administration affects the bioavailability and the rate at which a drug is absorbed. If the concentration of a drug over time (e.g., concentrations determined at 30-minute intervals) is plotted, a curve that is characteristic for the route of administration can be seen. If a drug is rapidly absorbed, the concentration curve tends to have a high peak concentration that drops fairly rapidly. A slowly absorbed drug's concentration curve increases slowly to a lower peak, then slowly declines. Figure 3-6 shows the different concentration curves for each route of administration. Blood concentrations of drugs are more correctly referred to as *plasma (serum) concentrations* because drugs mostly occupy only the fluid or water component of blood and not the fluid within the blood cells.

Figure 3-6 illustrates how intravenously administered drugs almost instantly achieve their peak concentration in the serum. As soon as the IV drug enters the systemic circulation, it begins to be excreted from the body and the concentrations begin to fall immediately after the peak until the entire drug has been excreted.

Drugs given intramuscularly show a similar pattern to IV administered drugs because they are rapidly, but not instantaneously, absorbed from the injection site. Figure 3-6 shows a rapid increase of drug concentrations between the time of injection and attainment of the peak plasma (blood) concentration. Because IM absorption is spread over a longer period, the peak plasma concentration is not as high as the IV administered drug. A difference also occurs if an IM drug is injected into muscle that is being exercised or a muscle that is inactive. IM drugs are absorbed rapidly from moving muscle, whereas drugs injected into unused muscles are absorbed more slowly because inactive muscles have less blood flow.

Drugs given by mouth or subcutaneously take longer to be absorbed. SQ drugs must

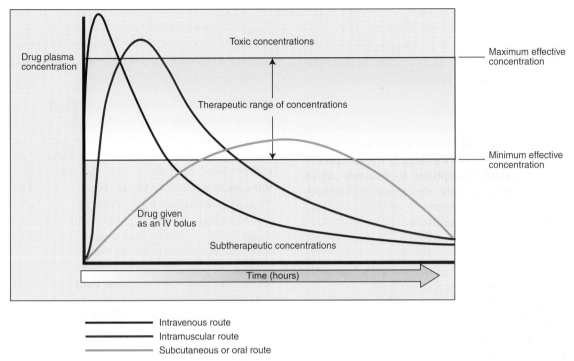

Figure 3-6 Plasma drug concentrations attained after IV, IM, SQ, and PO administration.

diffuse some distance to reach an open capillary and systemic circulation. PO drugs must dissolve and pass through several barriers before they gain access to systemic circulation. For these reasons, the concentration curves for PO and SQ drugs rise slowly, reach a peak that is much lower than IV drugs, and then decline slowly.

In emergency situations or in clinical circumstances for which the drug is needed "stat," the IV route is preferred because drugs given by other routes attain therapeutic concentrations more slowly than drugs given intravenously. Unfortunately, as explained in the previous chapters, some drug formulations may not be safe to give intravenously, requiring other routes of administration to be used.

Even though the IV route of administration has many advantages, the rapid, high peak concentration may, for a short period (few minutes), result in serum concentrations of drugs that are quite high and in some cases may exceed the therapeutic range. Signs of toxicity could

potentially develop during this time unless the IV administration is spread over several minutes as an IV infusion or IV drip. For example, injecting an animal with a bolus IV loading dose of digoxin (a widely used cardiac drug) might cause the animal to vomit or have serious cardiac arrhythmias (irregular heartbeats) as a result of the high concentration in those first few minutes after the injection. Veterinary professionals therefore need to be aware of these side effects for the specific drugs so they know to administer the drug by IV infusion to avoid the risk of short-term toxic concentrations caused by IV bolus administration.

EFFECT OF LIPOPHILIC AND HYDROPHILIC PROPERTIES ON ABSORPTION

As mentioned previously, drug molecules can exist in hydrophilic (water-loving) or lipophilic (fat-loving) forms, and these forms can affect the drug molecule's ability to dissolve in water or pass through a cellular membrane. Rapid absorption of drugs by different routes of administration depends on the drug molecule existing predominantly either in the hydrophilic or lipophilic form, whichever is most appropriate for reaching systemic circulation from the site of administration. For example, drugs injected subcutaneously or intramuscularly are deposited in the *extracellular fluid* (fluid outside the cells) and must diffuse through that fluid to reach the capillaries and be absorbed. Because extracellular fluid is an aqueous medium, drug molecules in the hydrophilic form will diffuse more readily through the fluid than will molecules in the lipophilic form. Thus a drug with molecules predominantly in the hydrophilic form will be more rapidly absorbed from the IM or SQ route than drugs that exist primarily in the lipophilic form.

In contrast to drugs given subcutaneously and intramuscularly, drugs given by mouth must pass through cellular membranes to be absorbed from the lumen of the intestinal tract. Unlike the more loosely organized cells of the muscle or connective tissue, where IM or SQ injections are given, the cells lining the intestinal tract are tightly adhered to their neighboring cells and form a continuous cellular barrier that separates the contents of the intestinal tract from the rest of the body. Therefore drugs given by mouth must be in a lipophilic form to dissolve in, and pass through, the cellular membrane barrier and be absorbed. Drugs that exist primarily in the hydrophilic form are poorly absorbed from the gut and may remain in the intestinal tract to be expelled with the feces.

In some cases a drug is purposely formulated to exist in a form that is not well absorbed. For example, deworming agents or antibiotics intended to work within the lumen (inner space) of the intestine are chemically formulated to exist primarily in the hydrophilic form to prevent their absorption from the intestine. Similarly, some drugs that are injected intramuscularly or subcutaneously are formulated to exist predominantly in a lipophilic form so that absorption of the drug

will be slowed and occur over hours to days. Some injectable antibiotics or hormone drugs are manufactured in this manner to provide concentrations of drug for several days after the drug is injected.

EFFECT OF pH OF THE ENVIRONMENT ON ABSORPTION

Acidic and basic (or alkaline) are terms used to describe the characteristics of a fluid as measured by its pH. pH is the measurement of the number of available hydrogen ions (H^+). The more hydrogen ions present in the liquid, the lower the pH. The term acidic generally refers to conditions in which many free hydrogen ions are available in the liquid, giving it a low pH. A pH of 1, 2, or 3 is considered acidic on the pH scale. A liquid with a high pH has few available hydrogen ions and is considered alkaline, or basic. A pH of 10, 11, or 12 is considered alkaline. No specific pH defines acidic because the term only indicates a relative direction on the pH scale. Thus a pH of 3 is more acidic than a pH of 6, but a pH of 6 is more acidic than a pH of 9.

As previously stated, a drug can exist as a ratio of hydrophilic (ionized) molecules to lipophilic (nonionized) molecules. This ratio can be affected by the pH of the liquid environment in which the drug is located. As shown below, the ratio of ionized to nonionized molecules for aspirin changes in a predictable manner as the drug is placed in environments with different pH levels.

ASPIRIN

pH	Ionized/Nonionized
1	1:100
2	1:10
3	1:1
4	10:1
5	100:1
6	1000:1
7	10,000:1
8	100,000:1

At a relatively *acidic pH* of 2 found in the stomach, aspirin exists at a ratio of 1 hydrophilic (ionized) molecule for every 10 lipophilic (nonionized) molecules (a 1:10 ratio). However, in the duodenum, which has a pH of approximately 6, the ratio shifts in favor of the hydrophilic form, with 1000 hydrophilic molecules for every 1 lipophilic molecule (a 1000:1 ratio). Because the lipophilic molecule form is required to diffuse across the cellular membrane of the intestinal tract, aspirin would be more readily absorbed in the acidic environment of the stomach than in the more alkaline (less acidic) environment of the duodenum.

Different drugs will vary in their ratios of ionized to nonionized at any individual pH and whether the ionized or nonionized form dominates as the pH becomes more acidic or more alkaline. As shown in Table 3-2, aspirin and sulfadimethoxine both increase in the relative number of hydrophilic (ionized) molecules as pH increases. However, the two drugs have different ratios from each other at each pH level. At a pH of 5, aspirin has more of its molecules in the ionized form (100:1), whereas sulfadimethoxine has more of its molecules in the nonionized form (1:10). In contrast to aspirin and sulfadimethoxine, lidocaine increases its relative number of lipophilic (nonionized) molecules as the pH increases. Thus the characteristic of each drug determines which way the ratio shifts as the pH changes from acidic to alkaline (and vice versa) and the pH at which the drug changes from predominantly ionized to predominantly nonionized. The two characteristics of drugs that determine their ratio of ionized to nonionized molecules at any given pH are the drug's acid/base nature and its *pKa*.

Acid Drugs versus Alkaline Drugs

The definition of an *acid drug* is not related to the definition of acidic conditions given previously, nor is the definition of an *alkaline drug* related to the definition of *alkaline pH*. An acid drug is defined as a drug whose chemical structure causes it to release a hydrogen ion (H^+, or proton) into the liquid environment as the drug is placed in increasingly alkaline environments (as the pH of the environment increases). By releasing a hydrogen ion from its chemical structure, the acid drug acquires a charge and thus becomes ionized. Therefore an acid drug becomes more hydrophilic as it is placed into a more alkaline or *basic environmental pH*.

In the example of aspirin, sulfadimethoxine, and lidocaine in Table 3-2, both aspirin and sulfadimethoxine are characterized as acid drugs because as the pH increases (the environment becomes more alkaline), the ratio of ionized to nonionized molecules increases, meaning that the drug is increasingly shifting to a more hydrophilic form.

Note that for an acid drug a decrease in the environmental pH favors the acid drug taking up H^+ from the environment, and in so doing the acid drug switches from an ionized form to an nonionized form. Therefore, as an acid drug is placed in increasingly acidic environments,

TABLE **3-2** Comparison of the Ionized/Nonionized States for Three Drugs at Different pHs

ASPIRIN		SULFADIMETHOXINE		LIDOCAINE	
pH	IONIZED/NONIONIZED	pH	IONIZED/NONIONIZED	pH	IONIZED/NONIONIZED
1	1:100	1	1:100,000	1	100:1
2	1:10	2	1:10,000	2	10:1
3	1:1	3	1:1000	3	1:1
4	10:1	4	1:100	4	1:10
5	100:1	5	1:10	5	1:100
6	1000:1	6	1:1	6	1:1000
7	10,000:1	7	10:1	7	1:10,000
8	100,000:1	8	100:1	8	1:100,000

the drug exists more in the lipophilic form. The example of aspirin and sulfadimethoxine shows that the ratio of ionized to nonionized molecules shifts increasingly in favor of the nonionized (lipophilic) form as the pH becomes more acidic.

A basic or alkaline drug behaves in a manner opposite to acid drugs. *Basic drugs* become more hydrophilic (ionized) as they are placed in increasingly acidic environments and become more lipophilic (nonionized) as they are placed in increasingly alkaline environments. As shown in Table 3-2, lidocaine is considered a basic drug because the ratio of ionized to nonionized shifts in favor of the ionized molecule form as the pH becomes more acidic. Thus the acid or base nature of a drug molecule determines the general shift in a drug's hydrophilic or lipophilic form as the environmental pH surrounding the drug changes. Box 3-1 explains some additional concepts related to the chemical differences between acidic and alkaline drugs.

The general change in the ratio of ionized/nonionized forms for acid and base drugs is summarized in Table 3-3.

pKa

As shown in Table 3-2, aspirin and sulfadimethoxine both act as acid drugs in that they both become increasingly lipophilic (nonionized) as the environment becomes increasingly acidic. Although both drugs shift toward the nonionized (lipophilic) form as they are placed in increasingly acidic environments, they do not have the same ratio of ionized (hydrophilic) to nonionized (lipophilic) molecules at each pH level. Aspirin switches from its predominantly hydrophilic form to its predominantly lipophilic form at a pH of 3. The

same switch occurs for sulfadimethoxine at a pH of 6. At a pH of 3 for aspirin and a pH of 6 for sulfadimethoxine, the ratio of ionized to nonionized molecules is 1:1 (equal numbers of ionized and nonionized drug molecules). The pH at which this occurs is called the drug's pKa. Thus knowing whether a drug is an acid or base and knowing its pKa, whether the drug will be predominantly in the ionized (hydrophilic) form or nonionized (lipophilic) form can be predicted at any pH.

For example, for any acid drug with a pKa of 7, the ratio of ionized to nonionized molecules is 1:1 at a pH of 7. Because it is an acid drug and acid drugs become more nonionized as they are placed in an acidic pH, it can be deduced that at any pH on the acidic side of a pH of 7 more of the drug molecules must be in the nonionized (lipophilic) form. Conversely, for any pH in the alkaline direction from a pH of 7, the acid drug must be more in the ionized (hydrophilic) form. For an alkaline drug with a pKa of 7, the opposite is true.

The ratio of ionized to nonionized molecules can be more precisely determined if the drug's acid/base nature, its pKa, and the pH of the environment are known. Notice that the ratio of ionized to nonionized molecules changes by a factor of 10 for each incremental change of pH. For an acid drug, a shift in pH of 1 unit to the acidic side of the pKa means the ratio of ionized to nonionized molecules will be 1:10 (10 times more nonionized than ionized). At the next pH unit, the ratio increases by 10 to 1:100, and at the next to 1:1000. To the alkaline pH side of the pKa, the ratio increases to 10:1, 100:1, and 1000:1 in favor of ionized molecules. Thus, by counting the increments between the pKa (pH at which the ratio is 1:1) and the environmental pH, the specific ratio

TABLE **3-3** Lipophilic and Hydrophilic States of Acid and Base Drugs as the pH Changes

	INCREASINGLY ACIDIC ENVIRONMENTAL pH	INCREASINGLY ALKALINE (BASIC) ENVIRONMENTAL pH
Acid drug	Becomes more nonionized (lipophilic)	Becomes more ionized (hydrophilic)
Alkaline (basic) drug	Becomes more ionized (hydrophilic)	Becomes more nonionized (lipophilic)

of ionized to nonionized molecules can be predicted.

In most basic chemistry courses the concepts of acid/base compounds, pKa, and pH are taught as a mathematic expression known as the Henderson-Hasselbalch equation. For those familiar with logarithms and comfortable with mathematic equations that express physiologic concepts, the Henderson-Hasselbalch equation may provide a convenient means of remembering the relation between the drug's characteristics and its environment. The two forms of this equation are shown below.

For acid drugs: pH = pKa + log (concentration of ionized/concentration of nonionized)

For basic drugs: pH = pKa + log (concentration of nonionized/concentration of ionized)

For example, the acid drug aspirin has a pKa of 3. At what pH does the ratio of ionized to nonionized molecules equal 10:1? By using the value of 10 as the concentration of ionized molecules and the value of 1 as the concentration of nonionized molecules, the following is determined:

pH = pKa + log (concentration of ionized/concentration of nonionized)

pH = 3 + log (10/1)

10/1 is equal to 10

pH = 3 + log (10)

The log of 10 is equal to 1 so

pH = 3 + 1

pH = 4

This correlates with the ratio given for aspirin at the pH of 4 in Table 3-2.

For purposes of veterinary technology pharmacology, it is enough to know that acid drugs become more lipophilic (hence more readily absorbed across cellular barriers) at pH values to the acidic side of a drug's pKa, whereas base drugs become more lipophilic at pH values to the alkaline side of the drug's pKa and that the opposite is true for alkaline or base drugs.

ION TRAPPING AND ABSORPTION OF DRUGS

Different compartments of the body have different pH environments. For example, the pH in the stomach is usually between 1 and 3, and that of the duodenum is between 6 and 7. Within cells and most body fluids, the pH remains a fairly constant 7.4. Therefore, as a drug molecule passes from one compartment to another compartment with a different pH, the ratio of ionized to nonionized molecules changes. If a drug molecule in a lipophilic (nonionized) form passes through a cellular membrane and enters a body compartment whose pH results in a significant shift from nonionized to ionized (hydrophilic) form, the drug molecule may not be able to exit the compartment through the cellular membrane because it now exists in a hydrophilic form. This phenomenon is called *ion trapping.*

An example of ion trapping is seen when aspirin is taken by mouth. In the acidic environment of the stomach lumen, the acidic aspirin molecules exist predominantly in the nonionized form, which readily penetrates the cellular membrane that constitutes the stomach wall (Figure 3-7). However, once reaching the interior of the cells where the pH is a more alkaline 7.4, most of the acid drug molecules shift to the ionized form, trapping them within the stomach cell membranes. As more lipophilic molecules pass through the cellular membrane and into the cell, changing into a hydrophilic form that becomes trapped, the aspirin molecules accumulate within the cells lining the stomach.

This does not mean an aspirin taken 3 weeks ago is still lodged in the cells of the stomach wall. The ratio of ionized to nonionized molecules in a compartment remains roughly the same. Thus, even at a pH of 7.4, some aspirin molecules remain in the nonionized form and are able to pass through the cellular membrane and out of the stomach cells. When a single nonionized molecule passes out of the cell

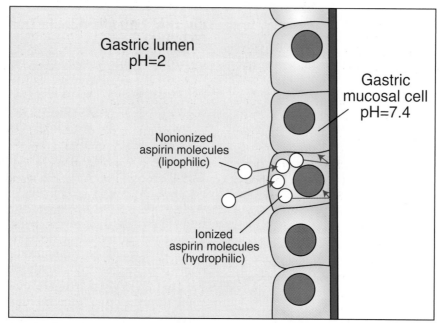

Figure 3-7 Ion trapping. The aspirin molecule in the lipophilic form at the acidic pH of the stomach (pH = 2) changes into primarily the hydrophilic form in the pH of the cellular fluid (pH = 7.4) and reduces the drug's ability to move out of the cellular compartment.

and into the blood, another ionized molecule within the cell is converted to the nonionized form to preserve the same ratio of ionized to nonionized molecules. When this newly converted nonionized molecule moves out of the cell, the cycle repeats until all the drug molecules trapped in the 7.4 pH fluid of the cell leave the stomach cells and are absorbed into systemic circulation. The net effect of ion trapping in this case is a temporary accumulation of aspirin molecules in the stomach cells (which can produce mild stomach discomfort) and a slower absorption of the drug from the stomach.

Sometimes ion trapping is used to remove excessive drug (as in an overdose) or absorbed toxic agents through the kidneys. Drug or toxin molecules are normally filtered out of the blood by the kidney but may be reabsorbed back into the body if these molecules exist in the lipophilic (nonionized) form. This *reabsorption* of the drug or toxin back into the systemic circulation can cause additional damage because the agent is recirculated instead of excreted in the urine. However, if the pH of the urine can be changed so that the nonionized lipophilic drug or toxin molecules become ionized, these hydrophilic molecules cannot passively diffuse through the renal tubular cell membranes to be reabsorbed back into the body. Thus the change in urine pH by urinary acidifiers or alkalizers could trap the molecule within the lumen of the renal tubule and allow it to be safely excreted from the body in urine.

EFFECT OF DISSOLUTION AND GASTROINTESTINAL MOTILITY ON ABSORPTION OF ORALLY ADMINISTERED DRUGS

Drugs given by mouth must be in the lipophilic form to penetrate the gastrointestinal mucosa and be absorbed. However, before a drug can diffuse across the membrane barrier, it must be small enough to dissolve in the membrane. Tablets, granules, and powders cannot be absorbed until they break apart into much smaller particles. Thus *dissolution,* or dissolving, of the drug form is a critical step in absorption of drugs given by mouth (Figure 3-8).

Drugs in liquid dose form, such as solutions and elixirs, do not have a dissolution step and thus are usually more rapidly absorbed by the oral (PO) route than are solid dosage forms such as tablets. Thus liquid forms of a drug may have a quicker onset of action in the body than the same drug in solid form. For example, digoxin elixir is more rapidly absorbed and has a higher bioavailability than the tablet form.

Chapter 1 describes sustained-release tablets as a special type of orally administered tablets. Sustained-release medications dissolve slowly over minutes to hours while releasing small amounts of medication for absorption. The advantage of sustained-release medications is that they provide a sustained concentration of drug over a period of time. However, the disadvantage of sustained-release formulations is that the concentrations achieved in the body have a lower peak concentration than the standard-release formulations. The higher peak concentration affects the movement of the drug from the blood to the tissues because most drugs distribute to the tissues by passive diffusion. Therefore a higher peak blood concentration of drug means a greater concentration gradient for moving drug molecules to the tissue, resulting in higher drug concentrations in the tissue. The typical drug concentrations in the blood for a sustained-release tablet and a standard-release tablet are shown in Figure 3-9.

Most drugs are absorbed from the small intestine; therefore a PO administered drug must be completely dissolved by the time it reaches the small intestine for it to be successfully absorbed with a high bioavailability. One disadvantage of sustained-release medications used in domestic animals is that the tablet may not completely dissolve in the domestic animal's intestinal tract before it has moved beyond the small intestine. Therefore the sustained-release medications may have

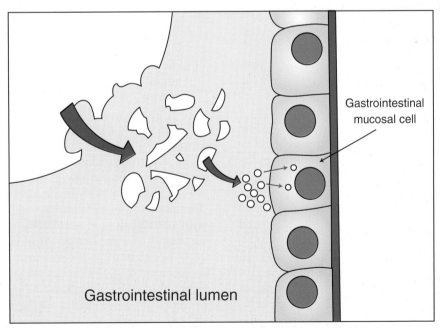

Gastrointestinal mucosal cell

Gastrointestinal lumen

Figure 3-8 Drugs administered in solid form must completely dissolve before they can be absorbed.

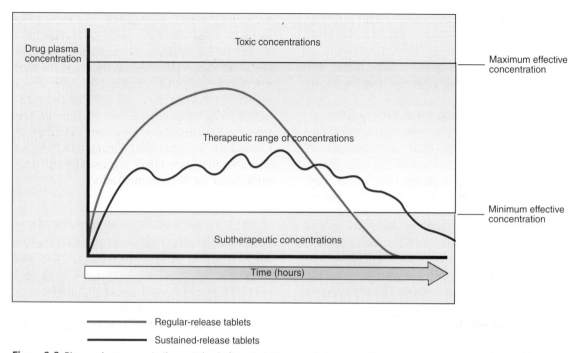

Figure 3-9 Plasma drug concentrations attained after administration of standard tablets and sustained-release tablets. The variability of the sustained-release tablet reflects the variability in the tablet dissolution.

a lower overall bioavailability than the same drug in a standard-release tablet formulation.

As illustrated with sustained-release tablets, whether the dose form has enough time to completely dissolve can affect the bioavailability of the drug. Alteration of the normal motility of the stomach and intestinal tract can affect how much time the solid dose form has available to dissolve. Therefore changes in motility of the gastrointestinal tract have the potential to alter the absorption of the drug.

Gastric motility refers to stomach contractions that mix stomach contents and move the contents from the stomach into the small intestine. Conditions or diseases that decrease gastric motility can delay the movement of drug from the stomach into the intestine and therefore delay the absorption and onset of action of orally administered drugs. Similarly, a spasm of the pylorus, the muscular ring controlling outflow of stomach contents into

the duodenum, also decreases gastric emptying and delays absorption of the drug by the intestine. Conversely, with increased gastric motility a drug may reach the intestine quicker and begin to be absorbed sooner than normal.

Intestinal motility is defined as the mixing and propulsive contractions of the intestine. Increased intestinal motility, as in hypermotile diarrhea, may move the orally administered tablet past the small intestine before it is completely dissolved, resulting in much of the drug passing out of the body in the feces. In contrast, decreased intestinal motility, such as occurs with constipation or antidiarrheal treatment, can result in complete absorption of a drug, even those that are not necessarily intended to be absorbed (e.g., antibiotics intended to work within the lumen of the intestine). When motility modifier drugs or disease alters gastrointestinal motility, the veterinary professional has to consider the possible impact the change in motility might have on orally administered medications.

FIRST-PASS EFFECT

Even if a drug in solid form has dissolved into small lipophilic molecules capable of diffusing readily across the gastrointestinal tract wall, one final barrier separates the drug from the systemic circulation. All blood that circulates to the small intestine (and part of the large intestine) must travel through the liver on its way back to the systemic circulation. The *hepatic portal system* conducts the blood from the intestine to the liver, where the materials from the intestine can be acted on. This system allows the liver to remove potential toxins and other substances before they reach systemic circulation. The liver recognizes some drugs as foreign substances *(xenobiotics)* and may remove certain drugs "absorbed" by the intestine, effectively preventing them from reaching the rest of the body. In dogs, for example, the tranquilizer diazepam is removed so extensively by the liver after "absorption" from the intestine that little of the tranquilizer makes it to the body to actually produce tranquilization. The phenomenon by which the liver removes so much of the drug that little reaches the systemic circulation is called the *first-pass effect*. Drugs that have an extensive first-pass effect are usually not recommended for PO administration.

EFFECT OF PERFUSION ON ABSORPTION OF PARENTERALLY ADMINISTERED DRUGS

As previously stated, when drugs are injected subcutaneously or intramuscularly they are placed in an aqueous environment in the extracellular fluid between cells. Therefore, to be most efficiently absorbed by these routes, the drug molecules should be predominantly

---

CLINICAL APPLICATION
Lidocaine With and Without Epinephrine

Preparations of the local anesthetic lidocaine come in two versions: lidocaine alone and lidocaine plus epinephrine. Epinephrine is a potent vasoconstrictor of superficial tissues such as subcutaneous tissues. In the body, epinephrine and norepinephrine are hormones and neurotransmitters released to cause the peripheral superficial vasoconstriction designed to raise arterial blood pressure (e.g., animals in shock from injury, animals with decreased blood pressure from blood loss).

Why would epinephrine be added to a local anesthetic? The presence of epinephrine at the SQ injection site would cause blood vessels in the area to vasoconstrict. The effect of this would be to decrease perfusion of blood into the area. Why would decreased perfusion in an area where a local anesthetic was placed be desired?

When a local anesthetic is injected to numb a superficial part of the body, the anesthetic only works as long as it stays where it is injected. Once the local anesthetic diffuses or is absorbed into systemic circulation, the anesthetic effect wears off. Therefore, by using epinephrine to artificially decrease the tissue perfusion around the area in which the local anesthetic was placed, the duration of anesthesia at the site can be prolonged.

What should be learned from this situation: Epinephrine plays an important role in decreasing local anesthetic absorption and prolonging its effect. In addition to its role as a local anesthetic, lidocaine is used without epinephrine to control irregular electrical activity of the heart called an arrhythmia. Epinephrine by itself will increase electrical activity in the heart and can worsen an arrhythmia associated with a diseased or damaged heart. Thus, if lidocaine plus epinephrine instead of lidocaine alone is mistakenly given to an animal with an arrhythmia the animal could suffer from a severe and potentially fatal arrhythmia due to the injection of the epinephrine. Therefore, if bottles of lidocaine and lidocaine plus epinephrine are kept in the clinic or hospital, the bottles should be clearly marked to prevent a staff member from accidentally picking up the wrong lidocaine during an arrhythmia emergency.

in the hydrophilic form so they may readily diffuse through the extracellular tissue fluid and reach a capillary to be absorbed.

If the capillary is farther away from where the drug was injected, it will take longer for the drug molecules to diffuse to the capillary and absorption will be slower. In addition, if fewer capillaries are present around the site of administration, the drug will take longer to be absorbed. The extent to which a tissue is supplied with blood affects its *perfusion*. Tissues that are well perfused with blood will absorb injected drugs much quicker than tissues that are poorly perfused. Fat is a tissue that is poorly perfused (notice in surgery how little cut fat bleeds); therefore drugs injected into a fat pad may remain there for an extended period without being absorbed. Muscle is much better perfused than subcutaneous tissue; therefore drugs injected intramuscularly are absorbed much quicker than those drugs injected subcutaneously.

Tissue perfusion can vary with physiologic conditions. For example, an inactive muscle is not as well perfused as an active muscle; consequently, drugs injected into inactive muscles (e.g., in an animal not moving because of anesthesia or a comatose state) will be absorbed at a slower rate than those injected into a muscle that is moving. Changes in environmental temperature can affect the perfusion of the subcutaneous tissue, resulting in changes in absorption of drugs administered subcutaneously. Cold environmental temperatures cause the precapillary sphincters (circular rings of smooth muscle located at the entrance of the capillary) in the subcutaneous capillaries to contract, thereby reducing blood flow to the area *(vasoconstriction)*. This constriction of superficial blood vessels protects the body from cold by shunting warm blood away from the surface. This same process of vasoconstriction also reduces perfusion of subcutaneous tissues and would decrease the rate of absorption of SQ injected drugs.

Vasodilation (dilation of blood vessels) enhances perfusion of tissues and therefore increases drug absorption in subcutaneous tissue and muscle. Vasodilation in the subcutaneous tissues is initiated by increased body temperature (such as from warm, ambient temperatures and exercise) or drugs (such as alcohol). Vasodilation of muscles occurs when the muscle is exercising or the animal is under conditions of "fight or flight" (sympathetic nervous system effect). Although fight-or-flight conditions increase the perfusion of muscles, the same sympathetic nervous system stimulation causes superficial tissues such as subcutaneous tissue to become vasoconstricted, reducing absorption of SQ administered drugs.

PHARMACOKINETICS: DRUG DISTRIBUTION

Once absorbed, most drugs are not beneficial unless they reach the target tissue for which they are intended. If a cardiac drug cannot reach the myocardium, it will not benefit the patient. If a tranquilizer is unable to reach the brain, the patient will not become tranquilized. This movement of a drug from the systemic circulation into tissues is called distribution.

BARRIERS TO DRUG DISTRIBUTION

Just as barriers to drug absorption exist, so do barriers to distribution. In tissues drugs enter and leave the bloodstream through the thin-walled capillaries. Although capillaries seem to be small, solid-walled "pipes" through which blood flows, in actuality they are more like leaky pipes. In most parts of the body capillary walls are one-cell thick and have small gaps, or *fenestrations* ("windows"), between adjacent cells. These fenestrations allow water and small drug molecules to move readily back and forth while keeping larger molecules, proteins, and red blood cells within the capillary (Figure 3-10). Distribution of the drug to the tissue occurs through these fenestrations.

Capillaries in the brain are different from capillaries in other tissues because the

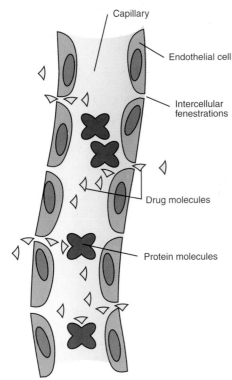

Figure 3-10 Both hydrophilic and lipophilic free drug molecules can pass through fenestrations in the capillary wall without having to dissolve in the capillary cell membrane.

Capillary

Endothelial cell

Intercellular fenestrations

Drug molecules

Protein molecules

endothelial cells abut closely with each other to form tight junctions similar to alignment of the cells lining the intestinal tract. Thus capillaries in the brain have no fenestrations through which drug molecules can pass. This continuous capillary wall forms a barrier to hydrophilic drugs, which cannot diffuse into and through the cellular membrane barrier. In addition to the continuous capillary wall, structural cells in the brain called astrocytes and glial cells surround the capillaries, providing additional membrane barriers through which drugs would have to pass to distribute successfully from blood to brain. The combination of continuous cell wall and the membranes of the supporting cells surrounding the capillaries forms the *blood-brain*

barrier. The blood-brain barrier provides an excellent defense against many toxins, but unfortunately it also prevents distribution of drugs that are not in the lipophilic form (Figure 3-11). Because of the blood-brain barrier, special consideration of drug distribution patterns must be made when attempting to select a drug to act on nervous tissue in the brain. Similar barriers to drug distribution occur in the prostate gland and the globe of the eye, which is why only selected antibiotics are effective for prostate infections and why many drugs meant to act within the globe of the eye must be injected directly into the globe itself.

Although the placenta is commonly thought of as being a protective barrier that guards the fetus against toxins or other damaging compounds, it is actually a poor barrier to drugs that circulate in the mother's bloodstream. The capillaries in the placenta have fenestrations and allow most drugs to pass easily from maternal to fetal circulation. The veterinary professional should always be aware of the potential for overdosing the fetus with drugs given to the mother. Some drugs that gain access to the developing fetus disrupt development, resulting in fetal death, spontaneous abortion, or fetal malformation. Therefore, unless proven otherwise, always assume that a drug given to the mother animal will also be distributed to the fetus.

EFFECT OF TISSUE PERFUSION ON DRUG DISTRIBUTION

Drugs are usually distributed most rapidly and in greater concentrations to well-perfused tissues such as exercised skeletal muscle, the liver, kidneys, and the brain. In contrast, inactive skeletal muscle and adipose (fat) tissue are relatively poorly perfused, so drug delivery to these tissues is delayed. This difference in perfusion can be clinically demonstrated by observing an animal injected with a short-acting barbiturate anesthetic such as thiopental. Thiopental is a lipophilic drug that will

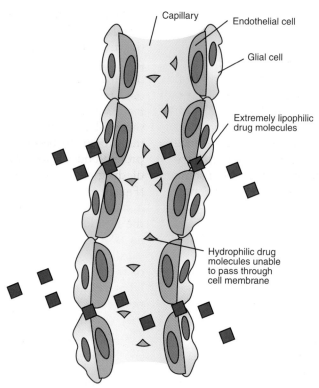

Capillary

Endothelial cell

Glial cell

Extremely lipophilic drug molecules

Hydrophilic drug molecules unable to pass through cell membrane

Figure 3-11 In the central nervous system, the blood-brain barrier allows only lipophilic drugs to distribute from the blood to the brain.

quickly distribute from the blood, through the blood-brain barrier, and into the brain, where it will produce anesthesia within seconds after it is given intravenously. The rapid onset of the anesthesia is a reflection of the lipophilic nature of the drug molecules and the high perfusion of the brain, both of which facilitate the distribution from blood to the brain. Within a few minutes of injection the animal begins to recover. This initial recovery is not due to removal of the drug from the body but from distribution of the drug.

When thiopental is first given intravenously, the high concentrations of drug in the blood distribute to highly perfused organs until concentrations between the blood and the well-perfused tissues, including the brain, are in equilibrium. As time goes on, the drug in the blood is still distributing to the poorer perfused tissues

(fat, inactive muscle) but at a much slower rate. As drug molecules continue to distribute to fat and muscle, the drug concentrations in the blood slowly drop. When drug concentrations in the blood drop below drug concentrations in the brain, the drug starts to move from the brain back into the blood along the concentration gradient. The decreasing thiopental concentration in the brain reduces the anesthetic effect (concentrations fall below the normal therapeutic range) and the animal begins to wake.

This movement of drug from the blood, to the tissue (brain), back to the blood, and then to a second tissue (fat) is called *redistribution*. In the example above, the redistribution of drug would have continued until all the tissues, including the poorly perfused fat tissue, were in equilibrium with the blood concentrations of drug.

EFFECT OF PLASMA PROTEIN BINDING ON DRUG DISTRIBUTION

The plasma of blood contains circulating proteins such as albumin and globulins as well as other proteins that bind to specific hormones or compounds used by the body. These proteins remain in the systemic circulation and do not normally distribute into tissue because they are too large to pass through the capillary fenestrations. The chemical properties of some drugs cause a percentage of the drug molecules to bind to these proteins. Those drug molecules attached to the protein are said to be protein bound and are unable to distribute

to the tissues; only the *free form of the drug molecules* is small enough to distribute through the capillary fenestrations. The protein-bound pool and the free-form pool of drug molecules in the blood are roughly in equilibrium with each other so that when free drug molecules leave the blood to distribute to the tissue, some protein-bound molecules will dissociate from the protein to become free. In this way, the protein-bound pool acts as a storage pool of drug molecules for possible distribution (Figure 3-12).

Because the *protein-bound drug* molecules are not distributed to the tissues to produce an effect, the protein-bound pool represents

CLINICAL APPLICATION
Highly Protein-Bound Drugs

A 5-year-old, terrier-X, male castrate dog was presented for a diagnostic workup for chronic diarrhea. The dog was diagnosed as having small intestinal disease that resulted in poor absorption of food and loss of protein through the gastrointestinal tract (protein-losing enteropathy). As a result of the chronic protein loss, the concentration of total blood proteins was below normal.

The dog was to be anesthetized with a short-acting barbiturate to perform further diagnostic procedures. The veterinary technician calculated the correct dose for the weight of the animal and administered half of the total dose as an IV bolus. Anesthesia was induced but the dog stopped breathing, suggesting that he had received an anesthetic overdose of the barbiturate. Although barbiturates normally cause some respiratory depression until the drug redistributes from the brain, this dog did not begin to breathe on his own and had to have his respiration assisted for several minutes.

The veterinarian checked the technician's calculations and found them to be correct. Only half of the dose was administered intravenously. Why did the dog become so profoundly anesthetized?

Barbiturates are normally highly protein-bound drugs. They bind to albumin, and thus dosages listed take into account the protein binding that will occur with a dose. However, in this case the dog had a low

albumin level because of the loss of proteins through the gastrointestinal tract. Because the plasma albumin level was low, more administered barbiturate was in the free form and available to distribute to well-perfused tissues such as the brain. The result was higher than normal drug concentrations in the brain and a more profound effect on the central nervous system (including the respiratory control centers). Thus a normal dose produced an overdose effect.

The dog survived. He was intubated (tracheal tube placed) and his breathing was assisted for 10 minutes before he started to breathe on his own.

What should be learned from this situation: Although no formula can predict how much a dose of a highly protein-bound drug should be reduced in a hypoproteinemic ("low protein in the blood") animal, the veterinary professional should be conservative in selecting doses of highly protein-bound drugs in hypoproteinemic animals. Barbiturates are an example of a highly protein-bound drug that should be administered very slowly to a hypoproteinemic animal to avoid giving too much drug.

As a general rule, the dose of highly protein-bound drugs should be reduced in animals with liver disease, protein-losing enteropathy (intestinal disease), protein-losing nephropathy (kidney disease), or any other condition that reduces the protein-binding capacity.

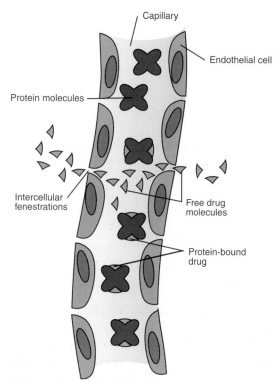

Figure 3-12 Drug molecules bound to large blood protein molecules cannot exit capillaries and so are not distributed to tissues.

the component of the drug dose that is largely inactive. The drug formulary dosages for highly protein-bound drugs take into account that a percentage of the dose given will become protein bound and not be available to produce a systemic effect. Therefore a change in the quantity of protein in the blood requires an adjustment of the dose for highly protein-bound drugs. For example, in severe or prolonged liver disease an animal may be unable to produce sufficient plasma albumin. In this circumstance, drugs normally highly protein bound to albumin would end up with more molecules available in the unbound form than normal. The result would be more molecules available for distribution and a concentration of drug molecules in the tissue that may exceed the normal therapeutic range for the tissue. To

compensate for the increased availability of unbound molecules, the overall dose would have to be decreased.

VOLUME OF DISTRIBUTION

The *volume of distribution (Vd)* is a pharmacokinetic value that provides an approximation of the extent to which a drug is distributed throughout the body. The Vd assumes that the drug is equally distributed throughout each compartment of the body and that the concentration in the blood is in equilibrium with the concentration in the rest of the body.

Generally, the larger the Vd listed for a drug, the more tissues the drug appears to be able to penetrate. Because a large Vd means the drug is distributed to more tissues, the drug concentration in the blood will be lower because the drug is being diluted by the fluid of many body compartments. For example, 100 mg of sugar is placed in a 1-L container of water (Figure 3-13). The same amount of sugar is then placed in a second container of water with a volume of 10 L. The 10-L container represents a larger volume of distribution for the sugar. As expected, the larger volume of distribution would have a lower concentration of sugar because it is diluted more. The 100 mg of sugar per 1 L of water yields a sugar concentration of 100 mg/1000 mL, or 0.1 mg/mL. The 10-L container with 100 mg of sugar produced a concentration of 100 mg/10,000 mL, or 0.01 mg/mL.

If a drug dose is properly calculated but the Vd is not normal, the resulting concentration in the body may be higher or lower than expected, resulting in drug concentrations above or below the normal therapeutic range. For example, an obese dog may have a very different volume of distribution than the same-sized lean dog because of the different relative amounts of fat and muscle in the two body types and the difference in the ability of the drug to distribute to fat and muscle. Because the fat tissue is poorly perfused, a significant portion of drug distribution in an obese dog

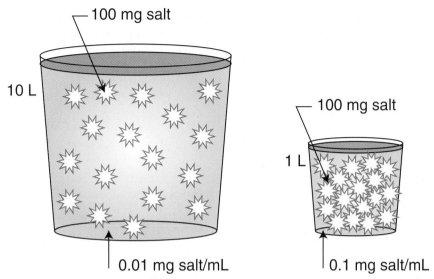

Figure 3-13 The larger the volume of distribution, the lower the concentration of a drug.

will be very slow. The initial volume of distribution of the drug in the obese dog may be much smaller (drug distributes to fewer compartments) than the initial volume of distribution in the lean dog with its low amounts of fat and higher percentage of well-perfused skeletal muscle. Because the drug would initially have a smaller Vd in the obese dog, resulting in a higher concentration of drug in the blood and the few tissues to which the drug is initially distributed, a lower initial drug dose (lower compared to the initial drug dose in a lean dog) should be used to avoid excessive drug concentrations in the perfused tissues.

The volume of distribution is more accurately called the apparent volume of distribution because it is a mathematically derived value as opposed to a value derived from an actual measurement of the volume into which the drug is distributed. The apparent volume of distribution may not always reflect what is actually happening to the drug in the body. As stated earlier, the apparent volume of distribution is estimated by knowing the dose of the drug that was given, examining the blood concentration of the drug, and then extrapolating backwards to determine the volume of fluid into which the drug would have to be diluted in order to result in the observed concentration in the blood. It would be similar to knowing that 100 mg of sugar was put in a container of unknown volume and that 0.01 mg of sugar was present in each milliliter of liquid.

$$100 \text{ mg} \times 1 \text{ mL}/0.01 \text{ mg} = 10,000 \text{ mL}$$
$$= 10 \text{ L for the Vd}$$

The apparent volume of distribution assumes equal distribution to all compartments, much like the container into which the sugar was placed. However, if a drug is sequestered (clustered or accumulated) in one compartment of the body, the apparent volume of distribution can be misleading. For example, the cardiac drug digoxin is highly bound to proteins in the heart and skeletal muscle. Distribution of the drug is primarily to these tissues for that reason, and these tissues may have concentrations that are relatively high compared with the blood and other tissues. However, the low concentration of digoxin that remains in the blood suggests that the digoxin is being distributed to many tissues and body compartments. In fact, so much of the digoxin is sequestered in the muscle and heart that the calculated volume of distribution, based on blood concentration, suggests that the drug is diluted in several liters of fluid more than the animal can possibly have in its body. With the exception of sequestering of drugs, however, the Vd still gives a general idea of the penetrability and distribution of a drug.

PHARMACODYNAMICS: THE WAY DRUGS EXERT THEIR EFFECTS

Pharmacodynamics is the study of how drugs interact with the body to produce their effect. Theoretically, if a drug is well absorbed and readily distributed in therapeutic concentrations to all tissues, it should have an effect on every tissue in the body. In reality this is not the case. Generally, for cells to respond to a drug molecule, the drug has to combine with a specifically shaped protein located on the cell's surface or within the cell. This specific protein is called a *receptor*. The shape or molecular structure of a receptor determines which drug molecules can combine with them. This concept may be compared to a key and lock; the receptor is the lock into which only the correct key (drug) will fit.

Once a drug molecule combines with a receptor, the receptor may trigger a cellular change, such as producing secretions, contracting muscle cells, or depolarizing neurons. The reason not all tissues respond to all drugs is that all cells do not have receptors for all drugs; only certain cells respond to certain drugs. For example, smooth muscle cells in the bronchioles of the lungs may have receptors to drug A, whereas smooth muscle cells in the uterus have no receptors to drug A. When drug A is administered, only the bronchiolar smooth muscle contracts even though drug A is present in the uterus at therapeutic concentrations. The number of drug receptors located on or in a cell also determines how sensitive a cell is to a drug. A cell with many

receptors to a drug will be much more sensitive to the drug than a cell with only a few. Cells can increase and decrease the number of drug receptors to change their sensitivity to drugs.

As shown in Figure 3-14, a cell's surface (or sometimes cell organelles such as the nucleus and lysosomes) may have multiple types of receptors on it, each capable of combining with different specific drugs and each drug having a different effect on the cell. For example, when drug A combines with its receptor, the cell produces a response such as secretion of a protein. When drug B is present in therapeutic concentrations and combines with its specific receptor, the cell does not secrete protein but instead may be stimulated to divide. Hence different drugs have different receptors and may produce different cellular effects.

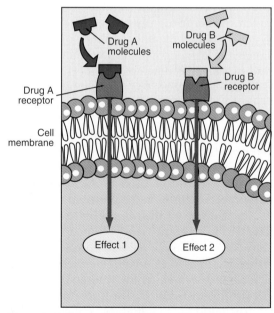

Figure 3-14 Drug molecules have specific shapes that allow them to combine with specific receptors on the cell membrane surface to produce an effect. Drug A Molecule combined with drug A Receptor produces Effect 1. A differently shaped drug Molecule B would not fit Receptor A combined but can combine with Receptor B to produce Effect 2 by the cell.

ANTAGONISTS AND AGONISTS

When drug X combines with its receptor, it produces a specific effect on the cell. Because drug X produces an effect on the cell, drug X is said to have *intrinsic activity* when it combines with this receptor. A drug with a molecular shape similar to drug X can combine with that same receptor but may not produce an effect because of some minor difference in the second drug's shape or the way in which it combines with the receptor. The second drug simply "sits" on the receptor and has no intrinsic activity. Because drug X produced a cellular effect and had intrinsic activity, it is called an *agonist*. The second drug molecule would be classified as an *antagonist* to drug X because when it combines with the receptor it produces an opposite effect; the second drug opposes, or is antagonistic to, the effects of drug X (Figure 3-15).

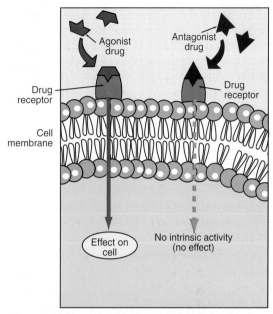

Figure 3-15 An agonist drug has intrinsic activity when it combines with its drug receptor. The antagonist occupies the same receptor site but does not produce an effect. Therefore, if the agonist is replaced on the receptor by an antagonist, the effect of the agonist would be reversed.

Competitive and Noncompetitive Antagonists

A drug's antagonist activity can be classified as competitive or noncompetitive. For example, if drug A is given to produce an effect and drug B is capable of completely reversing drug A's effect, then drug B is said to be a competitive antagonist of drug A (and vice versa; drug A would competitively antagonize drug B's effect). The reason this is classified as competitive antagonism is that drug A and drug B appear to have an equal opportunity to exert their effect on the cell. In competitive antagonism the cellular effect observed after administration of two competing drugs is determined by which drug is present in greater quantity at the receptor site. In the example above, drug A's effect can be reversed by drug B, which can then be reversed once again by drug A. For that reason, *competitive antagonism* is also called *reversible antagonism* or *surmountable antagonism*. The word inhibition can be substituted for the word antagonism when the effect of the antagonist drug stops the cellular effect of the agonist drug. In other words, if drug A produces anesthesia and drug B reverses that anesthetic effect so that the animal wakes up, drug B would be a competitive inhibitor of drug A.

Sometimes the agonist/antagonist relation between two drugs favors the effect of one drug over the other. For example, perhaps drug A is administered to produce smooth muscle contraction. But unlike the previous example, the effect of drug A cannot be easily reversed by administration of drug B even though drug B has the potential to combine with the same receptor. Drug A appears to have an advantage that prevents its effect from being reversed by drug B. The reason for this advantage may be that drug A has greater affinity (attraction) for the receptor than drug B and therefore combines more tightly with the receptor than drug B. Or perhaps drug A physically alters the shape of the receptor, reducing the ability of the antagonist drug B molecule to fit the receptor. Either way, the relation of drug A to drug B is an example of *noncompetitive, irreversible, or insurmountable antagonism.* In most cases the antagonism is not truly irreversible or insurmountable. But because the process of reversal is so slow or so much of the antagonist is needed to overcome the effect of the agonist drug, the drug interaction gives the impression of being irreversible.

Partial Agonist/Partial Antagonist

Up to this point the intrinsic activity of a drug and its receptor has been assumed to be an on/off relation; either the cell responds to the drug or it does not. However, two drugs attaching to the same receptor may have different levels of intrinsic activity. If drug A increases the heart rate 50% above baseline when producing its maximal effect but drug B, acting on the same receptor, only increases the heart rate 25%, drug B could be called a *partial agonist.* The partial agonist effect of drug B is in relation to the stronger intrinsic activity of drug A. Drug B is not as powerful an agonist as is drug A.

If an animal is given drug A and the heart rate increases 50% above baseline, then the animal is given drug B and the heart rate decreases to 25% above baseline, drug B has partially antagonized the effect of drug A. Drug B has not completely reversed the effect of drug A (the heart rate did not return to baseline); therefore drug B was a *partial antagonist.* Drugs such as drug B are called partial agonist/partial antagonist drugs because they partially

CLINICAL APPLICATION
Agonists, Antagonists, and Partial Agonists/Partial Antagonists in Anesthesia

A dog undergoes a painful surgical procedure to remove a front limb that has osteosarcoma, a serious cancer of the bone. The surgeon wants the dog to be comfortable after surgery, so she prescribes the strong narcotic analgesic (pain reliever) hydromorphone. She injects hydromorphone at the completion of surgery to smooth the dog's anesthetic recovery. The hydromorphone produces cellular changes that result in analgesia and is therefore an agonist in this situation.

As the dog is recovering from the anesthesia the surgeon notices that the dog appears to be comfortable regarding pain relief but is more sedated than desired and has some respiratory depression (both of which are common side effects of strong narcotic agonist drugs). She wants to reverse the respiratory depression and have the animal a bit less sedated, but she does not want to lose the analgesic effect for the patient's comfort.

Instead of using the competitive narcotic antagonist naloxone to reverse the effect of hydromorphone completely, she chooses to use the partial agonist/partial antagonist drug butorphanol. Butorphanol is a competitive antagonist of hydromorphone; given in sufficient quantities it will be able to displace hydromorphone from the receptor site, ending hydromorphone's analgesia, sedation, and respiratory depression. But butorphanol has some intrinsic analgesic activity of its own and is capable of producing some degree of analgesia, but less analgesia than hydromorphone. The less-powerful analgesia of butorphanol makes it an agonist, but relative to hydromorphone's stronger effect it is a partial agonist. The surgeon gives the butorphanol and sees the dog become more alert with less respiratory depression (partial antagonist effect) while still having some degree of pain relief (partial agonist effect).

What should be learned from this situation: All drugs do not act on the same receptor with the same degree of intrinsic activity. A potent drug may produce its maximal effect with very little drug administered. A less-potent drug requires a larger amount of the drug to be given to achieve its maximal effect or power. A powerful drug has a very strong maximal effect, whereas a weak drug has much less of an effect regardless of how much drug is administered. By understanding these terms and applying them to the concept of agonists, antagonists, and partial agonists/partial antagonists, medical therapies can be tailored more effectively to the specific need, and degree of need, of the veterinary patient.

reverse the effect of a more powerful drug but provide some cellular effect of their own.

NON–RECEPTOR-MEDIATED REACTIONS

Some drugs produce an effect without combining with receptors. For example, mannitol is a sugar compound used as a drug and classified as an osmotic diuretic. When administered by IV infusion, mannitol molecules are excreted into the urine, where they draw water from the body and into the urine by osmosis. Mannitol produces the increased production of urine (diuresis) without combining with a cellular receptor. This is an example of a *non–receptor-mediated drug reaction.*

Chelators are types of compounds used as drugs that physically combine with ions (e.g., calcium, chloride, magnesium) or other specific compounds in the environment to produce their effects. For example, penicillamine is a chelator that combines with lead in the body and facilitates excretion of the combined product in the urine. Another example of a chelator is the ethylenediamine tetraacetic acid (EDTA) anticoagulant compound included in blood collection tubes with lavender tops. EDTA combines with calcium in the blood sample and prevents the clotting mechanism from turning the sample into a clot.

Another non–receptor-mediated reaction occurs when calcium, aluminum, or magnesium antacid drugs (e.g., Tums, Rolaids) combine with the strong hydrochloric acid in the stomach to form a much weaker acid, thereby reducing stomach irritation. No cellular receptor is involved in these examples; thus they are described as non–receptor-mediated reactions.

PHARMACOKINETICS: BIOTRANSFORMATION AND DRUG METABOLISM

Many drugs are altered by the enzymes and chemical reactions in the body before they are eliminated. This process is referred to as *biotransformation,* or drug metabolism. The altered drug molecule is referred to as a *metabolite.* The majority of the enzymes involved in biotransformation are found in the liver, although other tissues such as the lung, skin, and intestinal tract may also have the capability to biotransform drug molecules. The biotransformation process usually results in a metabolite that is more hydrophilic and more readily eliminated by the kidney or liver.

Biotransformation is usually a two-step enzymatic process. In phase I metabolism of the original drug molecule is chemically transformed by the chemical processes of oxidation, reduction, or hydrolysis of the molecule. These processes most commonly add or remove oxygen, hydrogen, or other key molecules to transform the structure of the drug molecule chemically. In phase II metabolism, the metabolite from phase I is combined with another molecule such as glucuronic acid, sulfate, or glycine in a process called conjugation (to come together). The conjugated molecule is usually more water soluble (hydrophilic) and more readily excreted into the urine. (See Chapter 2 for a further explanation of why a hydrophilic molecule is more readily excreted in the urine.)

After phase I is complete, the resulting metabolite is typically less biologically active. However, sometimes phase I biotransformation does not diminish the activity of the original compound or yield a compound with more activity than the original drug. Drugs that require biotransformation to become active are called *prodrugs.* Once metabolized, the drug's metabolite is capable of producing a biologic effect. For example, prednisone is a commonly prescribed veterinary drug that is biotransformed by liver enzymes to its active antiinflammatory metabolite drug form, prednisolone.

DRUG INTERACTIONS AFFECTING BIOTRANSFORMATION

Very sick animals commonly receive several drugs at one time. Unfortunately, some drugs can interact with each other, altering their

CLINICAL APPLICATION
Cats Are Not Little Dogs

A client has an old German shepherd dog with longstanding degenerative hip disease (hip dysplasia) that has caused painful arthritic changes in the hip joint. Fortunately, the discomfort is controlled with a daily dose of 2 regular-strength aspirin tablets given with dog food to reduce stomach irritation.

When this client's 8-year-old cat developed a swollen paw, most likely caused by infection from a cat fight, she decided to administer aspirin to relieve his discomfort. Realizing that the cat weighed approximately one fifth of the weight of the dog, she decided to give half of an aspirin tablet daily to relieve the cat's discomfort (approximately one fourth of the dog's dose).

After 4 days the swelling of the paw had decreased but the cat was vomiting and acting lethargic. She took the cat to the veterinarian. On hearing the history, the veterinarian suspected aspirin toxicosis and began supportive therapy. The cat recovered and went home 3 days later with an owner who had learned an important lesson that "cats are not little dogs."

Why did the cat not tolerate a dose of aspirin that seemed close to a tolerable dose based on the dose that was working well in the dog?

Cats have a reduced ability to biotransform certain drugs; thus conversion to inactive metabolites and drug elimination occur more slowly in cats than in other species. One of the most important phase II biotransformations in mammals involves the conjugation (combining) of a molecule of a phase I

drug metabolite molecule with a molecule of glucuronic acid. This combination allows rapid removal of the drug from the body. Unfortunately, cats have a reduced ability to synthesize glucuronic acid, and therefore drugs that are normally metabolized by this conjugation pathway are shunted to other, less-efficient metabolic pathways, requiring more time for the drug to be metabolized and subsequently eliminated. Salicylate compounds, such as aspirin and bismuth subsalicylate (Pepto-Bismol), are drugs normally conjugated with glucuronic acid. By applying aspirin to the bucket analogy, the hole in the bottom of the bucket is smaller for cats than it is for other species.

This does not mean that aspirin should never be used in cats. Cats can still metabolize aspirin and other salicylate drugs. However, they must be given smaller doses than dogs, with longer dose intervals to allow enough time for the drug to be biotransformed between doses.

What should be learned from this situation: First, cats are not little dogs. Second, a dose of a drug in one species cannot necessarily be safely extrapolated to another species because of differences in species' ability to metabolize and excrete certain drugs. Drugs that do not depend on extensive biotransformation and conjugation by liver enzymes for elimination may be better tolerated by cats. However, whenever any doubt exists, the veterinary technician should always read the drug package insert closely, consult a drug reference, or ask the veterinarian.

---

metabolism and resulting in higher or lower drug concentrations or adverse effects. For example, two drugs may compete for the same limited number of biotransformation enzymes in the liver, causing both drugs to be metabolized at a slower rate. By using the bucket analogy, the decreased biotransformation capacity for each drug can be described as having two buckets of water draining out through the same small drain pipe. Unless one or both of the drug doses are decreased in this situation,

the drugs may accumulate in potentially toxic concentrations.

One of the most common biotransformation enzyme systems in the liver is the mixed function oxidase (MFO) system. The number of MFO enzyme molecules available for biotransformation may be increased when the MFO system is repeatedly exposed to certain drugs. The effect of the repeated exposure results in an increased rate of biotransformation for those drugs. This increased rate of metabolism is called metabolic induction, and metabolism of the drug is said to be *induced metabolism*. When a drug's metabolism has been induced, the active form of the drug is more rapidly converted to a less-active form, shortening the time in the body that the drug can be effective. This is seen clinically as a shorter duration of beneficial effect of the drug, a condition often referred to as tolerance. Metabolic induction and subsequent tolerance is why human beings and animals require increasing doses of drugs such as barbiturates, narcotics, and alcohol to produce the same effect.

When the MFO system has been induced by exposure to a particular drug, biotransformation of any other drug normally metabolized by the MFO system is also increased. For example, repeated use of phenobarbital, a barbiturate used for seizure control, also increases biotransformation of such drugs as phenylbutazone, digitoxin, estrogens, dipyrone, glucocorticoids, and others metabolized by the MFO system. For this reason the dose of any other drugs affected by enzyme induction must be increased to compensate for more rapid biotransformation.

SPECIES AND AGE DIFFERENCES IN DRUG BIOTRANSFORMATION

A drug that is safe to use in one species may produce severe side effects in another. Cats metabolize some drugs poorly or not at all. For example, certain drugs that are safe for use in dogs, horses, or pigs may produce toxicity in cats.

Very young animals and to a lesser extent older animals also have a decreased ability to biotransform drugs. In neonates (newborn animals) the liver may not be fully functional for several days to weeks depending on the species. In older animals, organ function declines as a part of the aging process. The amount of functional mass of the kidney or liver may decrease with age or with disease. For this reason, veterinary professionals should double check the dose and precautions for a drug

before administering it to any animal younger than 5 weeks old or older animals in which increased risk for reduced liver or kidney function exists.

PHARMACOKINETICS: DRUG ELIMINATION

Drug elimination or excretion is the movement of drug molecules out of the body. Generally this means that the drug is expelled in the feces or urine; released into the environment as exhaled air or sweat; or even incorporated into keratin of the hair, nails, or hooves. Elimination is the hole in the bottom of the bucket; as such, changes in elimination have the potential to markedly change the dose needed to achieve therapeutic concentrations. Changes in drug elimination occur with dehydration, age-related degeneration of the kidney or liver, and a variety of other physiologic and pathologic (disease) conditions that affect function of the kidney or liver. By understanding the factors affecting drug elimination, the veterinary professional can anticipate potential problems and adjust drug doses to avoid producing drug toxicity in their patients.

ROUTES OF DRUG ELIMINATION

The two major routes of elimination are by the kidney (into the urine) and the liver (into the bile and subsequently the feces). Inhalant anesthetics and other volatile agents are mostly eliminated by the lungs. Other less common routes of elimination include saliva, milk (in lactating animals), and sweat. Because of the concern about residues of drugs in milk, the veterinary professional needs to be aware of a drug's route of elimination when prescribing drugs to lactating dairy animals.

RENAL ELIMINATION OF DRUGS

In the kidney, circulating drugs are cleared from the blood through processes called *filtration* and *active secretion*. Filtration is a passive process that occurs as the blood flows from the renal arteriole through the specialized tuft of capillaries in the kidney called the *glomerulus.* The flow of blood into the glomerulus is regulated by smooth muscles around the renal arterioles such that blood pressure within the glomerulus forces water and small molecules from the blood into the first part of the renal nephron, called *Bowman's capsule.* The wall structure of the glomerulus and Bowman's capsule prevents blood cells and larger protein molecules from leaving the blood but allows the water and small molecules (including drug molecules) to become the glomerular filtrate that will be collected and modified to form urine.

Because proteins are too large to be filtered into the Bowman's capsule, drugs bound to plasma proteins remain in circulation and are not filtered. If, however, blood protein levels decrease, such as with hypoalbuminemia (low albumin protein in the blood) associated with chronic liver disease, more drug molecules will be in the free form and capable of passing into the glomerular filtrate and out the body in the urine. Under conditions of hypoalbuminemia or hypoproteinemia, highly protein-bound drugs are often eliminated more rapidly.

Changes in the degree of renal perfusion will also affect the renal elimination of drugs. In conditions of lowered blood pressure (hypotension), smooth muscle around the renal arterioles constricts as part of the body's protective mechanism for shunting blood to the brain and other critical organs. The vasoconstriction of the renal arteriole decreases blood flow into the glomerulus, resulting in decreased filtration pressure within the glomerulus, and decreases the force moving water and small molecules into the glomerular filtrate of the Bowman's capsule. The net result is decreased elimination of the drug and decreased urine formation.

Dehydration, blood loss, shock, or increased sympathetic nervous system stimulation result in renal arteriole vasoconstriction, decreased glomerular filtration, and decreased renal elimination of drugs. Conversely, the administration of intravenous fluids or the use of drugs that increase renal perfusion will increase flow through the glomerulus, increase glomerular filtration, and cause a more rapid removal of drug molecules from the blood flowing through the glomerulus.

After the glomerular filtrate has been formed in Bowman's capsule, it moves into the *proximal convoluted tubule* segment of the nephron. The proximal convoluted tubule of the nephron is an active segment that contains many active transport mechanisms for moving electrolytes, glucose, some drug molecules, and other essential molecules back and forth among the urine, the renal tubular cell, and the surrounding peritubular capillaries. Some drug molecules are actively transported from the peritubular capillaries into the urine by a process called active secretion. Because these selected drugs are moved by an active transport mechanism, the final concentration of drug in the urine does not depend on the concentration gradient from blood to urine. For that reason, drugs actively secreted into the urine can achieve very high concentrations in the urine. Penicillin antibiotics are one of the drugs actively secreted into the urine, which explains why penicillin drugs are often used to treat bacterial infections of the urinary tract.

The effect of plasma protein binding on drug elimination is more variable at the active secretion site than in the passive filtration site in the glomerulus. If the affinity, or attraction, between a protein-bound drug molecule and the transport molecule in the cell membrane is very high, the drug molecule may separate from the plasma protein and be transported into the proximal convoluted tubule. If, however, the protein-bound drug molecule has only a weak affinity for the carrier molecule, the drug molecule most likely will remain in the blood.

From the proximal convoluted tubule the filtrate moves into the *loop of Henle,* where some of the drug molecules may move from the filtrate back into circulation. This process is called reabsorption. Because reabsorption occurs by passive diffusion through the cells that comprise the renal tubule wall, reabsorbed drug molecules must be in the lipophilic form (nonionized). Hydrophilic (ionized) forms of the drug molecules remain in the urine and cannot be reabsorbed to any significant extent. As previously discussed, urinary acidifying or alkalinizing drugs can alter the pH of the renal tubule filtrate, causing drug molecules to shift between lipophilic and hydrophilic forms and affecting the degree to which the drug is reabsorbed.

Beyond the loop of Henle, the urine water and electrolyte composition is altered by the body, but only minor changes in the amount of drug in the urine generally occur. Although some lipophilic molecules may continue to pass out of the urine by passive reabsorption through the wall of the renal tubules and even through the wall of the urinary bladder, by the time the urine filtrate moves through the *distal convoluted tubule,* the *collecting ducts,* and into the renal pelvis and ureter, the drug is considered to have been eliminated or excreted from the body (Figure 3-16).

HEPATIC ELIMINATION OF DRUGS

Elimination of drugs by the liver is called biliary excretion, or *hepatic excretion.* The liver has a very rich blood supply that filters blood from the systemic circulation and the blood sent from the gastrointestinal tract by the hepatic portal system. As blood moves through specialized liver blood cavities called sinusoids, drugs excreted by the liver move by passive diffusion into the hepatocytes (liver cells), where they are either secreted directly into the bile unchanged or metabolized first and then secreted into the bile. The bile produced by the liver is collected in the bile duct, where it is transported to the duodenum.

If a drug excreted by the liver arrives in the duodenum in a lipophilic form, the drug molecule could be reabsorbed across the intestinal wall, transported by the hepatic portal circulation back to the liver, then either excreted again by the liver or reenter systemic circulation. This movement of drug from liver to intestinal tract and back to the liver is referred to as *enterohepatic circulation.* An unchanged drug excreted and reabsorbed in this way has the potential to exert its effect on the body for a much longer period than a drug either excreted as a metabolite or not reabsorbed. The extended duration of some drugs' action is caused by enterohepatic circulation of the unmodified drug.

If the liver is compromised by acute disease or chronic degenerative processes such as cirrhosis (replacement of functional liver cells by nonfunctional fibrous tissue), the liver's ability to metabolize and eliminate drugs is reduced. Therefore the dose of drugs eliminated by *biliary excretion* must be reduced to prevent drug accumulation in toxic concentrations.

HALF-LIFE AND CLEARANCE: MEASURES OF DRUG ELIMINATION RATES

The rate at which drugs leave the body is expressed as the drug's *clearance,* or *half-life of elimination.* Drug clearance is the measure of how fast a volume of blood is cleared of the drug and is typically expressed as a volume of blood cleared over time. A drug that is rapidly cleared means that it is quickly eliminated from the body. The kidney and liver are considered clearance organs because they remove drugs from the circulation. Therefore decreased function of either clearance organ can result in decreased clearance of a drug and decreased elimination from the body.

A drug's half-life of elimination is a time value that describes how long the drug concentration, usually measured in the blood, takes to decrease by 50%. Figure 3-17 shows how a drug's blood (plasma) concentration typically decreases over time in a predictable curve, not in a straight line. In the example shown, the drug concentrations drop by half every 2 hours until the drug is eliminated from the body. Therefore this drug has a half-life of 2 hours.

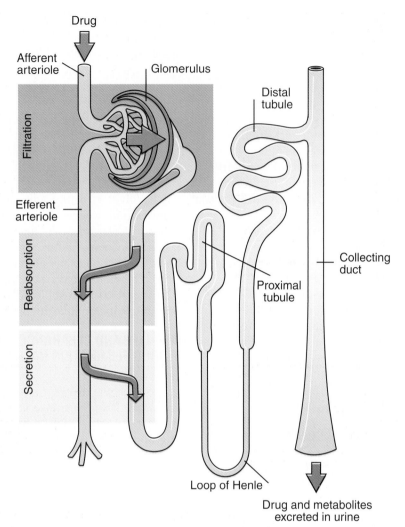

Figure 3-16 The renal nephron.

A drug's half-life may dictate how frequently the drug must be given (the dose interval) to maintain concentrations within the therapeutic range. For example, most antibiotics used in veterinary medicine have a half-life of 2 to 3 hours. With a half-life of 2 hours, 50% of the drug will be eliminated after 2 hours; after 4 hours only 25% remains, 12.5% remains at 6 hours, and 6.25% remains at 8 hours. Therefore the drug may have to be given several times daily to compensate for

the rapid elimination and to keep the concentrations within the normal therapeutic range. In contrast, phenobarbital, a commonly used anticonvulsant (seizure control) medication, has a half-life of approximately 2 days. Thus even within the span of 24 hours the drug concentration of phenobarbital does not decrease by half. This explains why phenobarbital is typically only given once daily.

A drug's half-life may also reflect how efficiently the clearance organs are functioning.

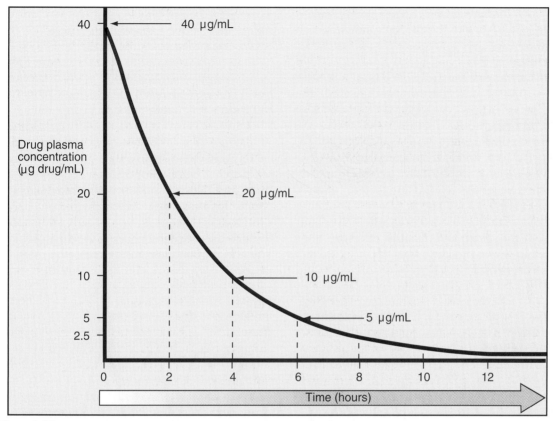

Figure 3-17 Decrease in plasma concentrations of a drug with a half-life of 2 hours. After 2 hours the concentration is 50% of the original concentration. In the next 2 hours the concentration drops again by half. This 50% decrease of drug concentration every 2 hours continues until the drug is completely eliminated.

If the kidney is damaged or not well perfused, the half-life of a drug excreted by the kidney increases (the concentrations take longer to drop by 50%). In dehydration, shock, or renal disease the half-life may double or triple, reflecting the decreased functioning of the kidney.

The half-life of drugs excreted by the liver would not change significantly if the kidney function was impaired because the hepatic elimination process is not directly affected by renal function. Therefore in animals with renal disease selecting drugs that are primarily excreted through the liver is important. The converse of this would be true for drugs excreted by the kidney in animals with liver disease. This point emphasizes why veterinary professionals must be aware of the route by which a drug is metabolized and excreted when selecting a drug or dosage regimen for animals with liver or kidney disease.

RELATION OF HALF-LIFE TO STEADY-STATE CONCENTRATIONS

As previously explained, when a drug is given repeatedly it accumulates to a plateau at which all the highest concentrations (the peak concentrations) and the lowest concentrations (the trough concentrations) are the same. When the concentrations reach this point, the drug is said to be at steady state.

How quickly a drug reaches steady state is determined mostly by the drug's elimination rate. A specific mathematic relation exists between a drug's half-life and its increase in concentrations toward a steady state. After the time of one half-life has elapsed, the peak and trough concentrations are 50% of the concentrations that they will be when they achieve steady state peak and trough. After two half-lives the concentrations are 75% (increased by another half) of the steady state concentrations, and after three half-lives the concentrations are 87.5% (50% + 25% + 12.5%) of the final concentrations. By five half-lives, the peak and trough concentrations are at approximately 97% (50% + 25% + 12.5% + 6.25% + 3.125%) of steady state and

considered, for practical purposes, to be at steady state (Figure 3-18). Therefore the time from the beginning of therapy to reach steady state is equal to 5 times the half-life. For example, an antibiotic with a half-life of 3 hours will reach steady state 15 hours (3 hours × 5) after the dosage regimen has begun. In contrast, a drug with a 30-hour half-life will take 150 hours, or approximately 6 days, to reach steady state after the dosage regimen is begun. For drugs with a long half-life, and hence a longer time to reach steady state, loading doses are often given to boost the concentrations close to steady state, after which the concentrations are then maintained by the regular dosage regimen (the maintenance dose).

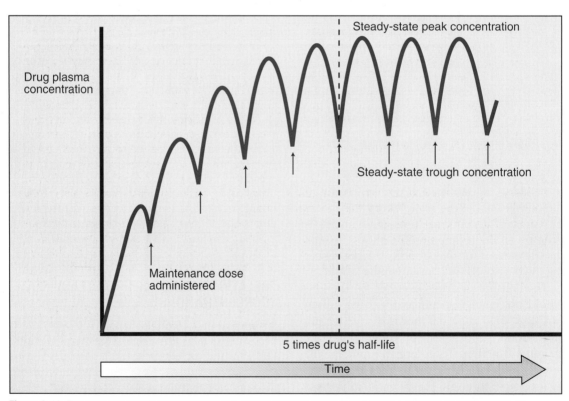

Figure 3-18 The peak and trough concentrations in a dosage regimen increase to a plateau at which all peak and trough concentrations are the same. At that point the drug is said to be at a steady state.

CLINICAL APPLICATION
Young Animals Are Special Cases

Three 5-day-old Springer Spaniel–mix puppies presented with enlarged mandibular lymph nodes caused by a severe localized bacterial infection ("puppy strangles"). The veterinarian's challenge was to select an antibiotic and an appropriate dose form that young puppies could take and tolerate. Why is selecting drugs for neonates (newborns) and very young animals often a challenge for the veterinary professional?

From birth to approximately 1 month of age, deficiencies in the neonatal liver slow the rate of drug biotransformation. Drugs that, in a mature animal, are normally oxidized, reduced, or conjugated with glucuronic acid as part of the biotransformation and excretion process will accumulate more readily in a young animal's liver because these metabolic pathways are more limited than in the adult liver, resulting in slower elimination of drugs. For that reason, ultra–short-acting barbiturates, some sulfonamide antibacterials, opioids, aspirinlike compounds (salicylates), some anticonvulsants, and local anesthetics (e.g., procaine) must be used with caution in neonates and very young animals. By 5 weeks of age, the liver of most neonates functions near adult capacity. The exception is young foals, which appear to develop important enzymes in their liver within a few days of birth.

Drug distribution is also different in young animals and can affect the selection of a drug and its dose. The blood-brain barrier in very young animals is more permeable to drugs than it is in adults. For this reason drug doses that normally do not produce therapeutic concentrations in adults may produce significant concentrations in a young animal's brain. The same is true for some toxic agents. For example, ingestion of even small amounts of lead can result in significant accumulations within the neonate or young animal's brain, leading to developmental problems in the central nervous system.

Plasma albumin levels are relatively low during the first 2 to 3 weeks of life. Therefore less protein is available to bind with highly protein-bound drugs, and free drug molecules are available for distribution to tissues. Doses of drugs that are normally highly protein bound must be reduced to compensate for a larger percentage of drug molecules free to distribute into the tissue.

The body composition of neonates and young animals contains a much higher ratio of water to fat than in adult animals. Therefore when a drug that normally distributes to the extracellular fluid is administered to a young animal, it is diluted in a larger volume of water than the same amount of drug in the same-sized older animal. Hence a 10-mg dose produces lower concentrations in a young animal than in an adult animal of the same weight.

Most drugs given by mouth to newborn ruminants (mammals with four-chambered stomachs) are absorbed in much the same way as in monogastric (single-stomach) animals. Therefore absorption patterns of drugs change over the 4- to 6-week period required for young ruminants to progress from a monogastric gastrointestinal tract to a tract of a functional ruminant. A functional rumen environment (fermentation vat) may degrade some orally administered drugs. The increasingly acidic pH in the abomasum may alter the ratio of ionized to nonionized drug molecules, reducing an alkaline drug's ability to readily absorb across the abomasal wall.

Because of these factors, veterinary professionals must review the package insert and other drug information closely before administering drugs to a neonate or young animal. The veterinary professional must remember that a young animal often cannot tolerate the same dose that an adult can because of differences in neonatal drug absorption, distribution, or biotransformation.

Can a drug be forced to reach steady state quicker by giving a larger maintenance dose (e.g., giving 100 mg t.i.d. instead of 50 mg t.i.d.)? No, the rate at which the drug reaches steady state still depends on time as expressed by the half-life of elimination. The half-life for 100 mg of a drug will be the same for 50 mg of that same drug. A larger dose will still achieve steady state in the same amount of time, but the peak and trough concentrations at steady state will be higher.

DRUG WITHDRAWAL TIMES

The presence of chemical or drug residues in beef, pork, lamb, chicken, and fish used for human consumption is a growing public health concern. Because of this, all drugs approved for use in food animals have mandated withdrawal times. The withdrawal time is the time (usually expressed as days) after drug administration during which the animal cannot be sent to market for slaughter and the eggs or milk must be discarded. Withdrawal times are based on the elimination half-lives of drugs. However, because most half-lives are considered to be the half-life of drug concentrations in the blood, they may not necessarily reflect the elimination of the drug in the tissues. Thus some drug withdrawal times may be quite long if the drug is normally sequestered (taken up or stored) by tissues.

Withdrawal times cause additional expense to the food animal producer because the treated animal cannot be sent to market or the animal products (such as milk or eggs) cannot be sold. Therefore the producer must continue to pay to feed and house the animal until the withdrawal time has elapsed. For that reason, some producers will attempt to cut corners by sending the animals, milk, or eggs to market, hoping that the carcass or products will not be checked for antibiotic residues. The government imposes fines and penalties on producers who attempt to sneak meat, milk, or egg products into the food chain that are contaminated with drug residues. For example, if a dairy producer sends antibiotic-contaminated milk to market and that contaminated milk is mixed into a holding tank with milk from several dairies, that producer will be required to "purchase" the entire tank of contaminated milk. The bottom line is that although a producer might consider cheating on withdrawal times for economic reasons, the economic penalty and potential impact on society (e.g., development of antibiotic resistance) far outweigh any marginal cost savings.

Veterinary technicians play an important role in helping educate and reinforce the intent of withdrawal times so that food animal producers view regulations pertaining to withdrawal times as directly related to public health and not as arbitrary government interference.

USING CONCEPTS OF PHARMACOKINETICS AND PHARMACODYNAMICS

This chapter discussed the factors that influence movement of drugs into, through, and out of the body and how drugs interact with a receptor to produce a cellular effect. By remembering the leaky bucket analogy and the fact that the amount of drug entering the body must balance the amount of drug leaving the body, veterinary professionals should be able to understand how these factors affect the daily care and treatment of veterinary patients. As the principles underlying good veterinary care become more familiar, situations in which the normal dose of a drug may not be safe or effective for a particular patient will become more apparent. A vigilant veterinary technician can help the veterinarian prevent animal illness or death from inappropriate administration of a drug.

Box 3-1 The Difference Between an Acid Drug and an Alkaline Drug

An acid drug is a drug molecule that is capable of donating a hydrogen ion (H^+, or proton) to the environment and in so doing changes from being nonionized to being ionized. Once in ionized form, if the acid drug molecule acquires a hydrogen ion, it reverts back to its nonionized form. Whether an acid drug donates or accepts a hydrogen ion is based on the pH of the environment. In the following chemical equation the compounds shown act as acids. *C* denotes a carbon atom, *O* denotes an oxygen atom, *S* denotes a sulfur atom, and *R* denotes the remainder of the drug molecule. The double arrows indicate that the forms can move back and forth depending on the environmental pH.

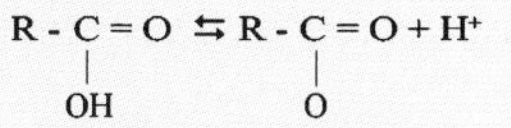

$$R - \underset{\underset{\text{OH}}{|}}{C} = O \quad \leftrightarrows \quad R - \underset{\underset{\text{O}}{|}}{C} = O + H^+$$

(nonionized form) (ionized form)

$$H_2SO_4 \quad \leftrightarrows \quad HSO_4^- + H^+$$
(nonionized form)   (ionized form)

The pH of a solution is a measurement of how many free H^+ ions are present in the solution. The more free H^+ ions, the lower the pH. Thus an acidic solution such as stomach acid contains many free H^+ ions. When an acid drug is placed into an acidic solution (low pH solution), the acid drug molecule tends to accept H^+ ions onto the drug molecule, shifting the drug molecule to the nonionized state. Therefore an acid drug placed in an acidic environment exists primarily in the nonionized (lipophilic) form.

In contrast to the acid drug molecule, when a molecule of an alkaline drug accepts or combines with a H^+ ion, it becomes ionized. As would be expected, when a molecule of an alkaline drug donates or loses a H^+ ion, it becomes nonionized again. Thus, in an environment that is rich with free H^+ ions (a low pH solution), alkaline drug molecules acquire H^+ ions and become ionized. This is illustrated below in the equation for an alkaline drug:

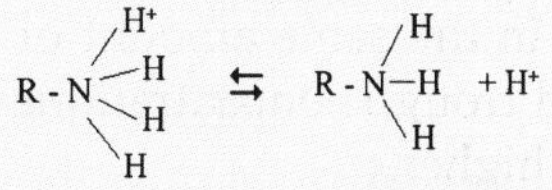

$$R - N \underset{\underset{\displaystyle H}{\diagdown}}{\overset{\overset{\displaystyle H^+}{\diagup}}{{-}H}} \quad \leftrightarrows \quad R - N \underset{\underset{\displaystyle H}{\diagdown}}{\overset{\overset{\displaystyle H}{\diagup}}{{-}H}} + H^+$$

Therefore the molecules of alkaline drugs placed in an acidic environment tend to become ionized, and more of the drug molecules are in the hydrophilic form. This is the opposite of what happens to a molecule of an acid drug.

Weak acids and *weak bases* are acidic or alkaline compounds that shift from a predominantly ionized form to a predominantly nonionized form (or vice versa) at pH ranges normally found within the body (referred to as physiologic pH). Weak acid drugs and weak base (alkaline) drugs may have their absorption characteristics altered when they enter body compartments with different pHs (e.g., stomach and duodenum). In contrast to weak acid and weak bases, the molecules of strong acids such as hydrochloric acid (HCl) or strong bases such as sodium hydroxide (NaOH) usually do not shift between ionized and nonionized forms at pH levels normally found within the body but remain primarily in one state.

RECOMMENDED READINGS

Boothe DM: *Small animal clinical pharmacology and therapeutics,* Philadelphia, 2001, WB Saunders.

Boothe DM: Principles of drug therapy for the practicing veterinarian. In Bonagura JD, editor: *Kirk's current veterinary therapy XII,* Philadelphia, 1995, WB Saunders.

Dowling PM: *Pharmacology and drug therapy: a cornerstone course.* In Proceedings of the Western Veterinary Conference, Las Vegas, NV, 2003.

Rowland M, Tozer TN: *Clinical pharmacokinetics: concepts and applications,* Philadelphia, 1995, Williams & Wilkins.

Trepanier L: *Avoiding adverse drug reactions.* In World Small Animal Veterinary Association World Congress Proceedings, Vancouver, Can, 2001.

Self-Assessment

REVIEW QUESTIONS

Fill in the following blanks with the correct item from the Key Terms list.

1. _____ hepatic effect in which some PO administered drugs do not make it to systemic circulation because they are removed by the liver.

2. _____ In a dosage regimen, the instructions "b.i.d." would be what component?

3. _____ movement of a drug molecule from an injection site to the systemic circulation.

4. _____ movement of a drug molecule into a compartment where it changes from a lipophilic state to a hydrophilic state and remains in that compartment.

5. _____ molecular process by which drugs move through fluid.

6. _____ form of a drug molecule that cannot readily penetrate a cell membrane.

7. _____ movement of drug molecules across a cellular membrane by using a carrier molecule and not requiring any energy expenditure by the cell.

8. _____ type of drug (not drug molecule form) that becomes more ionized as the environmental pH becomes more acidic.

9. _____ route of administration that typically reaches a peak almost as quickly as the IV route of administration.

10. _____ a smaller dose of a drug administered to keep drug concentrations in the therapeutic range after an initial, large dose of drug.

11. _____ movement of a drug from systemic circulation out of the body.

12. _____ movement of a drug from the blood into the brain would be an example of this movement of drugs in pharmacokinetics.

13. _____ where the first-pass effect occurs.

14. _____ conversion of a drug from active to inactive form by the liver.

15. _____ movement of drug from a tissue back to the blood and then to a second tissue.

16. _____ movement of drug from the intestinal tract, to the liver, to the blood and tissue, back to the liver, to the intestinal tract, and then reabsorbed back from the gastrointestinal tract to the liver.

17. _____ the point at which a t.i.d. administered drug achieves peak and trough concentrations that are the same from dose to dose.

18. _____ route of administration in which a drug is injected into the layers of the skin.

19. _____ a drug that combines with a receptor and causes a cell to produce a physiologic change.

20. The recommended total daily dose for a drug is 480 mg. What are the equivalent total daily doses for the following dosage intervals? From a practical point of view, which schedule provides the greatest chance for client compliance?

    _____ mg q12h   _____ mg q8h   _____ mg q4h

    _____ mg t.i.d.   _____ mg q24h   _____ mg q.i.d.

21. Which one of the following drugs is absorbed in the greatest amount?

    A. 100 mg of drug administered, bioavailability 0.7

    B. 150 mg of drug administered, bioavailability 0.5

    C. 200 mg of drug administered, bioavailability 0.4

    D. 250 mg of drug administered, bioavailability 0.2

22. Rank the following injection routes in order of the most superficial to the most deep: intramuscular, intradermal, subcutaneous.

23. If you were injecting a drug IP, in what body area would you inject it?

24. Drugs move through the body by a variety of mechanisms, including diffusion and active transport. Which mechanism of drug movement is described by each of the following scenarios?

    A. A local anesthetic injected subcutaneously produces a spreading feeling of numbness in the skin.

    B. Large drug molecules are taken up by macrophage scavenger cells in the alveoli of the lungs.

    C. The cells of the renal tubules accumulate concentrations of aminoglycoside antibiotic that greatly exceed drug concentrations in the plasma.

    D. A hydrophilic drug that moves down a concentration gradient into a cell.

25. Will ionized drug molecules dissolve more readily in water or fat? Which passes through membranes better: ionized molecules or nonionized molecules?

26. Which is the more acidic environment: a pH of 3 or a pH of 7?

27. Drug A is an acid drug. Is it more likely to be in the lipophilic or hydrophilic form when placed in a very acidic environment, such as the stomach?

28. Drug B exists in the ratios of nonionized molecules to ionized molecules at the following pH environments shown below:

    at a pH of 4, 1 nonionized molecule is present for every 100 ionized molecules

    at a pH of 5, 1 nonionized molecule is present for every 10 ionized molecules at a pH of 6, 1 nonionized molecule is present for every 1 ionized molecule

at a pH of 7, 10 nonionized molecules are present for every 1 ionized molecule

What is the pKa of drug B?

Based on how drug B reacts as the pH become more alkaline (basic) or acidic, determine if drug B is an acid drug or basic drug.

29. Indicate which of the following hypothetical drugs is most likely to have a predominance of drug molecules in the ionized form and which in the nonionized form.

    A. Acid drug   pKa of 3   Placed in a liquid with a pH of 6

    B. Acid drug   pKa of 2   Placed in a liquid with a pH of 9

    C. Acid drug   pKa of 5   Placed in a liquid with a pH of 2

    D. Acid drug   pKa of 7   Placed in a liquid with a pH of 5

    E. Acid drug   pKa of 7   Placed in a liquid with a pH of 7

    F. Alkaline drug   pKa of 6   Placed in a liquid with a pH of 9

    G. Alkaline drug   pKa of 9   Placed in a liquid with a pH of 8

    H. Alkaline drug   pKa of 5   Placed in a liquid with a pH of 2

    I. Alkaline drug   pKa of 5   Placed in a liquid with a pH of 8

30. Rank the following drugs in order from 1 to 4, with 1 being the most rapidly absorbed and 4 being the slowest to be absorbed from a subcutaneous tissue site with a pH of 7.4.

    _____ basic drug, pKa = 5.4

    _____ acid drug, pKa = 8.4

    _____ acid drug, pKa = 6.4

    _____ basic drug, pKa = 9.4

31. For each situation or condition below, state whether the dose should be *increased* or *decreased* to compensate for the condition and still achieve therapeutic concentrations in the body.

    A. the half-life for a drug is extended

    B. the metabolism of a drug has been accelerated by exposure to phenobarbital

    C. a hypoproteinemic animal is given a drug that is normally highly protein bound

    D. the volume of distribution for a drug is decreased

32. Answer the following questions by using the drug data listed below.

    Time after IV injection   Drug concentration (plasma)

       0 hr

       1 hr   160 μg/mL

2 hr	100 µg/mL
3 hr	_____
4 hr	_____
5 hr	40 µg/mL
6 hr	_____
7 hr	_____

A. What is the half-life?

B. What was the concentration at 4 hours?

C. What was the concentration at 7 hours?

D. What is the estimated peak concentration that occurred shortly after the IV bolus was given?

E. How long would it take multiple maintenance doses to reach a steady state for this drug?

33. Indicate whether the following statements are true or false.

A. If the metabolism of a drug has been induced, the dose of the drug should be decreased to compensate.

B. Excretion of a drug by the liver is called biliary excretion.

C. The neutralization of stomach acid by Tums or Rolaids is a non–receptor-mediated action.

D. An agonist would typically have little or no intrinsic activity on a receptor to which it binds.

E. If the Vd of a drug increases, the concentration of the drug decreases.

34. If a drug is in hydrophilic form when given subcutaneously, how is it able to enter the capillaries? Can it also exit the capillaries? Can it exit from all capillaries in the body?

APPLICATION QUESTIONS

1. The veterinarian asks you to administer four drugs. Each has a different route of administration. Drug A must be given PO, drug B must be given IV, drug C must be given SC, and drug D must be given IM. Assuming these drugs are given to normal animals, where should each of these drugs be administered, and which drug will reach its peak plasma concentration the fastest, second fastest, and slowest?

2. The veterinarian is reviewing a brochure for a new drug that says "Our drug reaches concentrations of 40 mg/mL within 2 hours of administration." The veterinarian comments that the drug concentration by itself does not indicate how effective the drug is. What is the reason for this comment, and what information is necessary to better assess the usefulness of this new drug?

3. A dosage regimen specifies 15 mg/kg IV for the loading dose followed by a maintenance dose of 5 mg/kg q12h PO. What is the advantage of using a loading dose?

4. Digoxin is a cardiac drug with a narrow therapeutic index. (Highest concentrations in the therapeutic range are close to the lowest effective concentrations.) Considering the plasma drug concentration curves for various routes of administration, why is IV administration not recommended for drugs with a narrow therapeutic range?

5. The veterinarian wants to lengthen the dosage interval from the 50 mg q6h PO being given now to 100 mg q12h PO. What will happen to the amount of swing between the peak (high) concentration and the trough (low) concentration when the interval is switched from q6h to q12h? Why might this be of concern?

6. A drug's package insert states that the drug can be given as an IV bolus or by IV infusion. What is the difference in these methods of administration? How do the systemic concentrations achieved differ?

7. A new drug's package insert has a caution statement that says "Do not give this drug extravascularly." What does this mean? How would you be able to tell if you had injected it extravascularly? What might be the hazard of giving such a drug extravascularly?

8. If a drug is given in aerosol form, where would you expect the largest drug concentration to be immediately after administration?

9. Why would an animal respond to injection of a drug directly into the carotid artery with severe central nervous system signs, whereas an IV injection of the same drug into the jugular vein in the same general area in the neck results in no adverse effects?

10. Why do facilitated diffusion and active transport have maximal rates at which they can transport drug molecules across a membrane and passive diffusion does not?

11. You are tired of fighting with a nasty stallion during his IM injections every 8 hours. Why not put the medication in a slurry and give it PO or sneak it into some sweet molasses for him to eat on his own?

12. Which would be more readily absorbed from the stomach (pH of 2 to 3): an acid drug or an alkaline drug, both with a similar pKa?

13. Aspirin causes stomach upset in people and animals a few hours after being taken PO because of the ion trapping phenomenon. Aspirin is an acidic drug. How does it get trapped and accumulate within cells lining the stomach lumen?

14. An animal has ingested a poison that is normally excreted by the kidneys. The poison is primarily an acid compound with a pKa of 6. To increase the rate of elimination of this drug, should the urine be acidified or alkalinized?

15. The manufacturer of an antibiotic claims that the enteric coating on the product enhances the drug's effectiveness compared with products without enteric coating. How might this be possible?

16. A cat with pylorospasm (contraction of the muscles surrounding the outflow tract from the stomach, which delays passage of stomach contents into the intestine) is given an alkaline

drug with a pKa of 6. What effect would pylorospasm have on the rate of drug absorption or the amount of drug absorbed?

17. Why would an orally administered antibiotic tablet not be well absorbed in an animal with diarrhea?

18. Why are some toxic materials not very toxic when ingested but are extremely lethal if accidentally injected?

19. Why are drugs injected subcutaneously absorbed more slowly on a cold day than on a hot day?

20. Diabetic animals are often overweight. Why should you be careful not to accidentally inject insulin (for control of diabetes mellitus) into the fat?

21. Why are many antibiotics effective for infections at other body sites often not effective against bacterial infections involving the brain?

22. You inject an appropriate dose of thiopental IV into a thin dog and the animal stops breathing, reacting as though it received an overdose. The veterinarian looks over your shoulder and says, "Don't worry, the redistribution will take care of it." What is the significance of that comment?

23. A very thin dog with chronic liver disease has low plasma protein levels. The dog requires treatment with a drug that is highly protein bound. Considering the dog's poor body condition and low plasma protein levels, should the standard drug dose be increased or decreased?

24. Which drug would probably better penetrate tissues: drug A, with a Vd of 1 L, or drug B, with a Vd of 3 L? If equal amounts of drug A and drug B were given to an animal, which would be present in greater concentrations in the plasma?

25. Digoxin is a cardiac drug with an apparent volume of distribution that seems to exceed the total volume of water possible within an animal's body. For example, in an animal with a body water volume of 3 L, the volume of distribution for digoxin may be 4 L. How is this possible? (Remember that digoxin selectively binds to sites in skeletal and cardiac muscle in high concentrations.)

26. In an animal with an increased volume of distribution as a result of ascites, would systemic drug concentrations resulting from a standard dose likely be higher or lower than normal?

27. A dog is hospitalized because of insecticide poisoning. The veterinarian is concerned and says, "We can't use an antidote to reverse the effect because the insecticide is a noncompetitive agonist." What is the significance of that comment?

28. What effect would a partial narcotic agonist/partial narcotic antagonist such as butorphanol have on an animal if it was given after administration of a strong narcotic such as hydromorphone? How would this effect be different than that of a true narcotic antagonist such as naloxone?

29. How can a chelating drug produce its physiologic effect when placed in a cell-free test tube of serum or within the lumen of the intestine where no cells, and hence no cellular receptors, are present for the drug to attach to?

30. Why must veterinary professionals be concerned about using hepatically biotransformed drugs in young animals and cats? Should they have similar concerns about administering drugs that are excreted unchanged through the kidneys?

31. A dog is being treated with phenobarbital to control epileptic seizures. Why must the dosage be adjusted 2 to 3 weeks after therapy begins? Is the dose likely to be increased or decreased at that time and why?

32. What effect would decreased renal perfusion have on blood concentrations of a drug excreted through the kidneys?

33. A particular dose of penicillin is quite effective against a specific bacterium when it is found in the urine. When the same bacterial strain is found in other tissues in the body, however, the same dose of penicillin is not nearly as effective. Based on what you know about penicillin from this chapter and how it is eliminated, explain why this could occur.

34. An animal has ingested a poison, and the veterinarian gives it activated charcoal repeatedly for several hours by a stomach tube because of enterohepatic circulation. Why must the charcoal be given repeatedly rather than only once or twice?

35. The veterinarian comments, "These fluids will increase drug clearance." What is the significance of that comment?

36. Why is a loading dose more necessary with a drug that has a long half-life than with a drug that has a short half-life?

37. Which food animal drug would require a longer withdrawal time: drug A, with a half-life of 30 minutes, or drug B, with a half-life of 5 hours?

Chapter 4

Drugs Affecting the Gastrointestinal Tract

outline

key terms

acetylcholine

adsorbents

alpha (α) adrenergic receptors

anticholinergic drugs

bloat (ruminal tympany)

centrally or locally acting emetics

chemoreceptor trigger zone (CRTZ)

chief cells

colonic

dopamine receptors

emetic

emetic center

enterotoxins

eructation

fermentative digestion

G cells

gastric

gastric glands

gastrin

gastritis

histamine

monogastric

mucins

mucous cells

narcotic (opioid) drugs

norepinephrine

parasympathetic nervous system

parietal cells (oxyntic cells)

prokinetic drugs

prostaglandins

protectants

ruminant

rumination

serotonin antagonists

serotonin receptors

sympathetic nervous system

tenesmus

vagus nerve

vestibular apparatus

objectives

objectives

After studying this chapter, the veterinary technician should be able to explain:

1. The basic physiology that controls the gastrointestinal tract

2. The mechanisms by which vomiting occurs and how drugs can modify it

3. The mechanisms by which gastrointestinal motility occurs and how drugs can modify it

4. The factors that increase the risk for gastrointestinal ulcers and how drugs may control them

5. How drugs modify the function of the ruminant gastrointestinal tract

Problems with the gastrointestinal (GI) tract of animals are a common occurrence in clinical veterinary medicine. Disease may directly or indirectly affect the GI tract, resulting in vomiting, colic (abdominal pain), bloat, diarrhea, and constipation. Although many of these functions are meant to be protective of the animal, when they occur in excess, therapeutic intervention is indicated. In addition to understanding how physiology of the GI tract is altered by prescription medications used to treat signs of GI disease, veterinary technicians should be aware of the potential for many over-the-counter (OTC) GI drugs to produce adverse effects in the veterinary patient. A listing of important GI drugs used in veterinary medicine can be found in Box 4-1.

FUNCTION AND CONTROL OF THE GASTROINTESTINAL TRACT

The diversity of anatomic differences among species is more pronounced with the GI tract than with any other organ system. Although the GI tracts of various domestic species appear different, they have many similarities in function and control. Functionally, the *monogastric* (single stomach) animal has three segments of GI tract: the stomach, intestines, and cecum and colon. Functions or diseases related to the stomach are identified with the adjective *gastric* (e.g., gastric ulcers, gastric blood flow, gastric emptying), those related to the duodenum, jejunum, or ileum are usually referred to as enteric, and those related to the colon are referred to as *colonic.*

Ruminants have a more elaborate "stomach" configuration than the monogastrics. The rumen, reticulum, and omasum constitute the forestomach, and the abomasum represents the "true" stomach similar to the monogastric stomach (Figure 4-1). These compartments physically break down and process the ruminant's herbivorous (plant) diet by a process known as *fermentative digestion.* Generally, the reticulum and rumen work together to receive and mix swallowed food. Coarse materials are regurgitated from the rumen back into the mouth for further mastication before being reswallowed in a process called *rumination* or "chewing cud." The rumen also acts as a large fermentation vat containing microbes (bacteria and single-celled protozoa) that produce enzymes of fermentative digestion to chemically break down foods into smaller components. The complex balance among food materials, the microbes of the rumen, and the products of fermentation can be easily upset by disease, requiring therapeutic intervention. Finally, the omasum and abomasum are concerned primarily with further mixing, some digestion, and absorption.

In addition to the monogastrics and ruminants, animals such as horses are classified as nonruminant herbivores, meaning they consume a plant diet but do not have rumens, as do cattle and sheep. The nonruminant herbivores have digestive enzymes secreted by glands as with the monogastrics, but they also have fermentative digestion by microbes located in the expanded colon and cecum. The increased size and complexity of the equine colon and cecum

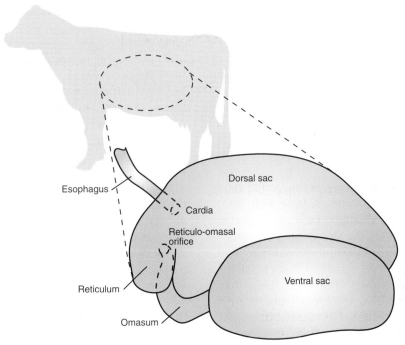

Figure 4-1 Anatomy of the ruminant GI tract. (From Colville T, Bassert JA: *Clinical anatomy & physiology for veterinary technicians*, St. Louis, 2002, Mosby, p. 242.)

contribute to colic problems that often require medical or surgical intervention.

AUTONOMIC NERVOUS SYSTEM CONTROL

The movement and release of secretions in the GI tract in all species are controlled by interactions among the nervous system, the endocrine system, and a variety of other compounds released by cells and intestinal microbes. The nervous system regulates GI function by the autonomic nervous system and local reflexes within the intestinal tract wall. The autonomic nervous system is the component of the nervous system that regulates bodily functions without conscious thought (e.g., digesting food does not require conscious effort). The autonomic nervous system is functionally divided into two opposing components, the *parasympathetic nervous system* and the *sympathetic nervous system*. The parasympathetic nervous system includes nerves that emerge from the central

nervous system (CNS) as cranial nerves and nerves in the caudal portion of the spinal cord. Parasympathetic nerves include the widely distributed *vagus nerve* (*vagus*, meaning vagabond or wandering), and parasympathetic effects are typically associated with the neurotransmitter *acetylcholine*. Stimulation of the parasympathetic nervous system, stimulation of the vagus nerve, and the use of drugs that mimic acetylcholine decrease heart rate, constrict the pupils, increase digestive secretions, improve blood flow to the GI tract, and increase gut (GI) smooth muscle tone and motility. The net effect of parasympathetic nervous system on the GI tract is increased digestion and absorption. Because digestion replaces bodily stores of nutrients that are normally lost or used up, the parasympathetic nervous system is sometimes referred to as the "rest and restore" system.

The sympathetic nervous system antagonizes or opposes the effects of the parasympathetic nervous system. At any given time the body is under the influence of both systems, with the observed net effect being a reflection of which system dominates at that moment. *Norepinephrine* is the neurotransmitter associated with the sympathetic effect. Sympathetic nervous system nerves emerge from the spinal cord at the thoracic and lumbar segments of the spinal column, where they synapse with a chain of ganglia (cluster of neuron cell bodies) that parallel the spinal cord before traveling to the rest of the body. The stimulation of the sympathetic nervous system or the use of drugs that emulate norepinephrine's effect results in increased heart rate, elevated blood pressure, and redirected blood flow from nonessential to essential organs and skeletal muscle. These responses allow an animal to fight or flee from a threatening situation. Hence, the sympathetic nervous system is known as the "fight or flight" system. Sympathetic nervous system stimulation of the GI tract results in decreased perfusion of the intestinal tract, reducing absorption of digested food, decreasing gastric (stomach) and enteric (small intestine) motility, and decreasing secretion of digestive juices. Therefore the net effect of sympathetic nervous system on the GI tract is decreased digestion and absorption of substances.

BIOLOGIC MEDIATORS OF GASTROINTESTINAL FUNCTION

Although the autonomic nervous system regulates the overall activity of the GI tract, a wide variety of locally acting hormones and other biologically active compounds also regulate GI motility and secretions. *Prostaglandins* are a group of compounds produced by many different tissues in the body to exert changes within the immediate area in which they are released. In the GI tract, the presence of prostaglandins E (PgE) and I (PgI) increases intestinal mucus and fluid production, decreases gastric hydrochloric acid production, increases intestinal motility, improves blood flow to areas in which prostaglandins are active, and

increases secretion of bicarbonate buffers in the mucus layer that protect the stomach from gastric acid. Drugs that mimic the effect of this class of prostaglandins also mimic these beneficial effects. Because other prostaglandins are involved in inflammation, antiinflammatory drugs that block prostaglandins in general also block these GI protective mechanisms (see Chapter 13).

Histamine is another biologic compound that affects GI tract function. Histamine is normally released by basophils and mast cells throughout the body during inflammation or allergic reactions. The released histamine diffuses through local tissue or is released into the blood from histamine-producing tumors (e.g., mast cell tumors) and produces cellular effects on those cells with histamine (H) receptors. Although most clinically observed responses to histamine are associated with H_1 receptors in the respiratory tract and skin, the stomach also contains histamine receptors in the form of H_2 receptors. These H_2 receptors, which are slightly different in structure from the H_1 receptors, are located on *parietal cells* (also called *oxyntic cells*) that produce hydrochloric acid in the stomach. Stimulation of H_2 receptors results in additional secretions of hydrochloric acid and increased gastric acidity (Figure 4-2). Overstimulation of H_2 receptors, such as occurs with the release of histamine from mast cell tumors, can produce a hyperacidity syndrome resulting in gastric or duodenal ulcers.

In addition to H_2 receptors, oxyntic cells also contain receptors for the parasympathetic system neurotransmitter acetylcholine and the hormone *gastrin*. Drugs that mimic acetylcholine or are capable of stimulating acetylcholine receptors on the parietal cells increase stomach acidity. Gastrin is a hormone normally released from the stomach wall in response to the presence of proteins in the stomach, distension of the stomach, or increased stimulation by the parasympathetic nervous system. The function of gastrin is normally to signal relaxation of the stomach (so more food can be stored) and, by

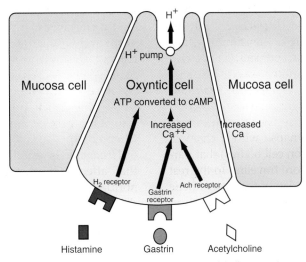

Figure 4-2 Parietal cell (oxyntic cell) with histamine (H$_2$), gastrin (G), and acetylcholine receptors.

stimulation of receptors on the parietal cell, to increase acid production in response to the presence of food. The acid-producing effect of gastrin and acetylcholine is enhanced by histamine.

Bacterial toxins, released by some types of bacteria in the intestinal tract, can stimulate secretion of electrolytes (sodium, chloride), which in turn osmotically draw fluids from intestinal cells, resulting in profuse diarrhea and dehydration. *Salmonella enteritis, Escherichia coli, Staphylococcus* spp., and other enteric bacteria often produce characteristic intestinal signs through this type of mechanism.

Many other biologically active compounds play a role in GI motility and secretion. However, for the veterinary technician, understanding these few will provide a manageable starting point for understanding the mechanisms behind GI therapeutics.

EMETIC DRUGS

Emesis (vomiting) is a normal, protective mechanism designed to remove substances the body perceives as toxic. An *emetic* is a drug that produces vomiting with the intent of removing an ingested toxic substance before it can be absorbed by the body. Because emetics are often used as emergency life-saving procedures, emetics must be consistently reliable and rapid acting.

VOMITING REFLEX

The complex, coordinated process of emesis is controlled by a group of neurons in the medulla of the brainstem, known as the vomiting center, or *emetic center* (Figure 4-3). The vomiting reflex may be triggered by input from five types of stimuli:

- Direct stimulation of neurons in the emetic center
- Direct stimulation of the *chemoreceptor trigger zone (CRTZ)*, located near the emetic center in the medulla
- Distension or irritation of the pharynx, stomach, duodenum, small intestine, peritoneum (as in peritonitis), kidney, gallbladder, or uterus
- Stimulation of nerves of the inner ear involved with balance (motion sickness)
- Stimulation of higher centers of the brain by emotional stimuli or intracranial trauma and swelling

The emetic center coordinates the muscle groups and autonomic functions that produce vomiting (in species capable of vomiting). The

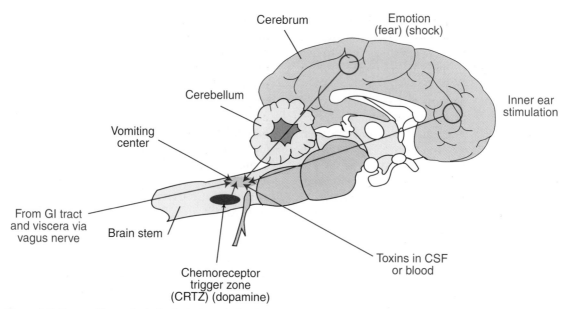

Figure 4-3 The vomiting center in the brainstem receives impulses from the chemoreceptor trigger zone, GI tract, and cerebrum.

neurons of the vomiting center have *alpha (α) adrenergic receptors,* which are a type of sympathetic nervous system receptor, and *serotonin receptors.* Drugs or toxins that stimulate these emetic center receptors evoke the vomiting reflex, whereas drugs that block these receptors reduce the emetic response. Cats seem to be especially sensitive to sympathetic nervous system stimulation of the α receptors and vomit from stimulation of the emetic center induced by natural stress or administration of drugs that stimulate the α receptors.

The CRTZ is a specialized area of receptors in the CNS that is capable of detecting toxic substances in the blood and cerebrospinal fluid (CSF). Unlike the emetic center, which is located within the CNS and therefore protected from the blood by the blood-brain barrier, the CRTZ has free nerve endings in direct contact with the cerebrospinal fluid and blood. Therefore vomiting associated with metabolic toxins from renal failure, excessive ketones associated with diabetes mellitus, bacterial toxemia (bacterial toxins in the blood), digoxin, narcotic analgesics, blood-borne ingested poisons, or some

emetic drugs work by stimulating these free nerve endings associated with the CRTZ. Sensitivity of the CRTZ to different drugs or chemicals varies among species and explains the reason some drugs produce emesis in one species but not another. For example, because the CRTZ of dogs contains more *dopamine receptors* than the CRTZ of cats, drugs or toxins that normally stimulate dopamine receptors, or drugs that normally stimulate release of dopamine more readily, produce emesis in dogs more often than cats. Conversely, dopaminergic antagonists, or antidopaminergic drugs, tend to decrease vomiting in dogs but have much less antiemetic effect in cats.

The CRTZ of dogs also contains more H_1 receptors than the CRTZ of cats. This correlates with histamine being a more potent emetic agent in dogs than it is in cats. In contrast, the CRTZ of cats is much more sensitive to drugs that stimulate α_2 receptors, which explains why α_2 sedative agonists such as xylazine (Rompun), and to a lesser extent detomidine and medetomidine, produce a strong emetic effect in cats and a much lesser emetic effect in dogs. Because of these differences in CRTZ sensitivity, dogs and cats often require different antiemetic drugs to counteract toxins or compounds that have stimulated vomiting through the CRTZ.

More recent evidence has shown that serotonin receptors (also called 5-hydroxytryptamine or 5-HT receptors) play an important role in vomiting through the CRTZ. In human medicine *serotonin antagonists* have been used to prevent vomiting associated with cancer chemotherapy. In veterinary medicine antiserotonin drugs have been used to decrease vomiting associated with nonresponsive vomiting from cancer chemotherapy or severe viral infections of the intestinal tract (parvovirus). 5-HT serotonin receptors may also be located in the GI tract itself and may help explain some of this drug's effectiveness in reducing vomiting associated with parvoviral enteritis.

The *vestibular apparatus* in the inner ear is the organ responsible for balance. Overstimulation of the sense organs in the vestibular apparatus is the source of vomiting associated with motion sickness and inner ear infections. The eighth cranial nerve (CN VIII—vestibulocochlear nerve) carries nerve impulses from the vestibular apparatus to the CRTZ and then onto the emetic center. Histamine (H_1) receptors appear to play an important role in stimulating vomiting from inner ear stimuli. Again, because of species' differences in the pathways from the vestibular apparatus to the emetic center and differences in types of receptors, drugs that control motion sickness in cats may not be as effective in dogs, and vice versa.

Inflammation or overdistension of abdominal organs, inflammation of the peritoneum, or stimulation of the pharynx can result in vomiting. When the GI tract becomes irritated by viral or bacterial infection, a foreign body, overdistension, or chemicals, impulses travel by the vagus nerve (a parasympathetic nerve) to the emetic center, where the vomiting reflex is initiated. The ninth cranial nerve transmits the stimulus for the vomiting reflex from the pharynx.

In human beings, vomiting can result from overstimulation of the cerebral cortex (a higher brain center) or the limbic system (the part of the brain involved with emotion) under circumstances of emotional shock, such as viewing surgery for the first time or experiencing an intense emotional situation. To what extent higher brain centers or the limbic system initiates vomiting in animals is uncertain, although some animals tend to vomit when stressed or excited, possibly as a result of release of sympathetic neurotransmitters and stimulation of receptors in the CRTZ and emetic center.

INDUCTION OF VOMITING

Emetics are most often used to induce vomiting in animals that have ingested toxic substances. They should not be used in all cases of ingested poisoning, however. In some situations, the risk of aspiration (inhalation) of vomited stomach contents into the lungs and subsequent death from aspiration pneumonia may outweigh the potential benefit of induced vomiting. In situations in which the aspiration risk is high, the veterinarian has to weigh whether the animal is more likely to die from the aspiration or from the ingested poison, and then act according to his or her clinical assessment and judgment.

Vomiting should not be induced if a corrosive substance such as alkali cleaning agents, acids, or oxalate products have been ingested. Corrosive substances will burn tissue and can extensively damage the oral and esophageal mucosa. The damaged esophagus may actually rupture or become perforated (form a hole through the wall), resulting in leakage of esophageal contents through the esophagus. Generally, if burns on the oral mucosa are observed in an animal that has ingested an unknown substance, the ingested compound should be assumed to be corrosive unless proven otherwise.

Emesis should not be induced in animals that have ingested volatile (easily evaporated) liquids such as gasoline, light petroleum products, and most oils. Because volatile liquids such as gasoline do not stimulate the normal gag reflexes, they are more readily aspirated into the lungs during vomiting. These compounds are highly irritating when introduced into the respiratory tree and quickly cause pulmonary edema.

The veterinary professional should not induce emesis in an animal that is comatose, extremely depressed, unconscious, or lacking a functional gag reflex because of the increased risk for aspiration of stomach contents. If a vomiting animal has to be heavily sedated, or an animal is semiconscious at the time of emesis induction, a cuffed endotracheal tube should be placed to reduce the risk of aspiration pneumonia. It is important to remember that even an inflated cuff on the endotracheal tube may not completely prevent aspiration of vomited stomach contents.

Induction of emesis in animals anesthetized or sedated with barbiturates, acepromazine, or other CNS depressant drugs is more difficult because these drugs suppress CNS activity, including activity of the emetic center in the brainstem. If an emetic has to be given to a sedated or anesthetized animal, the animal must be closely monitored for excessive or protracted vomiting as the anesthetic/sedative wears off because suppression of the emetic center will be lessened with the decreasing concentrations of the sedative in the circulation.

The veterinary professional should not induce emesis in an animal that is convulsing or showing preictal (preseizure) signs. This is especially true for poisons such as strychnine that cause full, tetanic seizures with almost any type of stimulation. The act of vomiting will often cause these animals to have full-blown seizures with the associated risk of aspiration.

Emesis should not be induced in an animal with bloat, gastric torsion, or esophageal damage because the weakened stomach or esophageal wall can perforate or rupture during vomiting. Finally, emesis should not be attempted in horses, rabbits, or many rodent species because these species either cannot

vomit or the act of vomiting may result in complications such as rupture of the stomach.

Timing of administration of the emetic is also important. If the emetic is administered too late, the poison may have moved out of the stomach and beyond the proximal duodenum. At that point, vomiting will not remove the poison and the risk for aspiration would outweigh the potential benefit from emesis. Most liquid toxins pass beyond this area or are absorbed into the systemic circulation within 2 hours of ingestion. Solid poisons, such as rat bait blocks and pelleted rodenticides, may still be in the stomach up to 4 hours after ingestion depending on the speed of gastric emptying.

Although the following statement should be obvious, in the haste to "do something" vomiting is often unnecessarily induced. If an animal has vomited several times after ingestion of a toxic material, the body has already removed as much as it can and additional emesis from an emetic drug is unlikely to produce any significant additional benefit. Therefore, the risk of aspiration would far outweigh the potential for benefit from additional emesis.

CENTRALLY ACTING EMETICS

Emetics are divided into two general categories: *centrally acting emetics* and *locally acting emetics*. Centrally acting emetics include drugs such as apomorphine and α_2 agonists such as xylazine. Apomorphine is an opioid (opium-like narcotic drug related to morphine) that directly stimulates dopamine receptors in the CRTZ to produce emesis. When given by intravenous or intramuscular injection, apomorphine quickly causes dopamine stimulation and emesis in dogs. Because cats have fewer dopamine receptors, apomorphine is a less effective emetic in cats.

Apomorphine is most readily available as a tablet. However, it is not consistently effective as an orally administered emetic. Although apomorphine stimulates the CRTZ, as an opioid it depresses the CNS overall, including the emetic center in the medulla. For apomorphine to work, it must stimulate the CRTZ before it depresses the emetic center. Apomorphine induces emesis if it rapidly achieves high blood concentrations. This is critical because the CRTZ has receptors in contact with the blood, whereas the emetic center, as part of the CNS, is behind the blood-brain barrier. Apomorphine in the blood will take some time to diffuse across the barrier to reach the emetic center and depress its function. Thus, if apomorphine achieves high blood concentrations quickly, the CRTZ can be stimulated to produce emesis before apomorphine exerts its depressant effect on the emetic center itself.

A slow rise in blood concentrations, such as would be observed with oral administration of apomorphine tablets, means that more time is available for apomorphine to diffuse across the blood-brain barrier and depress the emetic center before blood levels increase enough to stimulate the CRTZ. Although emesis is possible within 2 to 10 minutes after administration of apomorphine tablets, it is much less reliable than other routes of administration. If the first dose of orally administered apomorphine fails to produce emesis, subsequent doses are not likely to be any more effective because of previous emetic center depression from the first dose.

Intravenous or intramuscular injection of apomorphine rapidly establishes required concentrations in the blood to stimulate the CRTZ. Another method of apomorphine administration consists of placing the apomorphine tablet directly into the conjunctival sac of the dog's eye. The apomorphine tablet dissolves quickly and is rapidly absorbed through the mucous membranes of the conjunctiva to produce vomiting. After the desired effect is achieved, the tablet is removed and the remaining residue is flushed from the eye to prevent further absorption. This method of inducing emesis is advocated by some trainers of drug-sniffing dogs who, in their excitement at finding a "stash," sometimes ingest the contraband they find.

Because apomorphine is an opioid and depresses the CNS, it has the side effect of producing respiratory depression. Therefore apomorphine should not be given to animals that already have some degree of respiratory depression (e.g., breathing muscle paralysis, depression of respiratory center from poison). Although the respiratory depressant effects of apomorphine can be reversed with a narcotic antagonist such as naloxone, its emetic effects, which are mediated by dopamine receptors, are not affected by naloxone. Prolonged vomiting from apomorphine can be antagonized by dopaminergic antagonists such as phenothiazine tranquilizers (e.g., acepromazine, droperidol). As previously mentioned, if an animal is tranquilized with a drug such as acepromazine, subsequent administration of apomorphine will not produce the desired rapid and complete vomiting because the dopaminergic receptors on which apomorphine works are blocked by the acepromazine.

Another effective centrally acting emetic for cats is xylazine (e.g., Rompun, Anased, Sedazine). This commonly available sedative and anesthetic agent stimulates α_2 receptors in both the CRTZ and the emetic center in cats, producing emesis within minutes of injection. This emetic effect can be reversed by using α_2 antagonists such as yohimbine (Yobine). The dose used to induce emesis in cats (0.05 mg/kg) is generally lower than the dose used for sedation or preanesthesia. Xylazine produces emesis in dogs but at a much lower rate than in cats. Some sources state that xylazine administration will produce emesis in 50% of the dogs to which it is given compared with 90% of cats that will vomit with the drug.

LOCALLY ACTING EMETICS

Locally acting emetics typically produce their effect by irritating the GI tract, distending the stomach, and causing parasympathetic stimulation of the emetic center. The most commonly used locally acting emetic has historically been syrup of ipecac. Unfortunately, syrup of ipecac was pulled from the market in 2004 because of abuse from people with bulimia, anorexia, or compulsive eating syndromes. In addition, a study in a prominent pediatric journal indicated that use of syrup of ipecac at home did not reduce the need for subsequent emergency treatment.[1] This was followed by a position statement from the American Association of Pediatrics that recommended parents no longer keep syrup of ipecac in the house. These factors likely led to the withdrawal of this product in the United States.

Other locally acting emetics such as hydrogen peroxide, warm concentrated salt water solution, or a solution of powdered mustard and water may induce emesis, but these emetics do not work consistently and have some drawbacks. The use of hydrogen peroxide can result in a severe *gastritis* (inflammation of the stomach) because of the effect of the peroxide on the lining of the stomach. In cats, the response with hydrogen peroxide is quite variable, and many veterinarians state it does not work. The subsequent froth released from the hydrogen peroxide also increases the risk for aspiration. To enhance the emesis from hydrogen peroxide, the peroxide should be "fresh" (it loses its ability to fizz after a few months), the animal should be given a few pieces of dog food or bread to add bulk to the vomitus, and the use of hydrogen peroxide should be limited to ½ to 1 mL/lb with a maximum of 45 mL and no more than two doses used in a 15-minute period.

The administration of a concentrated salt solution may produce vomiting if it sufficiently stimulates the pharyngeal region of the throat. Placing a small amount plain table salt directly in the pharyngeal region may also produce this effect. If a salt solution is administered, the animal should be given water or intravenous fluids to reduce the risk of salt toxicity or dehydration. Some toxicologists state flatly that salt should not be given because of the risk of salt toxicosis producing tremors and seizures.[2] Inducing vomiting by forcing a finger to the back of an animal's throat usually results in a struggle and bitten fingers but seldom any vomiting because of the lessened sensitivity to inducing gagging in the parts of the animal's mouth and oral pharynx easily reached by the fingers.

ANTIEMETIC DRUGS

Antiemetic drugs prevent or decrease vomiting. The veterinary professional must remember that vomiting and diarrhea are naturally protective mechanisms that remove irritating or toxic substances from the intestinal tract. Prevention of vomiting by use of antiemetics may allow the offending substance to remain in the GI tract longer or may mask clinical signs that would help determine disease progression and recovery. Therefore antiemetics should only be used when the vomiting reflex is no longer beneficial to the animal.

Phenothiazine tranquilizers such as acepromazine and, to a lesser extent, chlorpromazine and prochlorperazine (human drug Compazine) are used to control vomiting caused by motion sickness. Some veterinary gastroenterologists also advocate chlorpromazine for controlling vomiting associated with acute gastroenteritis (inflammation of the stomach and intestines).

As mentioned previously, phenothiazine drugs block dopamine receptors in the CRTZ and the emetic center, thereby reducing vomiting. These drugs also have an antihistamine effect, which aids in prevention or control of the histamine-mediated motion sickness in dogs. Although phenothiazine drugs do have some anticholinergic activity (i.e., they block activity of the acetylcholine neurotransmitter effect of the parasympathetic nervous system), this antiemetic effect is not very potent and thus does not normally prevent vomiting caused by parasympathetic impulses entering the vomiting center from GI, peritoneal, pharyngeal, or other visceral stimulation. However, at higher doses phenothiazines may decrease some vomiting caused by stimulation of the parasympathetic nervous system.

Phenothiazine drugs have an α-adrenergic receptor antagonist activity and therefore block any attempt by the body to cause vasoconstriction by stimulation of α_1 receptors on the peripheral blood vessels. Vasoconstriction by stimulation of α_1 receptors is a compensatory mechanism by which the sympathetic nervous system attempts to maintain normal blood pressure after blood loss, during shock, or as the result of dehydration. For this reason, animals that are hypotensive (have low blood pressure) from any cause should have the hypotensive state corrected before phenothiazine antiemetic therapy is initiated. The role of α receptors in the regulation of blood pressure is discussed in greater detail in Chapter 5.

In normal animals phenothiazine drugs produce little tranquilization at the doses usually used for antiemetic effect. However, in depressed animals or those that have received other CNS depressant drugs, a tranquilizing effect may be evident. Seemingly in contrast to the CNS depressant effect, phenothiazine drugs lower the threshold for the onset of seizure activity in animals prone to seizures (e.g., epileptics) or those that have ingested seizure-producing toxins (e.g., strychnine, lead, organophosphate insecticides). This means that those animals already prone to seizure activity can have an increase in frequency or duration of seizures if given acepromazine or chlorpromazine. Normal animals are not likely to exhibit seizure activity.

Two drugs related to phenothiazine tranquilizers are droperidol and haloperidol. These powerful tranquilizers are seldom used by themselves in veterinary medicine for control of vomiting because of the side effects of hypotension and sedation. Additional effects of acepromazine are discussed in Chapter 8.

Antihistamines are the main ingredient in drugs used to control motion sickness in human beings. Veterinarians occasionally use dimenhydrinate (Dramamine) and diphenhydramine (Benadryl) to prevent motion sickness in animals. These drugs decrease impulses sent from the vestibular apparatus to the emetic center during continuous motion by blocking the H_1 receptors in the CRTZ. As previously mentioned, the larger number of H_1 receptors on the CRTZ in the dog makes the canine more responsive to the blocking effects of antihistamine than the cat. As with phenothiazine drugs, antihistamines are less effective in blocking the vomiting stimulus caused by intestinal vagus nerve stimulation (parasympathetic nervous system stimulation) and so are not very effective in blocking vomiting associated with gastroenteritis.

Antihistamines have a sedative effect on animals, similar to that observed in human beings, and thus may adversely affect the performance of working animals. These drugs can also decrease the wheal and flare reaction used to gauge the body's reaction to antigens in intradermal allergy testing. Antihistamines should not be used for at least 4 days before allergy testing.

As previously mentioned, *anticholinergic drugs* block the effect of the acetylcholine neurotransmitter. Because acetylcholine is associated with the effects caused by the parasympathetic nervous system, anticholinergic drugs are usually thought of as antiparasympathetic nervous system drugs. Anticholinergic drugs theoretically prevent vomiting by blocking the parasympathetic impulses traveling to the CNS by way of the vagus nerve and decrease the motor impulses traveling to the muscles involved with the vomiting reflex by the vagus nerve. Anticholinergic drugs also decrease secretions by the intestinal tract and overall gut motility. Anticholinergic drugs include atropine, aminopentamide (Centrine), isopropamide, and hyoscine (scopolamine; Donnatal as a human product).

Anticholinergic drugs usually do not completely block the vomiting response and may actually increase vomiting associated with gastric atony (lack of tone) or decreased intestinal motility. Many veterinarians still use anticholinergics as antiemetics, but many gastroenterologists do not recommend anticholinergics except for vomiting associated with irritable bowel syndrome or excessive stimulation of the parasympathetic nervous system. Some debate continues regarding their effectiveness, and the veterinary technician will likely find proponents for both sides of the argument represented within a practice.

Metoclopramide (Reglan) is a centrally acting antiemetic that also has local antiemetic activity. Its centrally acting effect is through blocking the dopamine and serotonin receptors on the CRTZ. Because dogs have more dopamine receptors on the CRTZ than do cats, this centrally acting effect of metoclopramide is more effective with canines. Metoclopramide is used to decrease vomiting caused by cancer chemotherapeutic agents.

Metoclopramide is considered a *prokinetic drug,* meaning that it increases GI motility. The prokinetic activities of increasing lower esophageal muscle tone, relaxing the pyloric outflow tract of the stomach, increasing gastric motility without increasing secretions, and increasing motility of the duodenum and jejunum all help decrease vomiting syndromes associated with gastric stasis (decreased or cessation of stomach contractions).

In addition to decreasing vomiting from chemotherapeutic agents and other blood-borne vomiting stimulants, metoclopramide has also been useful for intermittent vomiting of bile and mucus in otherwise healthy dogs. This syndrome is seldom enough of a problem to warrant a specific trip to the veterinarian because the animal has a good appetite and feels well otherwise. However, it is annoying to the pet owner because the yellow bile pigments stain fabric and carpeting. The cause of the vomiting is thought to be a reflux (reverse flow) of bile from the duodenum back into the stomach. Bile is irritating to the stomach and produces the subsequent vomiting. Because metoclopramide enhances gastric movement in the correct direction and reduces reflux, a dose of metoclopramide given to these dogs in the evening usually helps correct this situation.

Metoclopramide has other CNS effects in addition to its antiemetic effect. Like phenothiazine tranquilizers, it can produce sedation and should not be used in conjunction with phenothiazine tranquilizers because of the potential for an added sedative effect. Occasionally, cats given a dose of metoclopramide show frenzied behavior. Because metoclopramide relies on acetylcholine for gastric muscle contraction and much of its local antiemetic activity, use of anticholinergics such as atropine or narcotic analgesics can negate the local antiemetic effect.

Cisapride (Propulsid) is a prokinetic drug similar to metoclopramide but without its centrally acting, dopamine-blocking antiemetic effects. It does have serotonin antagonistic effects. The prokinetic activity of cisapride has been especially helpful in increasing smooth muscle tone in cats with a dilated colon condition called megacolon. Cisapride was taken off the market in the United States in 2000 because of incidents of fatal arrhythmias in people taking the drug with certain antibiotics, but it is available for veterinarians through compounding pharmacies. Similar cardiac problems in veterinary patients have not been observed.

The newest class of antiemetics to make its way from the human field to the veterinary field is the serotonin antagonists, also called the 5-HT receptor antagonists. As previously mentioned, stimulation of 5-HT receptors on the CRTZ can produce vomiting. This is the common mechanism for vomiting from chemotherapy in human beings. Ondansetron (Zofran) has been advocated by some veterinary gastroenterologists, oncologists, and internal medicine specialists for the dog with refractory vomiting that does not respond to other drugs. Severe parvoviral enteritis and vomiting associated with cancer chemotherapy are two examples in which ondansetron has been used with some success. Unfortunately, ondansetron is quite expensive. For short-term use the benefits may justify the cost. The recommended dose for this unapproved drug is

0.5 to 1.0 mg/kg PO s.i.d. to b.i.d. (some have advocated as often as t.i.d.) or 0.1 mg/kg IV.

Because vomiting is such a common complaint in veterinary patients, new antiemetics will continue to appear. When the use of human antiemetics, or any human drug, begins to appear in lecture notes from veterinary conferences or proceedings from national veterinary meetings, additional investigation and research are prudent before using such medications in the veterinary clinical setting. Always determine under what specific conditions and indications these "new" drugs should be used, what side effects are possible, and what clinical research has been done in veterinary medicine to justify the use of these medications in veterinary patients.

ANTIDIARRHEAL DRUGS

Antidiarrheals are drugs that change intestinal motility or reduce secretions that contribute to diarrhea. Like vomiting, diarrhea is normally a protective mechanism that helps remove irritating or toxic substances from the intestinal tract. Essentially, diarrhea occurs because the balance between fluid secretion into the intestinal lumen and fluid absorption from the intestinal lumen fluid has been upset, resulting in a net increase in fluid of the feces. For example, with secretory diarrhea caused by bacterial *enterotoxins* (toxins produced within the bowel lumen) or inflammation of the bowel, secretion of intestinal fluids into the lumen occurs at a rate that cannot be compensated by absorption of the fluid from the bowel. Diseases that decrease the absorption of fluid or intestinal contents (e.g., transmissible gastroenteritis in swine, parvovirus in dogs) also result in a net increase of fluid in the lumen. Exudative diarrhea occurs when increased permeability of the intestinal mucosa from inflammation or infection results in protein, fluid, serum, and even blood lost in the intestinal lumen. With maldigestion or malabsorption of food, such as occurs with exocrine pancreatic insufficiency (EPI) in young German shepherds, more fluid remains in the intestinal lumen because of the osmotic force the undigested food material has to hold fluid in the gut.

Diarrhea can also result from intestinal contents moving through the intestine so quickly that fluid has little chance to be absorbed. Laxatives produce loose stools by holding fluid in the intestinal lumen or causing water to move from the body to the intestine. Typically, most diarrhea syndromes are a combination of these mechanisms. Antidiarrheal drugs principally work by decreasing secretions, modifying intestinal motility, or decreasing the underlying problem (e.g., inflammation, infection) that produced the changes in secretions or motility.

ANTIDIARRHEALS THAT MODIFY INTESTINAL MOTILITY

Intestinal motility involves two types of contractions: segmental contractions, which mix the contents of the bowel, and peristaltic contractions, which propel the food along the tract (see Figure 4-3). Increased segmental contractions constrict the size of the intestinal lumen and slow movement of feces along the GI tract. Diseases that decrease segmental contractions or increase peristaltic movement result in more rapid movement of ingesta along the tract.

In many GI diseases a short period of hypermotility (increased movement of bowel contents by rapid peristalsis) is often followed by a longer period of hypomotility (decreased peristalsis) and atony (few or no segmental contractions). When the bowel loses smooth muscle tone, the decrease in segmental contractions still results in increased movement of feces even with weak peristaltic contractions. Thus diarrhea can also occur with decreased smooth muscle tone. Increased contractions in the colon caused by colonic or rectal inflammation and irritation can stimulate the defecation reflex, resulting in apparent straining to defecate called *tenesmus*.

Drugs can decrease diarrhea by decreasing peristaltic movements or increasing segmental contractions in the small intestine. The two most common groups of antidiarrheal drugs that work by modifying motility include anticholinergic drugs and *narcotic (opioid) drugs.*

Anticholinergic drugs work against the effects of the neurotransmitter acetylcholine. Acetylcholine is the neurotransmitter most commonly associated with parasympathetic effects and is the primary neurotransmitter involved with motility of the intestinal tract. Anticholinergic drugs are most effective at reducing spastic colonic contractions (antispasmodic effect) and diarrhea associated tenesmus. Although anticholinergics are effective in reducing colonic tenesmus, they can actually make small intestine diarrhea worse by decreasing segmental contractions and decreasing resistance to the flow of intestinal contents. Anticholinergics may have more potential to reduce diarrhea through their effect on intestinal secretions.

Anticholinergics used in veterinary medicine include drugs such as atropine, aminopentamide (Centrine), isopropamide, propantheline, and methscopolamine. Because of its wider range of side effects and its short duration of activity, atropine (one of the belladonna alkaloids) is used less often as an antispasmodic.

Anticholinergics, also called parasympatholytic drugs, block the parasympathetic effect and allow the sympathetic effect to dominate; therefore any condition in which sympathetic tone is already high is a contraindication for use of these drugs. For example, animals with cardiac arrhythmias, tachycardia (such as in cats with hyperthyroidism), or ileus (lack of intestinal motility) should not be treated with parasympatholytics. Decreased GI motility also prolongs contact of toxins or irritant substances with the bowel mucosa, prolonging their damaging effect on the bowel or increasing the degree of absorption into the body.

Narcotic or opioid antidiarrheals are schedule drugs (controlled substances) that decrease movement of feces through the GI tract by increasing segmental contractions. OTC versions of these drugs contain the same ingredients but at lower concentrations. These drugs are thought to have an antisecretory effect, which reduces the hypersecretory diarrheal effects of certain bacterial toxins and prostaglandins.

Narcotics commonly used to combat diarrhea include diphenoxylate (Lomotil) and loperamide (Imodium and Imodium A-D [OTC]). These narcotic antidiarrheals often contain a subtherapeutic dose of atropine designed to produce a slightly uncomfortable dryness in the mouth to dissuade abuse of the opioid. Paregoric (tincture of opium) is an older narcotic type of antidiarrheal that has been used for many years. It is still occasionally found to be used in veterinary medicine.

A disadvantage of some narcotic antidiarrheals is that they exert some analgesic effect that can mask abdominal pain that is used to monitor progression or resolution of disease. Because these drugs decrease gut motility and slow the transit time of intestinal contents, they also prolong the contact time between the bowel mucosa and pathogenic bacteria such as *Salmonella enteritidis* and enterotoxins, which could increase the damage caused by these agents. This is especially a concern in horses with bacterial enteritis. To avoid some of these detrimental effects, these compounds should not be given until sufficient time has passed for the infectious agent or enterotoxin to have been cleared from the bowel.

ANTIDIARRHEALS THAT BLOCK HYPERSECRETION

Secretion can result from enterotoxins, prostaglandins, and leukotrienes produced by inflammation of the GI tract as well as anything that increases the effect of acetylcholine or the parasympathetic nervous system. Stimulation of cells lining the GI tract can result in secretion of ions that osmotically pull water with them into the lumen of the gut. This type of diarrhea can be potentially dangerous because of the risk for life-threatening dehydration, especially in younger animals.

Secretory diarrheas can become exudative diarrheas when the GI inflammation also damages the tight junctions between cells lining the intestinal tract, allowing small-molecular-weight sugars, fluid, and protein molecules to be lost in the intestinal lumen. If inflammation or cellular destruction continues, the intestinal tract may become so porous that red blood cells escape into the intestinal lumen, resulting in bloody diarrhea.

Antisecretory antidiarrheal drugs used in veterinary medicine include the narcotic/opioid drugs and antiinflammatory drugs. Narcotics and opioids are effective antidiarrheals because they decrease the secretions while simultaneously increasing segmental contractions to slow the movement of feces through the gut.

Antiinflammatory drugs used as antisecretory antidiarrheals include aspirinlike compounds (salicylates), flunixin meglumine (Banamine, Flunixamine), and sulfasalazine (Azulfidine). Bismuth subsalicylate, the active ingredient in Pepto-Bismol and the new formulation of Kaopectate, breaks down in the gut to bismuth carbonate and salicylate. The bismuth coats the intestinal mucosa, protecting it from enterotoxins while producing some antibacterial activity. The major antisecretory effect, however, is probably from the salicylate, which decreases inflammation and blocks formation of prostaglandins that would normally stimulate fluid secretion.

Although bismuth is not well absorbed in the systemic circulation, the salicylate is absorbed in sufficient amounts to achieve potentially significant systemic concentrations. Therefore these compounds should be used with caution in cats because of their limited ability to metabolize and excrete salicylates. Some clinical investigators recommend limiting use of bismuth subsalicylate in cats to no more than 24 hours.

The bismuth that remains in the bowel can cause a dark, tarry appearance in the stool, resembling melena (stools darkened by digested blood). This color change can confuse the veterinarian who might mistake its presence as an indication of gastric or small intestinal hemorrhage. Bismuth, like barium, is used as a contrast material to better show the stomach and intestinal tract on radiographs and is a radiopaque compound that may interfere with visualization of organs on abdominal radiographs.

Veterinary patients commonly reject Pepto-Bismol because of its taste. Refrigerating the liquid form reduces the peppermint flavor, which may make it easier to administer. The tablet form greatly facilitates administration of the drug.

A potent antiprostaglandin that has been used in dogs and horses with GI problems is flunixin meglumine (Banamine). Although well tolerated in the horse, flunixin's use in dogs for diarrhea is limited because of the dog's predisposition to gastric or intestinal ulcers from the drug's antiprostaglandin effect. The same mechanism that allows flunixin meglumine to decrease inflammation also decreases the production of normal gastric mucus and the stomach's other self-protective mechanisms. Typically, within 72 hours most dogs on flunixin meglumine have evidence of blood in the stool. Therefore, although flunixin is a good drug for relief of colic pain in horses and to some degree for calf scours (diarrhea), it is not the drug of choice for treatment of diarrhea in other animals.

Sulfasalazine (Azulfidine) is a sulfonamide antibiotic (antimicrobial) linked chemically to a salicylate molecule called mesalamine (formerly called 5-aminosalicylic acid). Although the antibiotic component of this combination does little to relieve intestinal inflammation or infection, the mesalamine that is cleaved from the sulfa antibiotic by colonic bacteria decreases prostaglandin formation and thus acts as an antiinflammatory drug in the colon. Azulfidine has been successfully used in treatment of chronic bowel conditions such as ulcerative colitis. Because the salicylate, once cleaved from the sulfa antibiotic, is absorbed from the colon, the drug should be used with caution in cats because of the cat's reduced ability to metabolize salicylate drugs. The sulfonamide antibiotic is capable of producing side effects typically associated with sulfas, including vomiting (if given on an empty stomach) and decreased tear production leading to a condition called dry eye. Sulfonamide side effects are described in more detail in Chapter 10.

In the future, a number of other human products that contain mesalamine without the sulfonamide antibiotic are likely to find their way into veterinary use. These drugs are currently available for human use in slow-release tablet form and as enema preparations.

ADSORBENTS AND PROTECTANTS AS ANTIDIARRHEAL AGENTS

Bacterial enterotoxins and irritating substances cause hypersecretion and acute diarrhea by direct contact with intestinal mucosal cells. Any drug that prevents these agents from contacting the intestinal mucosa could theoretically reduce the diarrheal response. This is the underlying principle of *adsorbents* and *protectants*. An adsorbent drug molecule makes other substances adhere to its outer surface, thus reducing contact of that substance with the intestinal tract wall. In contrast, protectant-type compounds are designed to cover the intestinal wall to form a physical blanket or barrier that protects the intestinal wall from contact with irritating or disease-producing compounds. Although some of these adsorbents and protectants are widely used in human medicine for diarrhea, their effectiveness in veterinary patients is debatable.

The combination of kaolin and pectin is often used for symptomatic relief of vomiting or diarrhea in people and animals. The kaolin-pectin combination is thought to adsorb bacteria and their enterotoxins, reducing their hypersecretory effect on the intestinal tract. Whether kaolin-pectin has any significant effect in controlling diarrhea in veterinary patients is questionable. Because of their adsorbent qualities, kaolin-pectin combinations can decrease absorption of some antibiotics and the cardiac drug digoxin from the GI tract. Therefore if kaolin-pectin compounds are used with other oral medications, they should be given at least 2 hours before or 3 hours after the other orally administered drugs.

(Note: Kaopectate used to be a kaolin-pectin product. It was reformulated in late 2002 with bismuth subsalicylate, similar to Pepto-Bismol. Because of the addition of the salicylate and the reduced ability cats have for metabolizing salicylate compounds, owners familiar with using the old formulation of Kaopectate in their cats might trigger salicylate toxicosis if they use the new formulation in the same way. The new, regular-strength Kaopectate liquid contains 130 mg of aspirin per tablespoon and the extra-strength Kaopectate contains 230 mg of aspirin per tablespoon. A tablespoon of the extra-strength Kaopectate could produce salicylate toxicosis in a 5-pound cat. Veterinary professionals should educate their clients on the differences between the old and new formulation for this OTC antidiarrheal.)

Although not typically used as an antidiarrheal agent, activated charcoal adsorbs enterotoxins and many ingested poisons to its surface, preventing them from contacting the bowel wall and decreasing their ability to inflict damage or to be absorbed into the body. The charcoal and adsorbed poison or enterotoxin are then excreted in the feces. Because charcoal is messy to administer, it is seldom used as an adsorbent to decrease diarrhea.

The bismuth in bismuth subsalicylate (Pepto-Bismol and new Kaopectate) and the liquid barium used in contrast radiographic studies of the intestine both act as protectants. Animals with chronic diarrhea may improve for a while after oral administration of barium to provide radiographic contrast in the intestinal tract.

Bismuth is found in several human antidiarrheal products and has been shown to have antisecretory effects in diarrhea even if it is not combined with antiinflammatories such as subsalicylate. Whether this antisecretory effect comes from the adsorbent/protectant property or some other property of bismuth is not known. It is also debatable whether the course of the disease is shortened in veterinary patients on bismuth compounds. Still, veterinary technicians need to be aware of the public's perception of these drugs so that they may knowledgeably answer questions that owners have.

LAXATIVES, CATHARTICS, AND PURGATIVES

Laxatives, cathartics, and purgatives are used to increase the fluid content of the feces, making them softer and easing or promoting defecation. These types of drugs are used to control chronic constipation (common in some older cats), facilitate passage of trichobezoars (hairballs), evacuate the colon before radiographic procedures, and ease passage of stool after perianal surgery or in animals with severe pelvic fractures. The mechanisms and degree of aggressiveness in evacuating the bowel of these formulations may be different. Generally, laxatives are considered the most gentle of this class of drugs, whereas cathartics are more marked in their evacuating effect. Purgatives are the most potent in their actions. Although increasing the dose of some laxatives may produce a more pronounced diarrhea than a low dose of a cathartic, laxatives are generally used when the goal is to soften the stool and cathartics and purgatives are used when evacuation of the bowel is the goal.

LAXATIVES

Laxatives fall into two categories: emollient laxatives (lubricant oils and the so-called stool softeners) and bulk laxatives.

Emollient laxatives include lubricants such as mineral oil, cod liver oil, white petrolatum, and glycerin. Mineral oil is most commonly used for horses with impactions and is administered by stomach tube. The greatest danger associated with use of this oil is aspiration into the lungs with subsequent pneumonia. Because mineral oil has no distinct taste and does not readily stimulate swallowing, aspiration is a risk in all species if the oil is not given by stomach tube.

Cod liver oil and white petrolatum are common ingredients of laxatives used in cats and dogs. As with mineral oil, these oils dissolve lipid-soluble toxins and therefore are sometimes used to decrease absorption of certain ingested toxic substances. Controversy exists because some toxicologists believe that these oils may increase absorption of lipid-soluble toxins. Long-term use of nonabsorbable oils can decrease absorption of lipid-soluble vitamins such as A, D, E, and K from the bowel.

Glycerin is most commonly used as a suppository and therefore does not carry the risk of aspiration. Glycerin suppositories facilitate stool passing through the colon of animals with severe pelvic fractures or compression of the pelvic canal, through which the colon and rectum pass.

Besides the lubricant oils, another group of emollient laxatives includes compounds that change the surface tension of the fecal material, allowing water to penetrate the fecal material and softening it. Docusate sodium succinate (Colace) is a stool softener that acts as a wetting agent, or surfactant. Docusate sodium succinate and related calcium and phosphate compounds may also stimulate colonic secretions, resulting in increased fluid content of feces. These emollient laxatives are commonly used after anal surgery (for example, anal sacculectomy and perianal fistula surgery), when passage of a firm stool may be painful.

Bulk laxatives pull water into the bowel lumen by osmosis or retain water in the feces. Hydrophilic colloids or indigestible fiber (bran, methylcellulose, Metamucil) are not digested or absorbed to any degree and therefore create an osmotic force to produce their laxative effect. Psyllium is a hydrophilic compound that has gained popularity for its purported health benefits. It is successful as a bulk laxative but increases flatulence.

CATHARTICS

Cathartics fall into two categories on the basis of their mechanisms: osmotic cathartics and irritant cathartics. Osmotic cathartics are more aggressive than the osmotic bulk laxatives. Typically, osmotic cathartics are hypertonic salts such as magnesium (milk of magnesia, Epsom salts). These salts are poorly absorbed and create a strong osmotic force to attract water into the bowel lumen. In addition to the direct osmotic effect, magnesium also causes release of cholecystokinin, a hormone that increases peristalsis and thus facilitates movement of the fecal material. Large doses of hypertonic salts should be avoided because they can severely dehydrate an animal.

Although osmotic cathartic salts are poorly absorbed, if they are given in large doses or remain in the bowel for an extended period they may be absorbed in sufficient amounts to cause electrolyte imbalances. For example, absorption of excessive magnesium salt can cause muscle weakness and CNS alterations. Absorption of phosphate from phosphate and sodium phosphate salt laxatives or enemas can cause hypocalcemia to the extent of producing hypocalcemic tetany. Because cats are especially susceptible to these electrolyte imbalances, phosphate laxatives and sodium phosphate enemas, including soaps with a high phosphate content, should not be used in feline patients.

Lactulose is a poorly absorbed sugar osmotic cathartic used to treat cases of chronic constipation and reduce the ammonia absorbed from the colon. It is used in a condition called hepatic encephalopathy, a condition in which a poorly functioning liver or vascular shunts that bypass the liver result in increased levels of ammonia in the body, disrupting normal function of the CNS. The lactulose changes the pH of the colon, resulting in ammonia becoming more ionized and therefore less absorbed in the body.

Irritant laxatives, including castor oil and diphenylmethane compounds, work by irritating the bowel, resulting in increased peristaltic motility and some increased secretion by glands in the intestinal tract wall. Castor oil is converted in the duodenum to ricinoleic acid, which is a highly irritating compound. Because of their stimulant activity, these compounds should not be used in animals with suspected obstructed bowel or impacted feces or those with tenesmus resulting from colonic irritation or rectal/anal surgery.

ANTACIDS AND ANTIULCER DRUGS

PHYSIOLOGY OF STOMACH ACID SECRETION

The stomach is lined with *gastric glands* containing oxyntic or parietal cells, which produce hydrochloric acid; *chief cells*, which produce an enzyme precursor called pepsinogen; and *mucous cells*, which produce the protective mucus. The glands of the distal part of the stomach contain endocrine cells called *G cells*, which secrete the hormone gastrin. Gastrin is dumped into the blood and travels, among other places, to the gastric glands in the proximal part of the stomach and stimulates the release of hydrochloric acid from the parietal cells.

The mucus produced by the gastric glands is actually a complex of many substances that provides a gelatinous, protective coating for the stomach. *Mucins* are complex molecules produced by the goblet cells in the gastric glands and are the main constituent of the mucous coating. In addition to the mucin, bicarbonate ion is also secreted onto the surface, where it makes the mucous coat more alkaline. By alkalinizing the mucus, the hydrochloric acid contacting it will be neutralized to some degree. The mucous coating is essential to protect the stomach cells from the harsh acidic environment of the stomach (pH of 2 to 3). A pH of 2 would normally remove paint from many surfaces and etch metal.

Breaks in the surface of the mucus, epithelium, and underlying mucosa are called erosions or gastric ulcers. Inflammation of the stomach, called gastritis, often appears as a generalized reddening of the observed surface. The mucus itself is not digested by the pepsin but is fragmented by the hydrochloric acid in the stomach. For the stomach to be continually protected, all the components of the mucus must be continuously secreted. Failure to do so sets the stomach up for gastritis and gastric ulcers.

Hydrochloric acid secreted by the oxyntic or parietal cells is actually the process of secreting hydrogen (H^+) and chloride (Cl^-) ions. Once these ions are secreted into the stomach, they combine to produce hydrochloric acid, which accounts for the extremely acidic pH of the stomach. The secretion of hydrogen and chloride ions is an active process involving energy expenditure by the cell and an active transport mechanism. For that reason, the acid-producing process is capable of being tightly controlled by the body.

As previously mentioned, the parietal cell has three receptors on the blood side of the cell (as opposed to the stomach lumen side of the cell) that regulate acid production. These receptors are for gastrin, acetylcholine (the neurotransmitter of the parasympathetic nervous system), and histamine. Stimulation of all three of these receptors results in the optimal amount of hydrogen and chloride secretion (hence hydrochloric acid production). When the stomach is stretched by food entering the stomach or more acetylcholine from the parasympathetic nervous system is released at the G cells, gastrin is released from the G cells of the antrum, causing relaxation of the fundus and simultaneous production of increased amounts of hydrochloric acid.

DRUGS USED TO COUNTER ACIDITY AND ULCERS

Hyperacidity, reflux of bile from the duodenum into the stomach, accumulation of metabolic toxins (as in renal failure), stress from surgery or disease, or conditions that inhibit healthy prostaglandin type E (PgE) formation can all result in gastritis, erosion of the superficial epithelial layer, and possible ulcers. Increased ingestion of carbohydrates in ruminants, such as occurs with grain overload, can result in an overproduction of significant amounts of acidic byproducts by the rumen bacteria and protozoa. The change in the rumen pH kills the normal rumen flora and causes irritation or ulceration of the rumen and adjoining compartments of the intestinal tract.

Several drugs commonly used in veterinary medicine can also contribute to GI irritation and ulcer formation. Nonsteroidal antiinflammatory drugs (NSAIDs) such as aspirin, phenylbutazone, and flunixin meglumine (Banamine) all inhibit formation of PgE, resulting in the loss of its protective mechanisms and allowing the stomach acid to damage the stomach lining. Antacids and antiulcer drugs are used to reduce the stomach acid and enhance the mechanisms by which the stomach protects itself from its own acid.

Antacids are given to decrease stomach acidity (increasing the stomach or rumen pH by making it more alkaline), thus reducing gastric irritation caused by hyperacidity. Antacids are also used in cases of rumen acidosis to restore the proper pH for rumen microbes to function.

Antacids are classified as systemic or nonsystemic. Nonsystemic antacids are administered by mouth to neutralize acid molecules in the stomach or rumen directly by chemically converting the strong acid to a weaker acid. Nonsystemic antacids typically come in either liquid or tablet form and are composed of calcium, magnesium, or aluminum. OTC antacids such as Tums and Rolaids are nonsystemic antacids made primarily of calcium. Other nonsystemic antacids include magnesium products such as Riopan and Mylanta, aluminum products such as Amphojel, and combinations of magnesium and aluminum products such as Maalox.

Calcium and aluminum antacids often cause constipation, whereas magnesium products often trigger diarrhea. Products containing both aluminum and magnesium attempt to balance these constipating and diarrheal effects.

Calcium antacids are more prone to cause gastric acid rebound syndrome than the magnesium or aluminum antacids. The calcium carbonate in these antacids triggers the release of gastrin, with a subsequent increase in hydrochloric acid production. Unfortunately, this gastrin stimulation continues to occur after most of the calcium carbonate antacid has moved beyond the stomach. The result is an increased production of hydrochloric acid without the presence of the antacid to counter it. The acid content rebounds to levels that can be higher than they were previously. Fortunately, a normal stomach can tolerate this short-lived rebound, but a stomach with gastritis or an ulcer may become more inflamed.

The change in pH or the electrolytes in the nonsystemic antacids may interfere with absorption of other drugs from the bowel. The increased pH of the GI lumen may cause some drugs to shift to a predominantly hydrophilic form that is less able to be absorbed by the intestinal mucosa. Drugs may also become adsorbed to or chelated with the antacids, causing the drug to precipitate out of solution or otherwise have its absorption prevented. For example, tetracycline antibiotics combine with calcium antacids and precipitate out of solution. Absorption of digoxin (a cardiac drug), acepromazine (a tranquilizer), and corticosteroids (antiinflammatory drugs) given orally may be decreased by concurrent use of antacids. When these drugs must be used concurrently with antacids, the antacids should be given no closer than 2 hours before or 3 hours after the other drugs are administered.

Because of their high concentrations of calcium, magnesium, and aluminum, repeated use or large doses of nonsystemic antacids may cause electrolyte imbalances because of absorption of these electrolytes.

In contrast to the local neutralizing effect of nonsystemic antacids, systemic antacids must be absorbed, circulate, and attach to receptors on the cells of the stomach to produce their effect. Systemic antacids include cimetidine (Tagamet), ranitidine (Zantac), and famotidine (Pepcid) and are often referred to as H_2 antagonists or H_2 blockers because they block the H_2 histamine receptor located on oxyntic (parietal) cells in the stomach. By attaching to these receptors but not producing any effect (no intrinsic activity) the stimulus for gastric acid production is significantly decreased. These drugs are available in injectable and oral forms; cimetidine and famotidine are also available in OTC forms as Tagamet-HB and Pepcid-CD, respectively.

Cimetidine and ranitidine (less so famotidine) inhibit the hepatic enzymes responsible for metabolism and breakdown of some cardiac drugs (β blockers, calcium channel blockers, and quinidine), theophylline, and anticonvulsant drugs such as diazepam and phenytoin. Simultaneous use of systemic antacids with these drugs results in slowed metabolism, increased plasma drug concentrations, and potentially toxic drug concentrations unless the dose is reduced. Surprisingly, the metabolism of barbiturates is not significantly affected by cimetidine administration.

Omeprazole is described as an acid pump blocker. Unlike systemic antacids that block stimulation of acid production, omeprazole binds to the luminal surface of the stomach's oxyntic cells and inhibits the pump that normally transports hydrogen ions into the stomach lumen. Because pH depends on the concentration of hydrogen ions (more acidic pH = more H^+ ions), fewer hydrogen ions in the stomach means a less-acidic environment. Unfortunately, omeprazole comes in a capsule that is appropriate for use in adult human beings but contains too much drug for most veterinary patients that weigh less than 40 lb. To use this drug in patients smaller than 40 lb, one gastroenterologist recommends removing the powdered drug from the capsule and either putting it into a smaller gelatin capsule or mixing it with liquefied soft margarine, which is then refrigerated to solidify and later cut into smaller pieces for administration.

Sucralfate (Carafate) is an antiulcer drug that has been called a "gastric Band-Aid" because it forms a sticky paste in the stomach that binds with the proteins found in ulcers. Thus the gelatinous substance of the compound selectively adheres to the ulcer site, protecting it from the acidic environment of the stomach. In addition, sucralfate also stimulates prostaglandin release, which promotes gastric protective mechanisms such as increased mucus production.

Sucralfate requires the presence of an acidic environment to most effectively bind to the ulcer site. Thus theoretically sucralfate should not be used simultaneously with antacid drugs, which would make the stomach pH more alkaline. Whether this is truly a clinically significant interaction is still open to debate. However, avoiding the administration of sucralfate with antacids or other drugs that alkalinize the stomach environment is likely prudent.

In spite of the need for an acidic environment to adsorb to an ulcer site, clinical investigators have used sucralfate to treat esophageal ulcers by crushing the tablets and mixing them with warm water to form a slurry that is administered by mouth.

Misoprostol (Cytotec) is a synthetic PgE_1 drug. Just like the naturally occurring prostaglandins, misoprostol increases mucus production, decreases acid production, and facilitates the stomach's protective mechanisms for defense and healing. Although this drug has

been used with mixed results as an ulcer preventive (for example, in animals receiving large doses of nonsteroidal antiinflammatory drugs), it is more effective in healing existing ulcerations. Because it is a prostaglandin and because prostaglandins have so many functions throughout the body, it would be expected that misoprostol would stimulate many prostaglandin receptor sites, resulting in side effects. The most common side effects reflect GI stimulation and manifest themselves as diarrhea, abdominal discomfort, cramping, and colic. The drug is fairly expensive but is extremely effective in the treatment of animals that are prone to gastric ulcer formation, such as those that have received an overdose of nonsteroidal antiinflammatory drugs or those that are severely stressed from extensive surgery or debilitating disease.

RUMINATORICS AND ANTIBLOAT MEDICATIONS

When ruminant animals become sick, one of the side effects may be rumen stasis, a condition in which the normal motility of the rumen is halted. Because normal ruminal contractions are needed for processing food and the balance of gas and byproducts of rumen fermentation, rumen stasis can eventually result in a deterioration of the ruminant's health.

Ruminatorics are drugs that stimulate an atonic (no muscle tone) or flaccid rumen. In the past, many "barnyard" compounds have been used to "get the rumen started again." These compounds often were an integral part of a local livestock production community and were passed down as home remedies from generation to generation. Some of the more notable ruminatorics included mercury, strychnine, tartar, barium chloride, and various plant concoctions.

Although some of these ruminatorics may actually have stimulated the rumen, they obviously had their side effects and disadvantages.

Modern ruminatoric drugs are designed to stimulate the parasympathetic nervous system and thus increase motility of the GI tract. Neostigmine is a ruminatoric drug that combines with the enzyme acetylcholinesterase and prevents it from breaking down acetylcholine. Because acetylcholine is the neurotransmitter associated with parasympathetic stimulation, the prolonged effect of acetylcholine increases the parasympathetic stimulation, resulting in increased GI stimulation, increased bronchial secretions, bronchoconstriction, decreased heart rate, miosis (constricted pupils), and urination. Other drugs that block acetylcholinesterase or mimic the neurotransmitter acetylcholine would be expected to have similar effects.

Normal rumen and reticulum contractions allow partially digested plant food (the cud) to be regurgitated to the esophagus, where it is chewed and reswallowed (rumination) or to expel built-up carbon dioxide or methane gas from the rumen (a process called *eructation*). Eructation is essential for dispelling excessive gas created by the fermentation process, thereby reducing the risk of too much gas being trapped in the rumen (a condition called *bloat [ruminal tympany]*). The gas associated with bloat may be present either as a free gas pocket or within a froth of very small bubbles, a condition known as frothy bloat. Antibloat medications act either by reducing numbers of rumen microorganisms that produce the gas or by breaking up the bubbles formed in the rumen with frothy bloat. Just as home remedies were used as ruminatorics, in the past compounds such as oil of turpentine, pine oil, gasoline, creolin, and even formaldehyde have been used to kill rumen microorganisms and reduce the bloated condition. Obviously, many of these compounds carried the risk of tissue irritation, tainting of milk, and other potentially toxic side effects.

Most modern veterinary bloat medications act by decreasing the surface tension of foam in the rumen, causing the small bubbles to coalesce into much larger gas pockets that can be eructated (belched) from the rumen. Mineral oil or ordinary household detergents mixed with mineral oil are often used to decrease the viscosity of the rumen contents, decrease the stability of the bubbles, and remove the froth. Some commercial antibloat preparations contain vegetable oils and emulsifiers, and other products contain poloxalene. Dioctyl sodium succinate (DSS) also reduces the viscosity of rumen contents, which allows the foam to dissipate. The optimal use for these products is by oral administration or direct injection (into the rumen through the flank with a large-bore needle) in the early stages of bloat.

OTHER DRUGS USED FOR GASTROINTESTINAL PROBLEMS

ANTIMICROBIALS

Because many GI diseases are viral in nature, antimicrobials are not usually needed or indicated for most common GI problems. However, a few can be potentially useful in certain circumstances. Sulfasalazine (Azulfidine) is an antimicrobial mentioned under the antidiarrheal drugs that is broken down by GI bacteria into the sulfonamide sulfapyridine and the aspirinlike prostaglandin-blocking agent aminosalicylic acid (mesalamine). Sulfasalazine is typically used for its antiinflammatory effect instead of its antibiotic effect.

Tylosin (Tylan) is a macrolide antibiotic very similar to the antibiotic erythromycin, which is commonly used for respiratory infections. Tylosin is used in cattle and swine to treat GI infections by susceptible gram-negative and gram-positive bacteria, *Chlamydia* and *Mycoplasma* infections. Although tylosin can be used in an extra-label manner for enteritis and colitis in dogs and cats, its effectiveness has been quite variable. Veterinarians should not use tylosin in horses because the drug may

CLINICAL APPLICATION
"Brain Tumor" in a Dog

A veterinarian at a conference related a tale about an old dog that was having recurring diarrhea of several weeks' duration. The owners had fecal samples checked repeatedly, hoping to find either some intestinal worm parasites or protozoal organisms such as *Coccidia* or *Giardia* that could be treated. The clients went to several veterinarians to try to get an answer for the continual diarrhea. Along the way, radiographs were taken of the intestinal tract and a barium series was performed. The dog's diarrhea improved for several days after the barium series but then returned. A biopsy was done of the intestinal tract, but it came back as a nonspecific diagnosis of inflammation. After several weeks of dealing with the diarrhea and not wanting to spend any more money on diagnostics, the owners tried yet another veterinarian who put the dog on metronidazole as a "shot in the dark." In 2 days the diarrhea was remarkably better. By 4 days of metronidazole treatment the stools were firming up nicely. The owners were encouraged.

On day 8, the owners returned home from a weekend trip to find the dog wandering in a circle, staggering, and falling over. The owners feared that the dog had a brain tumor. After weeks of battling the diarrhea, this new development was too much for the owners to take. They feared their dog would never have a good quality of life again, so they took the dog to an emergency clinic where they requested euthanasia.

Unfortunately, with the history of metronidazole administration, the dog's clinical signs may have been related to the drug and not really indicative of a brain tumor. The circling behavior, the sudden onset, and the 8-day treatment with metronidazole (apparently at significant dose to correct the diarrhea problem) would be consistent with CNS side effects from metronidazole. Even at normal doses metronidazole has been reported to produce CNS signs in some canine patients. If the veterinarian was not aware of this side effect of metronidazole, the conclusion of a brain tumor or some acute cerebrovascular event would have been reasonable in an older dog. Therefore, it's important for veterinarians and veterinary technicians to be aware of effects of drugs such as this.

cause diarrhea potentially severe enough to cause death.

Metronidazole (Flagyl) is an antimicrobial that is effective against anaerobic colon bacteria and the protozoan *Giardia.* Sometimes metronidazole is used in dogs with prolonged or chronic diarrhea in which no agent (e.g., parasite, protozoal organism) has been identified. It may also be used to treat suspected cases of giardiasis in which no *Giardia* organisms have been identified on repeated fecal examinations. Metronidazole does have some significant side effects in some dogs even at concentrations in the normal therapeutic range if the drug has been used for an extended period. These side effects include CNS signs such as head tilt, staggering, disorientation, proprioceptive deficits (inability to sense the position of the limbs), and seizures. Fortunately, these neurologic signs typically disappear a few days after metronidazole is discontinued.

ORAL ELECTROLYTE REPLACEMENTS

Various liquid and powder products containing essential electrolytes (sodium, potassium, chloride) are administered orally to help replace ions lost with diarrhea or vomiting. These products are generally recommended for calves, lambs, and foals with scours or diarrhea for which the intravenous administration of fluids with electrolytes would be economically or logistically impractical. They are also sometimes used in practice for dogs and cats after they are able to take fluids orally. Electrolyte replacers are most likely to be helpful when the animal has secretory diarrhea without significant dehydration and no vomiting. Absorption of electrolytes may be impaired in animals with severe intestinal damage.

PANCREATIC ENZYME SUPPLEMENTS

Some dogs and cats may be affected by a syndrome in which the pancreas fails to produce sufficient amounts of the digestive enzymes lipase, which breaks down lipids; amylase, which breaks down starches; and various proteinases, which break down proteins. This condition, referred to as exocrine pancreatic insufficiency (EPI), causes a failure to digest food and results in maldigestion (inadequate digestion) and subsequent malabsorption (inadequate absorption) of nutrients. The presence of these undigested nutrients creates an osmotic force that retains water in the lumen of the GI tract and may actually pull water from the body like a bulk laxative. The undigested fats will be acted on by GI bacteria, resulting in rancid, malodorous fat that produces a voluminous, pale, greasy diarrhea and subsequent weight loss.

In animals with exocrine pancreatic insufficiency, pancreatic enzyme supplements such as Viokase and Pancrezyme are added to the animal's food before feeding. Unfortunately, commercially available enzyme supplements vary in their enzyme content. In addition, the supplemental enzymes are denatured by the acidic environment of the stomach, rendering the lipase and proteinases (to a lesser degree) largely ineffective. These enzyme products may be mixed with the food at least 15 to 20 minutes before the food is offered; however, the effectiveness of lipase in breaking down fats is minimal because it depends on the proper temperature and pH.

Because gastric acid inactivates these enzymes, it has been suggested that H_2 blockers such as cimetidine may decrease the breakdown of the enzyme supplement. Unfortunately, no significant improvement in fat digestion is observed when cimetidine is used concurrently with the enzyme supplement, and the cost of the H_2 blocker does not justify its limited benefit.

Most enzyme supplements are in powder form but are also available as tablets. The tablet form has been fairly ineffective in dogs. However, digestion is significantly increased when the tablets are crushed before administration. Enteric-coated enzyme tablets apparently have no advantage, even though the enteric coating protects the enzymes from the acidic environment of the stomach. The lack of efficacy with the enteric-coated enzymes may be related to insufficient dissolution of the coating or the relatively fast intestinal transit time in veterinary patients.

Thus, although many animals will show some resolution of the diarrhea and stabilizing of their weight, some animals with pancreatic exocrine insufficiency are likely to have subnormal digestion of fats and may not regain the weight that was lost before enzyme treatment.

CORTICOSTEROIDS

Corticosteroid use in GI disease is controversial because the beneficial antiinflammatory effect is offset by immunosuppression (decreased immune function), increased gastric acid production, suppression of normal gastric protective and healing mechanisms, and increased risk of infection. Some chronic inflammatory bowel problems such as eosinophilic gastroenteritis may respond quite well to corticosteroids. If corticosteroids are going to be used in GI disease (or any disease) the smallest dose necessary to control clinical signs should be used, the dose decreased as soon as possible to minimize side effects, and the animal monitored closely for signs of gastric problems or other adverse systemic effects. Corticosteroids are discussed in greater detail in Chapter 13.

Box 4-1 Gastrointestinal Drug Categories and Names

EMETICS

Centrally acting emetics
  Apomorphine
  Xylazine
Locally acting emetics

ANTIEMETICS

Phenothiazine tranquilizers
  Acepromazine
  Chlorpromazine
  Prochlorperazine (Compazine)
Antihistamines
  Dimenhydrinate (Dramamine)
  Diphenhydramine (Benadryl)
Anticholinergic drugs
  Aminopentamide
  Atropine
Prokinetic drugs
  Metoclopramide (Reglan)
  Cisapride
Serotonin antagonists
  Ondansetron (Zofran)

ANTIDIARRHEALS

Anticholinergics
  Aminopentamide (Centrine)
Opioid narcotic drugs
  Diphenoxylate (Lomotil)
  Loperamide (Imodium)
Antiinflammatory drugs
  Bismuth subsalicylate (Pepto-Bismol, Kaopectate)
  Flunixin meglumine (Banamine)
  Sulfasalazine (Azulfidine)
Adsorbents/protectants
  Activated charcoal
  Kaolin/pectin
  Bismuth

LAXATIVES AND STOOL SOFTENERS

Emollient laxatives
  Mineral oil

Cod liver oil
White petrolatum
Glycerin
Docusate sodium succinate (Colace)
Bulk laxatives

CATHARTICS

Osmotic cathartics
  Hypertonic salts (milk of magnesia, Epsom salts)
  Lactulose
Irritant cathartics
  Castor oil

ANTACID/ANTIULCER DRUGS

Nonsystemic antacids
  Magnesium products (Riopan, Mylanta)
  Aluminum products (Amphojel)
  Combination magnesium and aluminum
    (Maalox)
  Calcium products (Tums, Rolaids)
Systemic antacids or antiulcer drugs
  H_2 blockers
    Cimetidine (Tagamet)
    Famotidine (Pepcid)
    Ranitidine (Zantac)
  Misoprostol (Cytotec)
  Omeprazole
Sucralfate (Carafate)

RUMINATORICS AND ANTIBLOAT MEDICATIONS

Neostigmine
Dioctyl sodium succinate

OTHER GI DRUGS

Antimicrobials
  Metronidazole (Flagyl)
  Sulfasalazine (Azulfidine)
  Tylosin (Tylan)
Oral electrolyte replacements
Pancreatic enzyme replacements
Corticosteroids

REFERENCES

1. Bond GR: Home syrup of ipecac use does not reduce emergency department use or improve outcome. *Pediatrics* 112:1061-1064, 2003.
2. Casavant MJ, Fitch JA: Fatal hypernatremia from saltwater used as an emetic. *J Toxicol Clin Toxicol* 41:861-863, 2003.

RECOMMENDED READING

Boothe DM: *Small animal clinical pharmacology and therapeutics*, Philadelphia, 2001, WB Saunders.
Carlson GP: *New and old therapies for severe acute diarrhea*. In Proceedings of the International Veterinary Emergency and Critical Care Symposium, San Diego, CA, 2004.

Carlson GP: *Acute diarrhea in the adult horse: common causes and differential diagnosis.* In Proceedings of the International Veterinary Emergency and Critical Care Symposium, San Diego, CA, 2004.

Hughes D, Moreau RE, Overall KL, et al: Acute hepatic necrosis and liver failure associated with benzodiazepam therapy in cats. *J Vet Emerg Crit Care* 6:13-20, 1997.

Leib MS: *Diagnostic approach to acute diarrhea in dogs.* In Proceedings of the Western Veterinary Conference, Las Vegas, NV, 2004.

Leib MS: Chronic colitis in dogs. In Bonagura JD, editor: *Kirk's current veterinary therapy XIII,* Philadelphia, 2000, WB Saunders.

Plumb DC: *Veterinary drug handbook,* ed 5, Ames, IA, 2005, Blackwell Publishing.

Poppenga RH: My pet's been poisoned! A phone management primer. In Proceedings of the Western Veterinary Conference, Las Vegas, NV, 2002.

Tams TR: *Pharmacologic control of vomiting.* In Proceedings of the Atlantic Coast Veterinary Conference, Atlantic City, NJ, 2003.

Washabau RJ: *Difficult vomiting disorders: pathogenesis, diagnosis, and therapy.* In Proceedings of the Atlantic Coast Veterinary Conference, Atlantic City, NJ, 2004.

Willard MD: Chronic small bowel diarrhea: part II. In Proceedings of the American College of Veterinary Internal Medicine Annual Meeting, Minneapolis, MN, 2004.

Self-Assessment

REVIEW QUESTIONS

Fill in the following blanks with the correct item from the Key Terms list.

1. _____ pertaining to or associated with the stomach.

2. _____ pertaining to or associated with the intestine.

3. _____ pertaining to or associated with the colon.

4. _____ neurotransmitter associated with the parasympathetic nervous system.

5. _____ along with histamine and acetylcholine, the receptor found on acid-producing cells in the stomach (oxyntic or parietal cells).

6. _____ cells in the stomach that produce hydrochloric acid.

7. _____ cluster of neurons that coordinates the vomiting reflex.

8. _____ straining to defecate.

9. _____ a mostly parasympathetic nerve that innervates the GI tract and other organs in the abdominal cavity.

10. _____ "fight or flight" part of the autonomic nervous system.

11. _____ "rest and restore" part of the autonomic nervous system.

12. _____ specialized neurons that detect substances in the blood and in the cerebrospinal fluid (CSF) and stimulates the emetic center to produce vomiting.

13. _____ inflammation of the stomach.

14. _____ single-stomached animal.

Fill in the following blanks with the correct drug described in Box 4-1.

15. _____ adheres to open ulceration sites; needs acidic environment to act; stimulates local production of prostaglandins.

16. _____ adsorbent that turns stools a dark color.

17. _____ decreases gastric acid by being antagonistic to stimulation of histamine receptors on the stomach cells that produce acid.

18. _____ used in cattle with frothy bloat to break up bubbles or as a laxative drug that works by breaking down surface tension on dried fecal material, allowing water to penetrate.

19. _____ antibiotic used for treating giardiasis, a protozoa of the intestinal tract; known for producing neurologic side effects.

20. _____ given intravenously or as a tablet in the eye to produce emesis quickly in dogs by dopamine stimulation; less effective in cats.

21. _____ injectable sedative that is also an effective emetic in cats.

22. _____ antiemetic that blocks dopamine receptors in the CRTZ; also stimulates contractions and movement of the stomach in the normal direction; sometimes called a prokinetic agent.

23. _____ antidiarrheal that increases resistance to fecal movement by increasing the segmental contractions; also decreases GI secretions.

24. _____ decreases acid production in the stomach by blocking the pump on the oxyntic (parietal) cell that moves H^+ ions into the stomach.

25. _____ antibiotic for treating colitis that derives more beneficial effect from its antiinflammatory effect than its antimicrobial activity; is broken down into the antiinflammatory drug by the colonic bacteria.

26. _____ increases blood flow to the stomach, increases cell turnover, reduces stomach acid production, and is also a synthetic version of a natural compound.

27. _____ composed of lipase and proteinases.

28. _____ OTC antidiarrheal drug that turns stools dark like melena; decreases inflammation in the GI tract through "aspirin-like" activity.

29. _____ decreases gastric acid by being antagonistic to stimulation of H_2 receptors on the stomach cells that produce acid.

30. _____ phenothiazine tranquilizer; decreases stimulation of motion sickness receptors in dogs more than in cats.

31. What effect does the parasympathetic nervous system have on GI motility, GI secretions, and blood flow to the GI tract?

32. What type of enema should be avoided in cats? (hint: an electrolyte).

33. What effect do prostaglandins have on stomach mucus, stomach acid production, blood flow to stomach, and cell turnover?

34. Indicate whether or not induction of vomiting should be performed in the following situations:

    A. a dog that ingested a strong alkali liquid cleanser 3 hours ago.

    B. a cat that ingested pelleted rat bait 40 minutes ago.

    C. a horse that ingested insecticide-contaminated feed 25 minutes ago.

    D. a dog that ingested its owner's heart medication and has been vomiting since.

35. Indicate whether the following statements are true or false.

    A. Stimulation of dopamine receptors produces vomiting more frequently in cats than in dogs.

B. Histamine plays an important role in vomiting caused by motion.

C. Prostaglandins decrease the sodium bicarbonate content found in the mucus of the stomach.

D. Apomorphine works better in dogs when given orally than when given intravenously.

E. Ruminatorics are drugs or compounds designed to break up frothy bloat.

F. Cathartics are more aggressive than purgatives.

G. Antihistamines are generally more effective antiemetics in dogs than in cats.

H. Mast cell tumors can produce gastric ulcers because of the histamine they release and the gastric hyperacidity syndrome they cause.

APPLICATION QUESTIONS

1. When animals vomit they become dehydrated from the loss of fluid in the vomitus and because they are not ingesting food or water. Why should an extremely dehydrated animal not receive a phenothiazine tranquilizer as an antiemetic before its dehydration is corrected with intravenous fluids? Also, why are phenothiazines not the best antiemetic to use in an animal with a history of epileptic seizures?

2. Anticholinergic drugs were used for a number of years for diarrhea and sometimes for vomiting. Are these drugs effective antiemetics?

3. Metoclopramide (Reglan) is said to have an advantage over other antiemetics because it has centrally acting and locally acting antiemetic effects. What is meant by this?

4. You are caring for a dog with uncontrollable vomiting after administration of chemotherapy. The veterinarian is trying an expensive antiemetic drug that is a serotonin antagonist. What effect do serotonin antagonists have on the emetic response?

5. When you auscultated the abdomen of a dog that presented with a history of diarrhea of 2 days' duration, you did not hear sounds associated with intestinal movement. In fact, you heard only a few abdominal sounds suggesting the intestines have below-normal motility. How do hypomotility and hypermotility result in diarrhea?

6. Why are drugs such as Pepto-Bismol fairly effective in controlling hypersecretory diarrhea? Do they really decrease the diarrhea by "coating and soothing" the intestinal tract? What component of Pepto-Bismol is responsible for most of the antidiarrheal effect?

7. A client is concerned because her dog's stools have been a dark color for the past 2 days and she thinks the discoloration is caused by digested blood. She mentions that she has been giving the dog bismuth subsalicylate (generic) for the past 2 days. The doctor is unavailable to speak with the client. What reasonable explanation can you give the client to explain the stool discoloration?

8. A client telephones to ask about giving Pepto-Bismol to his cat. Can this drug be used in cats? Why is it not used in cats as often as in dogs?

9. Why should kaolin-pectin compounds be given 2 hours before or 3 hours after other orally administered drugs?

10. Mr. Jinx is a 14-year-old domestic long-haired cat. He has been on oil-based laxatives for 4 years because of hairballs and a predisposition toward constipation. Why might a patient like Mr. Jinx require supplemental vitamins if he is receiving long-term therapy with oil-based laxatives?

11. Some nonsteroidal antiinflammatory drugs have the potential to cause gastric ulcers. How does this happen?

12. Why might an animal or person taking a calcium-containing local antacid actually experience an increase in gastric acid production as a result of the medication?

13. What is the difference between a ruminatoric and an antibloat medication? Which category does neostigmine belong to? What about docusate sodium succinate (DSS)?

14. In what animals should the antibiotic tylosin not be used? Why?

15. The veterinarian stocks several bottles of oral electrolyte solutions. What are some indications for their use?

16. Why are the signs of pancreatic exocrine insufficiency often not completely alleviated by oral supplementation with pancreatic enzymes?

Drugs Affecting the Cardiovascular System

key terms

absolute refractory period
adrenergic drug
agonist
antagonist
aldosterone
α_1 receptor
angiotensin I and II
angiotensin-converting
enzyme (ACE)
arrhythmia
atrial fibrillation
atrioventricular (AV) block
atrioventricular (AV) node
automaticity
β_1 and β_2 receptors
β agonists

β antagonists
β blockers
bradycardia
bundle branches
cholinergic receptors
downregulation
ectopic focus
epinephrine
muscarinic receptors
negative inotropic drug
nicotinic receptors
norepinephrine
pacemaker
paroxysm
premature ventricular
contractions (PVC)

PR interval
Purkinje fibers
P wave
QRS complex
relative refractory period
renin-angiotensin system
repolarization
sinoatrial (SA) node
sodium-potassium-ATPase
pump
supraventricular arrhythmia
tachycardia
upregulation
ventricular fibrillation
ventricular flutter

After studying this chapter, the veterinary technician should be able to explain:

1. Normal cardiovascular anatomy

2. Mechanisms that control the amount and direction of blood flow through the heart and circulation

3. Types of antiarrhythmics and the way they exert their effects

4. Types of positive inotropic drugs and the way they exert their effects

5. Types of vasodilators and the way they exert their effects

6. Types of diuretics and the way they exert their effects

Treatment of cardiovascular problems is challenging for several reasons: cardiac drugs have complex mechanisms of action that can be difficult to understand; several cardiac drugs may be used simultaneously, so drug interactions must be considered; and many cardiac drugs have serious side effects that must be anticipated. In addition, impaired cardiovascular function may alter the normal absorption, distribution, metabolism, and elimination of these drugs. Box 5-1, listing cardiovascular drugs, can be found at the end of this chapter.

The veterinary professional must have knowledge of normal and abnormal cardiac physiology to understand the intended effect of a cardiac drug, determine whether the goals of the therapy are being met, and detect toxic side effects early enough to prevent serious consequences. Veterinary technicians often monitor hospitalized cardiac patients and listen to client descriptions of the animal's status at home and therefore must have a working knowledge of the effects of cardiac drugs and early signs of complications.

This chapter presents principles of cardiac drug use. Many specifics of individual cardiac drug mechanisms have been excluded for brevity and to focus on the key elements of each drug. Veterinary professionals should review the package insert or published information for any cardiac drug before administering it to a veterinary patient.

NORMAL CARDIAC FUNCTION

Many complex feedback mechanisms regulate function of the cardiovascular system. This chapter contains a brief review of cardiovascular physiology and pathology. More detailed information is contained in veterinary cardiology, physiology, and internal medicine textbooks (Figure 5-1).

CARDIAC ANATOMY AND DYNAMICS OF BLOOD FLOW

The mammalian heart acts like a two-pump system. A fairly small pump on the right side pumps blood to the lungs and back to the heart, and a larger, stronger pump on the left pumps blood throughout the remainder of the body and back to the heart. The vessels returning blood to the right side of the heart are the venae cavae (anterior vena cava from the head, posterior vena cava from the trunk). Blood flows from the venae cavae into the right atrium, through the tricuspid, or right atrioventricular (AV), valve, and into the right ventricle. From the right ventricle, blood is pumped through the pulmonic valve (pulmonary refers to the lungs) into the pulmonary arteries, to the lungs, and back to the heart by the pulmonary veins.

With few exceptions, arteries carry blood away from the heart and veins carry blood toward the heart. Blood from the pulmonary veins enters the left atrium, passes through the mitral, or left AV, valve, and into the muscular-walled left ventricle. Finally, blood is pumped out of the left

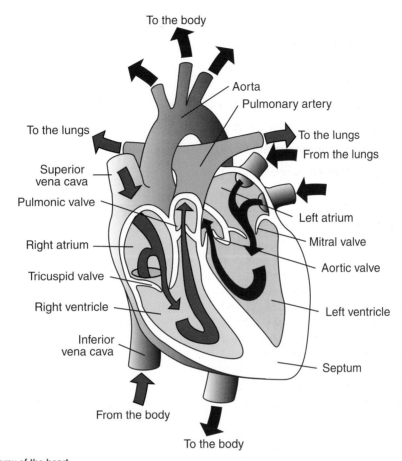

Figure 5-1 Anatomy of the heart.

ventricle, through the aortic valve, and into the aorta for distribution throughout the body.

The valves in the heart allow only one-way flow of blood and open and close passively. They swing like a one-way door in response to pressure changes between the atria and ventricles or between the ventricles and pulmonary arteries or aorta. The valves do not force blood from one part of the heart to another; they prevent reversal of blood flow.

ELECTRICAL CONDUCTION THROUGH THE HEART

The heart beats in a specific, coordinated manner. Special "wiring," or a conduction system, in the heart muscle ensures that the electrical

impulses, or waves of depolarization, that control heart contraction move through the heart in a specific sequence. These waves of depolarization can be recorded on an electrocardiogram (ECG).

Each heart muscle cell has the potential to depolarize (fire) spontaneously and independently, a property called *automaticity*. If a cardiac muscle cell were removed and placed in a special physiologic solution to keep it alive, the cell would spontaneously contract at a rate determined by that cell's physical and biochemical makeup. A specialized group of cardiac cells in the right atrium depolarizes more rapidly than any other cells in the heart. This group of cells is called the *sinoatrial (SA) node.* Cells in the SA node depolarize 50 to 150 times per minute depending on the species. Larger species generally have slower rates. The rate at which cells in the SA node depolarize determines the heart rate. For this reason the SA node is often referred to as the heart's *pacemaker* (Figure 5-2).

When cells in the SA node depolarize, a wave of depolarization spreads in all directions through the right atrium and then the left atrium. As the wave of depolarization passes from one cardiac muscle cell to another, each cell contracts. This wave passes so quickly that both atria contract almost simultaneously, pushing blood through the AV valves into the ventricles. On the ECG strip this atrial depolarization (and subsequent contraction of atrial muscle cells) is reflected as a small bump called the *P wave.* The wave components of the ECG shown in Figure 5-3 proceed in alphabetical

order, from P through T, as the strip is viewed from left to right.

The wave of depolarization spreads around the atria and is prevented from entering the ventricles by a cellular barrier to electrical impulses that acts like an electrical insulator. In normal animals the depolarization wave can reach the ventricles only through a specialized cluster of conducting cells called the *atrioventricular (AV) node.* The wave of depolarization enters the AV node and is delayed there for a fraction of a second before entering the ventricles. This short delay allows the atria to complete their contraction before the ventricles begin contracting and provides enough time for blood to move from the atria into the ventricles. Without this slight delay the atria and ventricles would contract at the same time and blood would not be pumped efficiently. On the ECG this period of conduction delay in the AV node shows up as a flat line after the

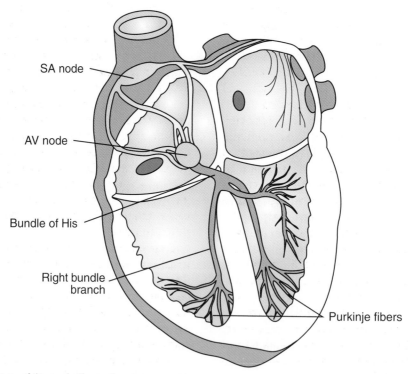

Figure 5-2 Anatomy of the conduction system.

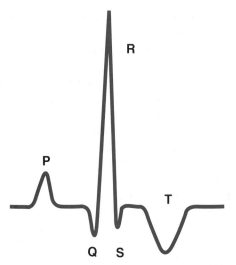

Figure 5-3 Basic components of the ECG: P wave, QRS wave, and T wave.

P wave and is referred to as the *PR interval* or the P-QRS interval.

After the depolarization wave passes through the AV node, it travels rapidly in the interventricular septum (wall between the right and left ventricles) along a specialized conduction pathway known as the *bundle branches.* The bundle branches conduct the electrical impulse to the *Purkinje fibers,* located at the apex (conical end) of the heart. The depolarization wave emerges from the Purkinje fibers at the apex and spreads rapidly throughout the ventricular muscle cells, causing them to contract from the apex toward the heart valves and push blood through the pulmonic and aortic valves and to the lungs and body.

Depolarization (and contraction) of the ventricles is reflected as a large wave on the ECG called the *QRS complex.* The QRS complex is composed of a small Q wave, a large R wave, and a small S wave all clumped together. After the ventricles contract, the ventricular muscle cells relax and repolarize (reset) in preparation for the next depolarization wave. This period of ventricular cell *repolarization* is displayed as the T wave on the ECG strip.

An ECG pattern shows the way electrical impulses travel through the heart. Any deviation from the normal pattern of cardiac depolarization or repolarization is apparent as abnormal P waves, bizarre QRS complexes, or skewed T waves. The ECG is not used to diagnose mechanical abnormalities of the heart (such as poorly functioning valves or weak cardiac muscle); it is only useful in identifying electrical abnormalities in the conduction pathway or in detecting an increase in overall mass of the heart (as reflected in enlarged P waves or QRS complexes).

DEPOLARIZATION, REPOLARIZATION, AND REFRACTORY PERIODS

Many cardiac drugs affect depolarization or repolarization, either as an intended effect or as a side effect; therefore the veterinary technician must have a basic understanding of the processes that take place within cardiac cells during depolarization and repolarization.

Depolarization and repolarization may be compared with the mechanics of a mousetrap. A mousetrap is set by moving the spring-loaded wire loop in place. After the trap snaps shut, it cannot fire again until it is reset. Cardiac cells, and all cells that depolarize, act in a similar manner. In its resting state a cardiac cell is much like the mousetrap, ready to snap shut. When the cardiac cell is stimulated by an adjacent cell, it fires, or depolarizes. Like the tripped (depolarized) mousetrap, the cardiac cell cannot depolarize again until it repolarizes (resets). Thus repolarization of the cardiac cell is like resetting the mousetrap, preparing it to fire again.

Depolarization and repolarization primarily involve movement of ions, specifically sodium (Na^+) and potassium (K^+), across the cardiac cell membrane (Figure 5-4). Although other ions such as chloride (Cl^-) and calcium (Ca^{++}) are involved, for simplicity this discussion focuses mostly on sodium and potassium.

In its resting state the cardiac cell is polarized; that is, it has two distinct poles, or segregated

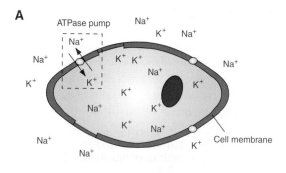

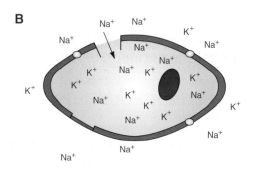

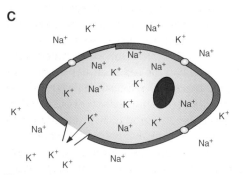

Figure 5-4 Changes in sodium (Na⁺) and potassium (K⁺) ion concentration during depolarization and repolarization. **A,** In the resting state, the Na⁺/K⁺ ATPase pump increases intracellular K⁺ concentrations while pumping Na⁺ out of the cell. **B,** During depolarization, the Na⁺ channels open, allowing Na⁺ to move into the cell along the concentration gradient. **C,** During repolarization, the Na⁺ channels close, the K⁺ channels open, and K⁺ moves out of the cell.

areas, of electrical charge. In resting cardiac cells the polarization is between sodium ions, which are found in high concentrations outside the cell membrane, and potassium ions, which are found in high concentrations inside the cell membrane. Although this polarized state is referred to as the resting state, the cell is actually expending energy to pump the Na⁺ out of the cell and the K⁺ into the cell to maintain polarization even if a stray ion leaks across the membrane. The pump itself is a specialized protein within the cell membrane called the sodium-potassium-adenosine triphosphatase (ATPase) pump. The enzyme ATPase is used to supply the sodium-potassium pump with energy stored in the cell's adenosine triphosphate (ATP). The pump can maintain polarization of these ions in the resting state because Na⁺ and K⁺ have difficulty crossing the cellular membrane except through specialized Na⁺ and K⁺ channels that are closed during the resting state.

The cardiac cell remains in this polarized resting state until the appropriate stimulus occurs. This stimulus is either the depolarization of adjoining cardiac cells or a change in electrical charge within the cardiac cell itself. When the stimulus occurs, the Na⁺ channels (sometimes called gates) open, allowing Na⁺ to move into the cell. The resting state concentration gradient of Na⁺ (high outside the membrane, low inside) and the slightly negative charge within the cell from negatively charged intracellular proteins cause the Na⁺ to move readily through the open channels into the cardiac cell. This influx of Na⁺ is known as depolarization because the two ion populations are no longer kept apart, or polarized.

As the positively charged Na⁺ flood into the cell during depolarization, the net charge within the cardiac cell becomes positive (phase 0 in Figure 5-5). When the charge within the cell becomes positive, the Na⁺ channels close and the K⁺ channels open. With the potassium channels open, the concentration gradient of K⁺ (high inside the membrane, low outside) and the increasingly positive charge within the cell

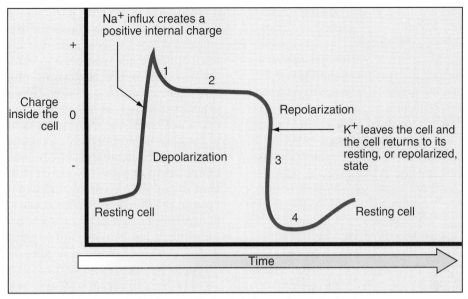

Na+ influx creates a
positive internal charge

+

1

2

Charge
inside the   0
cell

Repolarization

K+ leaves the cell and
the cell returns to its
resting, or repolarized,
state

-

Depolarization

3

Resting cell

4

Resting cell

Time

Figure 5-5 Phases of charge changes inside the cell with depolarization and repolarization.

cause the K+ to quickly leave the cell, taking with them their positive charges and causing the inside of the cardiac cell to become more negative (phases 1, 2, and 3 in Figure 5-5). This movement of K+ out of the cell is called repolarization because the ion populations are once again separated and the cell is polarized again.

When neurons depolarize, repolarization quickly follows. Cardiac cells, however, tend to have a plateau phase (phase 2 in Figure 5-5) between the influx of Na+ during depolarization and the efflux (outflow) of K+ during repolarization. During this plateau phase, Ca++ and Na+ continue to move into the cell through slow channels, thus maintaining the positive charge of the plateau phase. Once these channels close, repolarization rapidly occurs.

At the completion of K+ efflux of repolarization, the Na+ and K+ ions are located on the "wrong" sides of the cellular membrane, having passed through their respective channels during depolarization and repolarization. At this point the sodium-potassium pump begins to reestablish the correct location of Na+ and K+ by pumping the Na+ out of the cell and pumping the K+ into the cell.

The part of the line in phase 4 of Figure 5-5 moves gradually upward, reflecting a slow increase in positive charge within the cell. This gradual increase in positive charge is because most cardiac cells at the resting state are still somewhat permeable to Na+. As the Na+ ions leak in (faster than they can be pumped out), the charge within the cell becomes more positive until it reaches a point called the threshold at which depolarization spontaneously takes place. This phenomenon of Na+ leaking helps explain the mechanism by which cardiac cells depolarize spontaneously without stimulation (automaticity). How rapidly the slope rises determines how quickly a cell depolarizes and how often the cell automatically fires. The SA node, as the pacemaker of the heart, would be expected to have a relatively rapid rise to threshold, resulting in it depolarizing more frequently than other cardiac cells, thus setting the pace for contractions of the heart overall.

As mentioned earlier, after a cardiac cell has depolarized, it cannot depolarize again until it has repolarized. The time during the depolarization/repolarization cycle in which the cardiac cell cannot again depolarize is called the refractory period. The refractory period is divided into the *absolute refractory period* and the *relative refractory period.* A cardiac cell (or nerve) is absolutely refractory to depolarization in phase 0 of the cycle because no matter how strongly the cell is stimulated to depolarize, it cannot open the sodium channels to depolarize again because the Na^+ channels are already open and Na^+ is already entering the cell. As the sodium channels close and the cell begins to repolarize in phases 2 and 3, a sufficiently strong stimulus may be able to cause the sodium channels to open again and elicit a weak depolarization response. The cell is said to be relatively refractory to stimulus at this point because only a strong stimulus can evoke a depolarization response. As the cycle continues into phase 3, the cell becomes less refractory to depolarization stimuli and can produce a stronger depolarization response if given a sufficiently strong stimulus.

The refractory period is essential to prevent a wave of depolarization from traveling continuously from one end of the heart to the other and back again in an uncontrolled fashion. For example, when the SA node depolarizes and sends a wave of depolarization around the atria, the wave is stopped when it encounters depolarized cells that are in the refractory period of the cycle. If the refractory period of cells in the atria were shortened for some reason and the cells were capable of depolarizing again when the depolarization wave returned, the wave would be propagated (continue on) and the coordinated contraction of the heart would quickly turn into a continuous series of rapid, uncoordinated contractions. Such uncoordinated muscle contractions are called flutter or fibrillation of the atria or ventricles.

ROLE OF THE AUTONOMIC NERVOUS SYSTEM IN CARDIOVASCULAR FUNCTION

As mentioned in Chapter 4, the autonomic nervous system is composed of the sympathetic and parasympathetic branches and regulates many organ and system functions at an unconscious level. In the cardiovascular system, the sympathetic nervous system (also known as the "fight or flight" response system) increases the heart rate and force of contraction, elevates blood pressure, causes constriction of peripheral blood vessels, decreases perfusion of nonessential organs and tissues, decreases activity of the gastrointestinal (GI) tract, and dilates the bronchioles. All these functions improve the body's ability to survive a crisis. The increased heart rate delivers more blood to the muscles for movement, and vasoconstriction of peripheral vessels shunts blood away from the skin (resulting in less bleeding in the event of injury) and GI tract (negating the need to digest food during an emergency) and directs it to critical areas of the body. Bronchodilation allows more oxygen to reach the lungs and reduces accumulation of carbon dioxide. The combination of vasoconstriction and increased heart rate causes an increase in arterial blood pressure (much like blowing through one end of a rubber tube and squeezing off the other end would cause an increase in pressure within the tube).

To produce the sympathetic nervous system response, neurons of the sympathetic nervous system release the neurotransmitters *epinephrine* (adrenaline) and *norepinephrine.* These compounds bind to specific types of receptors called adrenergic receptors to produce the fight-or-flight changes. Drugs with intrinsic activity on these receptors can mimic the effects of epinephrine and norepinephrine and are called adrenergic *agonists.* In contrast, drugs that are able to bind to these receptors but have no intrinsic activity are called adrenergic *antagonists* because they block adrenergic molecules from combining with the receptors to produce the sympathetic effect.

Epinephrine, norepinephrine, and *adrenergic drugs* can bind to several different types of adrenergic receptors. These receptors, called alpha 1 (α_1), alpha 2 (α_2), beta 1 (β_1), and beta 2 (β_2) adrenergic receptors, are located on different types of cells in several different locations in the body. When stimulated, these receptors produce the physiologic effects associated with the sympathetic nervous system. β_1 *receptors* are located in the heart. They increase the heart rate, the strength of contraction by the cardiac muscle, and the speed of the depolarization wave through the heart's conduction system. Stimulation of β_1 adrenergic receptors by norepinephrine or adrenergic agonist drugs is responsible for the racing heart (*tachycardia*) experienced during exercise, fear, or excitement. An easy way to remember that β_1 receptors are responsible for this is to think of the β as standing for "beat."

β_2 *receptors* are found in smooth muscle surrounding blood vessels of the heart, skeletal muscles, arterioles, and the terminal bronchioles (smallest bronchioles) in the lungs. When stimulated, β_2 adrenergic receptors cause smooth muscle to relax (dilate). Therefore, β_2 receptor stimulation causes dilation of blood vessels in the skeletal muscle and heart (vasodilation) and dilation of airways in the lungs (bronchodilation).

If a drug is a nonspecific stimulator of β receptors, it may have some effect on both β_1 and β_2 receptors. Many drugs used to stimulate one type of β receptor often have stimulation of the other β receptor as a side effect. For example, bronchodilators commonly produce an increased heart rate as a side effect.

In contrast to the vasodilating effect of β_2 receptors, stimulated α_1 *receptors* cause smooth muscle surrounding blood vessels in the skin and intestinal tract to contract, decreasing blood flow (vasoconstriction). Thus in fight-or-flight situations, the α_1 vasoconstriction shunts blood away from the skin and digestive tract and toward the heart and skeletal muscles (β_2 effect) so that the pounding heart and rapidly moving skeletal muscles (fleeing or fighting) can receive more oxygen. α_2 receptors are located on the ends of adrenergic neurons, where they help regulate the release of norepinephrine. α_2 Receptors are discussed in greater detail in Chapter 8.

Although α_1, α_2 and β_1 receptors are all stimulated by sympathetic neurotransmitters and adrenergic agonist drugs, they are not necessarily stimulated equally. For example, epinephrine has a very strong α_1 effect (vasoconstriction of peripheral blood vessels) and a weaker β_2 effect (vasodilation of cardiac and skeletal muscle blood vessels). When epinephrine is released by the body or injected as a drug, blood pressure increases because blood is shunted away from the skin without increased flow to skeletal muscles. This selective stimulation of receptors is a common characteristic of drugs used in cardiovascular and respiratory therapeutics. Being able to use a drug that has the ability to combine with only one adrenergic receptor helps produce the desired therapeutic effect while decreasing undesirable side effects from stimulation of other adrenergic receptors.

The parasympathetic nervous system (the "rest and restore" system) antagonizes many effects of the sympathetic nervous system. The parasympathetic system slows the heart rate (opposite of the β_1-adrenergic effect), increases blood flow to the intestinal tract (opposite of α_1-adrenergic effect), and decreases the diameter of the bronchioles (opposite of β_2-adrenergic effect). The parasympathetic nervous system has little effect on peripheral blood vessels and thus does not antagonize the vasoconstriction of skin vessels caused by the sympathetic nervous system.

As described in Chapter 4, neurons of the parasympathetic nervous system secrete acetylcholine as the principal neurotransmitter. Acetylcholine combines with *cholinergic receptors* to produce parasympathetic effects. Just as there are different types of adrenergic receptors, there also different types of cholinergic receptors called *muscarinic receptors* and *nicotinic receptors*. Muscarinic receptors are typically found in neurons associated with the parasympathetic nervous system; thus drugs that stimulate muscarinic cholinergic receptors tend to produce clinical effects attributed to the parasympathetic nervous system (e.g., increased GI stimulation, slowed heart rate, pin-point pupils). The nicotinic cholinergic receptors are found in both the parasympathetic and sympathetic nervous system; therefore stimulation of these specific receptors often shows a mixture of both parts of the autonomic nervous system (Figure 5-6). Nicotinic cholinergic receptors are also found on the neuromuscular junction between the nervous system and skeletal (voluntary) muscles.

The parasympathetic and sympathetic nervous systems are always producing some effect on the body, often simultaneously on the same organ or tissues. Whichever of the two parts of the autonomic system produces the stronger effect at any particular moment determines whether the body shows sympathetic or parasympathetic signs. This is the reason that adrenergic antagonists (e.g., β_1 blockers) would cause parasympathetic nervous system signs as a side effect. Conversely, cholinergic antagonists allow the sympathetic nervous system to dominate, thus producing sympathetic nervous system signs.

ANTIARRHYTHMIC DRUGS

An *arrhythmia* is any abnormal pattern of electrical activity in the heart. As previously discussed, the waves of depolarization follow a specific sequence, starting in the SA node and ending with contraction of the ventricles. Sometimes, however, another area of the myocardium (heart muscle) or conduction system begins to depolarize out of sequence or more rapidly than the SA node, disrupting the normal electrical pattern. This abnormal site of depolarization is called an *ectopic focus*. Ectopic foci are often areas of damaged myocardial cells with membranes that allow leakage of Na^+ into the cell more rapidly than normal, resulting in quicker attainment of the threshold and more rapid spontaneous depolarization.

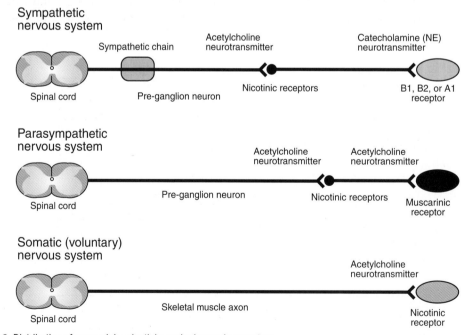

Figure 5-6 Distribution of muscarinic, nicotinic, and adrenergic receptors.

ECGs detect arrhythmias caused by ectopic foci or other abnormalities. An ectopic focus in the ventricles may be indicated on the ECG as a single, large, bizarre wave. This single wave is referred to as a *premature ventricular contraction (PVC)* because it represents depolarization of the ventricles out of the normal sequence, causing the ventricles to contract prematurely (Figure 5-7). Single, intermittent PVCs on the ECG do not significantly affect the heart's ability to pump blood and sometimes occur in healthy animals under general anesthesia. A short series of multiple PVCs is called a *paroxysm,* and a longer series of PVCs is referred to as *ventricular flutter.* If the conduction disturbance is severe, the ventricular contraction can become so uncoordinated that the heart simply quivers, a rapidly fatal condition called *ventricular fibrillation.* Similar changes of flutter and fibrillation can also occur in the atria. Antiarrhythmic drugs are used to control ectopic foci or reverse conduction abnormalities of the heart.

Different drugs must be used to control different types of arrhythmias. The veterinary professional must know which type of arrhythmia is present before choosing the appropriate antiarrhythmic drug. Arrhythmias are divided into two general groups: those that result in an increased heart rate (tachycardia) and those that cause a decreased heart rate *(bradycardia).* These arrhythmias are further subdivided according to location of the ectopic foci or lesion causing the arrhythmia. A *supraventricular arrhythmia* indicates that the source of the arrhythmia is above the ventricles and thus originates in the SA node, atria, or AV node. A ventricular arrhythmia indicates that the problem originates somewhere within the ventricles. The two terms are combined to describe the arrhythmia. For example, *atrial fibrillation* is a rapid heart rate caused by a problem in the atria and would therefore be classified as a supraventricular tachycardia.

Once the type of arrhythmia has been determined, an effective antiarrhythmic drug is used to reestablish a normal conduction sequence, or sinus rhythm (rhythm controlled by the SA node). The characteristics of the antiarrhythmic drug determine whether it will work in the atria or ventricles and whether the drug is capable of correcting bradycardia or tachycardia.

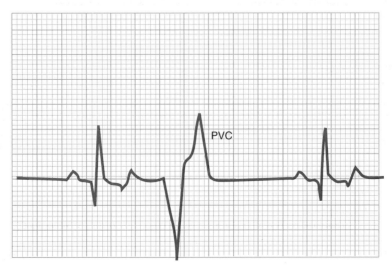

Figure 5-7 PVCs on the ECG.

ANTIARRHYTHMIC DRUGS THAT INHIBIT SODIUM INFLUX

Lidocaine, quinidine, and procainamide are antiarrhythmics that work primarily by decreasing the rate of Na^+ movement into the cell. Without normal Na^+ influx at depolarization, the steep phase 0 is retarded, resulting in less-effective depolarization. These drugs also slow the phase 4 leaking of Na^+ into the cell, which decreases the automaticity of bundle branch and Purkinje fiber cells as well as any abnormal ectopic foci in damaged tissue. Because the rate of automatic depolarization of an ectopic focus is slowed, the SA node should be able to regain control of the heart rate and reestablish a sinus rhythm.

Lidocaine is only available in injectable form. The extensive biotransformation by the liver (first-pass effect) and GI irritation lidocaine can cause if given by mouth preclude its use as an oral medication. The preferred route of administration of lidocaine for treatment of arrhythmias is by intravenous bolus or infusion. Because absorption after intramuscular injection is erratic, intramuscular injection is less preferred and used only in emergency situations.

Lidocaine is the major drug of choice for controlling PVCs and ventricular arrhythmias in canine cardiac patients or animals under anesthesia. Although lidocaine works well in controlling PVCs and ventricular ectopic foci, it has little efficacy against atrial ectopic foci, atrial fibrillation, or atrial flutter. For these arrhythmias, the other Na^+-blocking antiarrhythmics procainamide and quinidine are preferred.

Cats appear to be more sensitive to the side effects of lidocaine than other species. First- or second-degree AV block (decreased conduction of the depolarization wave through the AV node) becomes worse in cats given lidocaine. Large intravenous bolus doses of lidocaine have produced sinus arrest (the SA node stops depolarizing). Although debate about how sensitive cats are to lidocaine continues, reports of adverse reactions from lidocaine in cats do warrant caution in using this drug to treat this population.

Toxic CNS effects of lidocaine range from light toxicosis—as manifested by sedation, ataxia, and drowsiness—to excitement and seizures associated with larger overdoses. Lower dose lidocaine toxicity produces signs of CNS depression by inhibiting excitatory neurons, and higher dose toxicity signs of seizures result from inhibition of inhibitory neurons. Because lidocaine is so rapidly metabolized by the liver, lidocaine-induced seizure activity stops soon after lidocaine administration is halted and seldom requires treatment.

Veterinary technicians must realize that lidocaine is also packaged in vials with epinephrine for use as a local anesthetic. When injected as a local anesthetic, the epinephrine causes local vasoconstriction and decreased tissue perfusion, which reduces the absorption of lidocaine from the site of injection, thus prolonging the activity of the local anesthetic where injected. If the lidocaine with epinephrine is mistakenly used to treat an animal with an arrhythmia, the heart will be stimulated to beat faster and with greater force and will also become increasingly electrically unstable, resulting in worsening arrhythmias and possibly sudden collapse and death. Because most veterinary hospitals stock both forms of lidocaine, the bottles of the different forms should be clearly marked with colored tape or other distinctive marking so the wrong type is not picked up by accident during an arrhythmic emergency.

For animals with a lidocaine-responsive arrhythmia that require an oral drug for long-term maintenance, mexiletine is a lidocaine-like drug that is being used to control arrhythmias in dogs. Mexiletine has less first-pass effect than lidocaine; however, it may still produce GI and CNS side effects. Some veterinary cardiologists are advocating mexiletine as a first-choice PO administered antiarrhythmic drug in dogs with lidocaine-responsive arrhythmias.

Procainamide and quinidine are drugs that belong to the same general class as lidocaine. However, they differ from lidocaine in their ability to control both ventricular ectopic foci and atrial flutter or fibrillation (supraventricular tachycardia). In addition to decreasing the velocity of phase 0 depolarization and lengthening the phase 4 return to depolarization threshold (slowing the automaticity), these drugs also increase the refractory period. The increased refractory period helps control atrial fibrillation and flutter.

When the atria depolarize, the depolarization wave sweeps over the atria (think of the wave spreading across the surface of a ball). Normally the depolarization wave sweeps across the atria once, stimulating the AV node, and then stops when it encounters the first depolarized atrial cells that are in the refractory phase and unable to depolarize again. In atrial fibrillation the normal conduction pathway in the atria is disrupted by damaged cells, which slows or alters the depolarization wave's movement through the atria. Instead of the depolarization wave dying out when encountering refractory atrial cells, the wave reaches the first depolarized cells slightly later after they have completed the depolarization/repolarization cycle and are ready to depolarize again. The wave is therefore propagated again and continues on, resulting in continuous quivering muscular contractions throughout the atria. Procainamide and quinidine are effective in controlling arrhythmias by increasing the length of the refractory period so that when the depolarization wave returns to the initiating cells, they are still in the refractory phase. Thus procainamide and quinidine stop the wave from being continually propagated and the atrial fibrillation is controlled.

Quinidine and procainamide are most commonly administered by the PO route in veterinary medicine. This allows these drugs to be used for long-term maintenance of patients with ventricular or atrial arrhythmias.

Although quinidine frequently causes vomiting, diarrhea, and anorexia, procainamide appears to be well tolerated and causes fewer GI problems.

Even though quinidine prolongs the refractory period and slows depolarization, it may produce an increased heart rate. Quinidine has an antivagal effect, meaning that it decreases the effect of the vagus nerve on the AV node. Because the vagus nerve is a parasympathetic nerve and normally slows the impulses through the AV node (excessive stimulation would produce first- or second-degree AV block), blocking the vagus nerve effect would allow sympathetic stimulation to dominate, resulting in an increased rate of conduction of impulses through the AV nodes and a faster ventricular rate. This increase in heart rate despite a prolonged refractory period is called quinidine's paradoxic ventricular tachycardia effect.

Because quinidine and digoxin may be used together, veterinary professionals must be aware of the interaction between these two drugs. Digoxin is a drug that increases the strength of contraction of the heart. If quinidine is used to control arrhythmias while the digoxin is used to increase the force of heart contraction, digoxin toxicity may occur because quinidine displaces digoxin from its binding sites in cardiac and skeletal muscle cells while simultaneously decreasing digoxin elimination. These actions can double the plasma digoxin concentrations and produce clinical signs of digoxin toxicity (discussed below). Therefore digoxin doses should be decreased by half for animals being treated simultaneously with quinidine.

Procainamide is available in two forms of tablets. The standard tablet is usually given 4 times per day, whereas the sustained-release form (Procan-SR) is given only 3 times per day. The veterinary technician should not break sustained-release tablets in half to achieve a proper dose. Instead the technician should use a slightly smaller dose or the standard procainamide tablets. Because of the more rapid

GI transit time of dogs compared with people, owners should check the dog's stool to make sure that intact sustained-release tablets are not passing through the intestines and out the body with the feces.

β-BLOCKER ANTIARRHYTHMIC DRUGS

β_1 receptors are located primarily in the heart. When stimulated by the sympathetic nervous system or by sympathomimetic drugs (drugs that mimic the effects of the sympathetic nervous system), β_1 receptors cause the heart to beat more rapidly and with greater strength. Increased sympathetic nervous system activity occurs as a means by which the body attempts to increase cardiac output when the output is reduced by a weakened, diseased heart. Unfortunately, increased sympathetic stimulation of the heart can also make the heart more electrically unstable, allowing ectopic foci to appear and arrhythmias to develop. Thus decreasing β_1 sympathetic stimulation may help reduce the generation of ectopic foci and arrhythmias. Drugs that block β receptors are known as *β antagonists* or *β blockers.*

Normally, sympathetic stimulation of the β_1 receptor increases the speed of the depolarization waves through the cardiac conduction system. Therefore blocking these receptors should allow parasympathetic dominance on the SA and AV nodes, slowing conduction of impulses through the heart and decreasing the heart rate. These effects are evident on the ECG as a slowed heart rate (from decreased SA node depolarization) and as a prolonged interval between the P wave (which represents atrial depolarization) and the QRS complex (which represents ventricular depolarization), reflecting slower conduction through the AV node. The prolongation of the PR interval is referred to as first-degree *atrioventricular (AV) block.* If conduction through the AV node is delayed long enough by parasympathetic stimulation of the AV node, the depolarization wave may die out in the AV node and not reach the ventricles. This phenomenon

shows up on the ECG as a P wave without a corresponding QRS complex and is referred to as second-degree AV block. This might be detected on auscultation or pulse palpation as an intermittent missed beat.

Because parasympathetic stimulation slows the heart rate and decreases conduction speed, AV block or bradycardia from parasympathetic stimulation can be reversed with parasympathetic antagonist drugs such as atropine. As a general rule, when treating bradycardia or early heart block associated with the use of β_1-blocking antiarrhythmics, decreasing the β-blocker dose is better than using a β_1-stimulating drug. In cases of β-blocker overdose, atropine may be necessary to maintain adequate cardiovascular function and cardiac output.

Animals that have been receiving a β_1-blocking drug for some time may appear to become tolerant of the β blocker. The slower heart rate associated with the antiarrhythmic effect of the β_1-blocking drug may begin to reverse itself over time. In this case the resistance to the drug is not caused by induction of liver enzymes, as is observed with anesthetic agents or narcotics, but is the result of *upregulation* of the β_1-adrenergic receptors. Upregulation means that the cardiac muscle (and other tissues containing β_1 receptors) begins to produce more β_1 receptors on the surface of the cell to counteract the blocking activity of the β-blocking antiarrhythmics. These additional receptors make the tissues more sensitive to β_1-stimulating compounds such as epinephrine and norepinephrine and require more β-blocking drugs to produce the same antiarrhythmic effect.

Upregulation poses another hazard. In animals that have upregulated their β receptors in response to β-blocker drugs, administration of the β blocker must not be suddenly stopped. With all the additional receptors on the surface of cardiac cells induced by upregulation, the heart becomes very sensitive to β_1-stimulating drugs or endogenous compounds such as epinephrine.

If the β-blocker drug is suddenly stopped, even a normal release of epinephrine by the body may result in extreme tachycardia and possibly severe arrhythmias. Thus, if a patient is to be taken off a β-blocker antiarrhythmic after having been on it for a significant period, withdrawal should be done gradually over several days to several weeks to allow the body to "downregulate" the additional receptors. The rate of the withdrawal can be adjusted based on the resting pulse rate (which reflects the sympathetic and parasympathetic stimulation of the SA node).

Propranolol is a prototype β_1 antagonist. It blocks stimulation of β_1 receptors by the catecholamines such as epinephrine, norepinephrine, dobutamine, and other drugs that produce signs of sympathetic nervous system stimulation. Propranolol decreases the heart rate and prevents tachycardia in response to stress, fear, or excitement by blocking β_1 receptors on the SA node and AV node, thus depressing the automaticity of the SA node and slowing conduction of the depolarization wave through the AV node. Propranolol is also used to decrease the rapid heart rate associated with hyperthyroidism (increased thyroid hormone production) in cats. Automaticity of cardiac muscle cells and cells of the bundle branches is also decreased, reducing the chance of ventricular ectopic foci developing and producing cardiac arrhythmias.

One of the problems with propranolol, and to some degree all other β_1 antiarrhythmic drugs, is that these drugs may not be specific for blocking β_1 receptors but may also block β_2 receptors located on the smooth muscle of the terminal bronchioles (small bronchioles at the end of the bronchiole tree).

Stimulation of β_2-adrenergic receptors of the sympathetic nervous system normally causes bronchodilation as well as vasodilation in cardiac and skeletal muscle. Therefore blocking the β_2 receptors on the small bronchioles allows the parasympathetic nervous system to dominate, resulting in reflex bronchoconstriction. The newer β-blocker antiarrhythmic drugs such as carvedilol (one of the newest β blockers), metoprolol, and atenolol (which is also used to help control signs of cardiomyopathy in cats) are more selective for β_1 receptors, thus reducing, but not totally eliminating, the β_2 antagonist side effects on the bronchioles.

Because β blockers decrease sympathetic stimulation, they have the potential to cause the heart to contract with less force. Drugs that decrease the strength of contraction are referred to as *negative inotropic drugs* (negative inotropes). In animals with congestive heart failure (the heart is unable to pump sufficient blood for the body), the increased contractile force from increased sympathetic nervous system stimulation normally helps increase the contractility in the weakened heart. Therefore, although treatment with a β blocker decreases arrhythmias, its negative inotropic effect could worsen congestive heart failure by blocking the sympathetic stimulation that the body is using to keep the heart contracting with sufficient force to keep it alive. For this reason, β blockers must be used with caution in animals with myocardial failure.

CALCIUM CHANNEL BLOCKER ANTIARRHYTHMIC DRUGS

Calcium channel blockers occasionally used in veterinary medicine include verapamil and diltiazem. Although calcium channel blockers are not frequently used to treat arrhythmias in veterinary patients, verapamil and diltiazem have been used successfully for treatment of supraventricular tachycardia, atrial fibrillation, and atrial flutter. All these drugs combat arrhythmias by blocking calcium (Ca^{++}) channels of cardiac muscle cells, resulting in decreased conduction of depolarization waves and decreased automaticity of parts of the conduction system. Unfortunately, blocking the calcium channels can also decrease the strength of contraction and cardiac output. Therefore calcium channel blockers should be used with caution or not at all in animals with congestive heart failure because of their negative inotropic effect.

A more common use of diltiazem is in cats with hypertrophic cardiomyopathy, a disease in which the ventricular wall of the heart becomes very thickened and stiff such that the heart cannot contract efficiently. In these cats, diltiazem decreases the thickness of the left ventricular wall, increases the dilation of coronary blood vessels, and decreases arrhythmias. In one study the survival rate for cats with hypertrophic cardiomyopathy on diltiazem was three-fold greater than cats treated with propranolol, with many cats becoming asymptomatic after diltiazem therapy.[1]

POSITIVE INOTROPIC AGENTS

Positive inotropic drugs (positive inotropes) increase the strength of contraction of a weakened heart. Most positive inotropic agents work by directly or indirectly making more Ca^{++} available to the contractile proteins in the muscle cell or by increasing the affinity between Ca^{++} and contractile proteins.

Catecholamines (norepinephrine, epinephrine, and dobutamine) are the body's natural positive inotropic agents. Catecholamines are released in response to the body's need for sympathetic nervous system stimulation. Drugs that are either catecholamines or act like catecholamines are called adrenergic drugs in reference to the adrenal gland that is the source of catecholamine hormones. Adrenergic drugs are also called sympathomimetics because they mimic the effects of the sympathetic nervous system.

Adrenergic drugs and catecholamines produce a positive inotropic effect by stimulating β_1 receptors in the cardiac muscle. Although these drugs are strong positive inotropes, they improve cardiac contractility only for a relatively short period. Just as β-blocking drugs cause the myocardial cells to increase β_1 receptors, the increased stimulation of β_1 receptors by catecholamine-type drugs causes the myocardial cells to decrease the number of catecholamine receptors, thus decreasing the cells' ability to respond to stimuli. This phenomenon,

called *downregulation,* is the reason adrenergic drugs progressively lose their ability to produce significant positive inotropic effects over hours to days after initiation of therapy.

Catecholamines are used for short-term positive inotropic treatment, but digoxin is the drug of choice for maintaining long-term positive inotropic effects. Digoxin exerts its positive inotropic effect primarily by making more calcium available for the contractile elements within cardiac muscle cells. It does this indirectly by inhibiting the cell's *sodium-potassium-ATPase pump.* As previously discussed, the sodium-potassium-ATPase pump normally pumps Na^+ out and K^+ in to maintain depolarization. When this pump is inhibited by digoxin, Na^+ begins to accumulate within the cardiac cell. This relatively small increase of Na^+ displaces calcium from its "holding area" in the cardiac cell, making more calcium available to contractile elements and resulting in an increased force of contraction. However, increased Na^+ inside the cardiac muscle cell also increases the risk of spontaneous depolarization and ectopic foci. Therefore one of the side effects of digoxin therapy can be the appearance of arrhythmias associated with ectopic foci.

Digoxin improves the strength of myocardial cell contraction but has a very different effect on the SA and AV nodes. Digoxin enhances the parasympathetic effect on these nodes, slowing the heart rate (SA node effect) and delaying conduction of impulses through the AV node (first-degree AV block). This side effect on the AV node is used therapeutically to control supraventricular tachycardia caused by atrial fibrillation. In atrial fibrillation the danger is not from the quivering atria but from the very rapid contractions of the ventricles that result from continuous bombardment of the AV node by the uncoordinated atrial depolarization waves. If the ventricles beat too quickly, they don't have enough time to fill sufficiently with blood between contractions. The result is a decreased amount of blood ejected from the ventricles with each contraction and an overall decrease in cardiac output. The AV blocking side effect of digoxin decreases the number of depolarization waves that can pass through the AV node, subsequently slowing the ventricular rate and allowing more effective filling of the ventricles before contraction.

Digoxin is a cardiac glycoside, a group of poisons found in nature. Specifically, digoxin was originally derived from digitalis compounds naturally found in the foxglove plant. Because digoxin is a biologic toxin that produces its positive inotropic effect from poisoning the sodium-potassium pump, it would be expected that it would have a small therapeutic index (see Chapter 3). A small therapeutic index means that the dosages that achieve therapeutic concentrations are very close to the dosages that produce toxic concentrations. For that reason, digoxin toxicity is commonly seen in clinical medicine. The veterinary technician must be familiar with the signs of digoxin toxicosis and be able to clearly convey these signs to owners of animals on this drug. Early signs of digoxin toxicity reflect the drug's ability to directly stimulate the chemoreceptor trigger zone involved with the vomiting reflex (see Chapter 4). The first signs of digoxin toxicosis noticed by an owner or veterinary technician would include anorexia, vomiting, and diarrhea. Owners of animals receiving digoxin should be instructed to contact the veterinarian immediately if these early signs of toxicity occur.

As concentrations of digoxin accumulate further into the toxic range, the parasympathetic effect of digoxin slows the heart rate (SA node effect) and increases the PR interval on the ECG (first-degree AV block). As toxicity increases, bradycardia (slow heart rate) becomes more pronounced and the PR interval lengthens until occasional atrial impulses fade out in the AV node, resulting in a P wave without a QRS complex (second-degree AV block).

Third-degree, or complete, AV block is characterized by the ventricles' beating independently of the atria. This type of block is usually associated with severe myocardial disease

and physical changes within the conduction system but is not produced by AV-blocking drugs such as digoxin. Because the SA and AV node effects of digoxin are mostly through enhancement of the parasympathetic effect, most of the AV block and SA bradycardia can be reversed with atropine. Atropine combines with the acetylcholine receptors on the SA and AV node but does not stimulate the receptor. Because atropine occupies the receptor, the acetylcholine (parasympathetic nervous system neurotransmitter) cannot combine with the receptor and thus the parasympathetic effect is blocked or reversed (competitive antagonism; see Chapter 2).

Many of the signs of digoxin toxicosis (especially arrhythmias) appear at lower digoxin concentrations if the animal is hypokalemic (low blood potassium level) or has hypomagnesemia (low blood magnesium level). One of the most commonly used diuretic drugs (drugs that increase urine production) in cardiovascular disease works by increasing secretion of potassium that, over time, can decrease the amount of overall body potassium. The hypokalemia increases the ease at which digoxin toxicosis can occur; thus the dose of digoxin has to be decreased in animals with hypokalemia or hypomagnesemia.

Unfortunately, once digoxin toxicosis signs appear, they may persist for hours to days. Digoxin normally has a relatively long half-life (half-life for dogs of 15 to 50 hours, half-life for cats of 24 to 36 hours) and is eliminated primarily by the kidneys. Thus, if an animal vomits, has diarrhea, or stops eating and drinking as a result of digoxin toxicosis, the animal can become dehydrated. Dehydration decreases blood pressure, decreases renal perfusion, and subsequently decreases digoxin elimination even more. Generally, if an animal receiving digoxin suddenly shows anorexia or vomiting, digoxin therapy should be stopped and the animal examined by a veterinarian. If an ECG suggests digoxin toxicity (that is, shows bradycardia, increased PR interval, or second-degree

CLINICAL APPLICATION
"You Gave Him His Medicine Too?!"

A 9-year-old neutered male terrier mix was admitted with a history of the husband and wife both giving the dog its regular dose of digoxin, 0.125 mg tablet b.i.d. for two consecutive doses. The dog (Jake) began vomiting 1 hour after the morning doses were given (both doses were given approximately 15 minutes apart) and continued to vomit several times. Jake had not eaten anything that morning. The owners did not notice whether the tablets of digoxin were in the vomitus.

On presentation at the veterinary hospital Jake acted quite depressed. His heart rate was 60 beats/min (bradycardia). The ECG showed that the PR interval was increased to almost twice its normal interval (first-degree AV block) and ventricular QRS complexes were occasionally missing after the P wave (second-degree AV block). Ventricular premature contractions (VPCs or PVCs) were also evident on the ECG. The capillary refill time was 3 seconds, indicating decreased perfusion of peripheral tissues most likely caused by decreased arterial blood pressure from the decreased cardiac output.

Normally with oral ingestion of toxicant a clinician might automatically administer an emetic to remove the toxicant from the stomach and then follow it with activated charcoal to decrease absorption of any remaining toxicant. However, in this case Jake had already vomited repeatedly; therefore inducing vomiting with emetic drugs would provide no additional benefit. Activated charcoal was not administered because of the fear of stimulating additional vomiting.

The initial therapeutic regimen the clinician chose included atropine to treat the bradycardia and AV block and a low-flow intravenous infusion of lidocaine in fluids. Jake was closely monitored to prevent overhydration and pulmonary edema. Metoclopramide was administered to try to decrease vomiting from the digoxin stimulation of the CRTZ. The vomiting subsided 4 hours after metoclopramide treatment.

The plasma concentration of digoxin at the time of admission was 5.45 ng/mL (normal therapeutic range, 0.9 to 3.0 ng/mL). The blood urea nitrogen and creatinine levels were slightly elevated, suggesting poor perfusion of the kidney and reduced clearance function. Because digoxin is excreted by the kidneys, it would remain in the body much longer unless renal perfusion returned to normal. However, too-aggressive fluid therapy would result in pulmonary edema. Atropine was used in an attempt to return cardiac output to normal, and the low-flow intravenous fluids were administered to increase the arterial blood pressure sufficiently to increase renal perfusion without producing congestive heart failure. Over the next 24 hours Jake's attitude and condition improved. The PR interval remained prolonged, but the second-degree AV block seemed to resolve. The PVCs were well controlled.

The digoxin concentration at 24 hours after admission was 4.43 ng/mL. The clinician speculated about using a new therapy that involved administering digoxin antibodies to bind and render digoxin molecules ineffective. After consultation, the clinician decided against the therapy because of the cost (minimum of $250). More importantly, despite digoxin concentrations in the toxic range, Jake's clinical condition was stable. Jake continued to improve over the next 24 hours. Forty-eight hours after admission, Jake was interested in eating. Digoxin concentration 48 hours after admission was 2.88 ng/mL. Jake was sent home with instructions to his owners to not start the digoxin for another 24 hours.

What should be learned from this situation: "Treat the patient, not the toxin" should be the mantra regarding toxicosis. The clinician chose to treat those problems that were most potentially life threatening (decreased cardiac output and arrhythmia) and maintained body functions so that the body could clear the digoxin on its own. The clinician also did not treat the digoxin concentration values but adjusted therapy based on the animal's clinical condition.

Dr. Carl Osborne is often quoted as saying, "Don't just do something, stand there." Not overmedicating animals is important because of the potential for drug interactions. For example, the clinician paused before using metoclopramide because the vomiting

> ## CLINICAL APPLICATION—cont'd
> ### "You Gave Him His Medicine Too?!"
>
> was not especially life threatening by itself and meto-clopramide could potentially produce effects on the autonomic nervous system, which was already unbalanced. Fortunately, Jake tolerated the metoclopramide well and the drug had the desired effect of helping reduce vomiting. Jake went home because the clinician helped keep him functioning long enough to allow his body to remove the toxin with some help.
>
> The technician was helpful in this situation by keeping careful track of the cardiovascular parameters (e.g., heart rate, capillary refill time), charting the amount of urine production (to ensure IV fluid
>
> administered was balanced with urinary excretion), frequently auscultating the lungs to detect any suggestion of overhydration, and identifying and recording ECG abnormalities and their frequency so that the clinician could readily assess Jake's improvement.
>
> The technician also played an important role in helping the owners formulate a plan by which a mistaken double-dosing might be avoided in the future. She suggested the owners purchase a plastic "pill minder" that has seven compartments, each labeled with a day of the week, and into which the daily dose of digoxin could be placed.

AV block), digoxin use should be halted for at least 24 hours. In uncomplicated cases of digoxin toxicity, digoxin can usually be resumed after skipping only one or two doses and resuming with a slightly smaller dose. As mentioned previously, severe AV block or bradycardia can be treated with atropine.

Because digoxin is primarily excreted by the kidneys, animals with impaired kidney function (e.g., older animals with early renal failure) must use lower digoxin doses to avoid accumulating toxic concentrations. Monitoring plasma concentrations of digoxin is recommended for all dogs with marginal renal function or who show any early sign of digoxin toxicosis. Because therapeutic concentrations overlap the toxic concentrations, regular plasma drug concentration monitoring allows adjustment of the dosage regimen to avoid toxicity while maintaining effective concentrations.

Some clinicians prefer to dose cats and some prefer to dose dogs based on the surface area of the animal (milligrams of drug per square meter of surface area) on the premise that cats, small dogs, and very large dogs tend to be overdosed or underdosed if their dose is calculated by body weight (in milligrams per kilogram). Many texts or drug formularies contain tables for converting weight, in kilograms, to square meter (m^2) of surface area. The square meter

surface area can also be calculated by the following formulas:

$$\text{For dogs}: \quad m^2 = 10.1 \times \left(\frac{\text{weight in grams}}{10,000} \right)^{2/3}$$

$$\text{For cats}: \quad m^2 = 10.0 \times \left(\frac{\text{weight in grams}}{10,000} \right)^{2/3}$$

Digoxin is available in elixir and tablet form. As discussed in Chapter 3, elixirs are more rapidly and efficiently absorbed from the GI tract than tablets; therefore the dose of the elixir form of digoxin is different than the dose for the tablet form. The bioavailability of digoxin in tablet form is only 60% versus approximately 75% for the elixir. If the dosage form is switched from tablets to elixir or vice versa, the dose must be adjusted to prevent overdosing or underdosing. The following equation can help approximate a new calculated dose:

Dose in tablet form (mg) × 0.6
  = Dose in elixir form (mg) × 0.75

For example, if a dog is being treated with 0.1-mg tablets and needs to be switched to the equivalent dose of elixir, the following calculation would be performed:

0.1 mg in tablet × 0.6 = ____ mg of elixir × 0.75

$$0.06 \text{ mg} = \underline{\hspace{1cm}} \text{ mg of elixir} \times 0.75$$
$$0.06/0.75 = \underline{\hspace{1cm}} \text{ mg of elixir}$$
$$?? = 0.08 \text{ mg of elixir}$$

To check this, we know that the greater bioavailability of the elixir means that less drug needs to be administered to produce the same effect as digoxin tablets. Therefore a smaller elixir dose is required (0.08-mg elixir rather than 0.1-mg tablet) to reach concentrations equivalent to those attained with tablets.

VASODILATORS

Vasoconstriction of peripheral blood vessels is a normal physiologic response to a decreased arterial blood pressure. Vasoconstriction is a protective mechanism by which the body increases arterial blood pressure (e.g., what happens to air pressure in a rubber tube when the end is slightly pinched while blowing into it). Unfortunately, the narrowing of small arterial vessels increases the resistance to blood flow and increases the force required to push the blood through these constricted arterioles. Think about how hard it is to suck a milkshake through a small-diameter straw versus a large-diameter straw. Vasodilator drugs are used to relieve some of the cardiac workload by opening the constricted sphincters, decreasing resistance to flow, and making it easier for the heart to pump blood through these vessels.

VASOCONSTRICTION IN HEART DISEASE

Congestive heart failure means that the heart is not able to eject enough blood to maintain normal tissue perfusion. With a decreased cardiac output, the arterial blood pressure decreases. The decrease in arterial blood pressure is detected by special pressure receptors (baroreceptors) associated with the vasculature. These baroreceptors cause increased release of catecholamines and increase sympathetic nervous system stimulation of the heart and vasculature. As previously discussed, stimulation of the β_1 receptors causes the heart to beat more rapidly and with greater force, resulting in an increase in cardiac output.

Simultaneously, the catecholamines stimulate α_1 receptors on the small arterioles through which blood flows to the capillaries. The smooth muscle in these precapillary arterioles constricts in response to the α_1 receptor stimulation, narrowing the opening and causing vasoconstriction of the precapillary arterioles (Figure 5-8).

When the catecholamines caused vasoconstriction of peripheral arterioles by α_1 stimulation, they also caused vasoconstriction of the renal arterial blood supply to the renal tubules. This vasoconstriction decreases renal perfusion, decreases the force by which water and other molecules are filtered by the glomerulus, and reduces formation of urine. When cells in the renal tubules detect decreased urine formation, they release a compound called renin (Figure 5-9). Renin converts angiotensinogen to *angiotensin I,* which is then quickly converted by the *angiotensin-converting enzyme (ACE)* to *angiotensin II.* Angiotensin II is one of the body's most potent vasoconstrictors; therefore angiotensin II markedly increases the workload on the heart by trying to push blood through the peripheral constricted arterioles.

Angiotensin II further increases the workload on the heart by causing an increase of

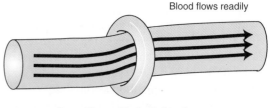

Blood flows readily

Precapillary sphincter (relaxed)

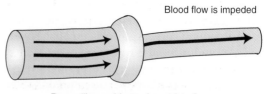

Blood flow is impeded

Precapillary sphincter (constricted)

Figure 5-8 Vasoconstriction of precapillary arterioles.

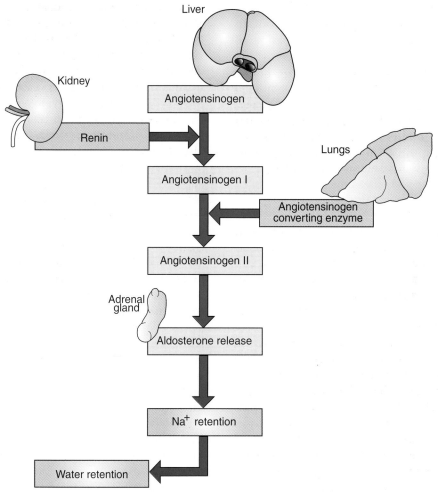

Figure 5-9 Renin-angiotensin cascade.

blood volume in circulation. In addition to its vasoconstriction effect, angiotensin II also stimulates release of the hormone *aldosterone* from the adrenal cortex. Aldosterone increases Na^+ resorption from the kidney, causing retention of Na^+ by the body. The increased sodium in the blood holds water in the blood by osmosis and thus causes expansion of blood volume. Although the increased fluid volume of the blood helps maintain arterial blood pressure, it also creates a larger volume of blood that the heart must pump, thereby increasing the workload of a failing heart.

VASOCONSTRICTION IN SYSTEMIC HYPERTENSION

A significant and prolonged increase in arterial blood pressure (systemic hypertension) is associated most commonly with cats with hyperthyroidism (increased production of hormones by the thyroid gland) and chronic renal disease. Other systemic diseases, such as diabetes mellitus (a lack of insulin production) and overproduction of aldosterone (which would increase sodium retention and increase blood volume), can also produce systemic hypertension.

The actual hypertension can be caused by a combination of increased cardiac output (increased heart rate, increased volume of blood, or both) and vasoconstriction. Think again about blowing into a rubber hose. Pinching the end (vasoconstriction) will increase the pressure within the hose, but the pressure will go much higher if you simultaneously pinch and blow harder (increased cardiac output).

The result of uncontrolled systemic hypertension can be retinal detachment, retinal bleeding and hyphema (bleeding into the interior chambers of the eye), or cerebrovascular accident (stroke). Note that strokes are fairly rare in veterinary patients. Treatment is targeted toward correcting any underlying problem (hyperthyroidism, renal disease), then using low-sodium diets, β blockers (to reduce heart rate and cardiac output), and vasodilators.

VASODILATOR DRUGS

Vasodilators reverse vasoconstriction associated with heart failure by causing relaxation of smooth muscle in the arterioles or veins, blocking the sympathetic stimulation of α_1 receptors, or blocking the *renin-angiotensin system* and preventing production of angiotensin II and aldosterone.

Vasodilators commonly cause a drop in blood pressure (hypotension) that may be manifest as ataxia (weakness), syncope (fainting), or lethargy. These signs may be most evident when the animal rises after being recumbent for some time. In response to the hypotension, the baroreceptors stimulate the sympathetic nervous system, producing an increased heart rate to attempt to bring the blood pressure back to normal. In animals being treated simultaneously with β-blocker antiarrhythmic drugs, this tachycardia response is less likely because β_1 receptors on the heart are blocked, making the hypotensive effect of the vasodilator much more significant. Vasodilators are more likely to produce hypotensive responses in animals on diuretics (drugs that increase water loss) because of the additive effect on hypotension that a decreased blood volume would have.

Because of the hypotensive effect of vasodilators, these drugs are usually given in small initial doses that are increased until signs of hypotension appear or an adequate clinical response is observed. If significant hypotension develops, use of the drug is discontinued for 12 hours and then resumed in slightly smaller doses. Mild hypotensive signs, such as lethargy, observed at the start of vasodilator therapy often disappear after a few days of the regimen.

Animals often adapt to a given dose of vasodilator because each vasodilator drug typically only affects one vasoconstrictive mechanism in the body (e.g., α_1 stimulation or angiotensin II vasoconstriction) while leaving the other vasoconstrictive mechanisms intact. Therefore, after a few weeks or months, these other vasoconstrictive mechanisms may compensate for the effect of the vasodilator drug, resulting in a return to the increased workload on the heart with a subsequent increase in signs of heart failure. In addition to these other compensatory vasoconstrictor mechanisms, the smooth muscle cells may become less sensitive to the drug because of fewer receptors for the drug (downregulation).

Angiotensin-Converting Enzyme Inhibitors (ACE inhibitors)

Enalapril (Enacard), captopril, benazepril (approved for use in dogs in Canada), and lisinopril are all vasodilators that exert their effects on arterial and venous vessels by blocking the angiotensin-converting enzyme (ACE) and thus preventing formation of angiotensin II (the potent vasoconstrictor) and aldosterone (the hormone that increases blood volume by causing sodium retention). Many veterinary cardiologists believe that stimulation of the renin-angiotensin system has profound effects on cardiac disease beyond the vasoconstrictive or increased blood volume effects. Therefore most cardiovascular therapeutic regimens routinely include ACE inhibitors.

ACE inhibitors are thought to have a positive inotropic effect on the heart; however, the mechanism of action for this effect is still unclear. Even though the mechanism is unclear, the beneficial effects of ACE inhibitors are well defined, so more ACE inhibitor–type drugs will continue to become available in human medicine and eventually veterinary medicine.

Although ACE inhibitors have a marked effect in animals with congestive heart failure, or even in animals with left heart disease without signs of failure, normal animals show little response to these drugs. Because these drugs work by blocking ACE, if no ACE is present to inhibit, the drug has little effect. In normal animals the renin-angiotensin system has not been activated and the vasoconstriction from angiotensin II is not present; therefore ACE inhibitors do not have much vasodilatory effect on the vasculature in normal animals.

Hyperkalemia (high concentrations of K^+ in the blood) may occur if ACE inhibitors are used simultaneously with potassium-sparing diuretics or K^+ supplements. Hyperkalemia results from the ACE inhibitors blocking aldosterone production. Aldosterone normally causes Na^+ and water reabsorption at the expense of K^+ excretion; therefore if aldosterone production is blocked by ACE inhibitors, normal K^+ excretion is decreased. Because aldosterone normally enhances Na^+ reabsorption from the urine and ACE inhibitors would block Na^+ reabsorption, ACE inhibitors should be used with caution in animals that are hyponatremic (with low Na^+ concentrations in the blood).

Drugs such as enalapril are considered balanced vasodilators because they relax the smooth muscles of arterioles and veins, so they are useful in treating animals with cardiac disease that involves either the right or left ventricle (or both), such as in severe cardiac valvular disease or cardiomyopathy. As with other vasodilators the initial doses of ACE inhibitors should start small and then be progressively increased to the most effective dose.

Hydralazine

Hydralazine is a vasodilator that directly causes arteriolar smooth muscle to relax, probably through inhibition of calcium movement into smooth muscle cells. Before the advent of ACE inhibitors hydralazine was used to relieve signs of congestive heart failure (CHF) by reducing arterial blood pressure and allowing more blood from the left ventricle to flow outward through the aorta instead of regurgitating back through the left AV valve into the left atrium.

Hydralazine has been shown to produce a slightly greater degree of dilation in the pulmonary arterioles than it does in the systemic (peripheral) arterioles. For that reason, hydralazine may have an advantage for use in right-sided heart failure as a result of vasoconstriction of the pulmonary vasculature.

One of the major drawbacks of hydralazine is the potential for stimulation of the renin-angiotensin system because of the decrease in arterial blood pressure and subsequent decrease in renal perfusion and filtration. Apparently hydralazine is more prone to this effect than the ACE inhibitors. An additional side effect is the drug's slightly positive inotropic effect. In animals with congestive heart failure, this additional stimulation of the heart may increase myocardial oxygen demand (the need the myocardial cells have for oxygen to work and survive) in an animal that already is compromised in its ability to circulate adequate oxygen in the blood. For these reasons, and because of the ready availability of ACE inhibitors, hydralazine is primarily used to treat congestive heart failure or systemic hypertension in animals that do not respond to ACE inhibitors.

Prazosin

Prazosin is an α_1 receptor blocker that causes vasodilation on the arterial and venous sides of the cardiovascular system. Unlike hydralazine, prazosin does not usually cause reflex tachycardia. Nor does prazosin significantly reduce renal perfusion; thus it does not stimulate activation of the renin-angiotensin system to the degree of other vasodilator drugs. Prazosin may be indicated in animals with congestive heart failure that are not responsive to other vasodilator medications.

Unfortunately, prazosin is difficult to obtain in dosage forms small enough for use in cats and small dogs and is therefore not used often in these animals. Prazosin does stimulate its own metabolism, and tolerance to the drug is said to develop rapidly. For these reasons, many veterinary cardiologists do not recommend prazosin because of greater success with other vasodilators and reports that patients receiving prazosin do not live any longer than untreated patients.

Nitroglycerin

Unlike hydralazine, which causes dilation of the small arterioles, nitroglycerin relaxes the primarily blood vessels on the venous side of the circulation. In addition to venodilation (dilation of veins), nitroglycerin may also help dilate coronary arterioles by relaxing the vascular smooth muscles. The drug is well absorbed through the skin and mucous membranes. People with angina pectoris (chest pain) take nitroglycerin by putting a tablet under the tongue. In animals, nitroglycerin cream and nitroglycerin in patch form are applied to the skin to improve cardiac output and reduce pulmonary edema and ascites (abdominal fluid accumulation).

Nitroglycerin cream is applied every 8 to 12 hours to the hairless inner aspect of the pinna of the ear or groin; the latter area is used less frequently because the animal can easily lick it. The nitroglycerin patch provides drug for 24 hours and can be cut into smaller pieces to adjust the dose for smaller patients.

The site of nitroglycerin application should be changed with each dose. Clients should be instructed to always wear gloves when applying this drug because it can be absorbed through their skin as well as the animal's. Children and others should be instructed not to pet the animal where the cream or patch has been applied. Although this compound is the same chemical used in explosives, danger of explosion does not exist because the drug has been diluted with several other compounds (mainly dextrose, lactose, and propylene glycol).

DIURETICS

Diuretics increase urine formation and promote water loss (diuresis). They are used for a variety of purposes that involve removing inappropriate amounts of fluid (e.g., pulmonary edema, cerebral edema), increasing removal of drugs or toxicants normally excreted by the kidney, reducing blood volume and hence arterial blood pressure, and decreasing the workload on a failing heart (congestive heart failure).

In animals with congestive heart failure, Na^+ retention from aldosterone secretion results in water retention in the blood and body tissues. Poor pumping capacity of the failing heart results in blood backing up or becoming congested in capillaries behind the failing side of the heart. In other words, right-sided heart failure results in congestion in peripheral capillaries of the body, increased pressure within the capillaries, and increased force to push water out of the blood into the tissues. Because the peripheral capillaries are affected, the fluid accumulates in the abdomen as ascites. In human beings, this type of congestion results in ascites and swelling of the ankles. Left-sided heart failure results in an increase in pulmonary capillary pressure, causing fluid to move into the pulmonary tissue and leading to pulmonary edema. For these reasons, water removal with diuretics is part of the therapeutic regimen for congestive heart failure.

All diuretics act by the same basic mechanism. Diuretics prevent reabsorption of Na^+ or K^+ from the renal tubules or they enhance their secretion into the tubules. The net increase of Na^+ or K^+ creates an osmotic force that draws water into or retains water within the renal tubules, thus removing water from the body as urine. Diuretics should be used cautiously in any animal with hypovolemia (low blood volume) or hypotension from any cause because the blood fluid volume decrease associated with fluid loss will further reduce blood pressure (Figure 5-10).

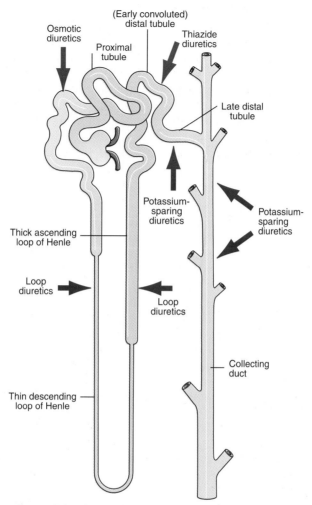

Figure 5-10 Anatomy of the nephron and site of action of diuretics.

LOOP DIURETICS

Loop diuretics such as furosemide (Lasix) are the most commonly used diuretics in veterinary medicine. The term "loop" refers to the way these drugs produce diuresis by inhibiting Na$^+$ reabsorption from the loop of Henle. Retention of Na$^+$ in the forming urine osmotically retains water in the urine, prevents water reabsorption back into the body, and results in water loss as urine.

Loop diuretics do not result in sodium loss even though they primarily work by preventing reclamation of sodium from the renal tubules and potentially a large sodium loss in the urine. Because sodium is so important to the body, the distal convoluted tubule (downstream from the loop of Henle) has an active transport mechanism by which sodium is reabsorbed and potassium is excreted in exchange for the sodium. Because the number of solutes (ions) in the urine remains the same and exerts the same degree of osmotic pressure to draw in or retain water, the diuretic effect continues in spite of the removal of sodium from the forming urine. Prolonged use of loop diuretics, which would result in continual potassium loss, may result in hypokalemia (low blood potassium) if the animal's diet is not supplemented with additional potassium. As previously mentioned, hypokalemia can significantly increase the risk of arrhythmias associated with digoxin toxicity.

Loop diuretics can be of some use in animals in the early stages of renal failure because they increase prostaglandin E_2, a naturally occurring vasodilator that increases renal blood flow. Because loop diuretics normally reach their sites of action in the loop of Henle by being actively transported (secreted) by the proximal convoluted tubule into the renal tubule lumen (upstream from the loop of Henle), in the advanced stages of renal failure the proximal convoluted tubule cannot actively transport furosemide from the blood into the renal tubule, significantly decreasing furosemide's effectiveness.

Furosemide and other loop diuretics have been implicated in ototoxicity (toxicity associated with hearing or the inner ear). Ion imbalances, especially with use of large doses of furosemide in cats, are believed to change the electrolyte balance in the inner ear, resulting in a loss of hearing. The risk of ototoxicosis is increased if other ototoxic compounds, such as aminoglycoside antibiotics (e.g., gentamicin, amikacin), are used concurrently with the loop diuretic. Unless permanent damage is done to the cochlea or other parts of the hearing apparatus, hearing apparently returns after diuretic use is discontinued.

THIAZIDE DIURETICS

Thiazide diuretics such as chlorothiazide, hydrochlorothiazide, and other thiazidelike diuretics are not often used by themselves in veterinary medicine for cardiac problems because of the safety and greater effectiveness of furosemide. After administration, thiazides are secreted by the proximal convoluted tubule, pass by the loop of Henle without causing any effect, and then move to the initial segment of the distal convoluted tubule where they decrease resorption of sodium and chloride. As with loop diuretics, the increased retained sodium in the urine is exchanged for potassium as it moves through the rest of the distal convoluted tubule. Thus thiazide diuretics can also cause a loss of K^+ with resultant hypokalemia.

Thiazides are less potent than loop diuretics because of the site of action in the distal convoluted tubule. Normally 90% of the sodium is resorbed in the loop of Henle, such that the urine arriving in the distal convoluted tubule contains significantly less sodium. Blocking reabsorption of Na^+ at that point only slightly increases the osmotic force within the urine, meaning that less osmotic force is available to retain water within the tubule and hence less diuretic effect. With long-term use of thiazides, the body seems to adjust to the thiazide-induced Na^+ loss, resulting in a further reduction of the diuretic effect. Thiazides may be used in early stages of congestive heart failure because they produce moderate diuresis without significantly altering the overall body balance of electrolytes (e.g., sodium, potassium). They may also be used in conjunction with furosemide when the kidneys become less responsive to furosemide alone.

POTASSIUM-SPARING DIURETICS

Spironolactone is a diuretic that is a competitive antagonist of aldosterone, the hormone that normally causes sodium reabsorption from the distal renal tubules and collection ducts. In animals with congestive heart failure, the decrease in arterial blood pressure stimulates the renin-angiotensin system and release of aldosterone to increase blood volume by body sodium retention. By blocking aldosterone, less sodium is reabsorbed from the renal tubule back into the body, more Na^+ remains in the lumen of the renal tubules, and water is osmotically held in the tubule, preventing its reabsorption and increasing diuresis.

Unlike the previous diuretics, spironolactone actually causes sodium ion excretion and potassium conservation by the body. Drugs such as spironolactone are called potassium-sparing diuretics. These drugs are likely not as effective as loop diuretics for the reasons described for the thiazide diuretics (90% of sodium is reabsorbed before the distal convoluted tubule).

Still, spironolactone can be useful for animals with excessive fluid retention associated with congestive heart failure that is unresponsive to furosemide or thiazide alone, or in situations in which hypokalemia is a concern.

OSMOTIC DIURETICS

Although not used for diuresis associated with cardiac problems, mannitol and other osmotic diuretics have their roles. Mannitol is a carbohydrate (sugar) and, unlike the other diuretics that work by inhibiting renal tubular resorption of Na^+ or K^+, mannitol retains water in the renal tubules by its physical presence within the lumen of the renal tubule. This sugar is freely filtered from the blood (glomerular capillaries) into the Bowman's capsule but is poorly reabsorbed from the renal tubule. Its presence provides a solute that osmotically retains water in the renal tubular lumen. Mannitol is primarily used to reduce cerebral edema associated with head trauma and as a diuretic for flushing absorbed toxins from the body.

CARBONIC ANHYDRASE INHIBITORS

Carbonic anhydrase inhibitors such as acetazolamide are not often used as diuretics in veterinary medicine but may be used to decrease production of aqueous humor in the eye, which reduces intraocular pressure in animals with glaucoma. Because of its relatively weak diuretic effect and the ready availability of more effective diuretics, acetazolamide is not used to treat cardiac problems in veterinary patients. Veterinary ophthalmology texts contain information on use of this diuretic in the treatment of glaucoma.

OTHER DRUGS USED IN TREATING CARDIOVASCULAR DISEASE

ASPIRIN

Aspirin (acetylsalicylic acid) inhibits formation of prostaglandins and thromboxanes. It reduces aggregation (clumping) of platelets among other actions. This reduces the chances of clot formation and subsequent occlusion of blood vessels. Use of aspirin has been advocated for the treatment of dogs with heartworm infection to reduce clot formation and retard the proliferation of pulmonary arterial endothelium that can decrease blood flow to the lungs (see Chapter 13). In cats, aspirin can reduce thrombus formation associated with hypertrophic or congestive cardiomyopathy. However, aspirin must be used cautiously in cats because they do not metabolize the drug as readily as other species. Aspirin is relatively safe to use in cats if the drug is given with a 48-hour dose interval to allow sufficient time to metabolize and eliminate the drug. Daily use of aspirin in human beings is advocated to decrease the risk of stroke or myocardial infarction by reducing the chance for clot formation in the coronary arteries or vessels in the brain.

BRONCHODILATORS

Aminophylline and theophylline dilate constricted bronchiole airways (see Chapter 6). These drugs may be used in animals with congestive heart failure and pulmonary edema to increase perfusion of the lungs and decrease the workload on the right ventricle. When bronchodilation allows increased oxygen to reach the alveoli, the vasculature associated with those alveoli dilates, easing the workload on the right heart by allowing blood to flow more easily through that portion of the lung.

SEDATIVES AND TRANQUILIZERS

Sedatives and tranquilizers are sometimes used to calm an anxious animal with aerophagia ("air hunger") because of pulmonary edema associated with advanced congestive heart failure. The combination of tachycardia from increased sympathetic tone caused by fear and anxiety and insufficient oxygenation of the stimulated heart can result in death from arrhythmia. Sometimes merely calming the animal reduces the heart rate and allows the weakened heart to pump sufficient blood to meet the physiologic needs, thereby reducing the risk of fatal arrhythmias.

Box 5-1 Cardiovascular Drug Categories and Names

ANTIARRHYTHMICS

Sodium influx inhibitors
  Lidocaine
  Quinidine
  Procainamide
  Mexiletine
β Blockers
  Propranolol (Inderal)
  Atenolol
Calcium channel blockers
  Diltiazem

POSITIVE INOTROPES

Adrenergic drugs/catecholamines
  Norepinephrine/epinephrine
  Dobutamine
Digoxin

VASODILATORS

ACE inhibitors

Enalapril (Enacard)
Captopril
Lisinopril
Benazepril
Hydralazine
Prazosin
Nitroglycerin

DIURETICS

Loop diuretics, furosemide (Lasix)
Thiazide diuretics, chlorothiazide
Potassium-sparing diuretics, spironolactone
Osmotic diuretics, mannitol

OTHER DRUGS

Aspirin
Aminophylline, theophylline
Sedatives, tranquilizers

REFERENCES

1. Bright JM, Golden AL: Evidence for and against efficacy of calcium channel blockers for management of hypertrophic cardiomyopathy in cats, *Vet Clin North Am* 21(5):1023-1034, 1991.

RECOMMENDED READING

Abbott JA: *Digoxin therapy,* Proceedings of the 18th American College of Veterinary Interval Medicine (ACVIM) Symposium, Seattle, WA, May 2000.

Boothe DM: *Small animal clinical pharmacology and therapeutics,* Philadelphia, 2001, WB Saunders.

Atkins CE: *Therapeutic strategies in feline heart disease.* In Proceedings of the American College of Veterinary Internal Medicine Annual Meeting, Charlotte, NC, 2003.

Ettinger SJ: Cardiac arrhythmias: diagnosis and treatment. In World Small Animal Veterinary Association Congress Proceedings, Rhodes, Greece, 2004.

Fox PR: Feline cardiomyopathies: new advances in diagnosis and treatment. Proceedings of the North American Veterinary Conference, Orlando, FL, January 2001.

Fox PR: Therapy for feline myocardial diseases. In Bonagura, editor: *Kirk's current veterinary therapy XIII,* Philadelphia, 2000, WB Saunders.

Moise SN: Ventricular arrhythmias. In Bonagura JD, editor: *Kirk's current veterinary therapy XIII,* Philadelphia, 2000, WB Saunders.

Plumb DC: *Veterinary drug handbook,* ed 5, Ames, IA, 2005, Blackwell Publishing.

Rishniw M, Thomas WPP: Bradyarrhythmias. In Bonagura JD, editor: *Kirk's current veterinary therapy XIII,* Philadelphia, 2000, WB Saunders.

Sisson D: Medical management of refractory congestive heart failure in dogs. In Bonagura JD, editor: *Kirk's current veterinary therapy XIII,* Philadelphia, 2000, WB Saunders.

Tilley LP: *A current cardiac formulary.* In Proceedings of the Western Veterinary Conference, Las Vegas, NV, 2004.

Ware WA, Keene BW: Outpatient management of chronic heart failure. In Bonagura JD, editor: *Kirk's current veterinary therapy XIII,* Philadelphia, 2000, WB Saunders.

Wright KN: Assessment and treatment of supraventricular tachyarrhythmias. In Bonagura JD, editor: *Kirk's current veterinary therapy XIII,* Philadelphia, 2000, WB Saunders.

Self-Assessment

REVIEW QUESTIONS

Fill in the following blanks with the correct item from the Key Terms list.

1. _____ pacemaker of the heart.

2. _____ delays the electrical impulses coming from the atria into the ventricles and allows the ventricles to fill with blood.

3. _____ ion that passes into the cardiac cell on depolarization.

4. _____ specific receptor that increases the heart rate.

5. _____ specific receptor that causes peripheral vasoconstriction.

6. _____ specific receptor that causes bronchodilation.

7. _____ part of the ECG representing movement of the depolarization wave through the AV node.

8. _____ two types of cholinergic receptors.

9. _____ neurotransmitter associated with the sympathetic nervous system.

10. _____ site from which the electrical activity of an arrhythmia originates.

Fill in the following blanks with the correct drug described in Box 5-1.

11. _____ drug of choice for controlling ventricular arrhythmias (ectopic focus); cannot be given orally because of GI upset and first-pass effect; cats are more sensitive to this drug than dogs.

12. _____ decreases arrhythmias by decreasing the stimulatory effect of the sympathetic nervous system on the heart.

13. _____ most commonly used positive inotropic agent; has a narrow therapeutic index and toxicosis is common.

14. _____ orally administered, sodium-blocking antiarrhythmic used to control lidocaine-responsive arrhythmias (hint: not procainamide or quinidine).

15. _____ positive inotropic drug; can only be used effectively for short periods before the heart muscle downregulates.

16. _____ diuretic of choice; very effective; called a loop diuretic because of its site of action in the kidney.

17. _____ potassium-sparing diuretic; not as effective as furosemide.

18. _____   current vasodilator of choice; is an ACE inhibitor.

19. _____   used to decrease spontaneous clot formation.

20. _____   topically applied vasodilator (cream).

21. _____   reverses first- or second-degree heart block.

22. Indicate whether the following statements are true or false.

   A. The QRS complex on the ECG represents atrial depolarization.

   B. Upregulation is the increased number of receptors produced by a cell that increases the sensitivity of the cell to a stimulus or drug.

   C. During the absolute refractory period, no amount of stimulus can cause the cell to depolarize again.

   D. Hypokalemia (low blood potassium) increases the risk for digoxin toxicosis.

   E. The early signs of digoxin toxicosis that the owner needs to be aware of (and watch for) are related to the GI tract (vomiting, diarrhea, anorexia).

   F. A positive inotropic drug is one that decreases the heart rate.

   G. Blood is pumped to the lungs from the left ventricle.

   H. The advantage of β-blocker drugs over other antiarrhythmics is that if problems arise after several weeks of therapy, the drug can be safely stopped immediately.

   I. When switching from the liquid form of digoxin to the tablet form, the dose has to be decreased to provide an equivalent amount of drug.

   J. A rapid heart rate (240 beats/min) caused by a problem in the atria would be classified as a supraventricular tachycardia.

   K. In severe digoxin toxicosis, a slow heart rate would be expected.

   L. Sympathetic nervous system stimulation of the heart causes an increase in rate and force of the heart contraction.

   M. Acetylcholine is the neurotransmitter associated with parasympathetic nervous system effects.

   N. Angiotensin II is a potent vasodilator.

   O. Peripheral vasoconstriction causes an increased resistance to blood flow.

   P. Aldosterone is a hormone that causes sodium to be reabsorbed from the renal tubules.

   Q. First-degree AV block with digoxin toxicosis is seen on the ECG as an increase in the PR interval.

   R. Nonspecific β receptor blockers can cause bronchodilation as a side effect.

23. What kind of noncardiac drugs do we use to help an animal that has aerophagia associated with congestive heart failure? _____

24. What drug slows the ventricular contraction rate in animals with atrial fibrillation without eliminating the atrial fibrillation itself?   _____

25. What organ of the body eliminates digoxin?   _____

APPLICATION QUESTIONS

1. If the veterinarian were to thread a catheter into the heart by way of the jugular vein into the anterior vena cava and then into the heart, what would be the first chamber of the heart the catheter would enter? What if the catheter were threaded up the femoral artery to the dorsal aorta and into the aorta itself?

2. Describe the path of a depolarization wave from the SA node to the ventricles. What physiologic purpose does the delay at the AV node serve?

3. What waveform on the ECG represents depolarization of the atria? Of the ventricles? Of the AV node?

4. Many drugs act by blocking movement of ions across cellular membranes. Describe the ionic movement into and out of cardiac muscle cells during depolarization and repolarization. At what stage of the depolarization cycle is a cell considered refractory?

5. If a drug is an adrenergic agonist, does it stimulate sympathetic or parasympathetic effects?

6. What are the two types of cholinergic receptors described in this chapter? What effect do drugs that stimulate these receptors have on heart rate, pupil size, and GI function?

7. Classify the following arrhythmias according to heart rate (tachycardia or bradycardia) and the location of the problem (supraventricular or ventricular):

   A. Arrhythmia in a dog with ventricular contraction rate of 200 per minute caused by atrial fibrillation

   B. Arrhythmia in a dog with a ventricular contraction rate of 40 per minute caused by inability of the SA node to depolarize normally

   C. Arrhythmia in a dog with a series of PVCs that increases the heart rate to 150 beats/min for approximately 30 seconds

8. What is the difference between ventricular flutter and fibrillation? What is a paroxysm of PVCs?

9. The veterinarian is looking at the cardiac monitor and mentions that the dog's heart is alternating back and forth between first- and second-degree AV block. What are first- and second-degree AV blocks? What is the difference between the two? What is the treatment of choice for reversing AV block?

10. A veterinary technician attempted to do a line block with lidocaine to anesthetize locally the side of a sheep for a surgical procedure. Unfortunately, she injected most of the lidocaine intravenously instead of subcutaneously. The sheep became ataxic, fell over, and began to seize. The seizures lasted a few minutes and were then followed by a period of ataxia and

depression, which lasted approximately 20 minutes. Why does lidocaine toxicity show signs of CNS depression and excitement (seizures) at different stages of toxicity?

11. The veterinarian in your practice labels two bottle of lidocaine with brightly colored tape. One color is for the lidocaine used to produce local anesthesia, and the other color for the lidocaine used to treat arrhythmias. What is the difference between these two forms of lidocaine?

12. A dog's medical chart indicates that the animal has been receiving digoxin to help increase contractility of the heart. The new associate veterinarian, a recent graduate, considers adding quinidine to the regimen to control the occasional PVCs seen on the ECG strip. What effect is quinidine likely to have in this dog because of the digoxin he is receiving?

13. The veterinarian asks you to dispense some sustained-release procainamide tablets for a client's dog. You calculate the required dose and determine that the dog needs 1½ of the sustained-release tablets per dose. The veterinarian tells you to label the vial and instruct the client to give only 1 tablet per dose rather than the 1½ tablets per dose that you calculated. Why did the doctor elect to reduce the dose to 1 tablet rather than instruct the client to give 1½ tablets per dose?

14. The veterinarian has you run an ECG strip on a dog with a history of ventricular arrhythmias that are responsive to a β-antagonist antiarrhythmic. You see that the PR interval is prolonged, suggesting a first-degree AV block. The veterinarian comments that the AV block may be caused by the β blocker that the dog is currently being given. How can a β blocker cause AV block? Why are these drugs dangerous to use in animals with poor cardiac contractility?

15. Why do β-blocker drugs begin to lose their effectiveness? Does the same thing happen to β agonists used to increase cardiac contractility?

16. Explain why propranolol, an antiarrhythmic drug, may contribute to dyspnea (difficult breathing) in animals with respiratory disease.

17. What are catecholamines? Why are catecholamine drugs not often used as a long-term treatment to increase contractility of a weakened heart?

18. What effect does digoxin have on the AV and SA nodes? Does third-degree AV block occur with drugs?

19. Why is using digoxin in animals with renal failure or animals with hypokalemia risky?

20. What changes on the ECG tracing occur with digoxin toxicosis?

21. Why might a veterinarian choose to dose digoxin on the basis of the animal's body surface area instead of weight?

22. An animal is treated with 0.2-mg tablets of digoxin, and you want to switch the dosage form to digoxin elixir. What would be the equivalent elixir dose? What would be the equivalent tablet dose if you wanted to switch from 0.5 mg of elixir to a tablet form?

23. Vasoconstriction is a natural physiologic response to certain changes in the body. It also plays a role in congestive heart failure. How does vasoconstriction occur as a consequence of heart failure, and how can it make heart failure worse?

24. What are the steps by which the renin-angiotensin system produces vasoconstriction and water retention?

25. Mrs. Jones' 14-year-old poodle has been put on a vasodilator. You are to inform Mrs. Jones of the signs of adverse reactions her dog might have to this drug. What are the signs of vasodilator overdose that pet owners should be warned about?

26. If the veterinarian prescribes nitroglycerin cream for use on a canine patient, what precautions should owners take to protect themselves when treating their animal with the topical nitroglycerin product?

27. Why does enalapril cause vasodilation in animals with heart failure but have little effect in normal animals?

28. Which diuretic drug seems to be most effective in veterinary patients? What is this drug's mechanism of action? How does this drug affect the body's electrolyte balance?

29. Why is furosemide considered a loop diuretic? How does this make furosemide more effective than spironolactone or the thiazide diuretics?

30. Mannitol is kept on the shelf for use as a diuretic. Why is mannitol not used in congestive heart failure to cause diuresis, as do the other diuretics such as furosemide, chlorothiazide, and spironolactone?

31. Why is spironolactone considered a potassium-sparing diuretic? What is the physiology behind that statement?

32. You overhear the veterinarian telling the owner of a cat with cardiomyopathy to administer aspirin. However, you remember that aspirin must be used with caution in cats. Is the doctor wrong to recommend aspirin for this cat?

33. Why can the judicious use of sedatives significantly help some animals in congestive heart failure?

Drugs Affecting the Respiratory System

key terms

aerosolization
aerosol therapy
α_1 receptor
β_1 receptor
β_2 receptor
bronchoconstriction
centrally acting antitussive

chronic obstructive
  pulmonary disease
cor pulmonale
dyspnea
H_1 receptors
inspissated
locally acting antitussive

metered-dose inhalers
mucociliary apparatus
nebulization
productive/nonproductive
  cough
opioid
serotonin

objectives

After studying this chapter, the veterinary technician should be able to explain:

1. The mechanisms by which the respiratory system protects itself

2. The mechanisms by which antitussives work

3. What mucolytics, expectorants, and decongestants do in respiratory disease and how they alter physiology to produce their effect

4. The types of bronchodilators and how they produce their effects

5. How corticosteroids and antihistamines are useful in respiratory disease and how they differ from each other in their mechanisms

6. The role of diuretics and oxygen in the treatment of respiratory disease

The body is quite effective at protecting the respiratory tract from injury or infection by either preventing foreign substances from reaching the alveoli or expelling offensive substances from the respiratory tract. The upper respiratory tract decreases entrance of materials or offensive substances by causing sneezing or excessive mucus secretions to expel or dilute the offending substances. If a substance makes it past the nose, any stimulation of the laryngeal area, trachea, or bronchial tree elicits a coughing response that can range from a deep, subtle cough to a retching gag. The vocal folds of the larynx can slam shut with a spasm if they are irritated or mechanically stimulated (e.g., laryngospasm when trying to place an endotracheal tube). In the trachea and larger bronchioles a sheet of sticky mucus traps particles. The mucus is then swept upwards by microscopic, hairlike cilia so that the mucus and trapped materials are coughed up and expelled. This combination of mucus and cilia constitutes the *mucociliary apparatus.* Because this apparatus moves mucus and trapped materials up the bronchi and trachea, it is sometimes referred to as the mucociliary escalator. Deep within the bronchial tree at the level near the alveoli the airways are surrounded by smooth muscle that can constrict and close off the alveolus, preventing foreign particles from entering and causing damage or inflammation *(bronchoconstriction).* Finally, if foreign particles do make it to the alveoli, macrophages (phagocytic cells) engulf the particles or bacteria.

When these protective mechanisms work effectively, the body and respiratory tree are healthy. But under certain conditions these protective mechanisms may become overstimulated or act when they are not needed for protection. In these situations the animal exhibits signs of disease that need to be controlled to some degree. For example, a *nonproductive cough* that continues for months may lead to changes in the airways that result in collapsing of the trachea or vascular changes in the lungs that can lead to heart problems (a condition called *cor pulmonale*). Another example of a protective mechanism causing disease or damage is bronchoconstriction associated with asthma. In these situations the veterinarian must intervene to prevent further tissue damage or death from an overzealous protective reaction. Whenever a cough, nasal secretions, or sneezing are treated, the benefit of the treatment must be weighed against the effect it has in decreasing the body's natural protective mechanisms. Box 6-1, listing respiratory drugs, can be found at the end of this chapter.

ANTITUSSIVES

Antitussive drugs block the cough reflex. The cough reflex is coordinated by the cough center, which is a cluster of neurons located next to the respiratory centers in the medullary area of the brainstem. The presence of irritation or stimulation of cough receptors in the larynx, trachea, bronchi, or bronchioles sends impulses to the brainstem, where the cough reflex causes contraction of the appropriate respiratory muscles to produce a sharp, forceful expiration (cough).

The nature of the cough is determined by the location of the cough receptors that are stimulated and whether mucus is brought up with the cough. When the larynx or pharynx is stimulated by irritation or pressure from food or other materials, receptors send impulses to the brainstem by way of the vagus nerve, resulting in a gagging, violent, retching type of coughing. Stimulation of these receptors can also produce a reflex constriction of the small terminal bronchioles (bronchoconstriction). This choking cough is observed when food is accidentally inhaled or anything irritates the pharynx.

Receptors lower in the trachea and those located in the bronchi respond to mechanical and chemical irritation or the release of histamine by producing a deep cough mediated by the cough center. Tachypnea (rapid breathing) and reflex bronchoconstriction may also accompany this type of stimulation. This deeper type of cough is associated with bronchitis, inhalation of irritating gases, allergic bronchoconstriction, or pressure of the bronchi from an enlarged heart.

The cough can also be classified as productive or nonproductive according to the amount of mucus associated with the cough. A *productive cough* produces mucus, whereas a nonproductive cough is dry and hacking, with no significant mucus brought up. A nonproductive cough may occur in the early stages of infection or inflammation when the mucous glands lining the respiratory tree have not yet increased production of mucus. A nonproductive cough may become productive as the disease progresses. A nonproductive cough may also be associated with chronic conditions such as chronic bronchitis, in which the mucus produced becomes *inspissated* (dry and sticky) and thus accumulates in the bronchi instead of being coughed up. A nonproductive cough may also occur in an animal that is significantly dehydrated because in this state the mucous glands are unable to produce liquid secretions.

Antitussives suppress the coughing mechanism that the body uses to remove mucus, cellular debris, exudates, and other products accumulating within the bronchi as a result of infection or inflammation. Therefore veterinarians should use antitussives cautiously and avoid large doses in animals with a very productive cough or a nonproductive cough in which the mucus is very sticky and not easily moved by the mucociliary apparatus (e.g., chronic bronchitis). In such situations, the mucociliary apparatus may not be able to clear the respiratory tree debris by itself, and the body may be relying on the cough to prevent obstruction of the airways by accumulation of excessive mucus and debris.

Antitussives are sometimes described as centrally acting or locally acting. A *centrally acting antitussive,* such as the codeine or hydrocodone found in cough syrups, reduces coughing by suppressing the cough center neurons in the brainstem. In contrast, a *locally acting antitussive,* such as a cough lozenge, reduces coughing by directly soothing the respiratory mucosal irritation that is initiating the cough. Centrally acting antitussives are the only type used in veterinary medicine because veterinary patients are unwilling to hold lozenges in their mouth long enough to be effective.

Antitussives are primarily used to treat animals with dry, nonproductive coughs that produce little or no mucus and are not associated with airway obstruction caused by inspissated mucus. Often these nonproductive coughs associated with tracheitis (inflammation of the trachea) or tracheobronchitis (inflammation of the trachea and bronchi) keep the pet and the owner from getting their proper rest and often delay resolution of the underlying cause of the cough (if an infectious or a short-term inflammatory process). One of the most common uses of antitussives is for treatment of uncomplicated tracheobronchitis in dogs, commonly called kennel cough. The retching type of cough associated with kennel cough is often punctuated by gagging of small amounts of mucus that the owner interprets as vomitus. The harsh coughing produces inflammation of the trachea, which stimulates more coughing, which further irritates the airway. This pattern can continue for weeks after the inciting agent has been removed or successfully treated unless the cough is treated. Cases of untreated tracheobronchitis can result in chronic bronchitis, secondary bacterial bronchitis or pneumonia, cardiac problems (cor pulmonale), or eventual weakening of the cartilaginous tracheal rings and subsequent tracheal collapse. In this situation the protective mechanism of the body is doing more harm than good and needs to be suppressed.

BUTORPHANOL

Butorphanol (Torbutrol) is a centrally acting *opioid* cough suppressant. Because it is an opioid (meaning *opiumlike*), is it considered a narcotic drug with potential for abuse and is therefore classified as a class C-IV controlled substance. Butorphanol is also commonly used as an analgesic (pain-killing) drug. Although all opioid drugs suppress the respiratory center as a side effect and as a means of suppressing the cough reflex, compared with codeine and hydrocodone butorphanol has fewer respiratory or cardiovascular depression effects. At antitussive doses, butorphanol causes less sedation compared with stronger opioid drugs but may still produce some nausea or appetite suppression.

HYDROCODONE

Hydrocodone (Hycodan) is a C-III narcotic available only by prescription from a veterinarian with a Drug Enforcement Administration clearance for writing C-III prescriptions. Hydrocodone is more potent as an antitussive than codeine, and sedation is often noted in animals treated with hydrocodone. Long-term administration of this drug can result in constipation because opioids slow gastrointestinal (GI) motility and decrease intestinal secretions (see Chapter 3).

An important rule to remember is that all potent opioids have the potential to mask pain in the animal. In animals with other disease, the perception of pain from the inflammation associated with the disease may be reduced, obscuring the clinical signs of the disease and allowing progression of the disease to occur unnoticed.

As with other controlled substances, hydrocodone has the potential for human abuse because of the psychologically and physiologically addictive qualities of opioids. Veterinary technicians should take notice of clients' repeated requests for strong opioid compounds to relieve their pet's cough. The technician should document these requests and inform the veterinarian.

CODEINE

Codeine, a relatively weak opioid and narcotic, is a component of many cough suppressant preparations. All products containing codeine are either prescription preparations with a C-II (pure codeine) or C-III (e.g., acetaminophen +

codeine) rating, or through the pharmacist as C-V (some cough and cold preparations with codeine). The sedative, nausea, and constipation effects of codeine are similar to those of hydrocodone.

DEXTROMETHORPHAN

Unlike the opioids from which it is chemically derived, dextromethorphan is an antitussive that is not a controlled substance and therefore is a common ingredient in over-the-counter (OTC) nonprescription cough, flu, and cold preparations. Dextromethorphan has a different chemical structure than the other more potent narcotics. This change in structure allows it to have antitussive activity without the addictive qualities of codeine or hydrocodone. The antitussive activity of dextromethorphan is not as effective as butorphanol or other prescription antitussives.

One of the reasons for veterinary technicians being aware of this drug is that owners may attempt to medicate pets for colds or cough by using human cold products containing dextromethorphan. Although dextromethorphan in OTC products is fairly harmless to animals, the other compounds in cold or flu preparations can cause significant harm. For example, acetaminophen (Tylenol) is a common ingredient in OTC cold and flu products with dextromethorphan and is very toxic in cats. For these reasons, OTC products should not be used to control coughing in pets.

MUCOLYTICS, EXPECTORANTS, AND DECONGESTANTS

Removal of materials or debris from the trachea and bronchioles is the function of the cough reflex and the mucociliary apparatus. Glands and mucus-producing cells line the respiratory tree where they produce the sticky mucus layer that traps particles that enter the lower respiratory tree. Ciliated columnar epithelial cells also line the respiratory tree from the larger bronchioles to the laryngeal area. The microscopic cilia sweep mucus and particulate matter up to the oropharynx, where it is coughed up and swallowed or expectorated (spit out). Some drugs are developed with the intent to enhance the activity of the mucociliary apparatus (Figure 6-1).

In severely dehydrated animals the mucous membranes become dry and the mucus layer becomes very sticky, impairing the action of the mucociliary apparatus. Dehydrated animals often exhibit a nonproductive cough, but after being rehydrated the mucus regains its normal fluid consistency and the cough may become quite productive. Thus the veterinary professional should correct for systemic dehydration before deciding whether an expectorant or mucolytic agent should be given.

MUCOLYTICS

The mucus in the respiratory tract can sometimes become difficult for the underlying cilia to move. For example, with infection or inflammation inflammatory cells move into the affected area to combat the infectious agent or to help clean up the cellular debris. During this process, the cells die and lyse, releasing their contents. When the cells die in the mucus, the DNA found in inflammatory cells or cellular debris chemically reacts with mucus, causing the mucus to become more viscous (thicker) and sticky. When this happens, the cilia cannot readily move the viscous mucus and the mucociliary apparatus becomes less effective. Mucolytic agents, as the name implies, are designed to break up, or lyse, mucus and reduce its viscosity so the cilia can more readily move it out of the respiratory tract. Acetylcysteine (Mucomyst) is a mucolytic agent that decreases the viscosity of mucus by breaking apart the disulfide bonds (S—S) that were contributed to the mucus by DNA strands and that contribute significantly to the viscosity of the mucus.

Acetylcysteine may be administered by *nebulization*, which is the inhalation of a fine mist containing the drug, or by mouth. If it is given by mouth, the unpleasant taste must be

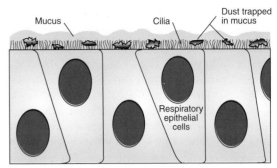

Figure 6-1 The mucociliary apparatus traps dust particles and other debris in a blanket of mucus.

masked with flavoring agents or the drug must be administered by feeding tube. Although nebulization provides the potential to deliver drug to the surface of the bronchi and bronchioles, it is not very effective for veterinary patients because the animals resist inhaling the mist deeply. Because acetylcysteine is also irritating to the respiratory tree, it may require the use of a bronchodilator before nebulization treatment to prevent reflex bronchoconstriction.

Acetylcysteine is also used as the intravenous antidote for acetaminophen toxicosis in cats. Acetylcysteine helps metabolize the hepatotoxic acetaminophen metabolite to a nontoxic metabolite and helps prevent acetaminophen's conversion of hemoglobin to nonfunctional methemoglobin.

Owners sometimes treat a coughing pet by placing the animal in a steamy bathroom. Although this practice increases the fluidity of secretions in the upper respiratory tract, it does not significantly increase the fluidity of the mucus in the lower airways because the comparatively large steam droplets precipitate in the trachea and are not inhaled deep enough to penetrate the lower airways.

When oxygen is administered to animals with respiratory problems or other disease, the very dry nature of the gas can dehydrate the mucociliary apparatus and decrease its efficiency. Therefore, in animals with a

---

CLINICAL APPLICATION
Metered-Dose Inhalers

One of the innovations borrowed from human medicine for delivering nebulized drug to the lungs of veterinary patients is the use of *metered-dose inhalers* (MDIs). MDIs are essentially the normal aerosolized delivery systems (inhalers) that have been used in human medicine for decades attached to a tube called a spacer that ends in a comfortable mask that fits over the nose and mouth of the animal. The point of the spacer tube is to allow the mist from the aerosol inhaler container to diffuse in a larger, but contained, air space, thereby allowing the animal to breathe in the medication with several breaths. Without the spacer, the animal would have to inhale the puffed drug directly and deeply, both of which are unnatural responses to breathing in a foreign mist that may have a funny taste or odor.

Dr. Paul Padrid, one of the champions of the MDI concept in veterinary medicine, claims that animals accept these MDIs quite well without tranquilization or sedation. In a recent study 20 cats were given a nebulized low-radiation drug by aerosol chamber and mask.[1] Nuclear scintigraphy, a means of imaging the location of the inhaled drug, showed that in all 20 cats the nebulized material was well distributed throughout the lung field. The conclusion was that the use of an inhalation chamber plus mask could be a viable means for delivering a drug to the airways.

What should be learned from this situation: *Aerosol therapy* or nebulization delivery of drugs may be more successful than previously thought if MDIs are used.[2]

---

compromised mucociliary apparatus, with respiratory disease, or on long-term oxygen, moisture should be added to the oxygen, usually by bubbling it through a container of water.

EXPECTORANTS

Expectorants also increase the fluidity of mucus in the respiratory tract and thereby improve the effectiveness of the mucociliary apparatus. As opposed to mucolytics, which reduce the viscosity of mucus by chemically altering it, expectorants increase the fluidity of mucus by generating liquid secretions by respiratory tract cells. To expectorate means to spit; therefore expectorants increase the amount of fluid moved up from the lower respiratory tract to a point where it can be spit out.

Although expectorants are commonly included in human OTC cold preparations, they are of questionable benefit in veterinary patients. A more effective expectorant-like effect can be achieved by maintaining proper systemic hydration and increasing the humidity of inspired air. The benefits of expectorants

must be weighed against the increased volume of fluid that would have to be removed from the respiratory tree by the mucociliary apparatus.

Guaifenesin (glyceryl guaiacolate) and saline expectorants such as ammonium chloride, potassium iodide, and sodium citrate are given by mouth and increase watery secretions in the respiratory tree. These drugs irritate the gastric mucosa and stimulate the parasympathetic nervous system, causing the parasympathetic nervous system to stimulate respiratory secretions. This link between GI tract stimulation of the parasympathetic nervous system and bronchiole secretions can be demonstrated after eating a large meal while having a cold. Within 5 to 15 minutes after eating, coughing will increase from the parasympathetic expectorant action caused by increased parasympathetic stimulation associated with increased GI function.

When animals accidentally ingest cold medications with these expectorants, they often vomit because of the irritant action of these medications on the gastric mucosa. Guaifenesin, often referred to as "GG" for glyceryl guaiacolate, is also administered intravenously to produce muscle relaxation in equine anesthesia protocols.

In contrast to expectorants that act by irritating the gastric mucosa, the volatile oil expectorants such as terpin hydrate, eucalyptus oil, and pine oil directly stimulate respiratory secretions when their vapors are inhaled or when the absorbed volatile oil is excreted by the respiratory tract.

Antitussives should not be used with expectorants because of the need to remove the increased fluid in the respiratory tree. However, most antitussives are not strong enough to suppress the cough reflex initiated by the increased secretions.

DECONGESTANTS

Many OTC human cold preparations that contain expectorants also contain decongestants such as pseudoephedrine, ephedrine, or phenylephrine for relief of nasal congestion. Decongestants reduce congestion (vascular engorgement) of swollen nasal tissues by stimulating the sympathetic nervous system's α_1 *receptors* on smooth muscle of blood vessels in the skin and mucous membranes. When stimulated, α_1 receptors cause vasoconstriction in the congested (swollen) mucous membranes of the nasal passages, reducing tissue edema and secretions by mucous glands.

Because the molecules in decongestants are not specific for α_1 receptors, most have some β_1 activity and therefore increase the heart rate as a side effect. In most animals this does not cause significant problems; however, if the animal has cardiovascular disease the additional oxygen demand by the β_1-stimulated myocardial cells could result in arrhythmia. If the animal has congestive heart failure with poor oxygenation of tissue because of poor circulation, the myocardial cells would not be able to get enough oxygen to meet the increased oxygen demand caused by β_1 stimulation.

Pet owners sometimes treat illness in their animals with their own drugs. Because veterinary professionals are often asked questions regarding use of OTC cold and flu preparations, they must understand the dangers involved with use of these products and be able to explain to pet owners the reasons these preparations should not be used in pets.

BRONCHODILATORS

Bronchoconstriction is the contraction of smooth muscles surrounding the small terminal bronchioles deep within the respiratory tree. Bronchoconstriction can be caused by many different mechanisms. For example, stimulation of the parasympathetic nervous system by drugs, insecticides, or toxicants causes both bronchoconstriction and increased respiratory secretions. Drugs that prolong the effect of the neurotransmitter acetylcholine by inhibiting acetylcholinesterase, the enzyme that breaks down acetylcholine, will also increase parasympathetic nervous system activity and result in bronchoconstriction and *dyspnea* (difficult breathing).

Histamine, a compound released by tissues during inflammation, causes bronchoconstriction by stimulating histamine type 1 (H_1) receptors on bronchiolar smooth muscle cells. The contraction of these smooth muscles produces the dyspnea often seen with allergic reactions in human beings. Other chemicals released by inflammatory cells may produce edema of the airways, excessive secretions, and migration of inflammatory cells onto the epithelial surface where they increase the viscosity of the mucus viscosity.

A third mechanism of bronchoconstriction involves blocking the sympathetic β_2 *receptors* found on smooth muscles and mast cells. Because β_2-receptor stimulation by the sympathetic nervous system neurotransmitters epinephrine and norepinephrine causes the bronchiolar smooth muscles to relax, they antagonize the bronchoconstricting activity

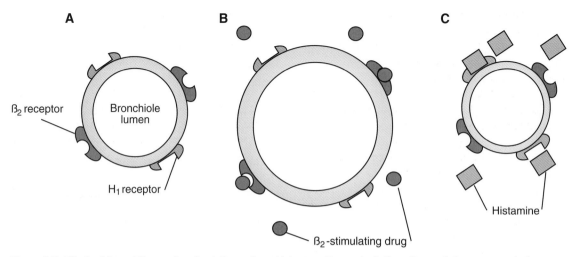

Figure 6-2 Effects of β_2 and H_1 receptor stimulation on bronchiolar smooth muscle. **A**, Smooth muscle layer surrounds the bronchiole. **B**, Smooth muscle relaxation and bronchiole dilation are caused by a predominance of β_2-stimulating drug. **C**, Smooth muscle contraction and bronchiole constriction are caused by a predominance of histamine.

of acetylcholine and the parasympathetic nervous system. Blocking the β_2 receptors results in dominance of the parasympathetic nervous system and a net bronchoconstriction (Figure 6-2).

β_2 receptors also produce vasodilation of coronary blood vessels and the vessels that supply blood to muscles (see Chapter 5). Additionally, stimulation of β_2 receptors also prevents mast cells from degranulating and releasing their mediators of inflammation (histamine, prostaglandins, and leukotrienes), which would contribute to bronchoconstriction. As mentioned in Chapter 5, β-blocking antiarrhythmic drugs such as propranolol are designed to block primarily the β_1 *receptors*. However, because they are not entirely specific for β_1 receptors, they may also block the β_2 receptors, allowing parasympathetic nervous system–mediated bronchoconstriction, excessive respiratory secretions, and edema within the airways.

Bronchoconstriction is actually a more complex response than illustrated above. The veterinary professional can expect to see new drugs being advocated, especially in equine and feline medicine, to control this reaction. For example, in the cat (but not human being) the inflammatory mediator *serotonin* causes bronchoconstriction in a similar fashion that histamines do in human beings. Because of serotonin's role in feline asthma, serotonin blockers such as cyproheptadine may begin to appear more frequently in veterinary literature.

β-ADRENERGIC AGONISTS

β-adrenergic agonists (β agonists) are drugs that stimulate β receptors in general. Because β_2 receptors are involved in bronchodilation and stabilization of mast cells, drugs that stimulate β_2 receptors are used as bronchodilators. Because many β_2 agonist bronchodilators also have some β_1-stimulating capacity, an increased heart rate is common with most β-adrenergic agonist bronchodilators. This can be risky if the heart is already hypoxic because of compromised respiratory airways and is stimulated by β_1 receptor stimulation to increase its contractility. Thus selective β_2 agonists are used to produce bronchodilation.

As opposed to the older bronchodilation drugs epinephrine, isoproterenol, and ephedrine, the newer drugs such as terbutaline and albuterol are selective β_2 agonists. These drugs produce some stimulation of the heart, especially with the first few doses; however, the degree of tachycardia (increased heart rate) decreases with repeated exposure to the drugs. Terbutaline has an additional value in the treatment of bronchoconstriction and general bronchial congestion because it reduces mucus viscosity, thereby allowing the mucociliary apparatus to work more effectively. Both drugs are available in oral form and as inhalers; terbutaline is also available for subcutaneous injection. The oral forms of these drugs require higher doses than the parenteral forms because of the extensive first-pass effect for the oral drugs (see Chapter 3).

Like β agonists, the β_2 agonist drugs can begin to lose their effectiveness as a result of downregulation of receptors. Downregulation is the phenomenon by which the cell begins to remove receptors from its surface as a means of compensating for the increased stimulation from the drug. Over time, the loss of receptors means the cell becomes less responsive to the drug.

METHYLXANTHINES

The methylxanthines include bronchodilators such as theophylline and aminophylline and the central nervous system (CNS) stimulants caffeine and theobromine (see Chapter 8). Aminophylline is essentially 80% theophylline plus 20% ethylenediamine salt. The salt facilitates absorption of aminophylline and allows the drug to be better tolerated by the GI tract. Because 100 mg of aminophylline contains 80 mg of active theophylline, the dosages of aminophylline and pure theophylline differ based on the amount of active ingredient (theophylline) in the compound. The conversion formula is shown below. Various aminophylline products may contain different amounts of theophylline; therefore the 80% value (0.80 in the conversion formula) may have to be changed to the percentage of theophylline in that aminophylline product

mg of theophylline = mg of aminophylline × 0.80

For example, a veterinarian wishes to switch a dog from 100 mg of theophylline to an equivalent dose of aminophylline. Following is how the veterinary technician calculated the conversion:

100 mg of theophylline
= __ mg of aminophylline × 0.80

100 mg of theophylline/0.80
= __ mg of aminophylline

125 mg = __ mg of aminophylline
(at the 80% theophylline preparation)

Methylxanthines cause bronchodilation by affecting some of the smooth muscle cell's biochemical functions. Normally, stimulation of the β_2 receptor results in production of cyclic adenosine monophosphate (cAMP), which promotes relaxation of the smooth muscle and subsequent bronchodilation. The smooth muscle relaxation of cAMP is normally terminated when the cAMP is broken down by the enzyme phosphodiesterase. Previously, it was proposed (and reported in earlier editions of this text) that methylxanthine bronchodilators inhibit phosphodiesterase, allowing relaxation of the smooth muscles. However, it has been determined that at normal therapeutic concentrations of theophylline, phosphodiesterase is not inhibited enough to explain the bronchodilation effect. The most likely mechanism for theophylline's action is by directly interference with calcium mobilization required for the contractile elements of muscle to connect and contract to produce smooth muscle contraction. By blocking this calcium-mediated step, the methylxanthines force the muscles to remain in a relaxed state.

A secondary benefit of theophylline in human beings includes an increased force of contraction of the respiratory muscles (greater ease in ventilating), a slightly increased force of contraction of the myocardium, and dilation of the coronary arteries. These increased contractility effects, in contrast to the smooth muscle relaxation of the bronchioles, are through other mechanisms (still debated) than those described for bronchial dilation. In most veterinary patients the increased contractility of respiratory muscles is considered clinically insignificant.

Many of the more widely known sustained-release theophylline products that prolong absorption of the drug over several hours have been discontinued in the United States. However, a few sustained-release oral products manufactured by small companies are still available. Sustained-release preparations generally achieve lower peak plasma concentrations, but drug concentrations remain in the therapeutic range for a longer time. As discussed in Chapter 3, various factors affect absorption of sustained-release preparations, including the rate at which the dose form dissolves and the GI transit time. These tablets are formulated for human GI transit times, but in animals the tablets may pass through the GI tract before all the tablet has dissolved. The dissolving rate may differ for tablets made by different manufacturers; therefore after an animal has initially been stabilized with a particular oral methylxanthine product, the animal should be maintained with that same manufacturer's product to ensure a more consistent clinical response.

Some CNS stimulation and GI upset may occur with use of methylxanthines. GI upset is more common with oral administration of theophylline than it is for aminophylline. Usually these effects are transient and resolve after a few days of administration. These drugs have a fairly narrow therapeutic index, meaning the therapeutic dose is quite close to dosages that produce toxicity. Signs of overdose may occur with overstimulation of the CNS, tachycardia, and nausea or vomiting.

Aminophylline and theophylline can interact with a wide variety of drugs. Always determine if aminophylline or theophylline can be safely used or administered with another drug. For example, aminophylline is physically incompatible with most intravenous fluids and therefore cannot be readily used in a fluid infusion. Theophylline is metabolized by the liver and therefore can increase or decrease the metabolism of other drugs, including phenobarbital, cimetidine, clindamycin, erythromycin, and lincomycin. Some of these drugs, if used concurrently with theophylline, will decrease the metabolism of theophylline, resulting in greater accumulation of the drug and greater risk for theophylline toxicosis. The veterinary professional should always take a few moments to refer to a pharmacology resource before treating an animal simultaneously with theophylline and another drug.

OTHER DRUGS USED TO TREAT RESPIRATORY PROBLEMS

ANTIMICROBIALS

Ideally the presence of a bacterial infection and the antibiotic susceptibility of the involved bacteria should be established before antimicrobials (drugs used to combat infection by microorganisms) are used in respiratory disease. Many respiratory infections are caused by viruses or allergens (allergy-producing substances) against which antimicrobials are completely ineffective. The repeated use of antimicrobials under such conditions does little to help the animal, creates a false sense of security ("we're doing something"), and creates opportunities for bacteria present to develop resistance to the antimicrobial.

Bacterial specimens can be obtained by a transtracheal wash, bronchoscopic wash, or other sampling techniques. Even if the specimens obtained are not submitted for culture identification and antimicrobial sensitivity testing, the sample can be stained to determine the general type of bacteria involved (e.g., gram negative vs gram positive, bacilli vs cocci). Based on the shape and gram stain of the bacteria, an antimicrobial can be selected that may be effective against that bacterial strain.

Although part of successful treatment of infectious respiratory disease depends on use of the appropriate antimicrobial, the other critical element is duration of therapy. Many animal owners stop giving their animal an antimicrobial after just a few days when clinical signs begin to subside and the animal feels better. Unfortunately, the improvement of clinical signs does not mean the infectious organism has been eliminated. If the owners fail to give the drug for the entire prescribed duration, do not give the drug in the prescribed amount, or skip doses, resistant bacteria can survive, then multiply, and become the predominant infectious bacteria in the respiratory tract. The next time the same antimicrobial is used for what appears to be the same respiratory infection the drug may be ineffective against the bacteria. Thus animals with respiratory infections should be treated with antimicrobials for at least 7 to 10 days, with some treatments for long-duration diseases such as chronic bronchitis lasting 4 to 6 weeks. A general rule is that antimicrobial use should be continued for 5 to 7 days after resolution of clinical signs.

The other challenge to using antimicrobials is the location of the bacteria. As described in Chapter 3, a drug is only effective if it reaches the site of action in sufficient concentrations to be in the therapeutic range. For bacterial infections the drug has to reach the bacteria at high enough concentrations to kill the bacteria. Unfortunately, instead of bacteria propagating within cells, bacteria may propagate on the luminal, or airway, surface of the bronchioles. Bacteria in this location are essentially outside the body, making it hard for an orally or parenterally administered antimicrobial circulating in the blood to reach this surface. Many otherwise effective antimicrobials may not be effective when administered systemically

because they do not reach the lumen infection site in concentrations sufficient to be bactericidal. Certain antimicrobials, however, are concentrated in the respiratory mucous and secretory glands and thus attain significant concentrations in the mucus secreted onto the surface of the respiratory tract.

In some of these cases the animal may benefit from administration of an antimicrobial by nebulization. Nebulization (also called *aerosolization* or aerosol therapy) is the process of administering a drug as a fine mist that the animal inhales into the airways. Properly performed, this technique deposits the drug directly on the surface of the bronchiolar epithelium. However, a significant disadvantage of nebulization in veterinary patients compared with human patients is that we cannot tell a dog or cat to breathe deeply to inhale the mist. Nebulized mist administered by a mask tends to precipitate in the upper respiratory tract and not deliver significant concentrations to the lower respiratory tract. Animals frequently fight having a mask placed over their face. Animals that are already hypoxic from airway compromise are at risk for potentially fatal cardiac arrhythmias if they become excited and stimulate the sympathetic nervous system. Sedation may be needed in animals that fight the mask, but sedation is not without risk to the compromised patient.

The use of nebulizing chambers reduces some of the animal's anxiety with having a mask placed over its nose; however, the same problem with precipitation of the mist exists. Nebulization can be carried out with an endotracheal tube; however, this requires anesthesia or heavy sedation with its inherent risks of depression of the respiratory centers and impaired cardiovascular function.

Poor-quality nebulizers result in relatively large droplets of moisture. Large droplets of moisture strike the wall of the upper respiratory tree and are swallowed, sneezed, or coughed out. Even fine-mist nebulizers lose a significant amount of mist in the trachea and upper parts of the main bronchi because the animal resists taking deep breaths.

Another potential problem with aerosol therapy is the risk of reflex bronchoconstriction in response to introduction of the mist into the respiratory tree. Thus a bronchodilator may be needed before nebulization if the aerosolized drug is irritating.

One of the advances in aerosol therapy in human medicine has been the use of MDIs. The drug is packaged in a pressurized container with a propellant and is released in a measured amount with each depression of the trigger or plunger. The resultant mist is then inhaled, theoretically delivering a set amount or dose. In equine medicine, specialized masks have been developed to accommodate MDIs in an attempt to use this technology to treat equine respiratory diseases. Considerable variability in dosing still exists with this method because of the nature of the animal, the temperature, the humidity, and the droplet size. Still, nebulization in various forms appears to remain a tool used by some veterinarians to treat selected respiratory conditions.

CORTICOSTEROIDS

Corticosteroid use in treatment of respiratory disease remains controversial. Corticosteroids are indicated in those situations in which the inflammation itself is potentially life threatening. For example, smoke inhalation triggers an acute inflammatory response that, if not held in check to some degree, can cause accumulation of fluid in and around the alveoli, causing pulmonary edema and interfering with the ability of oxygen to pass from the alveolus into the blood. If the degree of swelling and inflammation is suppressed by corticosteroids such as prednisone or methylprednisolone, the animal may have a greater chance of surviving.

Corticosteroids also stabilize the mast cells (inflammatory cells), thus decreasing their release of potent inflammatory mediators that cause swelling and edema of the bronchiolar tissues. Corticosteroids also help stabilize the integrity of the capillaries, thus reducing fluid loss in the tissues. Both effects decrease damage associated with inflammation. Allergic responses, aspiration of chemicals, inhalation of caustic fumes, and eosinophilic bronchitis all initially respond well to corticosteroids.

Corticosteroids have long been used as supplements for human treatment of asthma because they are believed to improve the activity of methylxanthine and β-agonist bronchodilators. They are used less often today because of the side effects of many corticosteroids (see Chapter 13). Cats with feline asthma syndrome appear to respond well to corticosteroid treatment. Horses with *chronic obstructive pulmonary disease* may be treated with aerosolized corticosteroids as part of their treatment.

Considerable debate exists about whether corticosteroids should be used in the treatment of chronic bronchitis or respiratory conditions involving a significant infectious component. Some veterinary internal medicine specialists who treat animals with chronic respiratory disease believe that corticosteroids are essential to maintain function of the respiratory tree; others are less adamant about the role of corticosteroids. Large doses of corticosteroids are known to impair the immune system response to infection and have the potential to delay healing. Corticosteroids also reduce cell-mediated immunity, a condition in which cells destroy the infectious agent. Cell-mediated immunity is required to destroy many fungal infections in the lungs; therefore the use of corticosteroids could result in a significant worsening of fungal infections in the lungs.

Note that nonsteroidal antiinflammatory drugs such as ibuprofen (Advil, Motrin), ketoprofen (Orudis KT), naproxen (Aleve), and aspirin are not often used in most respiratory diseases. As explained Chapter 13, these drugs block the formation of prostaglandins to relieve inflammation. Unfortunately, in the lungs prostaglandins play an important role in maintaining bronchodilation. Blocking of prostaglandins associated with inflammation would have the side effect of also blocking their benefits.

Because many positives and negatives exist to using corticosteroids in respiratory disease, the veterinary professional should carefully weigh the benefits and risks of corticosteroids before using them in a critically ill patient or one that could potentially become critical.

ANTIHISTAMINES

As previously discussed, histamine causes constriction of the bronchioles and is involved in the inflammatory response of the respiratory tract. Because allergic reactions cause mast cell degranulation and release of inflammatory mediators including histamine, antihistamines have been popular for use in people with hay fever and other allergies. However, histamine is less of a factor in small animal allergic respiratory problems because of the relative decrease in H_1 receptors; therefore antihistamines are usually much less effective in respiratory problems of small animals than they are in human beings.

In horses histamine release is involved in chronic obstructive pulmonary disease ("heaves") and other bronchial problems related to dust and particulate matter. Horses predisposed to respiratory problems from dust or airborne allergens may be kept on antihistamine continuously during the worst times of the year. However, therapy for heaves has shifted away from antihistamines and more toward the judicious use of corticosteroids by parenteral and aerosol routes of administration.

In contrast to corticosteroids, which can reverse or stabilize much of the damage caused by inflammation or allergic insult, antihistamines only prevent inflammation if they reach the H_1 receptors on bronchial or vascular smooth muscles in large quantities before the arrival of histamines. If histamine gets to the H_1 cell receptors first, antihistamine drugs do little to reverse the histamine effects. Theoretically the best use of antihistamines is either prophylactically before the histamine is released or when exposure to the allergic substance inducing release of histamine is continuous. This explains why antihistamines are used for heaves in horses that are continuously exposed to dust or molds in the barn environment.

DIURETICS

Diuretics are used to remove accumulated fluid from the lungs, such as in animals with pneumonia or congestive heart failure. As explained in Chapter 5, diuretics promote loss of body water through diminished reabsorption of water by the kidneys. The decreased water content of the blood increases the osmotic forces within the capillaries and consequently attracts water from body tissues into the bloodstream. Through this mechanism the fluid of ascites or pulmonary edema is slowly moved into the blood and then out the body through the kidneys. The use of diuretics can be thought of as therapeutic dehydration. A disadvantage of using diuretics to treat animals with respiratory disease is that they tend to dry the respiratory secretions, rendering the mucociliary apparatus less effective. This side effect must be measured against the potential benefits.

OXYGEN

Oxygen administration with an oxygen cage or a mask is indicated in animals that are transiently hypoxic. For an animal, the stress of having the oxygen mask applied or being placed in an oxygen cage can sometimes precipitate collapse. Some cats and dogs tolerate a small-diameter tube that is hooked to an oxygen source, placed into the nasal passages, and glued or taped to the hair of the head to hold it in place. Some veterinary professionals create a portable oxygen cage by placing an Elizabethan collar on the animal, partially covering the large end of the funnel with plastic wrap, and running an oxygen line to the inside of the collar. To allow heat to escape, the opening of the Elizabethan collar funnel head should never be totally covered with plastic wrap. Oxygen is very dry so it should be humidified to prevent severe drying of the mucous membranes and mucociliary apparatus.

Box 6-1 Respiratory Drug Categories and Names

ANTITUSSIVES

Butorphanol (Torbutrol)
Hydrocodone (Hycodan)
Codeine
Dextromethorphan

MUCOLYTICS

Acetylcysteine (Mucomyst)
Water (steam)

EXPECTORANTS

Guaifenesin (glyceryl guaiacolate)
Saline expectorants
Volatile oils (terpin hydrate, eucalyptus oil)

BRONCHODILATORS

β_2 Adrenergics
   Terbutaline
   Albuterol
Methylxanthines
   Theophylline
   Aminophylline

OTHER RESPIRATORY DRUGS

Antimicrobials
Corticosteroids
Antihistamines
Diuretics
Oxygen

REFERENCES

1. Schulman RL, Crochik SS, Kneur SK, et al: Investigation of pulmonary deposition of a nebulized radiopharmaceutical agent, *Am J Vet Res* 65(6):806-809, 2004.
2. Marcucci BA: Feline asthma: treatment and prognosis. *Veterinary Technician* 25(12):807-813, 2004.

RECOMMENDED READING

Boothe DM: *Drug therapy of the respiratory tract*. Proceedings of the North American Veterinary Conference, Orlando, Fla, Jan 2000.
Boothe DM: *Small animal clinical pharmacology and therapeutics*, Philadelphia, 2001, WB Saunders.
Dowling PM: *Using metered dose inhalers in veterinary patients*. In Proceedings of the Western Veterinary Conference, Las Vegas, NV, 2004.
Johnson L: Canine chronic bronchitis. In Bonagura JD, editor: *Kirk's current veterinary therapy XIII*, Philadelphia, 2000, WB Saunders.
Lavoie JP: Inhalation therapy for equine heaves, *Compendium of Continuing Education—Small Animal*, 23(5):475-477, 2001.
McKiernan BC: *Respiratory therapeutics*. In Proceedings of the 14th ECVIM-CA Congress, Barcelona, Spain, 2004.
Olsen JD: Rational antibiotic therapy for respiratory disorders in dogs and cats, *Vet Clin North Am Small An Pract* 30:1337, 2000.
Padrid P: Feline asthma. In Bonagura JD, editor: *Kirk's current veterinary therapy XIII*, Philadelphia, 2000, WB Saunders.
Plumb DC: *Veterinary drug handbook*, ed 5, Ames, IA, 2005, Blackwell.

Self-Assessment

REVIEW QUESTIONS

Fill in the following blanks with the correct item from the Key Terms list.

1. _____ administration a drug by a mist that is inhaled.

2. _____ mechanism that traps inhaled particles in a mucus layer and moves it up and out of the respiratory tree.

3. _____ pulmonary disease that in turn causes cardiac disease.

4. _____ type of drug that suppresses cough.

5. _____ type of drug that does not break apart mucus but increases watery secretions in the lungs.

6. _____ specific receptor that, when stimulated, causes bronchodilation.

7. _____ term meaning "difficult breathing."

8. _____ definition of MDI.

Fill in the following blanks with the correct drug described in Box 6-1.

9. _____ expectorant; works by irritating the gastric lining.

10. _____ centrally acting opioid antitussive; only Food and Drug Administration approved veterinary product for cough.

11. _____ same drug group as caffeine and theobromine in chocolate; a bronchodilator that contains 80% active ingredient and 20% salt.

12. _____ used in patients in which the inflammatory process is life threatening; not to be used with respiratory fungal disease; stabilizes cellular membranes more than antihistamines.

13. _____ mucolytic that breaks apart sulfhydryl (S—S) bonds.

14. _____ prophylactic antiinflammatory that decreases inflammatory response only if it is at the site of inflammation before the inflammation starts.

15. _____ potent narcotic antitussive; human product; C-III drug.

16. _____ type of drug used to decrease pulmonary edema.

17. _____ common antitussive ingredient in OTC cold preparations; not a controlled substance; not very effective in veterinary patients.

18. _____ also used as an intravenously administered muscle relaxant for equine patients.

19. _____   also used as an antidote in cats with acetaminophen toxicosis.

20. _____   active ingredient of aminophylline.

21. _____   used to dilate bronchioles by directly stimulating β_2 receptors.

22. Indicate whether the following statements are true or false.

   A. Inflammation and migration of inflammatory cells (e.g., neutrophils) cause the mucus to become more sticky or viscous.

   B. Rapid breathing is called dyspnea.

   C. Inspissated mucus means that the mucus is dried out.

   D. Use of a diuretic drug would decrease the efficiency of the mucociliary apparatus.

   E. Dextromethorphan is more effective than hydrocodone as an antitussive.

   F. In dehydrated animals the cough is usually nonproductive.

   G. A common side effect of most direct bronchodilators is decreased heart rate and force of cardiac contraction.

   H. If an animal is in distress from bronchoconstriction, antihistamine drugs should be used to dilate the bronchioles.

   I. Decongestants primarily work by causing vasoconstriction in the nasal mucosa.

   J. Prescribing dextromethorphan antitussive requires a controlled substance license or permit.

   K. Nebulization describes the process by which macrophages move into the alveoli and clean up debris that made it down that far.

   L. Stimulation of the larynx produces a more forceful and gagging cough than bronchiolar irritation.

   M. Theophylline is the active ingredient, and aminophylline is theophylline plus a salt.

   N. Stimulation of the parasympathetic nervous system in the bronchioles causes bronchoconstriction.

   O. Centrally acting cough suppressants work better in veterinary patients than locally acting ones.

   P. Overdose of the opioid narcotic antitussives causes respiratory depression.

   Q. Drugs that stimulate acetylcholine receptors in the respiratory tree cause bronchodilation.

   R. Stimulation of H_1 receptors on the bronchioles produces an effect opposite of what stimulation of β_2 receptors would do to the bronchioles.

   S. Butorphanol and hydrocodone are controlled substances.

23. Stimulation of which branch of the autonomic nervous system produces bronchodilation?

_____

24. Stimulation of which specific receptor causes vasoconstriction and is the receptor involved with the mechanism of action of decongestants?   _____

25. What effect do methylxanthines have on the CNS? _____

26. Which neurotransmitter is normally associated with the parasympathetic nervous system? _____

27. What substance is released by mast cells and causes inflammation and bronchoconstriction? _____

28. What type of cough brings up mucus? _____

29. What type of drug has a name that means "cause to spit"? _____

APPLICATION QUESTIONS

1. Different levels of the respiratory tree prevent foreign particles (e.g., food, dust, molds) from reaching the deepest levels of the respiratory system. What are the normal mechanisms by which the larynx protects the respiratory tract? How do they differ from the reactions of the bronchi and trachea? What about the protective mechanisms at the level of the terminal bronchioles and alveoli?

2. A dehydrated animal with a high temperature and a nonproductive cough is admitted to the clinic. The veterinarian wants to correct the dehydration and determine whether the character of the cough changes before using antitussives. Why does she do this?

3. A veterinary pharmaceutical sales representative is offering a special price on locally acting antitussives for your veterinary patients. Should you make such a purchase?

4. Why is inspissated mucus a bad thing as far as the respiratory tract protecting itself? How do expectorants and mucolytics help correct this? What is the difference in mechanism between expectorants and mucolytics?

5. What effect would an owner likely see if her cat lapped up several milliliters of the owner's spilled liquid decongestant?

6. What effect would stimulation or blocking of β_2 receptors have on the respiratory tree? Why is it that some β-blocking antiarrhythmic drugs such as propranolol also have an effect on the respiratory tree?

7. Why are terbutaline and albuterol used more commonly for bronchodilation than epinephrine even though they have similar mechanisms of action?

8. What are the differences among aminophylline, theophylline, and methylxanthine? If the veterinarian decides to switch the animal's treatment from 200 mg of theophylline to an equivalent dose of aminophylline, what would the equivalent dose be?

9. Why should the owner not stop antibiotics for a respiratory disease as soon as the pet seems back to normal?

10. What is the rationalization for using nebulization in animals with respiratory disease? What is the challenge with nebulizing an animal compared with nebulizing a human being? What techniques have been used to increase the effectiveness of nebulization?

11. Of what benefits are corticosteroids in respiratory disease? Why are they not used all the time?

12. What role might diuretics play in respiratory-related disease? Why do they decrease the effectiveness of some of the other respiratory-protective mechanisms?

13. Oxygen administration can be beneficial to hypoxic animals. Why does oxygen therapy often reduce an animal's ability to remove inflammatory products, cellular debris, or excess mucus from the respiratory tract?

Drugs Affecting the Endocrine System

outline

key terms

aplastic anemia
beta cells
carcinogenic
endogenous
estrous/estrus
exogenous
foal heat
follicular phase
gluconeogenesis
glycogenolysis
goiter

hyperthyroidism
insulin-dependent diabetes
  mellitus
luteal phase
myometrium
negative feedback
  mechanism
non–insulin-dependent
  diabetes mellitus
primary hypothyroidism
progestagen

progestational hormone
protamine
seasonal anestrus
secondary hypothyroidism
sulfonylurea compounds
tertiary hypothyroidism
thyroidectomy
thyrotoxicosis
type 1 diabetes
type 2 diabetes
U-40 and U-100 insulin

objectives

After studying this chapter, the veterinary technician should be able to explain:

1. The mechanisms by which the endocrine system regulates itself

2. The drugs used to treat thyroid diseases and how they work

3. The types of insulin used to treat diabetes and other diabetic therapeutic agents

4. The drugs used to regulate the estrous cycle and their mechanisms of action

5. The drugs and hormones that regulate pregnancy and how these are altered to produce an effect on reproductive functions

The endocrine system is composed of the thyroid gland, ovaries, testicles, pancreas, adrenal glands, and other glands that produce hormones. The proper balance of hormonal activity is essential to maintain normal physiologic functions. This balance is easily upset by disease or drugs that increase or decrease the amount or effectiveness of different hormones. Hormonal therapy, which is the therapeutic use of hormone or hormonelike substances, plays an important role in certain diseases and health conditions. Therefore veterinary technicians should understand the ways basic hormone mechanisms work and the effects specific hormonal therapies have on the body. Box 7-1, listing endocrine drugs, can be found at the end of this chapter.

THE NEGATIVE FEEDBACK SYSTEM

All endocrine systems are regulated by a feedback mechanism in much the same way as the temperature inside a house and a thermostat regulate the activity of a furnace. In a house, the furnace produces heat until the thermostat detects that the interior environment is warm enough and sends a signal that turns off the furnace. This signal from the thermostat to the furnace to stop, or inhibit, its heat production is called negative feedback. When the temperature in the house drops below a certain point again, the thermostat sends a signal that turns on the furnace, which in turn produces heat and the cycle repeats. The interaction between the thermostat controlling the furnace and the heat produced by the furnace keeps the temperature in the ideal range.

As shown in Figure 7-1, endocrine gland A is responsive to circulating levels of a hormone that it produces. When concentrations of that hormone fall below a certain level, endocrine gland A begins to produce the hormone again in a way that is similar to how the furnace produces heat when the

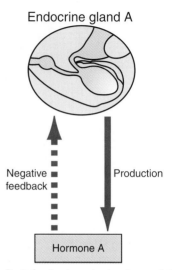

Figure 7-1 Basic feedback mechanism for regulation of endocrine glands.

temperature drops below a certain point. As concentrations of hormone increase to desired levels, the negative feedback from the presence of the increased hormone causes endocrine gland A to shut itself off. When the body metabolizes the hormone and concentrations drop below the critical concentration again, the negative feedback is removed from endocrine gland A and it begins to secrete hormone again.

Endocrine regulation and negative feedback are more complex than the simple mechanism illustrated above. Just as the thermostat is usually separate from the furnace, more than one endocrine gland is typically involved in the negative feedback loop. As shown in Figure 7-2, endocrine gland A produces a hormone that stimulates endocrine gland B to produce its hormone. The hormone from gland B circulates and has some intended effect on the body, but it also produces negative feedback on endocrine gland A. According to the furnace and thermostat analogy, endocrine gland B is the furnace that produces a hormone (heat) that has an effect on the body (increases the temperature in the house). When

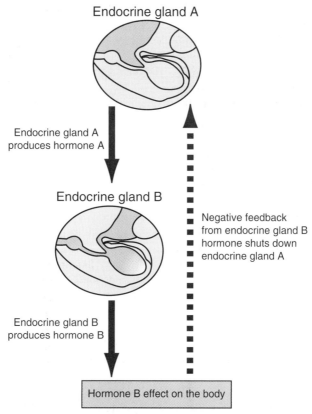

Endocrine gland A

Endocrine gland A
produces hormone A

Endocrine gland B

Negative feedback
from endocrine gland B
hormone shuts down
endocrine gland A

Endocrine gland B
produces hormone B

Hormone B effect on the body

Figure 7-2 Regulation of endocrine glands when more than one gland is involved.

sufficient gland B hormone (heat from the furnace) is circulating in the body (the house is warm enough), the negative feedback inhibition on endocrine gland A (heat's effect on the thermostat) decreases endocrine gland A's stimulating hormone (thermostat stops sending electrical impulse to the furnace to tell it to produce heat). Endocrine gland B is no longer stimulated and stops producing hormone (furnace stops producing heat) until endocrine gland B's hormone drops low enough and the cycle starts over again.

If an *exogenous* drug (a compound that originates outside the body) is chemically similar to an *endogenous,* or naturally occurring, hormone, it can produce similar physiologic effects and exert the same negative feedback effect as the natural hormone. For example, if a drug that did the same thing as endocrine gland B's hormone was injected, it would produce the same bodily effect as gland B's hormone plus inhibit endocrine gland A. Again referring to the furnace analogy, this action would be similar to bringing in a secondary heating source (e.g., sunshine, kerosene heater) to bring the temperature of the house up. With the temperature up, the thermostat does not turn the furnace on (the thermostat does not distinguish where the heat came from, it only responds to the temperature in the house). Similarly, if the drug injected imitated endocrine gland A's hormone, the drug would stimulate endocrine gland B, resulting in increased production of endocrine gland B's hormone (much like sending an electrical signal to the furnace from something other than the thermostat).

As illustrated above, endocrine systems are finely balanced to provide just the right amount of hormone that the body needs. Therefore exogenous hormone or hormone-like drugs can easily upset the balance and produce unintended effects. The veterinary professional must be very familiar with the effects, side effects, and mechanisms by which these hormone drugs work.

This chapter discusses thyroid, pancreatic, and reproductive hormones because these endocrine systems are the targets for most endocrine-related drugs used in veterinary medicine. Corticosteroids are also drugs that emulate natural endocrine hormones, but they are discussed in Chapter 13.

DRUGS USED TO TREAT THYROID DISEASE

DRUGS USED TO TREAT HYPOTHYROIDISM

When low concentrations of thyroid hormone are present in the blood, the hypothalamus releases a stimulating hormone called thyrotro-pin-releasing hormone (TRH) whose function is to stimulate the pituitary gland to release thyroid-stimulating hormone (TSH). Under the influence of the pituitary gland's TSH, fol-licular cells of the thyroid gland absorb iodine and incorporate it into tyrosine molecules to produce two thyroid hormones: triiodothyro-nine (T_3) and tetraiodothyronine, or thyroxine (T_4). The numbers 3 and 4 refer to the amount of iodine on the molecule: T_4 has four and T_3 has three. The T_4 and T_3 molecules are then released into circulation and taken up by cells in the body. Once taken up, T_4 is converted by tissues to T_3 by removing one iodine. The T_3 form is the physiologically active form of the hormone and causes the changes associ-ated with the thyroid hormones. Circulating T_4 levels provide the negative feedback to the hypothalamus and pituitary to decrease release of TRH and TSH (Figure 7-3).

Different species develop different problems with their thyroid glands. For example, dogs are prone to develop hypothyroidism (low production of thyroid hormone), whereas cats are prone to develop *hyperthyroidism* (an exces-sive production of thyroid hormone). Reports of hypothyroidism do occur in horses and cat-tle, but apparently these species are either less affected by hypothyroidism than are dogs or the condition is not recognized or treated to the same extent as in dogs.

Many endocrine diseases, including those of the thyroid, use the terms primary and secondary in their descriptions. The primary form of an endocrine disease means that the cause for the hormonal deviation is associ-ated with the organ that produces the final hormone. For example, *primary hypothyroidism* is a decrease in thyroid hormone production associated with disease or destruction of the thyroid gland. The secondary form of an endo-crine disease means that the end organ was secondarily affected by a problem in its regu-lating endocrine gland. For example, *secondary hypothyroidism* means that the pituitary gland cannot produce TSH for some reason. Without the stimulation of TSH, the thyroid gland does not produce thyroid hormones and hypothy-roidism results. In secondary hypothyroidism the thyroid gland itself is perfectly healthy, but it does not produce thyroid hormone because it has not been told to do so by the pituitary gland.

Another form of endocrine disease can be said to be tertiary, referring to a third-level problem. In *tertiary hypothyroidism* the thyroid gland is normal, the pituitary is also normal, but the hypothalamus is unable to produce TRH. No TRH means no stimulation of the pituitary to produce TSH, which means no stimulation of the thyroid to produce hor-mones, causing hypothyroidism. So the desig-nations of primary, secondary, and tertiary tell where the actual problem is that results in the deviation of hormones.

Canine thyroid tumors and immune dis-eases that attack the thyroid gland usually result in primary hypothyroidism because the

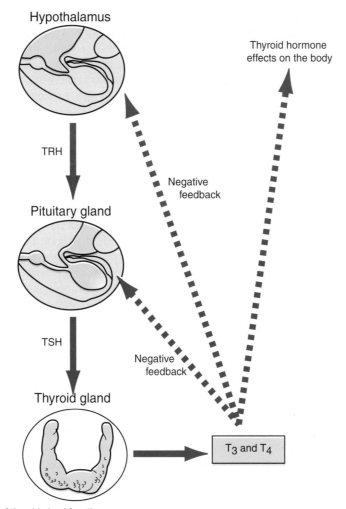

Figure 7-3 Regulation of thyroid gland function.

thyroid tumor cells are destroyed. The thyroid cannot produce T_4 and T_3 regardless of how much it is stimulated by TSH simply because it does not have enough functional cells left with which to respond. Secondary hypothyroidism may be caused by malformation of the pituitary gland, destruction of the pituitary gland by a tumor, or suppression of pituitary function by a variety of illnesses. Although primary and secondary hypothyroidism both result in decreased concentrations of T_4 and T_3, secondary hypothyroidism is considered

a more serious disease because of the potential for disruption of many hormonal systems regulated by the pituitary gland.

Goiter results in a hypothyroid condition caused by a lack of iodine in the diet. Without iodine the thyroid cannot manufacture T_3 or T_4 and thyroid hormone concentrations decrease. Unlike canine hypothyroidism, in which functional thyroid tissue is destroyed, in goiter the thyroid becomes enlarged with functional thyroid tissue. The increase in thyroid size is caused by excessive stimulation of the thyroid gland by TSH. Because the animal is hypothyroid, the hypothalamus and pituitary gland detect the low circulating levels of thyroid hormone and increase output of TRH and TSH in an attempt to raise T_3 and T_4 levels. In response to this stimulation from TSH, the thyroid cells proliferate and the gland increases in size to produce a goiter. In spite of the increased number of thyroid cells, without the required iodine the thyroid gland cannot manufacture thyroid hormones, and the hypothyroid condition remains uncorrected. Goiter is easily treated by feeding iodinated foods and is now rare because of the wide availability of commercially prepared, well-balanced animal feeds.

Because T_3 and T_4 are the main regulators of energy production and metabolism in the body, a lack of these hormones causes signs associated with a decreased basal metabolic rate. Signs of hypothyroidism include lethargy, weight gain despite normal consumption of food, heat-seeking behavior, bradycardia, decreased function of the *estrous* cycle, decreased growth in young animals, hair loss (alopecia), and dry and scaly skin (altered dermal metabolism). Contracted tendons and poor development of respiratory epithelium have been reported in foals of mares with hypothyroidism. These offspring often have poor central nervous system (CNS) development, resulting in lethargic, uncoordinated ("dull") young animals. Many of these signs are only evident when hypothyroidism has been chronic or has progressed to a fairly advanced stage. Early stages of hypothyroidism may have few signs or only subtle clinical signs.

The most common treatment for hypothyroidism is the use of thyroid drugs as hormone supplements. Drugs used to treat hypothyroidism include thyroid extracts, synthetic T_4 (levothyroxine), and synthetic T_3 (liothyronine). Thyroid extracts are no longer commonly used, but some products are still available through veterinary drug suppliers. Thyroid extracts are most commonly made from bovine or porcine thyroid glands acquired from slaughterhouses. The potency of these extracts is often based on the iodine content of the extract, not the actual amounts of T_3 or T_4; therefore the amount of thyroid hormone in an extract product may vary considerably among batches.

The synthetic T_4 product levothyroxine is the drug of choice for treatment of hypothyroidism. One of the key advantages of T_4 therapy is that it allows each tissue to individually convert T_4 to T_3 to meet its specific metabolic need. For example, the CNS has a high metabolic rate and therefore has an increased requirement for thyroid hormone. Thus the nervous system tissue normally uses all the T_3 presented to it and also converts any available T_4 to T_3 as needed. The drawback with using exclusive T_3 supplementation is supplying only T_3 bypasses the local tissue regulation of thyroid hormone conversion and essentially provides the same "dose" to all tissues. Another advantage of levothyroxine over T_3 is its ability to trigger the natural *negative feedback mechanism,* thus more closely emulating the normal regulatory mechanism for thyroid hormone production.

Some endocrinologists recommend initially using a well-known brand name of T_4 to initially regulate the animal because these products tend to achieve more consistent systemic concentrations of drug than some generic brands of T_4. Regardless of the brand of T_4 used, the dose should be regulated according to blood T_4 concentrations, and the product used should not be arbitrarily changed to another. Thyroid supplementations are typically given once daily, although some animals may respond more quickly when given levothyroxine twice daily initially.

The effects of T_4 overdose are generally not as severe in veterinary patients as they are in human beings because of the relatively wide therapeutic (safety) index of T_4 in the dog. Human beings being treated with

CLINICAL APPLICATION
Acute Overdose of Levothyroxine in a Dog

A six year old, male Keeshond was presented after being observed ingesting 850 of 0.2 mg levothyroxine sodium tablets. The owner initiated vomiting with hydrogen peroxide at home. Some of the dissolved tablets may have come up with the vomitus. At the time of admission, 3 to 9 hours after ingestion, the dog showed no significant clinical abnormalities. The rectal temperature was 102.4° F and the heart rate was 92 beats/min.

The National Animal Poison Control Center at the University of Illinois recommended treatment with activated charcoal (adsorbent) and diluted magnesium sulfate (saline cathartic). Blood was taken to determine T_4 concentration. The owner declined hospitalization.

The dog was reexamined and blood taken for T_3 and T_4 concentrations on days 3, 6, 9, 15, and 36 after ingestion. The initial T_4 concentration was 4900 nmol/L (normal range, 5.3 to 26.7 nmol/L). Although the concentrations of T_4 decreased significantly in the first 6 days (day 6 was less than 100 nmol/L), the concentrations did not return to normal until day 36. T_3 concentration at day 3 was 5.3 nmol/L (normal range, 0.4 to 1.4 nmol/L) but had returned to normal by day 6. The heart rate increased to 136 beats/min on day 3 and then to 156 beats/min on day 6. The owner reported no observable behavior changes.

Although problems with long-term overdose of thyroid supplements are cited in both the human and veterinary literature, seldom do acute overdoses of thyroid supplements produce severe degrees of tachycardia, hyperactivity, tachypnea (rapid breathing), abnormal pupillary light responses, or diarrhea. The veterinarian speculated that because only the non–protein-bound (unbound) form of levothyroxine is physiologically active and the very large capacity of protein binding of T_4 in the dog, perhaps not as much T_4 was physiologically available as the very high concentration would suggest.

What should be learned from this situation: A wide therapeutic index appears to exist for thyroid medications. Thus, when veterinarians try a therapeutic trial of thyroid supplementation in animals suspected of being hypothyroid, the risk of producing thyroid toxicosis is small. T_3 toxicosis would potentially be more of a risk for clinical toxicosis because of the direct cellular effect this hormone has. In human beings, overdose with T_3 typically produces signs sooner but of a shorter duration than T_4 toxicosis. Regardless of whether T_3 or T_4 toxicosis is the diagnosis, the animals at most risk for a fatal toxicosis would be elderly dogs that have concurrent heart disease.

Adapted from Hansen SR, Timmons SP, Dorman DC: Acute overdose of levothyroxine in a dog, *J Am Vet Med Assoc* 200:1512-1514, 1992.

thyroid supplements may have periodic thyroid storms, or *thyrotoxicosis,* in which even a relatively small overdose can cause hyperthyroidism signs such as tachycardia, agitation, nervousness, and polyuria. In contrast to human beings, most dogs are fairly resistant to thyrotoxicosis. However, thyroid drugs should still be used with caution in animals with cardiac disease because of the potential for increased cardiac stimulation and possible arrhythmias in dogs prone to arrhythmias.

Thyroid hormone normally increases the blood glucose concentrations by increasing glucose absorption from the gastrointestinal (GI) tract, converting protein to glucose (*gluconeogenesis),* and mobilizing liver glycogen stores to glucose (*glycogenolysis).* Therefore insulin requirements of diabetic animals that also are being treated for hypothyroidism may need to be increased after initiation of thyroid supplementation.

As previously mentioned, liothyronine (synthetic T_3) is generally not the first choice for treatment of hypothyroidism in dogs because T_3 supplementation bypasses regulation of local tissue conversion of T_4 to T_3. Theoretically the T_3 dose would be based on the T_3 needs of the CNS because that organ system has the highest demand for thyroid hormone. However, if an animal is given that dose, other organs with lesser requirements may be over-dosed with T_3. In addition, T_3 products are more expensive than T_4 products and most must be administered three times daily rather than once daily.

Occasionally liothyronine is used if levo-thyroxine therapy fails to produce adequate blood concentrations of thyroid hormone. Lack of T_4 efficacy may be related to the way it more readily combines with intestinal con-tents than T_3, thus reducing the amount of T_4 absorbed into the body. Normally T_3 has a bio-availability of 0.95, so 95% of T_3 is absorbed from the GI tract compared with only 40% to 80% absorption of T_4. However, consultation with a veterinary endocrinologist or internal medicine specialist is recommended before switching from T_4 to T_3.

A few products are available that contain both liothyronine and levothyroxine. The 4:1 ratio of T_3 to T_4 in these products is designed to meet the needs of human beings with hypothyroidism. Dogs require a slightly differ-ent ratio; therefore the human-formulated ratio would not provide the appropriate amount of thyroid hormones. Also, T_3 is metabolized more quickly than T_4; thus the ratio of T_3 to T_4 would continue to change over time after dos-ing. For these reasons, combination thyroid drugs are generally not recommended. The combined product can be used in dogs if the drug is dosed according to the T_4 component of the drug. As would be expected, the com-bination drug is considerably more expensive than the T_4 veterinary products.

DRUGS USED TO TREAT HYPERTHYROIDISM

Hyperthyroidism is an increase in circulat-ing concentrations of thyroid hormone. It is most common in cats and is associated with a hormone-secreting thyroid tumor. In contrast to hypothyroidism, hyperthyroidism is manifested by increased physical activity, diarrhea from increased GI motility, weight loss despite a voracious appetite, tachycardia (with heart rates exceeding 240 beats/min), polyuria (increased urination), and polydipsia (increased water intake). Owners of hyper-thyroid cats often do not bring their animals for treatment early in the course of disease because the animal appears healthy and fit (lean), is alert, and eats well.

Hyperthyroidism in cats is best treated by *thyroidectomy*, which is the removal of the thyroid gland, or by injection of radioactive iodine, which destroys the tumorous thy-roid tissue. However, some cats may not be a good surgical or anesthetic risk because of the effects of hyperthyroidism on the cardiovascu-lar system, or the radioactive iodine treatment may be unavailable or rejected by the owner because of the expense. As an alternative to surgery or radioactive iodine, these animals may be treated with antithyroid drugs, which decrease thyroid hormone production.

Methimazole (Tapazole) has been used to control hyperthyroidism in cats by blocking the thyroid tumor's ability to produce T_3 and T_4. These drugs block incorporation of iodine into the thyroid hormone molecule and thus prevent manufacture of a functional thyroid hormone molecule. Because methimazole only prevents hormone formation but does not destroy existing T_3 and T_4 molecules, signs of hyperthyroidism do not abate until body stores of thyroid hormones have been metabolized. Cessation of methimazole treatment results in recurrence of hyperthyroid signs because the mechanism for producing thyroid hormones is not permanently disabled by the drug. Cats with hyperthyroidism must take this drug for the rest of their lives to control the hyperthy-roid signs.

Side effects occur in approximately 20% of cats treated with methimazole. The most com-mon side effects are vomiting and anorexia; however, these signs may resolve after a few weeks of methimazole treatment. Although rare side effects such as liver problems, bleed-ing, and changes in white blood cell counts are seen in less than 3% of treated cats, when they do occur they are serious enough to require withdrawal of methimazole and reevaluation of the animal.

Some veterinarians choose to use methimazole in hyperthyroid cats for a few weeks to reduce the hyperthyroid signs that make the cat a poor surgical risk. Once these signs have resolved or the condition of the animal has improved, the cat can then have a thyroidectomy with less risk.

Radioactive iodine (^{131}I) is considered an effective means of removing the tumorous part of the thyroid gland that is producing the hyperthyroidism. ^{131}I can also be used if the patient is a poor surgical candidate and the owner is reluctant or unable to give oral medication on a daily basis for the rest of the cat's life.

The use of radioactive iodide is restricted to veterinary facilities that are designed to meet federal, state, and local regulations that govern the use of radioactive substances and radioactive waste generated by the patient. Fortunately for the general public, many veterinary facilities, including some specialized clinics that target cats needing ^{131}I treatment, are now available to administer the treatment.

The radioactive iodine is administered by intravenous injection. Because iodine is a normal component of thyroid hormone, the radioactive iodine is taken up and concentrated within the active thyroid tumor cells, causing them to receive a lethal dose of radioactivity while sparing the normal thyroid tissue. Generally, normal thyroid tissue is not destroyed by standard doses of radioactive iodine because the high levels of T_3 and T_4 produced by the tumor cells shut down TRH and TSH production, subsequently removing stimulation of normal thyroid tissue. Without TSH stimulation the normal thyroid tissue atrophies and does not take up much radioactive iodine.

Radioactive iodine kills the tumor cells as opposed to methimazole, which only controls hormone production without destroying the tumor itself. Radioactive iodine imposes less stress and risk on the patient than surgery and is less trouble for the owner than daily administration of oral drugs. However, ^{131}I treatment is significant because of the radioactivity and the need to keep the pet confined to a special containment area or unit for 1 to 3 weeks.

In hyperthyroidism the elevated levels of thyroid hormones produced by the thyroid tumor increase the number of β_1 receptors on cardiac cells, making the heart more sensitive to sympathetic stimulation. Thus normal sympathetic stimulation produces tachycardia, with heart rates in the cat often exceeding 240 beats/min. β_1 antagonists (see Chapter 5) such as propranolol decrease the effect of sympathetic stimulation by preventing the normal sympathetic neurotransmitter molecules of epinephrine and norepinephrine from combining with the β_1 receptors. Consequently, the heartbeat slows to a more normal rate and allows more efficient filling of the ventricles and has less myocardial oxygen demand.

ENDOCRINE PANCREATIC DRUGS

The pancreas plays a role in both endocrine (hormone) and exocrine (digestive enzyme) functions in the body. Insulin, glucagon, and somatostatin are the hormones normally produced by the pancreas. Of the three, insulin is the only pancreatic hormone that is used for therapeutic purposes with any regularity.

The major effect of insulin is to move glucose from the blood into tissue cells. Insulin also causes the liver to store glucose as glycogen and facilitates deposition of fat in adipose tissue. The net effect of insulin is to decrease blood glucose concentrations by enhancing distribution of glucose to body tissues. Lack of insulin results in diabetes mellitus, a disease characterized by high blood glucose levels, or hyperglycemia, and passage of glucose in the urine, or glucosuria.

The most common cause of diabetes mellitus in veterinary patients is destruction or lack of function of the pancreatic *beta cells,* which produce insulin. This type of diabetes is characterized by decreased insulin and is referred to as type 1, or *insulin-dependent diabetes mellitus* (IDDM). Whereas *type 1 diabetes* is related to the number of functional pancreatic beta cells, *type 2 diabetes,* or *non–insulin-dependent diabetes mellitus* (NIDDM), results from a decreased effectiveness of insulin even though the pancreatic beta cells are potentially capable of producing adequate insulin. A decreased number of insulin receptors on tissue cells, decreased sensitivity of insulin receptors present, or a decreased sensitivity of the pancreatic beta cells to hyperglycemia can all result in hyperglycemia classified as NIDDM.

Patients with IDDM require injections of insulin. Unfortunately, the administration of insulin by injection fails to mimic the body's normal production of insulin in response to elevated blood glucose concentrations. Therefore insulin administration must be scheduled and regulated in conjunction with the animal's diet and exercise 24 hours a day, 7 days week, 365 days of the year. Treatment of a diabetic patient requires a strong commitment from the pet owner.

Owners are often initially hesitant about giving injections to their animal and ask if they can give an oral medication. Because insulin is a protein, it would be destroyed (denatured) by the stomach's gastric acid and therefore cannot be given orally. Even if the insulin molecule was not denatured by the gastric acid, the insulin molecule is too large to be absorbed through the bowel mucosa. The technician's role in educating the client to properly administer the insulin and in explaining the dietary and lifestyle changes and the need for blood or urine glucose testing is very important in helping the client understand what is required to regulate the diabetic patient.

TYPES OF INSULIN

Various types of insulin are available, but the availability of certain insulins is in a constant state of flux. What is presented is an overview and guidelines of the types of insulin. Insulins are classified by their duration of activity (short-, intermediate-, and long-acting) and according to the species from which the insulin is derived (beef, pork, or genetically engineered human-type insulin).

Insulin derived from purified beef, pork, or a combination of beef and pork was the main type available to both the human and veterinary markets for many years. Differences in insulin structure between species are thought to have contributed to the development of insulin antibodies, which can lead to erratic control of blood glucose levels. Pork insulin is antigenically similar to canine insulin. The genetically engineered human insulin (recombinant human insulin), although not as close in structure to canine insulin as is pork insulin, is close enough to prevent significant antibody production. Bovine insulin structure, however, is different enough from that of the canine that antibody production against the foreign insulin can be significant.

Unfortunately, manufacturers of insulin (primarily for the wider human diabetic market) have moved from the beef, pork, or combination beef/pork insulin to the recombinant human insulin. However, in 2004 the U.S. Food and Drug Administration approved a porcine (pork) insulin zinc suspension product for treatment of diabetes in dogs.

As previously stated, insulins are also classified by the duration of effect they have in the body. The short-acting insulins include regular (crystalline) insulin, the intermediate-acting include isophane (NPH) and Lente insulins, and the long-acting insulins include Ultralente and *protamine* zinc (PZI) insulins. The manufacturer of PZI stopped producing it in 1991 but began producing it again in 2004 exclusively for veterinary use.

TABLE **7-1** Comparison of Types of Insulin Used for Dog and Cats

INSULIN TYPE	ROUTE OF ADMINISTRATION	ONSET OF EFFECT	DURATION OF EFFECT (DOG)	DURATION OF EFFECT (CAT)
Regular	IV	Immediate	1-4 hr	1-4 hr
crystalline	IM	10-30 min	3-8 hr	3-8 hr
	SC	10-30 min	4-10 hr	4-10 hr
NPH	SC	0.5-2 hr	6-18 hr	4-12 hr
Lente	SC	0.5-2 hr	8-20 hr	6-18 hr
Ultralente	SC	0.5-8 hr	8-24 hr	6-24 hr
PZI	SC	0.5-4 hr	NA	6-20 hr

Adapted from Feldman EC, Nelson RW: *Canine and feline endocrinology and reproduction,* Philadelphia, 2004, WB Saunders.

The duration of activity of insulin relates to the differences in absorption based on what the insulin is combined with and the solubility of the resulting insulin crystals. For example, NPH and PZI insulins are formed by mixing insulin, zinc, and a fish protein called protamine. The combination is allowed to precipitate into crystals that are poorly soluble and hence slow to dissolve and release the insulin when injected subcutaneously. The difference in length between NPH and PZI is from the different protamine and zinc ratios. The Lente family of insulins derives its duration from higher concentrations of zinc (no protamine) and the size of the crystals. Ultralente (long-acting) has the largest, least soluble crystals and Lente (intermediate-acting) has the smallest, most soluble crystals.

The most commonly used insulins for maintaining the health of diabetic dogs are the intermediate-duration insulins NPH and Lente. The pork form NPH and Lente are preferred over the recombinant human forms because they may have a longer duration of activity in dogs, sometimes allowing once-daily injections, which is more convenient and improves client compliance in treating the animal.

Controversy exists regarding which insulin to use in cats. Cats can vary widely in how they respond to insulin; some can be very sensitive to the insulin and others can be very resistant to the insulin effects. Also, cats may progress from type 2 to type 1 diabetes or go through periods where they appear to be in remission from diabetes. Thus blood glucose regulation in feline diabetic patients can be more of a challenge than in canine diabetics. Because insulin types in cats seem to have a shorter duration than in dogs, diabetic cats require the longer-acting PZI or Ultralente (Table 7-1).[1]

Regular insulin is not commonly used to maintain diabetic cats or dogs because its short duration of activity requires multiple doses during a 24-hour period. However, because regular insulin is the only type that can be given intravenously, it is used initially to stabilize the glucose concentrations of animals with severe, uncontrolled diabetes or diabetic ketoacidosis.

Insulin is administered in syringes marked differently than a typical 3-cc or 6-mL syringe. Unlike most drugs, which are measured in milligrams, insulin is measured in units. The bottles of insulin are listed as *U-40, U-100,* or U-500, meaning the bottle contains 40, 100, or 500 insulin units per milliliter. Likewise, the insulin syringes are calibrated for the different unit concentration bottles, meaning that U-40 syringes are different from U-100 syringes. The special insulin syringes help a client accurately measure the amount of insulin to give because the markings on the syringe are calibrated in units based on the unit rating of the insulin and matching syringe. Thus instead of the client having to calculate a dose in milliliters, they simply withdraw the required number of units from the appropriate insulin bottle.

Most of the insulins are suspensions, meaning that the insulin is not dissolved in the liquid but must be resuspended before each withdrawal of insulin from the bottle.

Resuspension of the insulin crystals should be done by rolling the bottle between the palms of the hands instead of vigorously shaking the bottle. Vigorous shaking can physically denature the insulin, rendering it useless. The veterinary technician should carefully show the pet owner how to resuspend the insulin crystals without causing physical destruction of the drug.

Because insulin doses are timed to have their maximal effect near the time when blood glucose concentrations are peaking after consumption of a meal, reliable patterns of absorption are important for the intermediate- and long-acting insulins. These insulins are administered subcutaneously, typically in the neck or lumbar area (although some authors may advocate other areas). The pet owner must administer the drug in areas that have consistent perfusion. As discussed in Chapter 3 the perfusion, and hence absorption, of drugs from well-perfused skeletal muscle is quite different from subcutaneous tissue and fat. If the client injects too deeply and administers the drug intramuscularly, the drug is likely to be absorbed quicker and the peak effect of the insulin may occur before the anticipated rise in blood glucose from eating a meal. At the other extreme, insulin injected into a poorly perfused fat pad may remain at that site for hours beyond what it would if injected subcutaneously. Proper depth and consistent location of insulin injection are essential for regulation of the diabetic patient by its owner.

Much research has been performed regarding the role of diet in controlling diabetic patients in human medicine as well as veterinary medicine. Many veterinary diabetic patients can benefit from diets that are lower in absorbable sugars or that reduce the amount of sugars available to be absorbed. At the least, semimoist dog and cat foods should be avoided because of the high concentrations of sucrose and fructose used to soften these products. If a food label lists sugars as some of the first ingredients, it should probably be avoided in diabetics.

OTHER DRUGS TO CONTROL DIABETES, AND DRUGS TO AVOID

The use of other drugs in diabetic patients can alter insulin requirements and may necessitate changing the insulin dosage. For example, corticosteroids (glucocorticoids) such as prednisone and dexamethasone mobilize glycogen stores, elevate blood glucose levels, and interfere with insulin receptors, all of which can produce significant hyperglycemia in a diabetic animal. Other drugs that elevate blood glucose levels include thiazide diuretics, phenothiazine tranquilizers (such as acepromazine), progesterone, and catecholamines such as epinephrine.

Clients often ask about use of human oral hypoglycemic agents for their pets as an alternative to daily injections of insulin. They know of relatives or friends who are type 2 diabetics who are well controlled with these oral drugs and do not require insulin injections. One of the most common of these hypoglycemic drugs is the *sulfonylurea compounds,* which include products such as glipizide. Although not totally understood, sulfonylurea compounds are thought to stimulate additional insulin production by pancreatic beta cells (the main effect), increase binding of insulin to peripheral tissue insulin receptors, or enhance the cellular response to insulin.

Because a relatively high incidence of NIDDM is believed to occur in cats, oral hypoglycemic agents such as glipizide may be able to increase insulin effectiveness, thus avoiding the use of insulin injections. Two studies by Nelson and Feldman[2,3] showed that fewer than 50% of untreated diabetic cats responded to glipizide. Cats that did respond usually did so by week 8 of therapy. Side effects occurred sooner than that (often by 30 days) and included transient vomiting and anorexia, increased liver enzymes on the serum chemistry profile, and some incidents of jaundice (yellowing of skin from the buildup of bilirubin from liver damage). The conclusion by one of the authors was that as many as one third of diabetic cats may respond to oral hypoglycemic therapy, thus avoiding insulin injections.[4]

Oral hypoglycemic therapy is not thought to be effective in dogs because dogs have very few functional pancreatic beta cells by the time diabetes mellitus is diagnosed. Therefore compounds that stimulate beta cells cannot significantly increase insulin production. In addition, dogs are at risk for hepatic injury if drugs such as glipizide are used. Cats that progress from type 2 (NIDDM) to type 1 (IDDM) are unlikely to respond to oral hypoglycemics. In both cats and dogs attempts to rule out nondiabetic underlying causes of hyperglycemia are important (e.g., drugs producing hyperglycemia, tumors of the adrenal gland).

DRUGS AFFECTING REPRODUCTION

Hormone drugs, either natural or synthetic, are used in food animals and horses to synchronize estrous cycles, terminate pregnancies, and induce ovulation. In dogs and cats, these drugs are used primarily to prevent pregnancy or alter the state of the uterus. Because the degree of response to reproductive hormone therapy varies among species, the dosage regimen or therapeutic protocol in one species should not be assumed to produce the same effect in another species. The following discussion describes some common ways drugs are used to treat reproductive problems. The reader is encouraged to review the literature to learn more about the ways these drugs are used in the treatment of specific reproductive problems in a particular species.

HORMONAL CONTROL OF THE ESTROUS CYCLE

In female animals, hormone therapies often block or enhance the effect of endogenous reproductive hormones. Because reproductive hormones increase and decrease at various times in the estrous cycle, the veterinarian must determine (before treatment) the animal's stage in the estrous cycle to ensure the presence of the required hormone or physiologic process on which the therapy acts. Hence reproductive hormone drugs can be effective or ineffective, indicated or contraindicated, at different stages of the estrous cycle (proestrus, *estrus*, diestrus, and anestrus).

The estrous cycle is sometimes described as having two phases: the *follicular phase*, in which hormones produced by the ovarian follicle exert predominant control, and the *luteal phase*, in which hormones of the corpus luteum on the ovary predominate. The follicular phase includes the proestrus and estrus stages, and the luteal phase usually includes diestrus (metestrus).

Early in the follicular phase the pituitary gland, under the influence of gonadotropin-releasing hormone (GnRH) from the hypothalamus, releases follicle-stimulating hormone (FSH), which in turn stimulates the ovary to produce follicles containing egg cells, or oocytes (Figure 7-4). Under the influence of FSH the follicular tissue also begins to produce estrogens. The behavioral and physical changes associated with estrus ("heat") are largely related to changes in estrogen levels.

Estrogen production usually peaks near the time of estrus, although considerable variation exists among species. A second hormone, inhibin, or folliculostatin, is also produced by the developing follicular tissue and serves as a negative feedback mechanism to decrease release of GnRH and FSH. By decreasing the release of FSH, inhibin allows only the most developed follicle to continue maturation until it can release an ovum. Thus inhibin helps prevent development of multiple follicles and decreases the potential for multiple births in animals that normally have only one or two offspring per birth.

The follicular phase terminates with the release of luteinizing hormone (LH) from the

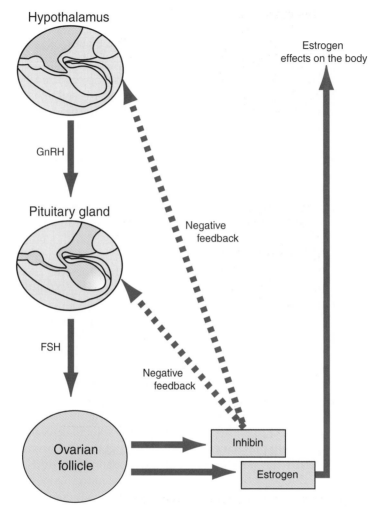

Figure 7-4 Hormones and glands involved in the follicular phase of the estrous cycle.

pituitary gland. LH lyses (aids in the rupture of) the mature follicles, releases the ova, and transforms the ruptured follicle into a corpus luteum (CL).

In the luteal phase of the estrous cycle (Figure 7-5), the principal hormone produced by the CL is progesterone, which is considered the hormone of pregnancy. Progesterone causes the lining of the uterus to thicken and secrete a nutrient-rich fluid in preparation for implantation of the ovum or ova. In addition, progesterone keeps the uterine smooth muscles

(myometrium) in a quiescent, noncontractile state and provides negative feedback to the hypothalamus and pituitary to inhibit further release of GnRH, FSH, and LH. If the released ova are not fertilized and do not implant in the receptive uterus within a certain time, the CL degenerates, causing a drop in progesterone production and subsequently reduced progesterone concentrations. This decrease in progesterone removes the inhibition on hypothalamic GnRH production and release of pituitary FSH and LH, resulting in initiation of a new estrous cycle.

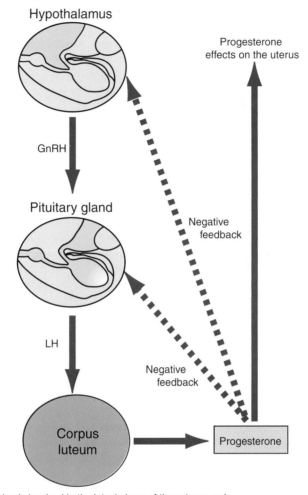

Figure 7-5 Hormones and glands involved in the luteal phase of the estrous cycle.

An important note: *estrus* is a noun referring to the state of being in heat. *Estrous* is an adjective, as indicated by *-ous,* and is used to describe the noun *cycle.*

HORMONAL CHANGES DURING PREGNANCY AND PARTURITION

A pregnant animal must have adequate levels of progesterone produced by the CL and the placenta to maintain the pregnancy. At the end of pregnancy the fetus initiates parturition (the birth process) by producing adrenocorticotropic hormone, which results in

elevated levels of cortisol (a natural corticosteroid) in both the fetal and maternal circulations. In response to the cortisol the uterus begins to produce estrogens and prostaglandins, both of which make the myometrium more prone to contraction and produce physical changes in the cervix and birth canal that favor passage of the newborn.

The prostaglandins produced by the uterus cause lysis (degeneration) of the CL, which terminates its production of progesterone. Together, estrogen and prostaglandins increase the number of oxytocin receptors on the myometrial cells, making these smooth muscle cells more sensitive to the powerful contracting effect of oxytocin. Stimulation of the cervix or vagina, such as from entry of the fetus into the birth canal, or stimulation of the nipples from a nursing animal causes the pituitary gland to release oxytocin, which produces the forceful uterine contractions associated with labor and postpartum contractions and release of milk (letdown) from the mammary gland.

TYPES OF REPRODUCTIVE DRUGS
Gonadotropin-Releasing Hormone and Synthetic Analogs

Synthesized GnRH drugs (GnRH analogs) have a similar structure as endogenous GnRH and stimulate release of LH and FSH. Because the natural endogenous GnRH is normally released in pulses from the hypothalamus, bolus injections or infusions of synthetic GnRH are usually not as effective as endogenous GnRH. Some GnRH analogs have several substitutions of the amino acids (components that make up protein) and if heavily substituted may act as antagonists to natural GnRH (prevent release of FSH and LH) by combining with the receptor for GnRH but having no intrinsic activity. These antagonists would be used to decrease progression of the estrous cycle by blocking endogenous GnRH stimulation of FSH and LH release.

GnRH analogs include commercial products available for cattle primarily indicated for lysis of persistent ovarian follicles. Although these products produce increased FSH and LH for a few days in cattle (primarily dairy cattle), the downregulation of receptors to GnRH (see Chapter 3) will result in a decreased effectiveness of the drug over the long term by a return of FSH and LH levels to baseline. Therefore the current use of GnRH analogs is mostly for short-term use to lyse persistent ovarian follicles.

Because the word fragment *-tropin* means *an affinity to,* the pituitary gonadotropins FSH and LH have an affinity for, and produce their effects on, the gonads (ovaries, testes). Gonadotropin drugs may be extracts from the pituitary glands of food animals and generally have more FSH effect than LH effect. In addition to pituitary gonadotropins, some species produce chorionic gonadotropins from the placenta. Human chorionic gonadotropin is a hormone produced by the human placenta and has LH-like effects with few or no FSH effects. Certain fetal cells in the horse produce equine chorionic gonadotropin, also known as pregnant mare serum gonadotropin, which has FSH and LH effects. These drugs are sometimes used in food animals to induce superovulation (release of ova from multiple follicles) and occasionally in dogs and cats to induce estrus. Chorionic gonadotropins have also been used to stimulate testicular descent in cryptorchid males with undescended testicles.

Progestins, Progestagens, and Progestational Hormones

Progestins are a group of reproductive hormones, with the prototype drug being progesterone. *Progestational hormones* are synonymous with progestins; the term *progestagen* refers to synthesized drugs that mimic progestins. Use of progestin or progestagen drugs during the follicular phase can slow or halt progression of the estrous cycle by inhibiting release of GnRH, FSH, and LH, further slowing development of the follicles. When used in this manner, progestins can prevent an animal from coming into full estrus. Use of progestins during the luteal phase can prolong diestrus beyond the time when the CL has regressed by providing exogenous progesterone to replace the declining progesterone concentrations that accompany CL regression. Progestin drugs used in veterinary medicine are often recognizable by the word fragment *-gest* in the nonproprietary (generic) name, such as altrenogest (Regu-Mate) or medroxyprogesterone (Depo Provera reposity injectable).

The veterinary professional should be aware of certain precautions when using progestins.

Progesterone causes the endometrium (uterine lining) to produce secretions ("uterine milk") that favor implantation of ova after fertilization. These progesterone-induced changes also provide an environment conducive for bacterial growth in the uterus. Thus use of progestins at higher than normal levels or for extended periods predisposes the uterus to infection, metritis, or pyometra. Pyometra is a uterine infection in which a great deal of pus is evident. If the cervix is relaxed, the purulent material (pus) produced within the uterus can escape and be evident as a purulent discharge, a condition called open-cervix pyometra. If the cervix is closed, the pus may accumulate within the uterus, creating a life-threatening condition called closed-cervix pyometra.

Even if the uterus does not become infected, prolonged treatment with progestins can produce a change within the lining of the uterus, resulting in cystic endometriosis with subsequent decreased fertility. Progestins may also cause mammary hyperplasia (increased proliferation of tissue), which may increase the risk of mammary tumors.

Progesterone and other progestins have an antagonistic effect on insulin and reduce its ability to move glucose into cells. This effect of progestins helps explain the hyperglycemia and a temporary diabetic-like syndrome (gestational diabetes) that is frequently seen in pregnant women and females in other species. Because of the insulin antagonism, progestational compounds should not be used in diabetic animals.

One of the most commonly used progestational agents is altrenogest. Because orally administered liquid forms of progestins can be readily absorbed through the skin, the manufacturer of Regu-Mate (altrenogest for use in horses) states that people with the following conditions should not handle this drug:

- women who are or suspect they are pregnant
- people with a history of thrombophlebitis (inflammation and clots within blood vessels) or thromboembolic disorders (spontaneous clot formation)
- people with cerebrovascular (brain blood vessels) or coronary artery disease (e.g., partial blockage, previous coronary bypass surgery)
- women with carcinoma (type of aggressive cancer) of the breast
- people with known estrogen-dependent neoplasia (e.g., some breast cancers)
- women with undiagnosed vaginal bleeding
- people who have developed any type of tumor while taking oral contraceptives or estrogen-containing products

Most of these conditions relate directly to the progestin effects; however, most progestational drugs also have some estrogen effect, hence the warnings related to estrogen stimulation. Because of the warnings associated with this drug, veterinary professionals should take extra steps to ensure they, their staff, and clients are protected from accidental exposure to this drug.

Estrogen

Estrogen drugs such as estradiol cypionate and diethylstilbestrol (DES) have been used for a variety of reproductive and nonreproductive functions. However, with refinement of medical treatments and the availability of newer drugs, fewer medical indications for estrogens are considered legitimate or state of the art. Injectable estradiol cypionate has been used to induce estrus in anestrual mares or used in conjunction with other drugs in cows to stimulate uterine contraction to expel purulent (pus, necrotic material) contents. DES is an estrogen compound that several years ago was used extensively in food animals as a growth-promoting, or anabolic, steroid. After DES was found to have significant *carcinogenic* (cancer-producing) potential in human beings, the drug was banned from use in food animals. DES is still available in an oral form, mostly from compounding pharmacies. The drug is still legitimately used to reduce urinary incontinence in dogs.

Estrogens in general are prone to some potentially serious side effects that every veterinary technician must know. These side effects have triggered the removal of estrogen from current treatment option lists. As with progesterone, estrogens can predispose the uterus to infection and pyometra. Estrogens increase the number of progesterone receptors on uterine cells; therefore a large dose of estrogen would make the uterus more sensitive to progesterone and increase the response of the uterus to the normal progesterone concentrations. Through this increased progesterone effect, estrogen may indirectly result in pyometra 3 to 6 weeks after a large dose of estrogen. Owners of animals treated with estrogen should watch for and report polyuria (increased urination), polydipsia (increased water intake), lethargy, anorexia, or any abnormal vulvar discharge because these constitute the early signs of open-cervix pyometra.

A second and potentially deadly side effect of estrogen, even when used at normal dosages, is suppression of blood cell production by the bone marrow. The resulting decrease in all bone marrow cells results in a condition called *aplastic anemia.* Estrogen-induced aplastic anemia usually appears 2 to 8 weeks after estrogen administration and is manifested as low platelet counts (thrombocytopenia), pinpoint hemorrhages in the skin or mucous membranes (caused by low platelet levels), evidence of bruising, leukopenia (low white blood cell count), and severe anemia. Aplastic anemia may slowly resolve after discontinuation of estrogen therapy; however, the anemia can continue to progress, resulting in death of the animal.

Prostaglandins

Synthetic prostaglandin drugs, most of which are derivations of prostaglandin $F_{2\alpha}$, are often used to lyse an active CL in an animal in the diestrus period of the luteal phase or to cause contractions of the uterus. By lysing the CL, prostaglandins terminate the major source of progesterone during the luteal phase, causing progesterone levels to drop and a new estrous cycle to begin. Obviously if prostaglandins are administered during the follicular phase when no CL is present, no clinical effect related to progesterone levels will be observed. Significant species differences exist in the susceptibility of the CL to prostaglandin lysis, with horses and cattle significantly more sensitive to lysis than dogs or cats. Also, a younger CL is more resistant to lysis than a more mature CL. This emphasizes the importance of knowing in which phase of the estrous cycle an animal is before administering drugs to alter the reproductive cycle.

Prostaglandins have a direct and indirect effect on the uterus. By decreasing progesterone through CL lysis, prostaglandins remove the hormone responsible for the quiescent state of the myometrium (uterine muscle), making the uterus more prone to contractions with time as progesterone levels decrease. Prostaglandins also have a more immediate effect by directly stimulating the myometrium to contract.

Prostaglandins are marketed under a variety of trade names. Most can be recognized by the stem -*prost* in the chemical or generic name. Common prostaglandin drugs include dinoprost tromethamine (Lutalyse) and cloprostenol (Estrumate).

Endogenous prostaglandins affect many body systems, and exogenous prostaglandins similarly cause a wide variety of effects. The most common side effects include unintended abortion in pregnant animals because of CL lysis; bronchoconstriction in animals with respiratory disease (such as horses with heaves); vomiting (in dogs and cats); colic and sweating (in horses); and, in larger doses, CNS effects such as anxiety, hyperpnea, and pupillary dilation.

Technicians who handle prostaglandins should be aware that these drugs are easily absorbed through the skin and can easily produce CL lysis and bronchoconstriction in people as well as animals. Technicians should take precautions such as wearing latex surgical gloves when handling these drugs. Women of childbearing age and those with asthma should completely avoid handling these drugs at any time.

USES OF REPRODUCTIVE DRUGS
Drugs Used to Control Estrous Cycling

Livestock breeders use estrus synchronization in female animals so that artificial insemination can be planned in advance and a number of animals can be inseminated at the same time. By synchronizing heat and insemination dates, all offspring are born at approximately the same time, which facilitates management at parturition and better neonatal care.

Injecting cows with prostaglandins during diestrus results in CL lysis, which subsequently causes progesterone concentrations to fall and the animal to return to estrus within 2 to 5 days of prostaglandin administration. Prostaglandins are used similarly in mares but with more variable results because, among other reasons, the equine CL is less sensitive to the lysing effects of prostaglandins for up to 5 days after ovulation and CL formation. Prostaglandins are not used in this manner in small animals because synchronizing groups of animals for breeding is not common, and the CL of cats and dogs tends to be resistant to the effects of exogenous prostaglandin for most of the luteal phase.

Another way to synchronize estrus in a herd of livestock in varying stages of diestrus is to administer progestins several times to prolong the luteal phase beyond its normal termination, then abruptly terminate treatment to mimic CL lysis and bring the animals back into heat. In mares, injectable progesterone in oil or oral progestin altrenogest (Regu-Mate) is administered for 2 weeks to mimic diestrus, suppress LH stimulation, and allow subsequent regression of the CL. When the exogenous progestin is withdrawn after 2 weeks, no CL is present to maintain progesterone levels, and the cycle returns to proestrus and estrus.

Estrogen is sometimes added to the progestin regimen in mares to suppress follicular development and provide a more predictable return to estrus. In some mares the CL persists beyond the 2 weeks of treatment with progestin, resulting in failure to return to estrus. Therefore prostaglandins may be used at the time of the progestin withdrawal to lyse any CL that has not already regressed.

Use of gonadotropins in an attempt to synchronize the estrous cycle by synchronizing follicle growth or ovulation has not been consistently successful. Equine chorionic gonadotropin has been used to stimulate follicle growth because of its FSH and LH effects. In contrast, human chorionic gonadotropin, because of its predominantly LH effect, has been used to lyse normal, developed follicles or those that persist, such as occur in cows with prolonged estrus (nymphomania), thus bringing the animal back into proestrus.

Drugs Used in Foal Heat

Mares that come into heat soon after foaling generally have a significantly lower conception rate than mares that come into heat at a later time. Many breeding managers delay this *foal heat* to increase the chances of conception at a later breeding. Because progesterone inhibits release of FSH and LH by negative feedback, administration of exogenous progestin drugs halts progression of the estrous cycle, delaying the onset of foal heat. This delay facilitates recovery of the uterus from the recent pregnancy so that it can support the embryo of the next pregnancy. A second technique to increase conception rates in mares that have recently foaled is to shorten the diestrus phase of the first cycle by using prostaglandins to lyse the CL and initiate a new cycle.

Drugs Used to Treat Anestrus

As the days grow shorter in autumn and the photoperiod decreases, the reproductive hormones decrease to minimal amounts, causing the mare to stop cycling and enter a period of *seasonal anestrus.* Because equine breed registries encourage birth of foals as soon as possible after January 1, breeders often ask veterinarians to help mares conceive during the spring, when the animals are in transition from seasonal anestrus to full reproductive capacity. During this period of transitional estrus, several follicles normally grow and regress, causing periods of estrus that are frequently long and during which the exact time of ovulation is unknown. To stimulate more predictable ovulation, progesterone or a progestin drug is administered for 10 to 14 days to mimic diestrus and then halted to mimic CL lysis.

This technique is only successful if multiple, large follicles are on the ovaries. In this technique, the progesterone drug blocks release of LH from the pituitary gland for the 10 to 14 days but does not significantly decrease production of LH, causing LH to accumulate in the pituitary gland. When progesterone administration is halted (mimicking CL lysis), the stored LH is released in sufficient quantities to lyse the large follicles, thereby releasing the ova. Concomitant use of estrogens seems to enhance this effect on LH. Human chorionic gonadotropin may also be used in conjunction with the drop in progesterone to aid lysis of follicles because of its predominant LH activity. Such hormonal therapy is often coupled with exposing the mares to artificial lighting in the stalls to lengthen the perceived photoperiod and to emulate the longer daylight hours of summer.

Drugs Used to Maintain Pregnancy

Because progesterone is the normal hormone that maintains pregnancy, progestagens and progesterone have been advocated for use in maintaining pregnancy in mares prone to abortion. These drugs may help if the problem is related to low progesterone levels because of a poorly functioning CL. Altrenogest has been used with varying success in mares to prevent premature parturition. Because altrenogest is slightly different from progesterone, it does not produce negative feedback on endogenous progesterone production and thus can be given as an oral progesterone supplement. Unfortunately, because abortion and premature parturition have multiple causes, the success of progestin therapy in maintaining pregnancy varies considerably.

Drugs Used to Prevent Pregnancy

Pregnancy can be prevented by suppressing the estrous cycle or preventing implantation of the fertilized ova in the uterine wall. Megestrol acetate (Ovaban) is an orally administered progestin used for contraception in female dogs and cats. The drug is similar to progesterone and is thought to suppress release of GnRH and subsequent release of FSH and LH, causing cessation of cycling. Because megestrol is a progestin, it causes endometrial changes such as thickened, increased secretions consistent with progesterone stimulation. Use of megestrol increases the risk of cystic hyperplasia of the endometrium, endometritis, or pyometra, although the risk of pyometra appears to be fairly low. Prolonged use of megestrol can result in mammary hyperplasia (proliferation of mammary tissue). For these reasons, megestrol acetate is contraindicated in animals with any disease of the reproductive organs, mammary tumors, or mammary growth. Megestrol is contraindicated in pregnant females because the drug can have a masculinizing effect on female fetuses and can delay parturition.

As with progesterone and other progestins, megestrol has an antagonistic effect on insulin and reduces its ability to move glucose into cells. Long-term therapy with megestrol may predispose female dogs and cats to diabetes mellitus.

The adrenal gland in cats is apparently sensitive to the suppressive effects of megestrol acetate. Plasma cortisol levels in cats treated with megestrol can drop well below normal, producing a syndrome resembling hypoadrenocorticism. Most cats treated with megestrol do not show severe signs with this effect; however, administration of prednisone or other corticosteroids should be considered if such cats are to have surgery, be hospitalized, or be subjected to other stress.

Mibolerone is another contraceptive previously used in female dogs. This is an androgen hormone similar to testosterone and interrupts estrous cycling by inhibiting LH release. Follicles develop to a point but do not lyse and consequently do not release their ova. Because mibolerone is a testosterone analog and therefore has a similar structure to testosterone, it produces effects similar to those of high levels of endogenous testosterone. These include increased production of anal sac secretions, masculinization of developing female fetuses, and increased vulvar discharge. Mibolerone is contraindicated in dogs with perianal adenoma or perianal adenocarcinoma because these types of tumors are stimulated by androgen (male) hormones such as testosterone. Some dogs develop icterus (jaundice) while receiving this drug; therefore mibolerone should not be used in dogs with a history of liver disease. Female dogs treated for longer than 8 months should have tests to monitor liver function. Although mibolerone is relatively effective in female cats, it is generally contraindicated in this species because of reports of liver toxicosis and thyrotoxicosis. Commercially prepared mibolerone is no longer available in the United States; however, compounding pharmacies are still able to provide this product.

Drugs Used to Terminate Pregnancy

Several drugs are used to induce abortion or initiate parturition. These drugs are used in animals carrying a dead fetus, mares carrying twins, or heifers that have been bred too young to safely deliver a live calf. Prostaglandins are the most commonly used drugs for termination of pregnancy. Prostaglandin administration causes CL lysis, resulting in a decrease in progesterone levels and subsequent fetal death.

The effectiveness of prostaglandin $F_{2\alpha}$ and its analogs varies among species because of the resistance of some CLs to prostaglandin and the placenta's role in providing some progesterone necessary to maintain pregnancy. In cows the CL continues to produce progesterone for the entire pregnancy; however, the placenta can produce sufficient progesterone to maintain pregnancy without the CL after the fourth or fifth month. Therefore prostaglandins are only effective in cows if given before the fourth month of pregnancy.

In dogs the CL is relatively resistant to the lytic effects of prostaglandins during the first 2 to 4 weeks of pregnancy. Canine CL sensitivity to prostaglandin increases after this time. Although prostaglandins are quite effective in terminating pregnancy, they often cause side effects such as panting, salivation, respiratory distress, GI stimulation (vomiting and diarrhea), tachycardia, and increased urination. If side effects occur, they last only approximately 20 minutes. If needed, the GI stimulation and respiratory distress can be alleviated by giving the animal atropine.

Dinoprost tromethamine (Lutalyse) is approved for termination of pregnancy in mares. As in dogs, side effects include increased respiratory and heart rates, sweating, transient fever, and some abdominal discomfort. These signs usually disappear approximately 1 hour after administration.

The use of misoprostol (prostaglandin E; see Chapter 4) in conjunction with prostaglandin $F_{2\alpha}$ has been advocated.[5] Prostaglandin type E is thought to be involved with the opening of the cervix; therefore when used in conjunction with prostaglandin $F_{2\alpha}$ it may provide a more complete evacuation of the uterus.

Dopamine agonists are a group of compounds that, as the name implies, bind with and stimulate dopamine receptors. Dopamine agonists can indirectly cause a series of changes that result in premature parturition or abortion. One of the other effects of dopamine is to inhibit release of prolactin, a hormone produced by the anterior pituitary gland. Prolactin helps maintain the CL. If a dopamine agonist drug is used, prolactin is inhibited and the CL may degenerate, resulting in a decline of progesterone necessary for maintaining pregnancy. Bromocriptine is a drug that has been advocated in various protocols, but because of the high incidence of vomiting its use has not gained acceptance. Two other dopamine agonist drugs that have been investigated are metergoline and cabergoline.

Corticosteroids may induce abortion in mares or cows by mimicking the elevated levels of cortisol that occur at the beginning of normal parturition. In dogs, corticosteroids such as dexamethasone have been reported to cause intrauterine death and fetal resorption if given after 30 days of gestation (pregnancy) and abortion if given during the last 3 weeks of gestation. When used as abortifacients (drugs that induce abortion), corticosteroids are unpredictable in their efficacy. Corticosteroid use in cows is associated with a fairly high incidence of retained placenta. Because prostaglandins are usually much more effective, corticosteroids are not used often for inducing parturition or abortion. However, the inadvertent administration of a significant dose of a corticosteroid in a pregnant animal for a problem unrelated to pregnancy, such as joint inflammation or immune-mediated disease, can induce unintended abortion.

OTHER USES OF REPRODUCTIVE DRUGS

Oxytocin is an endogenous hormone released from the pituitary gland that causes contraction of the myometrium (muscles of the uterus). Just before parturition the increased concentrations of prostaglandins and estrogens cause increased numbers of oxytocin receptors to appear on the smooth muscle cells of the uterus, making them more sensitive to the effects of oxytocin. When the entrance of the fetus into the birth canal stimulates oxytocin

release, the uterus contracts to expel the newborn. Exogenous oxytocin is most commonly used to increase uterine contractions in animals with dystocia (difficult labor) related to a weakened or fatigued uterus. Calcium gluconate is sometimes given in conjunction with oxytocin to facilitate uterine contraction in dystocia. Veterinarians may also give an oxytocin injection to increase expulsion of placental materials after birth and to decrease uterine hemorrhage. Controversy exists regarding whether this is of any significant benefit. Administration of oxytocin causes both contraction of mammary smooth muscles and milk letdown and therefore may also result in dripping of milk from the teats after administration for uterine contraction.

Many reproductive hormones such as testosterone and progesterone have anabolic effects (enhance production of muscle and body tissue). Corticosteroids have catabolic effects (favor breakdown of muscle and tissue). Anabolic steroids such as forms of testosterone and progesterone have been used in the past in the food animal industry to increase the weight and conditioning of feedlot cattle. The use of anabolic steroids to increase muscularity in food animals is controversial because of the potential for introduction of these steroids into the human food chain. Anabolic steroids are also used to improve the appetite and condition of dogs or cats subjected to surgery or stress. In human beings, some anabolic steroids are used to improve muscle tone and conditioning of geriatric patients. But because of the abuse potential of anabolic steroids by athletes, many anabolic steroids are now labeled as controlled substances.

Treatment of urinary incontinence in spayed dogs with low doses of estrogen is one of the few uses of estrogen still considered to have medical benefit that outweighs the risk. Estrogen (usually DES from a compounding pharmacy) is thought to increase the sensitivity of α receptors (sympathetic nervous system receptors) on the urinary outflow tract, thus increasing the smooth muscle tone and decreasing dribbling of urine. Often the estrogen is combined with an α agonist such as phenylpropanolamine (also from a compounding pharmacy) to enhance the effect.

USES OF REPRODUCTIVE DRUGS NO LONGER CONSIDERED LEGITIMATE

In the past estrogens were used in large doses to prevent implantation of fertilized ova. They were thought to prevent pregnancy by increasing the number and thickness of folds within the oviducts, thereby preventing passage of the ova from the ovary to the uterus. The estradiol cypionate injection had to be given after the egg was released from the follicle but before it had arrived in the uterus. For this reason, injections of estradiol cypionate prevented pregnancy in approximately half of the treated females. Because of the high risk for potentially fatal side effects and better alternatives, estrogen can no longer be recommended in any form for preventing conception after mismating. In fact, the use of estrogen for this purpose is considered by many to be grounds for malpractice.

Estrogens can no longer be recommended for benign prostatic hyperplasia in intact male dogs. In addition to the side effects previously mentioned for estrogen, the hormone may increase the risk for bacterial infection in the prostate and prostatic cyst formation. Likewise, the use of estrogens as a supplement to castration in male dogs with perianal adenomas and perianal adenocarcinomas has decreased significantly.

The use of megestrol acetate for behavior modification is no longer recommended. Because of its side effects as a progestin, its nonspecific effect on behavior modification, and the advent of many other psychotropic drugs (see Chapter 9), the benefits cannot be considered to outweigh the risks. Megestrol may still find occasional use as an adjunct drug for behavior modification; however, as we become more familiar with psychotropic drugs, its use will likely fade out completely.

Box 7-1 Endocrine Drug Categories and Names

THYROID HORMONES

Thyroid-stimulating hormone
Triiodothyronine (T_3)
Tetraiodothyronine, thyroxine (T_4)
Levothyroxine (Soloxine)
Liothyronine

DRUGS USED TO TREAT HYPERTHYROIDISM

Methimazole (Tapazole)
Radioactive iodine (^{131}I)
Propranolol

ENDOCRINE PANCREATIC DRUGS

Regular crystalline insulin
NPH insulin
Lente insulin
Ultralente insulin
PZI insulin
Recombinant human insulin
Glipizide (sulfonylurea compound)

REPRODUCTIVE DRUGS

GnRH analogs
Gonadotropins
 FSH
 LH
 Equine chorionic gonadotropin
 Human chorionic gonadotropin
Progestins, progestagens, progestational hormones
 Altrenogest (Regu-Mate)
 Medroxyprogesterone (Depo Provera)
 Megestrol acetate (Ovaban)
Estrogen
 Estradiol cypionate
 DES
Prostaglandins
 Dinoprost tromethamine (Lutalyse)
 Cloprostenol (Estrumate)
 Fenprostalene
Mibolerone
Dopamine agonists
Corticosteroids
Oxytocin

REFERENCES

1. Feldman EC, Nelson RW: *Canine and feline endocrinology and reproduction,* Philadelphia, 2004, WB Saunders.
2. Feldman EC, Nelson RW, Feldman MS: Intensive 50-week evaluation of glipizide administration in 50 cats with previously untreated diabetes mellitus, *J Am Vet Med Assoc* 210:772-777, 1997.
3. Nelson RW, Feldman EC, Ford SL, et al: Effect of an orally administered sulfonylurea, glipizide, for treatment of diabetes mellitus in cats, *J Am Vet Med Assoc* 203:821-827, 1993.
4. Feldman EC: *Successful management of nonresponsive diabetic cats.* In Proceedings of the North American Veterinary Conference, Orlando, FL, 2002.
5. Davidson AP: Infertility in the queen. In Bonagura JD, editor: *Kirk's current veterinary therapy XIII,* Philadelphia, 2000, WB Saunders, pp. 929-931.

RECOMMENDED READING

Boothe DM: *Small animal clinical pharmacology and therapeutics,* Philadelphia, 2001, WB Saunders.
Feldman EC, Nelson RW: *Canine and feline endocrinology and reproduction,* ed 2, Philadelphia, 1996, WB Saunders.
Plumb DC: *Veterinary drug handbook,* ed 4, Ames, IA, 2002, Iowa State University Press.

Thyroid Drugs

Behrend E, Grauer G: *Hypothyroid: to be or not to be.* In Proceedings of the North American Veterinary Conference, Orlando, FL, 2004.

Feldman EC: *Hyperthyroidism in cats: current treatment options.* In Proceedings of the Western Veterinary Conference, Las Vegas, NV, 2004.
Green RW: *The hyperthyroid cat and I-131 treatment.* In Proceedings of the Western Veterinary Conference, Las Vegas, NV, 2004.
Mooney CT, Thoday K: CVT update: medical treatment for hyperthyroidism in cats. In Bonagura JD, editor: *Kirk's current veterinary therapy XIII,* Philadelphia, 2000, WB Saunders.
Nelson RW: *Diagnosis and management of feline hyperthyroidism.* In Proceedings of the Western Veterinary Conference, Las Vegas, NV, 2004.

Endocrine Pancreatic Drugs

Feldman EC: *Successful management of nonresponsive diabetic cats.* In Proceedings of the North American Veterinary Conference, Orlando, FL, 2002.
Nelson RW: *Management of the newly diagnosed diabetic cat.* In Proceedings of the North American Veterinary Conference, Orlando, FL, 2004.
Norsworthy GD: *Feline diabetes.* In Proceedings of the Western Veterinary Conference, Las Vegas, NV, 2004.
Schulman RL: *Endocrine emergencies.* In Proceedings of the American College of Veterinary Internal Medicine Conference, Charlotte, NC, 2003.

Reproductive Drugs

MacIntire DK: *Reproductive emergencies II: mastitis, pyometra, prolapses, and mismating.* In Proceedings of the Western Veterinary Conference, Las Vegas, NV, 2004.
McCue PM: *Hormone therapy: new aspects.* In Proceedings of the Western Veterinary Conference, Las Vegas, NV, 2003.

Self-Assessment

REVIEW QUESTIONS

Fill in the following blanks with the correct item from the Key Terms list.

1. _____ structures in the pancreas that produce insulin.

2. _____ type of hypothyroidism caused by a disease in the pituitary gland.

3. _____ state of being in heat.

4. _____ Of the terms exogenous and endogenous, the one applied to drugs.

5. _____ part of the estrous cycle that runs from the development of the follicle to lysis of the follicle.

6. _____ part of the estrous cycle controlled by the CL.

7. _____ thyroid condition caused by a lack of iodine and not a malfunction with the thyroid gland.

8. _____ muscular layer of the uterus.

9. _____ creation of glucose from amino acids.

10. _____ can cause cancer.

11. _____ disease treated by sulfonylurea compounds.

12. _____ breakdown of glycogen stores in the liver.

Fill in the following blanks with the correct drug described in Box 7-1.

13. _____ lyses the corpus luteum.

14. _____ stimulates secretion of T_3 and T_4.

15. _____ hormone secreted by the developing follicles on the ovary.

16. _____ this hormone that predisposes the uterus to pyometra (two possible answers).

17. _____ hormone that triggers development of cells that hold the ovum (egg).

18. _____ side effects in the mare include bronchoconstriction, colic, and premature abortion.

19. _____ used to treat urinary incontinence in spayed female dogs.

20. _____ used to bring cattle in the luteal phase of estrous cycle back into estrus; not effective in the follicular phase.

21. _____ hormone naturally produced by the CL.

22. _____ hormone that naturally lyses the mature follicle and releases the egg.

23. _____ form of thyroid drug most commonly used to treat hypothyroidism.

24. _____ level is decreased in cats with primary hyperthyroidism.

25. _____ drug of choice for maintaining control of diabetes mellitus in the dog; considered to be an intermediate-acting insulin.

26. _____ short-term treatment of choice for hyperglycemia in dogs with uncontrolled diabetes mellitus; brings the glucose levels down quickly; given intravenously.

27. _____ hormone that maintains pregnant state of the uterus.

28. _____ hormone associated with the behavioral signs of heat.

29. _____ given to help a flaccid, pregnant uterus contract during labor.

30. _____ given to transitional estrus mares over several days to imitate diestrus, then stopped to simulate the normal regression of the CL and hopefully initiate the follicular phase.

31. _____ used to decrease hyperglycemic condition in some cats with diabetes; given orally.

32. _____ sometimes given to mares to attempt to maintain pregnancy; rarely successful other than in mares that are naturally lacking this hormone.

33. _____ hormone that directly stimulates the thyroid to produce and release hormones.

34. _____ thyroid hormone that actually causes the changes inside the cell.

35. _____ thyroid hormone that allows local tissue regulation of its thyroid hormone need.

36. _____ hormone that causes release of FSH and LH to start the follicular phase.

37. _____ hormone that causes development of ovarian cells that produce estrogen.

38. _____ hormone that stimulates the development of the CL from follicular cells.

39. _____ hormone released by the pituitary when the fetus enters the birth canal; causes forceful uterine contractions.

40. _____ hormone released by the fetus to begin the steps leading to parturition.

41. _____ a control, not a cure, for hyperthyroidism; keeps the thyroid from synthesizing thyroid hormones.

42. _____ only compound on the list that destroys the feline thyroid tumor in feline hyperthyroidism.

43. _____ used to decrease the heart rate of a hyperthyroid cat but does not affect the excessive concentrations of T_3 and T_4.

44. _____ was used to prevent pregnancy in the dog by suppressing release of GnRH, FSH, and LH.

45. _____ prevents a mare from coming into foal heat by inhibiting the follicular phase of the estrous cycle; is a progestin.

46. _____ can cause open-cervix pyometra in the dog 2 to 4 weeks after administration; can also cause aplastic anemia.

47. _____ long-lasting insulin.

48. _____ used to synchronize the estrus cycle of animals in the luteal phase by terminating the luteal phase and bringing them back into the follicular phase; can cause abortion in pregnant human beings who inject or spill it on themselves.

49. _____ used to terminate pregnancy in mares; much species variation in its effectiveness; does not work well in dogs in early pregnancy; many side effects (GI colic signs, sweating).

50. Indicate whether the following statements are true or false.

    A. An overdose of insulin will result in hypoglycemia.

    B. Compared with human beings, dogs are very susceptible to thyrotoxicosis.

    C. As a general rule, cats need a longer acting insulin than dogs.

APPLICATION QUESTIONS

1. An endocrine gland A secretes hormone A, which causes gland B to produce hormone B. Hormone B produces an effect on other body tissues. What effect will hormone B likely have on gland A and hormone A?

2. If an animal has primary hypothyroidism, would you expect the serum T_3/T_4 level to be increased or decreased? What about serum TSH and TRH levels? What if the hypothyroidism was secondary or tertiary?

3. What are the clinical signs associated with hypothyroidism? Do they occur more commonly in the cat or the dog? Which species tends to have hyperthyroidism? How do the signs of hyperthyroidism differ from the signs of hypothyroidism?

4. Why is T_4 the supplement of choice for treating hypothyroidism? Why not T_3 or a combination of the human form of T_3 and T_4?

5. Why might a diabetic dog be more at risk with oversupplementation of T_4 than a normal, healthy dog? Why might a cardiovascular patient with arrhythmias also be more at risk?

6. What are the treatment options for any cat with hyperthyroidism? What are the advantages and disadvantages of each option? Which drugs are used to treat hyperthyroidism in cats? Why are they not used more often? Why would propranolol be used?

7. In which species does NIDDM more frequently occur? Is NIDDM (type 2 diabetes) treated the same way as IDDM? Why or why not? How do these two diseases differ physiologically?

8. Which type of insulin is most likely to be dispensed to a client for home treatment of a diabetic cat?

9. Why are special syringes used for insulin administration? What does the designation "U-40" on an insulin bottle or syringe mean? Why should insulin be resuspended carefully in the bottle?

10. In what species have oral hypoglycemics been used? Under what conditions might this therapy work? Why can't insulin be given by mouth instead?

11. Mr. Smith has found the ideal location to give insulin to his diabetic dog, Spot. He finds that if he injects it into the fat over the hip, Spot does not complain. Is this acceptable? Why or why not?

12. What is the difference between estrus and estrous? What is the difference between mucus and mucous?

13. Why can a veterinarian potentially lose his or her license if he or she administers DES to a cow?

14. How do dopamine agonists terminate pregnancy?

15. A horse owner calls to say her pregnant mare is slightly lame in a front leg. The injury does not appear to be serious, but she asks whether giving some dexamethasone intramuscularly to reduce the swelling and inflammation would be safe. What is an appropriate response?

16. What previous uses of estrogen are no longer considered legitimate?

Chapter 8

Drugs Affecting the Nervous System: Analgesics, Anesthetics, and Stimulants

outline

Analgesics
   The Pain Pathway
   Opioid Analgesics
   Clinical Application: Dangers from Fentanyl
      Patch
   Opioid Antagonists
Tranquilizers and Sedatives
   Acepromazine
   Benzodiazepine Tranquilizers: Diazepam,
      Zolazepam, Midazolam, and Clonazepam
   α₂ Agonists: Xylazine, Detomidine,
      and Medetomidine

Anesthetics
   Barbiturates
   Propofol
   Dissociative Anesthetics
   Inhalant Anesthetics
   Other Anesthetic Gasses
Central Nervous System Stimulants
   Methylxanthines
   Doxapram
   α₂ Antagonists: Yohimbine, Tolazoline,
      and Atipamezole

key terms

α_2 receptor
analgesic
anesthesia
apnea
baroreceptors
bradypnea
catalepsis
compound A
disinhibition
dysphoria
euphoria
γ-aminobutyric acid
general anesthesia

hyperalgesia
hypoproteinemia
local anesthesia
minimum alveolar
   concentration
mixed agonists and
   antagonists
mixed-function oxidase
   enzyme system
modulation (of pain)
narcosis
narcotics
neuroleptanalgesic

opiate
opioid
opioid receptors (μ, κ, δ)
partial agonists and
   antagonists
sedative
somatic pain
tachypnea
transduction
tranquilizer
visceral pain
wind-up (pain)

objectives

After studying this chapter, the veterinary technician should be able to explain:

1. Different types of tranquilizers and sedatives, mechanisms, and indications for their use

2. Different types of analgesics, mechanisms, and their effects

3. Different types of anesthetics, their basic mechanisms of action, and their effects on the body

4. Drugs used to stimulate respiration

Numerous drugs used in veterinary medicine alter the function of the nervous system. The categories of these drugs include anesthetics, *tranquilizers, sedatives, analgesics*, anticonvulsants, and stimulants. Texts of anesthesiology provide a more complete description of the uses of anesthetic agents. This chapter provides an overview of the anesthetic, tranquilizing, sedating, and analgesic drugs, their mechanisms of action, and problems encountered when using these drugs. Box 8-1, listing nervous system drugs, can be found at the end of this chapter.

ANALGESICS

Analgesics are drugs that reduce the perception of pain without significant loss of other sensations.

THE PAIN PATHWAY

As more research has been done in veterinary medicine to gain a better understanding of pain, its causes, and its transmission, a better understanding of how to control it in veterinary patients has resulted. One of the simpler means of understanding the means by which a stimulus produces pain is what some authors call the pain pathway (Figure 8-1). Essentially, pain can be thought of as having four steps. Step one is the stimulus of sensory nerve endings to the painful stimulus, whether it be a cut, a burn, pressure, chemical irritation, or inflammation. This process, called *transduction,* is the translation of the physical stimulus into excitation of the receptor (depolarization). Pain can be blocked at this point by local anesthetic drugs, which can prevent depolarization of the receptors and hence block the first step of the pain transmission process.

Step two is the transmission of the depolarization from the receptor to a sensory nerve and along that nerve toward the spinal cord and eventually up to the brain. However, the transmission of this sensory depolarization wave along the nerve can be modified in the spinal cord or brain by other neurotransmitters, naturally occurring pain killing compounds (e.g., natural opioids such as enkephalins or endorphins), or other nerve pathways. This third step of the pain pathway is called *modulation* and explains why the sensation of pain during the first few minutes of the injury is different from that felt hours later. By preventing or reducing transmission of the pain impulse along the pain pathway through modulation, the perception of pain at the brain level can be decreased even though the pain receptor in the periphery continues to initiate the pain signal.

The fourth step in pain perception is the actual perception of the pain impulse at the conscious level; that is, being aware of the pain. In human beings a traumatic event may emotionally overwhelm an individual to such a degree that he or she is unaware (does not perceive) that a severe physical injury has occurred. In this case, the pain is being successfully transmitted to the brain, but the brain is unable to process this perception at a conscious level because of so many other sensory signals and the emotional state. *General anesthesia* produces unconsciousness, which in turn prevents conscious perception of pain. However, pain transmission in the unconscious patient still occurs at all levels below the brain.

As mentioned above, pain perception changes over time, as anyone who has had an injury knows. The pain may progress from an acute, focal pain to a more diffuse, throbbing pain. This change in perception has a physiologic explanation. When a tissue is injured, the inflammatory process is initiated by the arachidonic acid pathway (see Chapter 13). One of the side effects of all the inflammatory compounds liberated during this process is the increased ease at which the pain receptors in and around the site of inflammation can depolarize. In other words, the inflammation makes pain receptors in the adjacent area much more sensitive to any stimulation. Decreasing inflammation early on can decrease this increased sensitivity to pain, or *hyperalgesia.*

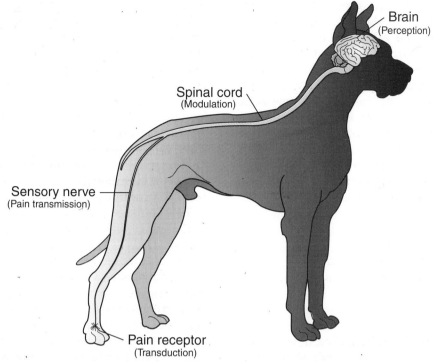

Figure 8-1 The pain pathway. A painful stimulus is converted into a depolarization wave by the pain receptor (transduction) sent along the sensory nerve to the spinal cord (transmission), where it may be modified in intensity (modulation) before ascending the spinal cord and reaching the conscious areas of the brain (perception).

In addition to this local hyperalgesia caused by inflammatory mediator compounds, the spinal cord becomes more sensitive to pain impulses coming from an injured area over a fairly short period. Some of the pain impulses initially reaching the spinal cord may have been dampened or modulated, resulting in less perception of pain, but over time (hours) this dampening effect is significantly reduced and pain is more effectively transmitted up the spinal cord to the brain. Thus, even though a patient may be unconscious during a surgical procedure and hence unable to perceive the pain at a conscious level, the spinal cord may be changing in its ability to transmit pain sensations, resulting in the patient having a higher level of pain perception once it wakes up from the anesthesia. This process of increasing sensitivity of the spinal cord is sometimes referred to as *wind-up*. If drugs can be used to prevent or reduce spinal cord wind-up, pain perception can be more effectively controlled for an animal in postoperative recovery. This is also the basis for the argument of using selected analgesics before the surgery.

OPIOID ANALGESICS

Typically the most potent analgesics used in veterinary medicine are the opioids. *Opiates* are derived as extracts from poppy seeds, whereas *opioids* are chemically synthesized, opiatelike drugs that bind specifically to *opioid receptors*. Opioids are often called *narcotics* because of the *narcosis*, or stuporous state of disorientation, they produce. Opioids are often used as part of a preanesthetic or general anesthetic regimen to reduce the need for other anesthetic agents. In addition, opioids are used alone as analgesics for animals in pain or before painful surgeries or procedures. The administration of analgesics in human beings before a painful procedure reduces the overall need for analgesics compared with administration of analgesics once pain has begun.

Opioids act by binding to opioid receptors in the central nervous system (CNS) (both brain and spinal cord), gastrointestinal (GI) tract, urinary tract, and smooth muscle. Three major types of opioid receptors are recognized in mammals: mu (μ) receptors, kappa (κ) receptors, and delta (δ) receptors. The actions from sigma (σ) receptors may actually be functions of the μ, κ, and δ opioid receptors, thus suggesting that σ receptors may no longer be recognized as a separate receptor. The different classes of opioid receptors may be distributed selectively to various parts of the nervous system, and the distribution pattern of receptors may vary from species to species. In addition, opioid drugs vary in their ability and affinity to combine with each of the opioid receptor types and the degree of intrinsic activity they will have once bound to the receptor (the drug can be an agonist, a *partial agonist,* or an *antagonist*). The variation in distribution of the receptors and the different receptor effects of each opioid drug help explain the wide variation observed in patient responses to different opioid drugs and why the same drug may produce quite different responses across species. Because each opioid drug has inherent characteristics that vary from species to species, the veterinary professional must thoroughly understand the side effects and monitoring peculiarities of the individual opioid drugs in the particular species to which the drug is given.

μ Receptors are found on nerves associated with the pain pathways throughout the brain and spinal cord and therefore are primarily responsible for the strong analgesia observed with selected opioid drugs. Because μ receptors decrease nerve impulse transmission, stimulation of μ receptors also produces the sedation associated with narcosis. μ Receptors are located on the cells of the respiratory center, and opioids that are μ agonists can therefore also be antitussive (cough) medications. Strong μ stimulation can produce the respiratory depression characteristic of most strong opioid drugs. These μ receptors are also thought to be associated with the pleasant hallucinogenic *euphoria* of opioids and the side effect of hypothermia.

Stimulation of κ receptors produces a milder degree of analgesia than the μ receptor response and contributes to sedation without as much respiratory depression as seen with μ receptor stimulation. The roles of κ and μ receptors continue to change as further research provides additional knowledge of how opioid receptors work. For example, κ receptor stimulation has been suggested to partially inhibit some of the beneficial μ receptor effects, resulting in less analgesia. κ Receptor stimulation is now identified as the principal receptor involved with unpleasant hallucinogenic effects called *dysphoria.*

The δ receptors are thought to provide some spinal cord analgesia and perhaps some degree of motor stimulation, cardiac stimulation, and dysphoria. Most opioid drugs used in veterinary medicine primarily work by stimulation of μ and κ receptors, with minimal identified effects through the δ receptors.

Partial, Mixed, and Full Opioid Agonists

The terminology used to describe opioid analgesic drug mechanisms of action can sometimes be confusing. Several different receptors each have different activities, and each opioid drug can react with the receptor in a different way. As explained in Chapter 3, drugs are generally either agonists (produce an effect when combined with a receptor; are said to have intrinsic activity) or antagonists (do not produce an effect when combined with a receptor). A partial agonist may be thought of as an opioid drug that produces some effect on the cell when it combines with the opioid

TABLE **8-1** Agonist/Antagonist Activity of Commonly Used Opioid Drugs in Veterinary Medicine

Strong agonists	Morphine (μ, κ), fentanyl (μ), hydromorphone (μ, κ), meperidine (μ)
Partial agonists	Butorphanol (μ partial agonist, κ agonist), buprenorphine (μ partial agonist, κ antagonist)
Strong antagonists	Naloxone (μ, κ)
Partial antagonists	Nalorphine (μ partial antagonist, κ agonist)

receptor, but not as much as a strong or full agonist. Administration of a partial agonist drug produces a weaker degree of analgesia than that observed after administration of a strong agonist regardless of how much of the weaker drug is given.

The term *mixed agonist and antagonist* means that an opioid drug may have an agonist activity at one type of opioid receptor while simultaneously producing an antagonist activity against another type of opioid receptor. For example, buprenorphine is an agonist of the μ receptor but an antagonist of the κ receptor. Therefore each receptor activity for a drug needs to be described to understand and predict the action of the opioid drug (e.g., buprenorphine is a partial agonist of the μ receptor and an antagonist of the κ receptor).

As described in previous chapters, a partial agonist opioid drug can reverse some of the effect of a stronger full agonist when it displaces the strong agonist molecules from the receptor site. In this situation, the strong analgesia and strong respiratory depression caused by μ receptor stimulation might be replaced with a weaker degree of analgesia, but also a lessening of the respiratory depression.

Commonly used opioid drugs in veterinary medicine are classified by their agonist/antagonist activity (Table 8-1). Many of the drugs are mixed in their degree of agonist and antagonist activity.

Adverse Effects of Opioids

The most profound adverse effect of opioids is respiratory depression caused by μ receptor stimulation of the respiratory area of the medulla. Stronger μ receptor stimulating opioids (morphine, hydromorphone, fentanyl) can produce more profound respiratory depression than the partial μ agonists (buprenorphine, butorphanol). The decreased respiratory reflexes (including cough reflexes) result in less response to carbon dioxide (a major stimulus for increased respiratory activity), a slowing of breathing, and a subsequent accumulation of carbon dioxide in the body. Death from opioid overdose is usually related to respiratory depression.

Another effect of the elevated carbon dioxide level is the reflex vasodilation of blood vessels in the brain. The increased perfusion of CNS tissue increases the pressure within the skull (intracranial pressure). Under normal conditions this is not a life-threatening side effect. However, when head trauma has occurred and swelling or hemorrhage is already present within the brain, the increased intracranial perfusion from opioid analgesia can further increase brain swelling or hemorrhage, with potentially life-threatening results.

As mentioned in Chapter 4, opioids have an effect on the digestive tract. Opioids cause vomiting by stimulation of the chemoreceptor trigger zone (CRTZ) and emetic center (varies with species), but, as described with apomorphine, opioids may also have a depressant effect on the vomiting reflex. Generally, opioids increase segmental contractions of the intestines and contractions of sphincters such as the pylorus. Some authors report that such constriction can make passage of an endoscope from the stomach to the small intestine quite difficult for up to 12 hours after administration of an opioid.[1]

Central stimulation of the cardiovascular center in the brainstem results in some degree of bradycardia. Generally, the bradycardic effect is not as profound as the degree of respiratory depression. However, this decrease in heart rate and subsequent decrease in cardiac output would be of concern in animals with existing heart disease in which cardiac output is already compromised (e.g., congestive heart failure).

Opioids produce analgesia through their action on opioid receptors, but most opioids do not induce anesthesia. Therefore animals given opioids may still respond to sound, cold, heat, taste, and visual stimuli. Some animals medicated with opioids may appear to become hypersensitive to sound, resulting in an exaggerated response to noise. Animals recovering from significant doses of opioids should be placed in a quiet room to avoid a stormy recovery.

Although the concept of "morphine mania" in cats has been disseminated widely in veterinary literature, some anesthesiologists are now stating that these effects are largely from excessive dosages of opioids. Unlike dogs and human beings, in whom opioid administration causes pupillary constriction (miosis), opioids cause pupillary dilation in cats (mydriasis), which makes the cat sensitive to light and more readily startled because it cannot see as well when the pupil is widely dilated. The combination of these factors has probably given rise to the idea that cats are more prone to manic effects from opioids.

Still, cats, horses, pigs, and ruminants are reported to be more susceptible to μ receptor–mediated motor excitation, muscular rigidity, and explosive behavior as the result of *disinhibition* (inhibition of inhibitory neurons) associated with the centers in the brain that regulate emotions and emotional responses. Although morphine mania in cats is probably a misnomer, remembering the potential for startle responses or excitement in cats to which opioid drugs have been given is in the technician's best interests.

Opioids depend on hepatic conjugation of the drug molecule with glucuronic acid for metabolic breakdown and renal elimination. Because of this, the rate of opioid metabolism may be reduced in neonates and animals with severe liver disease. Because the conjugated opioid metabolites are subsequently eliminated by the kidney, animals with kidney disease or decreased perfusion of the kidney may accumulate metabolites. If the metabolite suppresses function of the respiratory control cells in the brainstem (as one of the metabolites of morphine metabolism does), an accumulation of the metabolite because of poor renal function could exacerbate the opioid's respiratory depression effect.

Neuroleptanalgesics are opioid drugs combined with a tranquilizer or *sedative* (e.g., butorphanol opioid with diazepam tranquilizer). The intent of these drugs is to use the tranquilizer effects to decrease some of the excitement and emetic effects of the opioids. When using these types of drugs the veterinary technician needs to be aware of the side effects of both drugs used in the neuroleptanalgesic combination.

Because opioids are powerful drugs regarding their individual actions and side effects, the veterinary technician should become very familiar with the specific characteristics of any opioids they are asked to administer for preanesthetic, anesthetic, or analgesic purposes.

Morphine is the prototypical opioid drug against whose potency all other opioids tend to be measured. For example, hydromorphone is said to have 5 times the analgesic potency of morphine. Morphine primarily stimulates μ receptors and has some activity with κ receptors. Therefore morphine is an effective drug for visceral (organ-related) and somatic (superficial tissues and skin) pain. Morphine is commonly used in combinations with tranquilizers as part of the preanesthetic regimen and as a postsurgical analgesic. In animals who receive fentanyl patches (see below), morphine may also be used to supplement the analgesic effect. Morphine is also used as an epidural drug (drug injected into the space surrounding the spinal cord) to provide regional analgesia for painful procedures involving the hind limbs, pelvis, perineal area (under the tail), or posterior abdomen.

Dogs injected parenterally with morphine often salivate and vomit; however, the vomiting is typically limited to one or two instances. Protracted vomiting is uncommon at normal analgesic doses of morphine. Because of its strong μ receptor effect, morphine produces significant respiratory depression and requires the veterinary technician monitoring the patient to pay particular attention to the respiratory parameters (e.g., respiratory rate and depth of breathing).

Morphine stimulates the nucleus of cranial nerve III (oculomotor nerve) that controls the muscles that regulate the size of the pupil. In dogs, the presence of morphine results in pupillary constriction (miosis), whereas in cats and horses morphine administration results in pupillary dilation. The depth of analgesia does not appear to correlate well with the degree of mydriasis observed in the cat.

One of the side effects of morphine (seen less with other opioids) is the release of histamine after intravenous injection. Among its other effects, histamine causes vasodilation. The combination of histamine vasodilation, some depression of cardiac output by slowed heart rate, and some vasodilation by CNS activity can result in systemic hypotension (decreased blood pressure). Thus morphine should be used with caution in animals that have lost blood, are severely dehydrated, or have other conditions that would cause decreased arterial blood pressure.

Hydromorphone

Oxymorphone, a potent opioid that was used frequently in veterinary medicine, became unavailable in the United States as of 2001. Because of this many veterinary anesthesiologists switched to a chemically related opioid, hydromorphone, because of its similar degree of analgesia and side effects. Hydromorphone is a strong μ agonist and provides a greater analgesic effect than morphine sulfate. Another advantage of hydromorphone over morphine is that hydromorphone does not stimulate vomiting or defecation to the same degree as morphine. Because hydromorphone causes less release of histamine than morphine and some of the other opioids, it is less likely to produce systemic hypotension as a result of histamine-mediated vasodilation.

Hydromorphone depresses the respiratory center as do all opioids; however, the veterinary technician may notice that dogs treated with hydromorphone or fentanyl may pant, giving the impression that the respiratory rate is actually increased. In this case, however, the panting is caused by the lowering of the temperature set point, essentially causing the body to activate mechanisms by which it would normally get rid of excess heat (e.g., panting). Panting results in shallow movement of air in and out of the airways, meaning that the amount of ventilation and oxygen/carbon dioxide exchange at the alveolus level could still be inadequate in spite of the appearance of rapid breathing.

Hydromorphone causes bradycardia; however, the bradycardic effect can be blunted by the use of atropine before hydromorphone administration. Hydromorphone does appear to cause increased sensitivity to auditory stimulation (loud sounds). Animals lightly sedated with this drug might suddenly jump from a treatment table in response to a sudden loud sound. Therefore veterinary technicians should be aware of this response and take measures to decrease the chance of such noise when working with a patient sedated with this drug.

Fentanyl is a potent opioid with an analgesic effect 100 to 250 times greater than that of morphine. Its short duration of action means that the drug is most useful if used as a continuous rate infusion (IV infusion) or as a patch (e.g., Duragesic) applied to the skin.

As with hydromorphone, fentanyl is a respiratory depressant, it increases sensitivity to auditory stimuli, and it produces bradycardia that should be pretreated with atropine. Some dogs will show panting as a result of lowering of the thermoregulatory set point, similar to what is observed with hydromorphone.

TABLE **8-2** Fentanyl Patch Size for Patient

TYPE OF PATIENT	PATCH SIZE (DOSE)	AMOUNT OF FENTANYL IN PATCH
Dogs <5 kg and cats	25 µg/hr	2.5 mg
Dogs 5-10 kg	25 µg/hr	2.5 mg
Dogs 10-20 kg	50 µg/hr	5 mg
Dogs 20-30 kg	75 µg/hr	7.5 mg
Dogs >30 kg	100 µg/hr	10 mg

Adapted from Plumb DC: *Veterinary drug handbook,* ed 5, Ames, IA, 2005, Blackwell, p. 472.

Fentanyl is increasingly being used in veterinary medicine as an analgesic administered by a dermal patch (skin patch) applied to a clipped and cleaned area on the body. Because the amount of fentanyl dosed to the animal is based on the surface area of the patch applied to the skin, small patches are used in cats and small dogs and increasingly larger patches are used in larger dogs. Studies have shown that fentanyl takes between 12 and 24 hours to reach steady-state concentrations in the dog but only 6 to 12 hours in cats. For that reason, the patch may be applied the day before surgery or an opioid injectable may be used until the full effect of the fentanyl patch is reached. The patch should not be cut, as this will alter the rate at which the drug is released and cause evaporation of the alcohol-based gel in which the fentanyl is dissolved. Differences in skin thickness based on species or location on the body will also affect how quickly the drug is able to enter the body, thus making the actual analgesic response somewhat unpredictable for all animals (Table 8-2).

Generally, the fentanyl patch delivers drug for up to 72 hours; thus patches should be replaced after approximately 3 days. Occasionally the adhesive on the patch irritates the skin, so the veterinary technician should monitor the animal if in the hospital or the owner should monitor the animal at home for any signs of the patient trying to remove the patch. Owners should be cautioned about preventing young children from playing with the patch or making sure a patch that falls off does not end up in the hands of a child.

Butorphanol (Torbutrol, Torbugesic) is a synthetic opioid with partial µ receptor agonist activity. It is considered a mild analgesic with more analgesic effect on *visceral pain* (e.g., equine colic) than superficial, *somatic pain*. Butorphanol is considered to have an analgesic effect three to five times greater than morphine. Although it has less respiratory depression than the stronger opioids, it has a strong cough suppression activity and is approved for use as an antitussive in small animals. Because butorphanol is a partial µ agonist, giving additional doses of butorphanol will not increase the depth of analgesia or degree of respiratory depression (ceiling effect) but will only prolong the duration of drug activity.

Larger doses of butorphanol have been reported to occasionally cause excitement in high-strung horses if not administered with a sedative such as xylazine or detomidine. Stronger opioids have the potential to produce this same effect in horses at lower doses. Because butorphanol is a partial agonist, it can be used to reverse some degree of the respiratory depressant effects of such drugs as hydromorphone while providing some level of analgesia and sedation of its own.

Buprenorphine (Buprenex) is a partial µ agonist with moderately strong analgesic properties that appears to be gaining popularity with some veterinary anesthesiologists. It is most commonly combined with sedatives or tranquilizers such as acepromazine, xylazine, and detomidine as parts of anesthetic protocols; however, its strong affinity

CLINICAL APPLICATION
Dangers from Fentanyl Patch

Two Canadian adolescents died after using a transdermal fentanyl patch. A 15-year-old girl was found in respiratory depression and unresponsive 21 hours after the first application of a Duragesic 25 patch. In the other case, a 14-year-old boy was found in respiratory arrest 14 hours after the patch had been first applied. Duragesic has been marketed in Canada for use in controlling chronic pain; however, the patch is not recommended for use in children younger than 18 years of age because of the risk of life-threatening respiratory depression.

What should be learned from this situation: Veterinary technicians must caution owners regarding the proper use and disposal of this patch medication.

From Canadian Adverse Reaction Newsletter 14(4), 2004 and reported in Off label perils, *Compendium on Continuing Education for the Practicing Veterinarian* 26(11):834, 2004.

for μ receptors, longer duration of activity (8 to 12 hours), and degree of analgesia (30 times the analgesic potency of morphine) make it a useful drug for postsurgical or posttraumatic analgesia. As with butorphanol, buprenorphine has a ceiling effect for analgesia and therefore can partially reverse the analgesic and respiratory depression effects of stronger opioids. Also like butorphanol, buprenorphine does not cause any significant vomiting or GI side effects.

Other opioids are sometimes used in veterinary medicine, and veterinarians may be asked about their use in veterinary medicine by their colleagues in human medicine. For that reason, the veterinary technician should be aware of some of them and the reasons why they are not currently used (even though some have been used in the past). Meperidine (Demerol) is used as an oral medication in human medicine but has significant abuse potential. In veterinary medicine the side effects of meperidine, the availability of better opioids, and the concern over diversion of abuse drugs means that meperidine is not used to any great extent. Codeine is an opioid used in human medicine for mild analgesia and cough suppression. Although codeine with acetaminophen or another nonsteroidal antiinflammatory drug occasionally surfaces as a suggested oral medication for use in dogs (acetaminophen is highly toxic to cats), the analgesia from codeine is less than morphine. Thus codeine use in veterinary medicine is limited to cough suppression and occasionally to reduce diarrhea. Pentazocine is an older drug that was originally approved for use in veterinary medicine but is no longer available in the veterinary form. Its side effects, short duration of activity, and relatively weak analgesia (said to be one third that of morphine) have caused it to largely disappear from veterinary use. Hydrocodone (Hycodan) is a human antitussive that is a more potent antitussive than codeine. Hydrocodone is occasionally mentioned for use as an analgesic; however, better opioids are available for analgesic purposes. Oxycodone (Percodan, OxyContin) is a relatively strong analgesic in human medicine; however, the widespread publicity of diversion of oxycodone makes keeping it within a veterinary practice attractive to those who would divert or abuse the drug as well as subject to questioning about the legitimate use of the drug within veterinary practice when other opioid drugs are available and more commonly used.

OPIOID ANTAGONISTS

An advantage of using opioids for analgesia or in anesthetic regimens is that their effects are reversible with narcotic antagonists. These drugs reverse some of the effects of opioid narcosis by competing for sites on the μ and κ receptors. Naloxone (Narcan) is considered a pure narcotic antagonist because when it combines with μ and κ receptors, it has no intrinsic activity (meaning when the drug combines with the cell receptor it produces no effect on the cell). If an animal has been sedated with an opioid agonist, then naloxone, if given in sufficient quantity to compete against the agonist for available receptor sites, should almost completely reverse the sedation, analgesia, and respiratory depression of potent opioids such as hydromorphone without producing sedation of its own. Naloxone has a more difficult time reversing the effects of buprenorphine because the buprenorphine molecule adheres tightly to the μ receptor, making it hard for the naloxone to displace it.

Although naloxone can reverse sedative and analgesic effects, it cannot reverse the emetic effects of apomorphine because the emetic effect is stimulated through dopamine receptors, not opioid receptors. The complete reversal of an opioid can result in the animal suddenly becoming very aware of painful conditions or stimuli. Therefore pure opioid antagonists such as naloxone are best used to reverse an opioid overdose situation. In cases in which the veterinarian wants to partially reverse the respiratory depression without losing all the analgesia, a partial agonist/partial antagonist such as buprenorphine or butorphanol is a better choice.

TRANQUILIZERS AND SEDATIVES

Tranquilizers and sedatives produce a relaxed state usually without producing significant analgesia (unless the drug specifically has analgesic properties). The veterinary technician should realize that a tranquilized animal in a relaxed state is still quite capable of feeling pain and responding quickly and viciously to manipulations that elicit pain. Only if the animal is sedated so deeply that it begins to approach narcosis (a state of sleep from

which an animal is not readily aroused) or anesthesia will the animal's response to pain be decreased.

ACEPROMAZINE

Acepromazine maleate is a phenothiazine tranquilizer that is often used to calm animals for physical examination or transport. Unlike some of the sedatives such as xylazine, detomidine, or medetomidine, which relieve pain to some degree, phenothiazine tranquilizers have no analgesic effect. In addition to its tranquilizing effect, the antidopaminergic (antidopamine receptor activity) effect of acepromazine makes it a commonly used drug to decrease vomiting associated with motion sickness or to reduce stimulation of the CRTZ by drugs such as cancer chemotherapeutic agents or narcotic analgesics. Acepromazine and other phenothiazines have little effect in preventing vomiting caused by irritation or direct stimulation of the GI tract.

Although phenothiazine tranquilizers are generally safe, in some situations they should be used with caution or not at all. The action of acepromazine on the CNS reduces the threshold for seizures in animals with epilepsy. Acepromazine is therefore contraindicated for use in animals with a history of seizures. Acepromazine also should generally be avoided in animals undergoing myelography, a radiographic procedure in which a contrast dye is injected into the cerebrospinal fluid surrounding the spinal cord for a radiographic contrast study. The presence of the contrast material in the cerebrospinal fluid predisposes the animal to seizures, and concurrent use of acepromazine could potentially increase that risk.

In addition to their other activities, phenothiazines also block the α_1 receptors found on smooth muscle cells of peripheral blood vessels that cause vasoconstriction of the precapillary arterioles (small arteries that pass blood into the capillaries). Blocking these receptors results in relaxation of smooth muscle. If the animal is attempting to maintain arterial blood pressure by stimulating vasoconstriction, this α_1 receptor blocking activity, combined with acepromazine's direct relaxation of vascular smooth muscles and depression of some normal blood pressure regulatory mechanisms, has the potential to produce a marked drop in blood pressure. For this reason, phenothiazines should be used with caution or not used in animals with hypotension (decreased blood pressure) associated with shock, blood loss, or dehydration.

A common but harmless effect of phenothiazine tranquilizers is protrusion of the nictitating membrane (third eyelid) over the surface of the eye. The appearance of this fleshy membrane can be alarming to clients using the drug for the first time to control their dog's motion sickness. Obviously the appearance of the membrane also makes ophthalmologic examination more difficult.

Animals having intradermal skin testing for allergy sensitivities should probably not be given phenothiazine tranquilizers before the procedure. Drugs such as acepromazine have an antihistamine effect and therefore may interfere with the histamine response (flare reaction) needed to identify those substances to which an animal is allergic.

For reasons not completely understood, some cats, and occasionally dogs, exhibit frenzied behavior when given acepromazine. Reports of cats becoming aggressive and hyperactive have been observed anecdotally (reported orally but not written up) and in veterinary literature. Predicting which animal will react this way to acepromazine is not possible because this is considered an idiosyncratic reaction (not necessarily dose related).

In stallions, phenothiazine tranquilizers may produce transient or permanent penile prolapse, reducing or preventing the animal's use in breeding.

Another type of tranquilizer that is very similar in effect to the phenothiazine tranquilizers but that belongs to another class of drugs called the butyrophenones is droperidol. As with acepromazine, it has an α-adrenergic–blocking effect and should be used with caution in animals that are hypotensive. It has much more potent sedative and antiemetic effects than most phenothiazine tranquilizers. Droperidol is seldom used in the United States in veterinary medicine but is packaged with fentanyl, a strong opioid, and marketed in other countries as a combination tranquilizer/analgesic for veterinary use.

BENZODIAZEPINE TRANQUILIZERS: DIAZEPAM, ZOLAZEPAM, MIDAZOLAM, AND CLONAZEPAM

Diazepam (Valium), zolazepam (in Telazol), midazolam (Versed), and clonazepam (Klonopin) are benzodiazepine tranquilizers often used for their calming and muscle-relaxing effects. Benzodiazepines (often recognized by their -*epam* suffix) produce their calming effect by enhancing the activity of γ-*aminobutyric acid* (GABA), an inhibitory neurotransmitter in the CNS. The benzodiazepine molecule attaches to the GABA receptor and causes enhanced binding of the GABA molecule with its receptor and thus enhancing its effect. By increasing GABA's inhibitory activity, the brain becomes less active and the animal appears to become less agitated and more relaxed. This same CNS inhibitory effect makes benzodiazepines effective anticonvulsants.

Benzodiazepines do not produce analgesia; however, they are often used in conjunction with anesthetics or analgesics to ease induction of anesthesia or smooth recovery. Zolazepam is a benzodiazepine tranquilizer marketed in combination with tiletamine, a dissociative anesthetic, as the short-acting sedative-analgesic Telazol. Diazepam is often combined (compounded by the veterinarian) with ketamine to produce a similar sedative-analgesic effect. Midazolam is a slightly more potent benzodiazepine and is sometimes used as an alternative to diazepam. Clonazepam is not commonly used as a preanesthetic drug but has been used as anticonvulsant therapy for seizure control.

Unlike the phenothiazine tranquilizers, benzodiazepines have little effect on the brain's CRTZ and therefore are not useful in preventing motion sickness. In contrast to phenothiazines, which potentially increase the frequency or strength of seizures, benzodiazepines' enhanced GABA effect inhibits seizure foci (areas of origin for seizure activity) and the potential spread of seizure waves of depolarization throughout the brain.

One advantage of the benzodiazepines in a preanesthetic or anesthetic regimen is their muscle-relaxing ability and minimal depressant effect on the respiratory and cardiovascular system. For that reason, some anesthesiologists prefer to use diazepam in their anesthetic regimens for animals with cardiovascular disease. Another advantage is that the benzodiazepines can be reversed with the antagonist flumazenil if need be.

Because of their stimulatory effects on the appetite center in the brain, diazepam and midazolam have been used to increase the appetite in anorectic cats. However, because hepatic failure has been reported in cats given repeated oral dosages of diazepam, this practice is becoming less common.

α₂ AGONISTS: XYLAZINE, DETOMIDINE, AND MEDETOMIDINE

Xylazine (Rompun, Anased, Sedazine), detomidine (Dormosedan), and medetomidine (Domitor) are grouped together as α_2 agonists and are most commonly used in dogs, cats, and horses. The α_2 designation refers to the mechanism by which these drugs act. When these drugs attach to and stimulate α_2 *receptors* located on the terminal bouton of norepinephrine-secreting neurons (Figure 8-2), they decrease norepinephrine release from the neuron both within the CNS and in the peripheral nervous system. Because norepinephrine is part of the sympathetic nervous system and plays a role in maintaining general alertness, inhibition of norepinephrine release by xylazine, detomidine, or medetomidine

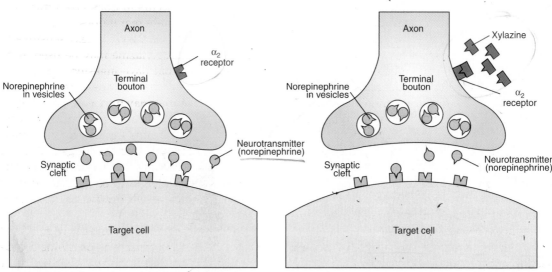

Figure 8-2 Mechanism of action of α_2 agonist drugs. **A,** Normally, norepinephrine is released and travels across the synaptic cleft to receptors on the target cell. After norepinephrine is released, some norepinephrine released provides negative feedback to prevent further release by attaching to the α_2 receptor on the terminal bouton. **B,** When xylazine is present, it attaches to the α_2 receptors on the terminal bouton. This stimulates the α_2 receptor's negative feedback effect on the release of norepinephrine, decreasing its release and decreasing CNS excitation.

results in sedation. The degree of sedation with α_2 agonists is said to be more predictable than the benzodiazepines or phenothiazine tranquilizers.

α_2 Agonists are classified as sedative/analgesics; therefore, in addition to the sedation described, they also decrease perception of painful stimuli. In addition, this class of drugs also produces some degree of muscle relaxation, which makes them helpful when used in conjunction with dissociative anesthetics (ketamine), which have poor muscle-relaxation capabilities.

Analgesia from α_2 agonists wears off before the sedation effect dose. Thus an animal sedated with xylazine may begin to respond to painful stimuli if the procedure continues for more than 20 minutes even though the animal appears to be comfortable. This illustrates an important safety point: a sedated animal may be quite capable of responding rapidly and violently to painful stimuli.

Xylazine and detomidine have a shorter duration of analgesia and sedation than the newer drug medetomidine. However, the duration of analgesia can be significantly increased by using these drugs in combination with opioid analgesics such as butorphanol. Stress or fear in the animal before administration of the α_2 agonist may decrease the ability of these drugs to produce significant sedation quickly. Under such conditions the α_2 agonists cannot reverse the existing high levels of norepinephrine already circulating in the body in response to the stress; therefore the onset of sedation from the drug is delayed until these levels of norepinephrine drop. Only at that point will the drug's inhibition of further norepinephrine be noted clinically.

In horses, xylazine and detomidine are used to relieve pain associated with GI conditions such as colic. Although these drugs can be used to control visceral pain associated with intestinal disease, their analgesic effect on skin and superficial tissue (somatic, or nonvisceral pain) appears to be less effective.

Some authors have observed that the analgesia in horses appears to wear off in the hind limbs before the front limbs.

Once sedation has been achieved with α_2 agonists, further dosing will not produce further depth of sedation or analgesia but will only prolong the duration of the drug and increase the incidence of side effects.

Although α_2 agonists are widely used in veterinary medicine, they do have significant physiologic effects on many body systems and therefore require the veterinary technician to evaluate the patient carefully before, during, and immediately after using these drugs. Generally, most veterinary references state that α_2 agonists should be used only in relatively young and/or healthy patients. Even so, the side effects in healthy animals can be potentially serious if the veterinary professional is not anticipating them.

One disadvantage of xylazine is that sedative doses produce vomiting, or emesis, in a significant percentage of cats by directly stimulating α receptors in the CRTZ. Vomiting frequently occurs in dogs given this drug but not to the extent that it does in cats in part because the canine CRTZ is less sensitive to α-agonist drugs. Xylazine may be used as an emetic in cats that have ingested a poison or as a means of evacuating the stomach contents of a dog or cat that may have eaten before surgery. Although this latter procedure is done in practice, it still runs the risk for aspiration of stomach contents into the lungs and is not as safe as postponing the surgical procedure. Vomiting associated with α_2 agonists can be reduced to some extent by the use of phenothiazine tranquilizers.

In deep-chested dog breeds (e.g., Great Danes, Doberman pinschers) or canine breeds predisposed to gastric distension, the use of xylazine has resulted in an increased incidence of gastric distension. The mechanism is not understood but may be related to multiple factors, including the atonic effect (lack of tone) α_2 agonists have on the stomach.

Dogs predisposed to bloat or with a previous history of gastric dilatation should generally not receive this drug.

The cardiovascular effects of α_2 agonists make them a risk drug for older animals. Even in younger animals, the veterinary technician must understand the basic physiology behind these cardiovascular changes to better interpret the clinical signs they are observing in a patient that has received these drugs. After injection of these drugs, blood pressure initially increases in response to α_1 receptor stimulation and vasoconstriction of precapillary arterioles (see Chapter 5). This response illustrates that these drugs are not specific for α_2 receptors, although medetomidine is more selective for α_2 receptors than xylazine or detomidine. Generally, medetomidine has fewer cardiovascular side effects than xylazine or detomidine.

The increased arterial blood pressure is detected by *baroreceptors* (*baro*, meaning pressure) in the major vessels of the body that, in turn, stimulate the parasympathetic nervous system and subsequently slow the heart rate through parasympathetic stimulation of the sinoatrial node. The parasympathetic effect dominates the body because the drug's α_2 agonist effect on neurons secreting norepinephrine (the sympathetic nervous system's neurons) prevents the sympathetic nervous system from antagonizing the parasympathetic effect. Thus, in addition to the bradycardia (some sources say the heart rate drops by 50%), the electrocardiogram also shows evidence of first-degree (prolonged PR interval) or second-degree (an occasional P wave without a corresponding QRS complex) atrioventricular block caused by parasympathetic stimulation of the atrioventricular node. As mentioned in Chapter 5, atrioventricular block and bradycardia caused by parasympathetic stimulation can be reversed by parasympathetic blocking drugs such as atropine.

The resulting decrease in norepinephrine caused by α_2 agonists means less sympathetic stimulation of the precapillary arterioles that were directly stimulated by xylazine, detomidine, and medetomidine. Thus the initial hypertension from the initial α_1 stimulation is countered by an overall decrease in sympathetic stimulation and some vasodilation may begin to appear. The combination of the decreased vasoconstriction plus bradycardia means that the arterial blood pressure returns to near normal. When monitoring an animal given one of these drugs, the initial firm pulse should be replaced by a slower than normal heart rate with near-normal blood pressure (felt as a slow, but normal strength, pulse).

The species variations seen in response to α_2 agonists emphasize the general principle that what is good in one species is not necessarily good in another. Compared with horses, cattle are quite sensitive to the effects of α_2 agonists such as xylazine. Cattle only require 10% of the equivalent equine dose to produce an equivalent degree of sedation. Like dogs, cattle are predisposed to rumen stasis (decreased rumen motility or rumen atony), which may result in subsequent development of gas bloat or tympany. In contrast to cattle's sensitivity to xylazine, swine appear to be quite resistant to its effects and require much higher dosages to produce any sedative effect. For this reason, α_2 agonists are usually not used in swine.

In cattle and other ruminants, xylazine increases the contractility of uterine smooth muscle. If given to pregnant ruminants in high doses, xylazine could have the potential to induce premature onset of parturition. This effect has not been noted in horses or small animals, although a similar increase in contractility of uterine smooth muscle has been noted with high doses of medetomidine in the pregnant bitch.

Some of the effects of medetomidine, xylazine, and detomidine sedation can be reversed with α_2 antagonist drugs such as yohimbine, atipamezole, and tolazoline. Yohimbine and atipamezole are marketed as the veterinary formulations Yobine and Antisedan, respectively, and tolazoline is available as a human formulation Priscoline. Atipamezole is specifically indicated for reversal of medetomidine.

ANESTHETICS

Anesthesia means "without sensation." A fully anesthetized animal or person cannot feel stimulations of pain, cold, heat, pressure, or touch. General anesthesia is the reversible loss of these sensations associated with unconsciousness, and *local anesthesia* is the reversible loss of sensation in a regional area of the body without loss of consciousness.

Anesthetics should not be confused with analgesics, which are compounds that decrease pain perception but do not necessarily cause total loss of all sensations. For example, opioid narcotics are analgesics because they decrease the perception of pain; however, they are not anesthetics because animals can usually still feel sensations. However, a higher dose of an analgesic drug may induce narcosis, a state of sleep from which the patient is not easily aroused; and that higher dose may act as an anesthetic.

Sedatives or tranquilizers are not anesthetic agents; however, they enhance the effect of anesthetic drugs and decrease the amount of anesthetic drug needed by calming the animal or putting it into a state of relaxation or light sleep.

BARBITURATES
Types of Barbiturates

Barbiturates are frequently used in veterinary medicine to produce short-term anesthesia, induce general anesthesia, control seizures, and euthanize animals. Barbiturates are classified accordingly to their duration of action or anesthetic period. Ultrashort-acting barbiturates have a duration of action measured in minutes. Thiopental sodium is the most commonly used ultrashort-acting barbiturate in veterinary medicine. Its short duration of action

makes it ideal for induction of general anesthesia and placement of the endotracheal tube, which then allows the anesthesia to be maintained as a gas. Methohexital is also classified as an ultrashort-acting barbiturate but is not used as widely as thiopental. Pentobarbital is the prototype for the short-acting barbiturates. Because pentobarbital's duration is longer than that of thiopental, it has been used in veterinary medicine as an anesthetic agent for short procedures when gas anesthetic agents are either unavailable or impractical. The long-acting barbiturates are represented by phenobarbital. Although phenobarbital has been used successfully for anesthesia in veterinary patients under conditions described for pentobarbital, a more common use of phenobarbital is as an anticonvulsant (antiseizure) medication.

Barbiturates are also divided into thiobarbiturates, which contain a sulfur molecule on the barbituric acid molecule, and oxybarbiturates, which contain an oxygen molecule. Thiopental is a thiobarbiturate; pentobarbital and phenobarbital are oxybarbiturates. Thiobarbiturates are more lipid soluble than are oxybarbiturates and therefore penetrate the blood-brain barrier more readily and have a more rapid onset on anesthesia but a shorter duration of action than oxybarbiturates.

Clinical Effects of Barbiturates

Because barbiturate drugs are quickly distributed and easily penetrate the blood-brain barrier, the onset of anesthesia is rapid. However, when ultrashort-acting barbiturate anesthetics are used, the rapid onset of anesthesia decreases within a very short period and the animal appears to partially recover. This partial recovery shortly after induction of anesthesia is caused by redistribution of the barbiturate from the brain to the blood and to lesser-perfused tissues such as adipose (fat) tissue or inactive muscle. As the drug moves into the lesser perfused tissues, the blood concentration decreases, creating a concentration gradient for the barbiturate to move from the brain back into the blood. The decreased barbiturate brain concentrations result in a lessening of anesthesia and the animal appears to partially recover from the anesthetic. The decreased anesthetic depth observed in the first few minutes after administration of thiopental anesthesia is largely caused by redistribution as opposed to metabolism or elimination of the drug.

When the initial recovery occurs shortly after induction, a second dose of barbiturate is given to reestablish an adequate level of anesthesia. The second dose must be smaller than the first because the second dose will not redistribute to fat or other poorly perfused tissues to the same extent that the first dose did. Because the second dose of barbiturate does not redistribute, concentrations in the blood and brain remain higher, anesthesia is reestablished, and the animal remains anesthetized until the drug is metabolized or excreted from the body.

Although barbiturates are used to depress the CNS, animals given an IV bolus injection of ultrashort-acting barbiturates often are observed to have a momentary excitatory phase before passing into unconsciousness. If the dose of ultrashort-acting barbiturate is insufficient to induce anesthesia fully, the animal may become agitated, excited, or frenzied in its semiconscious state.

Dosing Barbiturates

Different species metabolize and eliminate barbiturates at different rates. Cats generally have a reduced ability to metabolize barbiturates; therefore, a lower dose is used in cats than in dogs. To control seizure activity, cats typically require lower concentrations of barbiturate than dogs.

An obese animal will also require a different barbiturate dose than a similar-sized lean animal. In this case, the obese animal has a higher percentage of poorly perfused tissue (fat) than the lean animal. For example, if a 20-lb obese animal is given a dose based on body weight, the majority of the initial barbiturate

dose will be delivered to the brain and other well-perfused tissues, resulting in high concentrations in the brain and profound anesthesia. Because a lean 20-lb animal will have less fat and more well-perfused tissue, the wider initial distribution of barbiturate in the lean animal will result in lower concentrations in the brain than those achieved in the brain of the obese animal. For this reason, obese animals should be given several small doses based on their estimated lean weight (actual weight less estimated weight of excess fat) so that the drug has time to enter poorly perfused adipose tissue and the brain is not overly affected.

Unfortunately, because the barbiturates enter poorly perfused tissues slowly, they also leave poorly perfused tissues slowly, resulting in a continuing infusion of anesthetic from fat into blood and prolonging barbiturate anesthesia recovery in obese animals.

As discussed in Chapter 3, repeated use of barbiturates induces accelerated liver metabolism of phenobarbital and all other drugs that use the *mixed-function oxidase (MFO) enzyme system* of metabolism. Animals anesthetized with a multiple doses of barbiturate over several days will require increasingly larger doses to produce an equivalent depth or duration of anesthesia. This is the mechanism that produces drug tolerance associated with barbiturate drugs. Long-acting barbiturates appear to induce enzyme activity more than short-acting barbiturates. Because this induced metabolism also speeds up metabolism of any other drugs that also use the same metabolic pathway, development of tolerance to phenobarbital is often accompanied by a greater tolerance to corticosteroids, chloramphenicol, propranolol, doxycycline, and quinidine.

Barbiturates are highly protein bound drugs. Barbiturate dosages are determined by taking into account the high percentage of barbiturate molecules that will be bound to blood proteins and unavailable to distribute to the tissue. Therefore anything that decreases the protein binding of the barbiturate molecules makes more drug molecules available as unbound or free drug molecules that can distribute to tissue and produce an effect. Increased distribution of barbiturate occurs with *hypoproteinemia* (low plasma protein levels) or decreased protein binding caused by blood pH more acidic than 7.4 (acidosis or, more accurately, acidemia). A lower than normal dose of barbiturate must be used to prevent an overdose under these circumstances. A general rule of thumb under such conditions is to administer the barbiturate slowly and titrate the dose to the desired effect, realizing that less drug is needed to produce the desired level of anesthetic.

Side Effects of Barbiturates

The CNS depressant effects of barbiturates account for their major side effect: respiratory and cardiac depression. Because barbiturates produce unconsciousness before they cause respiratory and cardiac arrest, they are commonly used as euthanasia solutions. Even when barbiturates are used for anesthetic purposes, animals often have a transient period of *apnea* (cessation of breathing) that reflects high concentrations of barbiturate distributed to the brain. This effect is seen especially with thiopental because of its high lipid solubility and easy distribution into the CNS. Fortunately, within a few minutes the initial dose of barbiturate redistributes to fat and less-perfused tissues, lowering the concentration in the blood and brain, lessening CNS depression and allowing spontaneous breathing to resume.

Methohexital, the other ultrashort-acting barbiturate, has a similar anesthetic pattern as thiopental. However, methohexital is metabolized very rapidly (more rapidly than thiopental); thus the observed recovery from methohexital anesthesia is within a few minutes of administration more because of the metabolism of the drug than redistribution of the drug to fat.

Thiobarbiturates can only be administered intravenously because they are extremely

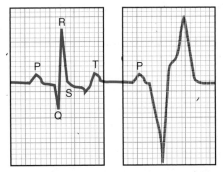

Figure 8-3 Bigeminy is characterized by normal QRS complexes alternating with premature ventricular contractions.

irritating to tissue. If accidentally injected perivascularly (in the area surrounding the vein), thiobarbiturates can produce severe inflammation, swelling, and necrosis (tissue death). After accidental perivascular injection, the area should be infiltrated immediately with lidocaine (local anesthetics) and sterile saline to dilute the drug and prevent tissue sloughing. Injection of additional saline into the site, injections of corticosteroids or nonsteroidal antiinflammatory drugs, and application of cold packs and later hot packs also have been advocated to reduce tissue inflammation and necrosis.

A common side effect of ultrashort-acting barbiturates is cardiac arrhythmia (abnormal heart rhythm). The risk for cardiac arrhythmia is increased by concurrent administration of xylazine, halothane, or epinephrine. Excitement before anesthetic induction also predisposes an animal to cardiac arrhythmias from release of norepinephrine. On an electrocardiogram monitor, one of the most common abnormalities is bigeminy, in which a normal QRS complex alternates with an abnormal complex (Figure 8-3). Generally, bigeminy is not life threatening and spontaneously disappears or is lessened with administration of oxygen or lidocaine. As long as the animal is otherwise healthy and adequately oxygenated during anesthesia, this arrhythmia poses no significant risk.

Greyhounds, whippets, and other thin-bodied sight hounds metabolize thiobarbiturates much more slowly than other canine breeds. For this reason, some anesthetists may use methohexital rather than thiobarbiturates because of the more rapid metabolism of methohexital. Surgical anesthesia with methohexital is usually maintained for 5 to 15 minutes after the initial injection. Recovery is rapid but is often accompanied by paddling, excitement, and muscle tremors. Therefore methohexital is probably better used as an induction agent for gas anesthesia rather than as the sole anesthetic agent.

Because appropriate barbiturate anesthesia must be modified to reflect changes in physiology, body conformation, or breed, the veterinary technician needs to carefully assess the whole patient before determining the dose and using this class of injectable anesthetic drugs.

PROPOFOL

Propofol is an injectable anesthetic agent chemically unrelated to barbiturates. Because propofol is so poorly dissolved in water, it is produced as a drug dissolved in an emulsion of drug, egg lecithin, and soybean oil. Because of the organic nature of this emulsion, bacteria can readily grow and produce endotoxins if the propofol emulsion becomes contaminated. For this reason, unused propofol either in single-dose glass ampules or a multidose vial should be discarded within 24 hours after being opened.

Propofol is usually injected as an IV bolus and provides rapid induction of anesthesia and a short period of unconsciousness. Care should be taken not to inject the IV bolus too rapidly, which results in apnea. Some authors recommend giving the IV dose in 25% increments every 30 seconds until the desired effect is achieved. If apnea does occur, the animal may need to be intubated and ventilated until the drug is metabolized or redistributed.

Recovery time after a single bolus injection is approximately 20 minutes for dogs and 30 minutes for cats. The IV dosage is 3 to 8 mg/kg depending on whether the animal has been premedicated with a tranquilizer, sedative, or opioid. Propofol provides sedation and only minimal analgesic activity at dosages that do not induce full anesthesia. Even in an unconscious state, animals often respond to painful stimuli unless other analgesics such as xylazine and hydromorphone also are administered.

People receiving propofol sometimes report pain on injection; this may also occur in veterinary patients. This discomfort can be minimized by first using an analgesic such as xylazine or injecting the propofol into the larger veins. Fortunately, propofol, unlike thiobarbiturates, does not cause tissue inflammation or necrosis if injected perivascularly.

Propofol has the potential to enhance arrhythmias caused by epinephrine release associated with fear or stress, but it does not seem to generate arrhythmias alone. Because propofol is a phenol type of chemical, cats cannot effectively conjugate and metabolize it and therefore have the potential to develop Heinz-body anemia if given repeatedly.

DISSOCIATIVE ANESTHETICS

Ketamine and tiletamine (a component of Telazol) are short-acting injectable anesthetics that produce a rather unique form of anesthesia in which the animal feels dissociated (apart) from its body. A veterinary technician in a university veterinary teaching hospital accidentally received a dose of ketamine while attempting to inject a cat. She described feeling as though she were walking down the hall ahead of herself, in effect, dissociated from her body.

This dissociative effect is thought to be associated with overstimulation of the CNS, resulting in a cataleptic state. *Catalepsis* is characterized by a heightened emotional response, maintenance of many reflexes (laryngeal, pharyngeal, and corneal), a general lack of muscular relaxation (often increased muscle tone or rigidity), and an increased heart rate. The lack of muscular relaxation makes ketamine or tiletamine unsuitable as a sole anesthetic agent for major surgery. Both drugs are commonly used with a tranquilizer or sedative to reduce some of the CNS stimulation effects during induction or recovery.

Ketamine and tiletamine produce good somatic (peripheral tissue) analgesia and are suitable for superficial surgery; however, they are much less effective in blocking visceral pain and should not be used alone as anesthesia for internal procedures.

More recent research into pain management has shown that ketamine may have an additional effect that helps prevent postoperative pain. Typically, when an animal has a surgical or traumatic injury, the local pain receptors and the pathway to conduct the pain impulses become hypersensitized (which refers to the sensitivity of the receptors as opposed to a hypersensitivity reaction, which typically refers to an allergic reaction to a drug). An animal whose pain receptors and pain conduction pathway have become hypersensitized more readily feels pain with a smaller amount of stimulation. Part of this hypersensitized change occurs at the pain receptors in the tissue and part of it occurs at synapses with the neurons in the spinal cord. A specific receptor in the spinal cord (N-methyl-D-aspartate, or NMDA receptor), whose stimulation is part of the increased hypersensitization process, has been found to be antagonized by ketamine. Thus the use of ketaminelike drugs may decrease some of this increased hypersensitization process and decrease the reaction the animal has to pain in the period after the initial injury.

In cats given ketamine, the eyes remain open and unblinking, which can dry the cornea. When using ketamine in cats, the veterinary professional should apply an ophthalmic lubricant or ointment to prevent corneal damage.

Some cats recovering from ketamine anesthesia develop seizures. Such seizures can be controlled with IV diazepam (Valium). Most animals recovering from ketamine or tiletamine anesthesia often appear delirious. The term "tennis match cats" is sometimes used to describe the rhythmic back-and-forth, head-bobbing motion of cats recovering from ketamine anesthesia. These recovering animals are best placed in areas with little visual or auditory stimulation; loud noises or bright lights may precipitate violent reactions or even seizures.

Ketamine is well absorbed through the mucous membranes of the mouth and nasal cavity. The drug is sometimes squirted through the cage bars into the mouth of a hissing, fractious cat to subdue the animal enough to properly anesthetize it.

Ketamine and tiletamine are chemically related to another potential abuse drug with hallucinogenic activity called phencyclidine (also known as PCP, angel dust, and several other street names). Because of its similarity to phencyclidine, ketamine has gained popularity and is known on the streets as "special K." Stolen or diverted ketamine is evaporated to a white powder and then inhaled by the abuser. Ketamine is now classified as a C-III controlled substance and because of its abuse potential should be stored and inventoried according to federal and state controlled substance storage laws and guidelines.

Tiletamine is commercially packaged with the benzodiazepine tranquilizer zolazepam (Telazol). Like ketamine, tiletamine is a C-III controlled substance. The zolazepam tranquilizer reduces some of the CNS excitation and side effects produced by tiletamine. The product is used for restraint or anesthesia for minor procedures lasting less than an hour in cats and less than 30 minutes in dogs. As with ketamine, animals given tiletamine have open eyes (with the potential for corneal drying), poor muscle relaxation, and analgesia insufficient to prevent visceral pain. The zolazepam in Telazol reduces CNS excitation and provides some degree of muscle relaxation. Tiletamine anesthesia lasts longer and produces better analgesia than ketamine; however, even when tiletamine is combined with zolazepam in Telazol, the drug should be used for restraint or minor surgical procedures only.

INHALANT ANESTHETICS

Inhalant, or gas, anesthesia is the administration of a drug by the lungs that is absorbed from the alveoli and distributes to the brain to produce unconsciousness. Generally, injectable anesthetics are used initially to induce sedation or anesthesia that is then maintained with gas anesthesia. The most common gas anesthetics include halothane, isoflurane, and sevoflurane. These anesthetics are listed in order from slowest induction (onset of anesthesia) and recovery. Each anesthetic gas has a *minimum alveolar concentration*, which is the concentration that must be achieved in the alveoli to produce a safe level of anesthesia. The lower the minimum alveolar concentration (MAC) the less gas it takes to produce anesthesia and the more potent the anesthetic gas is considered.

Because gas anesthetics are delivered by breathing, the suppression of breathing by injectable or gas anesthetics can affect the amount of drug delivered to the body. Therefore the veterinary technician must be familiar with the effect each anesthetic gas has on respiratory rate, blood pressure, and other observable signs that indicate the depth of anesthesia.

Halothane

Of the three anesthetics listed above, halothane is the oldest of the so-called precision vaporizer anesthetics (as opposed to the older "wick" vaporizer anesthetics such as methoxyflurane). Halothane (Fluothane) is a nonflammable, nonirritating inhalant anesthetic that can be used in all species. Although most of halothane is excreted from the body by the lungs (breathing out the gas), fluoride and bromide metabolites of halothane have been implicated in producing hepatotoxicity in human patients repeatedly anesthetized for extended periods with halothane. Although the potential for this exists in veterinary patients, similar syndromes have rarely been reported in the veterinary literature.

A more common disadvantage of halothane is that it sensitizes the heart to epinephrine and predisposes to arrhythmias caused by excitement or stress associated with fear or struggling during anesthetic induction. The effects of stress and fear can be reduced by administration of tranquilizers or sedatives before induction of anesthesia.

While other anesthetic drugs cause slowing of the breathing rate *(bradypnea)* halothane often produces *tachypnea* (an increased rate of breathing) by a mechanism that is not well understood. If the tachypnea is accompanied by a normal to deep degree of inspiration (as opposed to panting, which is tachypnea with shallow breathing) more halothane will be taken into the body, producing a deeper plane of anesthesia. Therefore halothane anesthesia needs to be monitored closely to prevent an anesthetic depth that is too deep for the need of the surgery or too deep to allow proper oxygen exchange.

Halothane decreases cardiac output (amount of blood pumped from the heart), resulting in a drop in arterial blood pressure. This will decrease force of the blood going into the capillaries, resulting in a longer capillary refill time. Thus the veterinary technician can roughly monitor the anesthetic depth by noting the length of time return of the color of the gums takes after pushing against them with a finger and releasing (capillary refill time). The deeper the anesthetic depth, the longer the blanched gums take to regain their color.

An abnormal thermoregulatory response has been reported in human beings, horses, pigs, and occasionally dogs and cats anesthetized with halothane. This condition, called malignant hyperthermia, occurs in a small number of animals and is characterized by sudden onset of an extremely elevated body temperature that can result in brain damage or death. Rapid recognition of the condition and aggressive treatment to lower the core body temperature can save some animals with this condition. The more common effect of halothane on body temperature is hypothermia, or subnormal body temperature, which is caused by halothane's inhibition of the thermoregulatory centers in the brain, reducing the normal reflexes that maintain body temperature such as shivering and vasoconstriction.

Halothane should not be used in animals with head trauma or any condition in which the brain is swelling from injury. Halothane anesthesia causes the brain blood vessels to dilate, resulting in an increase in pressure within the brain itself. The combination of pressure from injury plus increased intracranial pressure from the halothane could be potentially life threatening. As of 2005, manufacture of halothane in the United States has been discontinued.

Isoflurane

The inhalant anesthetic isoflurane (IsoFlo, Forane) has gained increasing popularity over halothane in veterinary practices because of its rapid, smooth induction of anesthesia and short recovery period. Unlike the newer inhalant anesthetics such as sevoflurane, isoflurane has a somewhat pungent, musty odor, which can make anesthesia induction with a mask on a conscious animal difficult because the animal may fight the mask and odor.

Unlike halothane, isoflurane is not metabolized to any significant amount and therefore does not produce potentially toxic metabolites. Isoflurane produces much less sensitization of the myocardium to epinephrine or similar sympathomimetic compounds than halothane. Some anesthesiologists have stated that halothane-related arrhythmias may resolve if the anesthesia is switched to isoflurane. Nonetheless, reducing excessive stress, which produces sympathetic nervous system stimulation, and avoiding the use of catecholamine drugs such as epinephrine, norepinephrine, and dopamine before or during isoflurane use are prudent.

Isoflurane induction, recovery, and changes within anesthesia are more rapid than seen with halothane. Respiratory depression can be profound with isoflurane anesthesia, especially in horses and dogs. Respiratory rate and heart rate decrease and capillary refill time increases as anesthetic depth increases. However, the respiratory rate and heart rate depression can vary from accumulating carbon dioxide with respiratory depression or stimulation from surgical manipulation. Between the rapid responses to small changes in isoflurane flow rates and the variable heart and respiratory rates, isoflurane anesthesia must be more closely monitored and anticipated than halothane.

The rapid recovery from isoflurane anesthesia in cats has sometimes resulted in delirium and a somewhat stormy recovery. Use of a tranquilizer or sedative before anesthetic induction with isoflurane can smooth the recovery period. If an animal is likely to have significant postsurgical pain, narcotic/opioid analgesics should be used to decrease thrashing about during the recovery period from isoflurane.

Sevoflurane

Sevoflurane (SevoFlo) is the newest of the three anesthetic gases. It has a very rapid induction and recovery (even faster than isoflurane), good cardiac stability (does not predispose the myocardium to arrhythmias), and respiratory depression similar to isoflurane. Generally, sevoflurane produces less cardiac output suppression than isoflurane; therefore the heart rate may not decrease as predictably with anesthetic depth.

The rapid induction and recovery make sevoflurane a good anesthetic for outpatient procedures. Sevoflurane would also be good for cesarean sections because any anesthetic gas absorbed by the fetuses would be eliminated quickly and not depend on their livers to metabolize the drug. Because anesthetic recovery is so rapid with sevoflurane, the judicious use of tranquilizers and analgesics is important to smooth the transition from anesthesia to full awareness of all body sensations, including pain.

Like isoflurane, sevoflurane is minimally metabolized by the liver. However, sevoflurane does react with the carbon dioxide scavenger compounds commonly used in anesthetic machines (e.g., soda lime). The resulting chemical is called *compound A* and has been show to be nephrotoxic in rats. Controlled studies in dogs administered sevoflurane for 3 hours a day, 5 days a week for 2 weeks (30 hours total) showed no evidence of nephrotoxicity. Although no reports of nephrotoxicity have appeared in cases of human or veterinary patient exposure to sevoflurane, this is a topic on which the veterinary professional needs to continually remain current.

OTHER ANESTHETIC GASSES
Nitrous Oxide

Also referred to as "laughing gas," nitrous oxide is safe when used properly and has much weaker analgesic qualities than other inhalant anesthetics. The major role of nitrous oxide is to decrease the amount of the more potent inhalant anesthetics needed to achieve a surgical plane of anesthesia.

The gas diffuses through the body very rapidly and enters gas-filled body compartments such as the stomach, rumen, and loops of bowel. When a gas diffuses into a compartment, it increases the overall pressure within that compartment. Under normal conditions, this causes no ill effects. However, if the animal has a distended rumen, twisted necrotic bowel, dilated stomach (gastric dilation), or gas-filled thoracic cavity (pneumothorax), the increased pressure from nitrous oxide diffusion can rupture devitalized tissue or compress adjoining structures. Therefore nitrous oxide is contraindicated under these conditions.

At the end of surgery when the flow of inhalant anesthetic gas is stopped, 100% oxygen should be administered at a high flow rate, as the animal recovers with the endotracheal tube in place. When the flow of nitrous oxide ceases at the end of a surgical procedure, nitrous oxide rapidly diffuses out of tissues, into the blood, and then into the alveoli, diluting the oxygen concentration within the alveoli. If the flow of 100% oxygen has been turned off and the animal is receiving oxygen only from room air, which contains 15% to 17% oxygen, the oxygen concentration in the lungs can be diluted enough by the nitrous oxide to produce hypoxia. This phenomenon, called diffusion hypoxia, or the second-gas effect, is the reason for maintaining a high rate of oxygen flow for at least 5 to 10 minutes after the end of nitrous oxide administration.

Desflurane

Desflurane is an anesthetic gas similar in activity to isoflurane and sevoflurane. It has a very pungent smell and requires a special thermoregulated (heated) vaporizer to ensure proper delivery of the anesthetic gas. Because of its expense and the requirement for special vaporizers, this anesthetic gas has not been widely used in veterinary medicine.

CENTRAL NERVOUS SYSTEM STIMULANTS

CNS stimulants are occasionally used to stimulate respiration in anesthetized animals or to reverse CNS depression caused by anesthetic or sedative agents. Therapeutic stimulants or toxic compounds that produce CNS stimulation act by any of the following mechanisms:

- Promote release of excitatory neurotransmitters such as acetylcholine and norepinephrine
- Delay separation of excitatory neurotransmitters from their receptors
- Inhibit release of inhibitory neurotransmitters such as GABA and adenosine
- Facilitate the breakdown or removal of inhibitory neurotransmitters after their release

• Inhibit processes that prevent release of excitatory neurotransmitters such as by blocking α_2 receptors

The latter three processes are often referred to as disinhibition because the compound inhibits an inhibitory process, resulting in CNS stimulation. Common toxicants that operate by one of these mechanisms include strychnine, which blocks GABA activity; theobromine, the component in chocolate that increases norepinephrine release and inhibits adenosine activity; caffeine, which has a mechanism of action similar to that of theobromine and is commonly found in diet pills; and amphetamines or cocaine.

METHYLXANTHINES

Caffeine and theobromine belong to a broad group of drugs known as methylxanthines, which include the respiratory drugs theophylline and aminophylline (see Chapter 6). Because chocolate toxicity in dogs has been a popular topic in magazines and newspapers, veterinary technicians should be aware of facts surrounding this syndrome. The active ingredient in chocolate is theobromine. A dosage as low as 90 mg/kg (41 mg/lb) can produce toxicity in dogs. The toxic dose for theobromine is estimated by the LD_{50}, which is the dose at which half of the dogs given that dose would be expected to die. The LD_{50} for theobromine in dogs is 250 to 500 mg/kg (114 to 228 mg/lb).

A typical chocolate bar contains 2 or 3 oz of milk chocolate, and 4 oz of milk chocolate contain approximately 240 mg of theobromine. A 10-lb dog would have to ingest two or three candy bars to produce toxicity. Fortunately, ingestion of that much chocolate by such a small dog would likely produce vomiting, thus decreasing the amount of theobromine absorbed.

A greater danger comes from ingestion of unsweetened baking chocolate, which usually contains 390 mg of theobromine per ounce. Thus a single ounce of baking chocolate could be enough to produce toxicity in a susceptible 10-lb dog. An additional source of theobromine intoxication in horses is cocoa bean hulls, which are sometimes used as stall bedding.

Treatment of chocolate toxicity is by induction of emesis and supportive care. Animals that ingest amounts of milk chocolate sufficient to cause toxicity usually vomit spontaneously and develop diarrhea. Removal of a large mass of chocolate by gastric lavage using a stomach tube can be difficult because the soft chocolate tends to form a ball within the stomach.

DOXAPRAM

Doxapram (Dopram, Dopram-V) is a CNS stimulant that works primarily at the medulla of the brainstem to increase respiration in animals with apnea (cessation of breathing) or bradypnea (slow breathing). Because many anesthetic, sedative, and analgesic drugs depress the medullary respiratory centers as part of their overall CNS depression effect, doxapram is most often used in animals that have received large amounts of these respiratory depressant drugs. For example, doxapram is occasionally used when opioids have been used as part of the anesthetic regimen for cesarean section or dystocia. The neonates, who receive the opioid drug by way of the placenta, usually have depressed respiratory function. After removal from the dam, the neonates can be given doxapram by the umbilical vein or sublingually (under the tongue). Of course, narcotic antagonists could also be used in this situation.

Doxapram also stimulates other parts of the brain in addition to the medullary area, but this stimulation is significantly weaker. Still, when combined with the effects of such drugs as xylazine, this stimulation of the cerebral cortex or emotion and behavior areas of the brain may produce aggressive behavior, muscle tremors, catatonic rigidity, and symptoms that have been attributed to hallucinogenic behavior. These effects are fortunately transient and subside within a few minutes after administration of doxapram.

Doxapram should be used with caution in animals that are predisposed to seizures. Overstimulation of the CNS by doxapram may precipitate seizures in susceptible animals.

α_2 ANTAGONISTS: YOHIMBINE, TOLAZOLINE, AND ATIPAMEZOLE

Yohimbine (Yobine), tolazoline (Priscoline), and atipamezole (Antisedan) are α_2 antagonists that bind to α_2 receptors on the terminal bouton of norepinephrine-releasing neurons and prevent the negative feedback that normally decreases release of more excitatory neurotransmitter. The net result is more release of excitatory neurotransmitters such as norepinephrine.

Because α_2 receptors are found in the cardiovascular system, GI tract, and genitourinary system, yohimbine, tolazoline, and atipamezole may cause increased heart rate, increased blood pressure, and an antidiuretic effect from sympathetic tone, causing vasoconstriction of renal arteries and thereby decreasing urine formation. Respiration is increased through stimulation of respiratory centers in the CNS. Although the effects of yohimbine, tolazoline, and atipamezole on animals predisposed to seizures are not well documented, cautious use of these drugs in these animals is prudent.

Box 8-1 Drug Categories and Names

ANALGESICS

Opioid analgesics
  Morphine
  Hydromorphone
  Fentanyl
  Butorphanol (Torbutrol, Torbugesic)
  Buprenorphine (Buprenex)
  Other opioids (meperidine, codeine, oxycodone)
Opioid antagonist
  Naloxone

TRANQUILIZERS AND SEDATIVES

Acepromazine maleate
Benzodiazepine tranquilizers
  Diazepam (Valium)
  Zolazepam (Telazol)
  Midazolam (Versed)
  Clonazepam (Klonopin)
Benzodiazepine antagonist
  Flumazenil
α_2 Agonists
  Xylazine (Rompun)
  Detomidine (Dormosedan)
  Medetomidine (Domitor)
α_2 Antagonists
  Yohimbine (Yobine)
  Atipamezole (Antisedan)
  Tolazoline (Priscoline)

ANESTHETICS

Barbiturates
  Thiopental (Pentothal)
  Pentobarbital
  Phenobarbital
  Methohexital (Brevital)
Propofol
Dissociative anesthetics
  Ketamine
  Tiletamine (Telazol)
Inhalant anesthetics
  Halothane
  Isoflurane
  Sevoflurane
Other anesthetic gas agents
  Nitrous oxide
  Desflurane

CNS STIMULANTS

Methylxanthines
  Caffeine
  Theobromine
Doxapram (Dopram)
α_2 Antagonists
  Yohimbine (Yobine)
  Tolazoline
  Atipamezole (Antisedan)

REFERENCES

1. Boothe DM: *Small animal clinical pharmacology and therapeutics*, Philadelphia, 2001, WB Saunders.

RECOMMENDED READING

Maddison J, Page S, Church D: *Small animal clinical pharmacology*, Philadelphia, 2002, WB Saunders.

Mathews KA: Management of pain, *Vet Clin North Am* 30(4):703-967, 2000.

Mathews NS: Clinical anesthesia, *Vet Clin North Am* 29(3):611-831, 1999.

Mosby's drug consult, St. Louis, 2002, Mosby.

Pfizer Animal Health: *Managing pain in cats, dogs, small mammals and birds*, Wilmington, DE, 2003, Gloyd Group.

Plumb DC: *Veterinary drug handbook*, ed 5, Ames, IA, 2005, Blackwell.

Robertson SA, Duncan B: *Safe and effective acute pain relief for cats*, in the Proceedings of the North American Veterinary Conference, Orlando, FL, 2003.

Tranquilli WJ, Grimm KA, Lamont LA: *Pain management for the small animal practitioner*, Jackson, WY, 2000, Teton New Media.

Self-Assessment

REVIEW QUESTIONS

Fill in the following blanks with the correct item from the Key Terms list.

1. _____ type of drug that directly relieves the perception of pain without loss of other sensations.

2. _____ type of drug that causes relaxation in the animal without a loss of consciousness; animal may be sleepy but is easily aroused.

3. _____ type of drug that relieves anxiety but produces no real analgesia; animal is relaxed but not necessarily sleepy.

4. _____ type of drug that removes perception of touch, pain, temperature, and pressure.

5. _____ pain associated with or originating from the organs or tissues inside the body.

6. _____ pain associated with a specific location on the surface of the body.

7. _____ translation of physical stimulus into depolarization of a receptor.

8. _____ means "increased sensitivity to pain."

9. _____ refers to the increased sensitivity the spinal cord acquires to pain as the result of pain signals being transmitted up the spinal cord.

10. _____ group of analgesics derived from poppy seeds.

11. _____ group of chemically synthesized, opiatelike drugs.

12. _____ pleasant hallucinogenic effects.

13. _____ unpleasant hallucinogenic effects.

14. _____ type of drug that produces some analgesic effect when combined with an opioid receptor; the effect is not as strong as other opioid agonist drugs.

15. _____ type of opioid drug that has activity at one type of opioid receptor and a blocking effect on another type of opioid receptor.

16. _____ opioid drugs combined with tranquilizer or sedative drugs.

17. _____ stimulation of this catecholamine-type receptor causes decreased release of norepinephrine from the neuron.

18. _____ means "low blood protein."

19. _____ nephrotoxic (in rats) chemical produced by the reaction of sevoflurane and carbon dioxide scavenger compounds commonly used in anesthetic machines (e.g., soda lime).

Fill in the following blanks with the correct drug listed in Box 8-1.

20. _____ injectable anesthetic agent; ultrashort acting; initial recovery is from redistribution of the drug to less-perfused tissues.

21. _____ drug that produces sedation by decreasing the release of norepinephrine.

22. _____ one of the drugs that can reverse xylazine overdose in the cow.

23. _____ barbiturate used in greyhounds because of its rapid metabolism.

24. _____ fastest gas anesthetic for induction and recovery of veterinary patients.

25. _____ tranquilizer with antiemetic properties; third eyelid comes up (prolapses) with this drug.

26. _____ anesthetic gas usually used as an additional agent; not used in pneumothorax or bloated patients.

27. _____ tranquilizer that has no inherent antiemetic properties.

28. _____ classified as a short-acting barbiturate not as long in duration as phenobarbital injectable; adequate for short surgical procedures.

29. _____ agent associated with malignant hyperthermia.

30. _____ dissociative anesthetic; visceral analgesia not as good as somatic analgesia; muscle relaxation is poor.

31. _____ Nonbarbiturate injectable drug used for intubation; has weak anesthetic and analgesic properties; comes in a single-use ampule or vial.

32. _____ drugs that make animals hypersensitive to sound.

33. _____ injectable anesthetic agent that produces a cataleptic state in cats; reflexes for swallowing stay intact; use requires ophthalmic ointment to keep eyes from drying.

34. _____ tranquilizer that can produce penile prolapse and should not be used in hypotensive animals because of α_1 antagonist effect.

35. _____ partial agonist/partial antagonist opioid narcotic; also the ingredient of a centrally acting cough medication approved for use in dogs.

36. _____ strong opioid narcotic analgesic administered as a patch (Duragesic).

37. _____ CNS stimulant found in chocolate.

38. _____ CNS stimulant used to reverse general respiratory depression such as might occur with inhalant anesthesia in pups delivered by cesarean section; stimulates the brainstem in a general way.

39. Indicate whether the following statements are true or false.

    A. The normal dose of barbiturates should be decreased in a dog with low plasma protein levels.

    B. Ketamine can result in dried corneas if the eyes are not medicated.

    C. The two drugs in Telazol are tiletamine and zolazepam.

    D. Typically the respiratory rate increases with opioid analgesic drugs.

40. What species is highly sensitive to the effects of xylazine? _____

APPLICATION QUESTIONS

1. Which would you rather administer to an animal with a broken pelvis that needs to be positioned for radiographs: a sedative, a local anesthetic, a general anesthetic, or an analgesic? What would be the advantages or disadvantages of each type of drug in this situation?

2. How are pentobarbital, thiopental, and phenobarbital classified? Which is an oxybarbiturate? Which would be used to induce anesthesia for purposes of intubating?

3. What is the physiology behind the rapid recovery from an initial injection of thiopental? Why must the second dose given be smaller than the first?

4. Why are cats dosed with barbiturates differently than dogs? Why is a 30-kg obese animal dosed differently than a 30-kg lean animal?

5. Is recovery from barbiturate anesthesia quicker in a lean dog or an obese dog? Why?

6. Explain how a person or animal becomes "tolerant" of barbiturates after repeated dosages.

7. Why do many animals become apneic when given thiopental intravenously? Does the apnea last long? Is oxygen therapy or artificial ventilation needed to keep the patient from dying in this situation?

8. What are the consequences of accidentally injecting a thiobarbiturate outside the vein? What can be done to prevent or reduce these consequences?

9. An animal is anesthetized with an injectable agent and the ECG is being monitored. The doctor comments about the bigeminy arrhythmia. What is bigeminy? What is the most appropriate action with regard to heart function in this anesthetized animal?

10. Is propofol appropriate to use as a light anesthetic for animals experiencing painful diagnostic or therapeutic procedures? Does extravascular injection of propofol cause tissue sloughing?

11. Why can't the ampules of propofol simply be kept around until they are completely used up? Why are they supposed to be discarded shortly after they are used for the first time?

12. The veterinarian comments that Telazol is basically a commercial preparation of Valium plus ketamine. What is the therapeutic significance of that comment? Is he correct?

13. Why are ketamine and tiletamine not used as sole anesthetics for surgical procedures such as a spay operation or the removal of an intraabdominal mass?

14. Why is applying an ophthalmic ointment to the eyes of a cat injected with ketamine or tiletamine important?

15. The veterinarian has told you to keep the ketamine locked up with the narcotic injectables. The label of the ketamine vial does list it as a controlled substance. Why is ketamine of special concern for keeping controlled substances carefully locked away?

16. Which of these drugs is fastest at inducing and recovery from anesthesia: sevoflurane, isoflurane, or halothane?

17. If you had two gas anesthetic drugs, which do you suppose would produce the onset of its activity more rapidly, the gas with the low MAC or the gas with the higher MAC?

18. Why should cardiac function be monitored during halothane anesthesia? Why is a tranquilizer a good idea as a preanesthetic agent prior to halothane anesthesia? Is this a concern with isoflurane or sevoflurane?

19. What is malignant hyperthermia? What causes it and how is it treated?

20. Why should halothane not be used as an anesthetic in animals with head trauma?

21. How does acepromazine compare to xylazine or detomidine for analgesia?

22. By what mechanism does acepromazine have an antiemetic effect?

23. What special considerations are there for dogs on acepromazine that are going to be skin-tested for allergies?

24. What is the relationship between benzodiazepine tranquilizers and GABA in the brain?

25. How effective are benzodiazepine tranquilizers as analgesics? How effective are they as antiemetics? Do they have much of a muscle relaxant effect?

26. Why is diazepam no longer used as an appetite stimulant in cats?

27. Which wears off sooner for xylazine: the analgesia or the sedation? Why is it important for the veterinary technician to remember this? If an animal still appears to be in pain after a full dose of an α_2-agonist drug, will additional doses increase the degree of analgesia?

28. Under what conditions is the use of xylazine contraindicated in dogs?

29. Explain the physiology behind the initial increase in blood pressure, the slowing of the heart, and the returning of blood pressure to near normal after the injection of an α_2-agonist drug.

30. What are the three principal opioid receptors? Which contribute to analgesia? Which contribute to euphoria or dysphoria?

31. What is the difference between an opioid agonist, a partial agonist, and an antagonist? How is a mixed agonist antagonist different from a partial agonist?

32. Why should animals recovering from deep sedation with opioids be placed in a dark, quiet room?

33. If we are monitoring the depth of anesthesia for an animal that has received morphine as part of its preanesthetic/anesthetic cocktail (mixture of drugs), what effect would we expect to see on the pupil size as a result of the morphine in dogs? In cats?

34. Why do some dogs pant when on hydromorphone or fentanyl? Are they hypoxic (low oxygen)?

35. What can be given to the dog on hydromorphone to decrease the bradycardia caused by the opioid?

36. Butorphanol and buprenorphine both experience a "ceiling effect" in their depth of analgesia. What is the pharmacologic basis for this ceiling effect?

37. Oxycodone is a very potent analgesic. Why is it generally not used in veterinary medicine?

38. What would be the advantage of reversing hydromorphone's respiratory depression with butorphanol or buprenorphine versus naloxone?

39. A drug reference describes a particular drug as a CNS disinhibitor. What effects will this drug have?

40. A client telephones and asks if his 65-lb Siberian Husky will become ill from the half of a chocolate bar it just stole off the kitchen table. Is this a potential health threat?

Drugs Affecting the Nervous System: Anticonvulsants and Behavior-Modifying Drugs

key terms

anticonvulsant

antidepressant

antipsychotic

anxiolytics

convulsion

drug-induced hepatopathy

epilepsy

γ-aminobutyric acid

generalized seizure

grain (measurement)

ictus

idiopathic epilepsy

induced

limbic system

major tranquilizers

monoamine oxidase
  inhibitors

partial seizure

polydipsic

polyphagic

polyuric

postictal phase

preictal phase (aura)

seizure

selective serotonin reuptake
  inhibitors

status epilepticus

tricyclic antidepressants

objectives

After studying this chapter, the veterinary technician should be able to explain:

1. The different types of anticonvulsants drugs, their indications, and their precautions

2. How the behavior-modifying drugs work

3. Some commonly used behavior-modifying drugs and what type of problems they are used for

In addition to the central nervous system (CNS) effects associated with drugs used to calm animals, manage pain, or stimulate the CNS, two other groups of CNS-related drugs also are used in veterinary medicine. This chapter focuses on the mechanisms of action and problems encountered when using *anticonvulsant* drugs and drugs for modifying behavior. Box 9-1, listing anticonvulsants and behavior-modifying drugs, can be found at the end of this chapter.

ANTICONVULSANTS

Seizures are periods of altered brain function characterized by loss of consciousness, increased muscle tone or movement, altered sensations, and other neurologic changes. *Convulsions* are seizures that manifest themselves as spastic muscle movement caused by stimulation of motor nerves in the brain or spinal cord. Some seizures can result in no apparent convulsive activity but may appear more like the animal is in a state of semiconsciousness (absence seizures). Unless stated otherwise, the term seizure in this text typically implies the presence of convulsions.

Seizure activity can be caused by various pathologic states such as hypoxia (low tissue oxygen tension), hypoglycemia (low blood sugar level), hypocalcemia (low blood calcium level), and toxicity such as that caused by lead, strychnine, and organophosphates. Infectious diseases such as canine distemper or conditions such as hydrocephalus, brain neoplasia, and parasitic migration involving the CNS may also precipitate seizures.

Recurrent seizures are referred to as *epilepsy,* whereas recurrent seizures of unknown cause are referred to as *idiopathic epilepsy. Status epilepticus* refers to the state of being in the seizure activity and often is used to describe the condition of animals with prolonged seizure activity.

Seizure activities associated with epilepsy typically have three phases. The *preictal phase*

(aura) occurs before a seizure begins and may be characterized by pacing, panting, anxiety, apprehension, and other behavioral changes. This phase may last for minutes or hours before a seizure. The seizure, or *ictus,* may be partial (involving only a limited area of the brain and manifesting itself in a localized response, such as one limb), or generalized (involving the whole brain and affecting the entire body). In some cases, the aura may actually be a *partial seizure* that does or does not lead to a full-blown *generalized seizure.* The older terms "grand mal" and "petit mal" are no longer used in human medicine to describe epilepsy and are being replaced in veterinary medicine with the terms partial seizures and generalized seizures. The *postictal phase* occurs after the seizure activity has subsided. During this phase, which can last from seconds to hours, the animal may appear tired, confused, anxious, or even blind depending on the nature and location of the seizure activity within the CNS and the type of seizure experienced.

Drugs used to control seizures are called anticonvulsants. Most seizures associated with epilepsy, although frightening to the animal's owner, are usually not life threatening. However, prolonged seizure activity, such as occurs with toxicity or brain pathology, can result in hyperthermia (elevated body temperature) from prolonged muscle activity, hypoxia from the inability to expand the chest because of muscle contractions, or severe acidosis (pH of the blood becomes acidic) from the release of lactic acid from overworked muscles. Once status epilepticus is controlled with anticonvulsants the veterinarian must identify or rule out the cause of the seizure activity. Idiopathic epilepsy is often the default diagnosis after other causes have been ruled out.

Seizures associated with idiopathic epilepsy are often emotional issues for the pet owner. The goal of seizure control in these cases is to find a level of control that is comfortable for both the animal and owner. For example, a dog that has minor seizures twice a year with

6 months of normal behavior between episodes may not be a candidate for daily anticonvulsant therapy. On the other hand, if the client or family members are upset by the seizures and they are willing to medicate the animal daily to prevent them, the goal may be to use daily medication to reduce seizures to very mild ones with relatively long periods between seizure activity. Seizure activity in a horse or livestock animal usually warrants euthanasia because of the potential for injury to animal handlers and others near the animal during a seizure.

PHENOBARBITAL

Phenobarbital is still the drug of choice for long-term control of seizures in dogs and cats. This barbiturate is inexpensive and, because of its long half-life, may be given orally once or twice a day. Although the mechanism of phenobarbital is not completely understood, it is fairly well established that phenobarbital acts by decreasing the likelihood of spontaneous depolarization in brain cells and the spread of electrical activity throughout the brain from this seizure focus (point of seizure origin). The end result is a decrease in frequency of seizure activity and a lessening of the seizure severity.

For phenobarbital to be effective, concentrations of the drug must continuously remain in the normal therapeutic range. Fortunately, phenobarbital is relatively slowly removed from the body, which allows daily or twice-daily dosing of the medication to maintain therapeutic concentrations. This dosing schedule is reasonable for client compliance on a long-term basis.

Although the therapeutic range for phenobarbital is fairly well established for dogs and cats, the dosages required to achieve and maintain those therapeutic concentrations vary widely. The range in dosages is explained by the wide variability in how the individual animal metabolizes the drug.

Phenobarbital is biotransformed by mixed-function oxidases, a family of enzymes found primarily in the liver. Mixed function oxidases can be *induced* by the repeated administration of phenobarbital, meaning that the number of enzymes increases, thus metabolizing phenobarbital at a more rapid rate. The net result is that for a given dose, the drug concentrations in the blood will decrease as the body becomes more efficient at metabolizing the drug. This is the basis behind the drug tolerance observed with barbiturates.

The metabolites of phenobarbital and some nonmetabolized phenobarbital molecules are eliminated by the kidney. The half-life of elimination for these drugs varies widely in dogs and cats, reflecting the differences in hepatic conversion of the drug to the more readily excreted metabolite. Canine half-lives from various studies range from 30 to 90 hours, with feline studies showing a similar wide range. Because of this wide range in metabolism and elimination half-life, two dogs of the same weight, age, and breed can require very different dosages to achieve the same drug concentrations in the blood.

Cats have a lower therapeutic range for phenobarbital than dogs. Consequently, phenobarbital dosages in cats are approximately half those used in dogs. Because plasma phenobarbital concentrations achieved with any given dose vary considerably, the concentrations should be checked periodically by a veterinary diagnostic laboratory. Without such monitoring, some veterinarians continue to increase a phenobarbital dose if seizures are not well controlled without knowing whether the dosage previously used was inadequate or whether the poor control is associated with underlying disease that is resistant to barbiturate. The only way to determine this is to measure the plasma concentration of the barbiturate.

Because the mixed function oxidases are also responsible for metabolism of a number of other commonly used veterinary drugs, phenobarbital induction of this enzyme system can result in other drugs also being broken down more rapidly with a subsequent decrease in concentrations. Therefore epileptic animals treated with phenobarbital may need to have the dose of any other drugs using the same metabolic pathway increased to compensate for their accelerated metabolism.

As with most other barbiturates, phenobarbital is highly protein bound. When plasma protein levels are decreased, such as from liver disease or protein-losing kidney or GI disease, more phenobarbital becomes available in the free form and therefore more phenobarbital molecules are free to diffuse in the brain to produce the clinical effect (see Chapter 3). Thus, animals with hypoproteinemia may require lower dosages of phenobarbital than normal. Use of salicylates such as aspirin or sulfonamide antimicrobials also increases the amount of free phenobarbital by displacing the barbiturate from sites on plasma proteins.

Adverse Effects of Phenobarbital

Many animals, when started on phenobarbital tablets for control of epileptic seizure activity, show signs of sedation and ataxia (they may wobble or stagger when walking). Owners need to be advised that this side effect is usually temporary and should diminish over the first 2 to 3 weeks of therapy. Severe sedation or ataxia may be a sign of phenobarbital overdose; however, a plasma concentration of the drug should be submitted to determine if the observed ataxia is truly an overdose or merely reflects the transient initial effect of the drug.

The dog or cat may become *polyphagic* (increase in appetite), *polydipsic* (increase in drinking), or *polyuric* (increase in urination) while taking phenobarbital. Phenobarbital appears to have an inhibitory effect on the release of antidiuretic hormone, a hormone that normally helps the body conserve water. With decreased effect of antidiuretic hormone, the animal excretes more water (polyuria) and subsequently needs to drink more water to compensate. The polyuria and polydipsia tend to diminish with time, although some animals may show these signs to some degree the entire time they are on phenobarbital.

Serum activity of liver-associated enzymes such as alkaline phosphatase (ALP) and alanine aminotransferase (ALT) may be increased after an animal has received phenobarbital for a few days. Serum activity of ALP may be increased fourfold above normal ranges. As long as the activity of other liver enzymes is not markedly increased and other parameters such as bile acids remain normal, these elevations of ALT and ALP are not indicative of liver disease but reflect a normal increase that is expected with phenobarbital administration. ALP does not appear to increase in cats as much as it does in dogs. Actual hepatotoxicity has been reported with phenobarbital; however, this is relatively rare unless the animal is also on other potentially hepatotoxic drugs (e.g., primidone anticonvulsant) or other hepatotoxic compounds (e.g., toxicants in the environment). The concentrations of ALT and ALP in animals that have had benign increases as a result of phenobarbital administration will return to normal a few weeks after phenobarbital therapy is discontinued.

Occasionally a dog receiving phenobarbital becomes excitable or hyperactive instead of lethargic or sedated. This may occur at a subtherapeutic dose, and an increase in the dose of phenobarbital does not necessarily seem to decrease this effect until very high concentrations of phenobarbital are achieved. This idiosyncratic reaction to phenobarbital is not predictable and is not dose dependent. That is, as the dose increases, signs do not necessarily increase in severity. Often these animals need to be switched to a different anticonvulsant.

The dose of phenobarbital is often measured in *grains*, with 1 grain equaling approximately 60 mg. The apothecary scale conversion of grains to milligrams is technically 1 grain = 65.8 mg; however, today that conversion is typically rounded to 1 grain = 60 mg. Tablets are usually available in ¼-, ½-, 1-, and 2-grain sizes, which roughly correspond to 15, 30, 60, and 120 mg, respectively.

DIAZEPAM

Diazepam (Valium) is a benzodiazepine tranquilizer and the drug of choice for emergency treatment of animals in status epilepticus. Benzodiazepine tranquilizers such as diazepam and clonazepam control seizures by rapidly penetrating the blood-brain barrier and enhancing the inhibitory effect of the CNS neurotransmitter *γ-aminobutyric acid* (GABA). Because GABA helps counter the effect of stimulatory neurotransmitters in the brain such as acetylcholine and norepinephrine, enhancing the GABA effect quiets the activity of the CNS.

Diazepam comes in oral and intravenous dose forms. Although diazepam is quite effective when given intravenously, it is poorly effective when given by mouth. Only approximately 2% to 5% of the diazepam given orally to dogs actually makes it to the systemic circulation because of the significant first-pass effect (see Chapter 3). The first-pass effect occurs when drugs absorbed from the intestinal tract pass by way of the hepatic portal system to the liver and are rapidly metabolized before they reach the systemic circulation. Because the metabolites of diazepam have much less anticonvulsant activity, the first-pass effect essentially renders the diazepam ineffective. This rapid hepatic metabolism also explains diazepam's fairly short duration of activity when it is given intravenously.

In addition to the first-pass effect, the body develops tolerance to the drug very quickly. This plus the first-pass effect and quick half-life limit diazepam's use in the dog to treatment of status epilepticus. Animals with underlying conditions that continue to produce seizures may be treated with a continuous-rate infusion of diazepam. However, these animals may be more practically treated with IV pentobarbital or phenobarbital because these drugs control the seizures for a longer time than diazepam. If diazepam is added to a drip bottle or bag as part of a continuous-rate infusion, the mixture should be inverted several times to more evenly distribute the diazepam in the solution because it does not mix well with most fluids. In addition, diazepam tends to adhere to the polyvinyl plastic that makes up most IV lines. To keep the diazepam from the IV fluid bag from sticking to the inside of the IV tubing, the IV line is first flushed with diazepam to "saturate" the inner lining.

Cats are less efficient at metabolizing diazepam than dogs; therefore diazepam theoretically should be more effective as an anticonvulsant for maintaining control on a long-term basis. However, a fatal idiosyncratic *drug-induced hepatopathy* (liver disease caused by drugs) has been reported in cats receiving low-dose diazepam for treatment of behavior disorders. In one study only 1 of 11 cats with diazepam-induced liver failure survived. For this reason, most clinicians are leery about long-term use of diazepam in cats, and phenobarbital is still the drug of choice for maintaining long-term control of seizures in cats just as it is in dogs.

If diazepam cannot be given intravenously for some reason during status epilepticus, the drug can be administered per rectum. This has been suggested as a way an owner can safely administer diazepam to an animal that is showing preictal signs of an epileptic episode. A gel formulation of diazepam (Diastat) is available in the United States for per rectum administration.

Side effects of diazepam are usually minimal compared with barbiturates or opioids. Because benzodiazepine tranquilizers are muscle relaxants, ataxia and weakness unrelated to sedation may occur. Diazepam also may unmask certain learned behaviors, resulting in an animal becoming more aggressive when its learned controlled behavior is inhibited by diazepam. Veterinary technicians must always remember that a relaxed animal from benzodiazepine tranquilizer is still quite capable of responding in an aggressive and dangerous manner if it chooses.

POTASSIUM BROMIDE

Potassium bromide is a very old drug. Bromides were used in the 1800s to treat a wide variety of "nervous disorders." Today, potassium bromide is one of the most commonly used adjunct therapies for animals whose seizures are not well controlled by phenobarbital alone.

Bromide is more of a chemical reagent than a drug. It is combined with sodium, potassium, or ammonia and compounded in water or corn syrup (for sweetness) by veterinary pharmacies for use in veterinary patients. The mechanism of action of the drug is not clearly defined; however, it may act like chloride ions do to change the resting membrane potential of neurons, making them more difficult to depolarize (fire). The net effect is a nervous system that is less likely to spontaneously discharge and produce a seizure.

Like phenobarbital, potassium bromide has a long half-life. Whereas phenobarbital's half-life is measured in hours, potassium bromide's half-life in the dog is 21 to 24 days. Clinically this is important because of the amount of time it takes for potassium bromide to reach steady-state concentrations (see Chapter 3). By using the formula of Steady state = 5 × Half life, potassium bromide will not reach equilibrium in the body for 3 to 5 months.

To avoid this lag time between when the drug is first given and when it reaches therapeutic concentrations, a large loading dose can be given to establish concentrations within the therapeutic range. A smaller maintenance dose is then given to keep the concentrations within range. The disadvantage to using the loading dose is the variable response of animals to potassium bromide. Potassium bromide has a narrow therapeutic index, meaning that the dose producing therapeutic effects is quite close to the dose causing toxicity. Therefore, if a loading dose overshoots the therapeutic range and produces toxicity (anorexia, vomiting, diarrhea, sedation, stupor, coma), the long half-life means that the side effects are going to be present for hours to days.

Vomiting may occur even if the dose of potassium bromide is within an acceptable range. This appears to be a direct effect of the salt on the stomach, which produces gastric irritation. Vomiting can be reduced by using a liquid formulation instead of a capsule, by dividing the prescribed dose into twice-daily or three times daily doses, and by trying different foods to be given with the potassium bromide to see which are tolerated the best.

Laboratory tests that measure serum electrolytes may report an elevated chloride concentration in animals that are taking potassium bromide. This is a false reading caused by the interference of bromide ions with many of the chloride ion analyzers used to measure chloride concentrations.

Although some neurologists are trying potassium bromide as a solo anticonvulsant, most often it is used in conjunction with phenobarbital when phenobarbital by itself fails to adequately control seizure activity. Because high therapeutic concentrations of potassium bromide and phenobarbital are likely to produce an unacceptable level of sedation or ataxia, the phenobarbital dose needs to be decreased as the potassium bromide concentrations begin to produce clinical response. During this period of transition, the veterinary technician plays an important role in helping educate the client regarding the reason for the drug dose changes, the need to check blood concentrations of the anticonvulsants, the expected side effects, and the increased risk for breakthrough seizure activity as dosages are adjusted.

In addition to potassium bromide, sodium bromide is also used as an adjunct anticonvulsant.

OTHER ANTICONVULSANTS

Primidone is an approved drug for use as an anticonvulsant in dogs. Although primidone has some anticonvulsant activity, most of its efficacy is attributable to phenobarbital

CLINICAL APPLICATION
Use of Propofol for Seizures

The anesthetic agent propofol has been used in human medicine as a continuous-rate infusion (constant IV drip) for treatment of status epilepticus that is unresponsive to traditional anticonvulsant therapy. Can this drug be used in veterinary medicine for the same purposes?

Propofol (Rapinovet, PropoFlo) is a short-acting drug with label indications for induction of anesthesia, maintenance of anesthesia for up to 20 minutes, and induction of general anesthesia when maintenance is provided by inhalant anesthetics. It has been described for use in managing seizures in dogs after surgical closure of portosystemic shunts. Portosystemic shunts are abnormal blood vessels that allow blood coming from the intestinal tract to bypass the liver and flow directly into the systemic circulation, delivering toxins from the gastrointestinal tract (e.g., ammonia, short-chain fatty acids) into systemic circulation. Even though the existence of the shunt often results in abnormalities in the CNS from increased ammonia and other compounds, surgical closure of portosystemic shunts occasionally results in seizure activity that is difficult to control.

A report in the *Journal of Small Animal Practice* described the use of propofol to control seizures after correction of a portosystemic shunt in four cats and one dog (Table 9-1).[1] In this report, the seizures in each of the five animals were controlled with IV propofol, including two animals that could not be controlled by the use of other anticonvulsants.

A number of reasons exist why propofol is not the first choice for controlling status epilepticus. Respiratory depression is common with propofol, and apnea can occur if too much drug is administered too rapidly. However, the apnea and respiratory depression are fairly short lived and therefore clinically manageable. Propofol is thought to have a depressant effect on the heart, but these effects, typically observed as a drop in arterial blood pressure, occur mostly at higher doses.

Paradoxically, seizurelike activity has been associated with propofol. The cause is still not well understood; however, clinicians dealing with an animal in status epilepticus that is refractory to diazepam, phenobarbital, or pentobarbital appear to believe the potential risk for additional seizure activity is offset by the greater potential for control of the seizures.

What should be learned from this situation: Propofol can be used extra label for control of refractory seizures, but it is not without its own problems. Because of this, it is considered a back-up drug and not a drug of first choice for seizure control.

produced by its metabolism. The other primidone metabolite, phenylethylmalonamide, has weak anticonvulsant activity in dogs. Because the efficacy of primidone largely depends on its metabolism to phenobarbital, many clinicians simply give phenobarbital rather than primidone. The side effects and drug interactions of primidone are similar to those seen with phenobarbital. Long-term use of large doses of primidone, especially if used in conjunction with the anticonvulsant phenytoin (Dilantin), has been implicated in drug-induced hepatopathy. This syndrome is characterized by diffuse inflammation and destruction of the liver. Unfortunately, once the signs become apparent, the prognosis for recovery is poor.

If a veterinarian is considering switching anticonvulsants from primidone to phenobarbital, a reasonable dosage conversion rate is 60 mg of phenobarbital for each 250 mg of primidone. Plasma concentrations of phenobarbital should be measured in treated dogs 1 to 2 weeks after conversion to phenobarbital to determine the plasma concentration relative to the normal therapeutic range.

Phenytoin (Dilantin) is a human anticonvulsant that was once popular for use in treating epilepsy in animals. The major disadvantage of phenytoin is that maintaining therapeutic plasma concentrations of drug is difficult in dogs. The drug is poorly and erratically absorbed from the gastrointestinal tract and,

TABLE **9-1** Use of Propofol to Control Seizures After Correction of a Portosystemic Shunt

	BOLUS DOSE OF PROPOFOL USED	CONTINUOUS-RATE INFUSION DOSE OF PROPOFOL USED
Cat 1	1 mg/kg bolus followed by CRI	0.1 mg/kg/min for 12 hr
Cat 2	1 mg/kg bolus followed by CRI	0.1 mg/kg/min for 12 hr
Cat 3		0.25 mg/kg/min for 48 hr
Cat 4		0.2 mg/kg/min for 48 hr
Dog 1	Periodic boluses 3-5 mg/kg + CRI	0.2 mg/kg/min for 48 hr

CRI, Continuous-rate infusion.
From Heldmann E, Holt D, Brockman DJ, et al: Use of propofol to manage seizure activity after surgical treatment of portosystemic shunts, *J Small Anim Pract* 40:590-592, 1999.

once absorbed, is rapidly eliminated by the liver. Phenytoin must be given at least three times daily to maintain therapeutic levels in plasma. Another disadvantage of phenytoin is that at doses necessary to achieve and maintain therapeutic plasma concentrations, the enzyme system that eliminates phenytoin becomes saturated. At the point of saturation, the elimination system, which is working at its maximum rate, is overwhelmed, resulting in accumulation of the drug in the body. As with primidone, phenytoin has also been implicated in drug-induced hepatopathy, usually when the drug is used in conjunction with primidone. Because of its poor absorption, short half-life, saturation kinetics, and risk of liver damage, phenytoin is not generally recommended for use in controlling idiopathic epilepsy. However, because physicians and nurses who treat human beings may ask about the use of this drug in their epileptic pet, the veterinary technician should have at least some knowledge of the drug and why it is not used in veterinary medicine.

Other benzodiazepine tranquilizers considered for use as anticonvulsants include clonazepam (Klonopin), lorazepam, and clorazepate. Like diazepam, all these drugs have problems with bioavailability and the need to use multiple doses to maintain therapeutic concentrations. In addition, these human dose formulations are often not very convenient for use in veterinary medicine. For example, an 88-lb German shepherd on the recommended dose of clonazepam at 0.1 to 0.5 mg/kg PO q8h would require between 4 and 20 mg of clonazepam three times a day. Clonazepam is available only in ½-, 1-, and 2-mg tablets, requiring administration of 6 to 30 tablets a day in this large dog. For smaller dogs, some of these benzodiazepines might theoretically be reasonable adjunct therapies for phenobarbital. Unfortunately, most animals develop a significant tolerance to the benzodiazepine drugs within a relatively short period, limiting their long-term use.

Other human anticonvulsant drugs will continue to emerge and be considered for use in veterinary medicine. Most will have mechanisms similar to those described above. The veterinary technician should remain current on anticonvulsant therapies and be able to answer questions related to the drugs and their side effects.

BEHAVIOR-MODIFYING DRUGS

Personality, emotions, and fears are the result of a complex, integrated balance (or imbalance) of a wide variety of chemical neurotransmitters. This complexity shows how readily normal brain function can be altered by even minor changes in concentrations of various neurotransmitters. Chapter 8 discussed how several of these neurotransmitters (e.g., acetylcholine, epinephrine, GABA) were altered to produce changes in brain function that resulted in the beneficial effects of anesthesia, sedation, tranquilization, or analgesia. Activity in the brain can be decreased by suppressing the release of norepinephrine (e.g., xylazine acting on α_2 receptors to decrease norepinephrine release), enhancing the effect of glutamate (e.g., ivermectin toxicosis), or enhancing the activity of GABA (e.g., diazepam or the other benzodiazepine tranquilizers). Brain activity can also be increased by the use of methylxanthine compounds such as caffeine from coffee or theobromine in chocolate. Thus seeing how an imbalance of neurotransmitters can result in clinical depression, behavior changes, old-age memory changes, self-destructive activities, or anxiety/fear reactions is not difficult. As society has come to recognize that signs of some of these human behavioral syndromes seem to occur in pets, an interest in using the human mood-altering medications to control what are perceived to be similar syndromes in pets has developed.

Without a doubt, behavior modification drug therapeutics is a complex study of pharmacology and is full of dissenting opinions about the best course of action for approaching pet behavioral problems. This section provides some basic terminology and mechanisms so that the veterinary technician may gain an entry-level understanding of what these drugs do and how they are proposed to modify behaviors of the animal.

WHAT ARE BEHAVIOR-MODIFYING DRUGS?

Essentially, behavior-modifying drugs change the concentrations of selected neurotransmitters in the brain with the intent of decreasing or enhancing specific mental (neuronal) activity. These drugs all work by one of the following general mechanisms:

- Enhancing the release of neurotransmitters (either inhibitory or excitatory neurotransmitters)
- Enhancing the binding (affinity) of neurotransmitters to their receptors
- Imitating the natural neurotransmitter and combining with the neurotransmitter's receptor to stimulate the receptor (agonist effect)

- Imitating the natural neurotransmitter and combining with the neurotransmitter's receptor but producing reduced or no stimulation of the receptor (antagonist effect)
- Prolonging the action of the neurotransmitter by decreasing the breakdown or slowing the rate of termination of the neurotransmitter itself
- Shortening the action of the neurotransmitter by enhancing its breakdown or termination

The net effect of these mechanisms is to either increase or decrease the action of a neurotransmitter and thus the activity in specific regions of the brain.

A variety of terms are used to describe behavior-modifying drugs. *Antipsychotic* drugs are also called *major tranquilizers* and include phenothiazine tranquilizers such as acepromazine. Even though veterinary patients do not express specific, identified psychoses, these drugs still play a role in treating behavior disorders in pets. *Antidepressant* drugs, as the name implies, are mood-elevating drugs used in human therapy. In veterinary medicine, antidepressants are used for a number of behaviors in pets that are not necessarily associated with what we would call "depressed" behaviors. *Anxiolytics* are drugs that "lyse" anxiety or decrease fear responses.

Other descriptor terms are used to describe drugs used in behavior modification; however, these three terms capture the basic mechanisms behind some of the more popular behavior-modification drugs in veterinary medicine.

ANTIPSYCHOTIC DRUGS

Antipsychotic drugs include the phenothiazine tranquilizers acepromazine and chlorpromazine and more potent tranquilizers such as haloperidol and prochlorperazine. Generally, this class of drugs in veterinary medicine is used to decrease inappropriate behavioral responses to stimuli but has the disadvantage of reducing both normal and abnormal responses to the environment. In other words, these drugs are not very specific in their mechanism of action and produce their beneficial effects at the cost of calming all behaviors, including those behaviors that are not necessarily desirable to decrease.

As was discussed in Chapter 4, phenothiazines block dopamine receptors that, by blocking dopamine receptors in the CRTZ, decrease vomiting. Increased dopamine and the stimulation of dopamine receptors in parts of the brain thought to control emotion (the *limbic system*) have been shown to result in abnormal behaviors tied to emotions. Thus blocking dopamine receptors in this area of the brain allows other neurotransmitters to dominate and decreases the incidence of the abnormal behaviors. This mechanism as described is simplified for purposes of gaining a basic understanding. Phenothiazine tranquilizers are also known to have a variety of effects on other receptors that may or may not contribute to a particular behavior. However, the dopamine-blocking (antagonist) effect does help explain the change in emotional behavior observed with animals on phenothiazine tranquilizers.

Phenothiazine tranquilizers are not without side effects. Animals and people on these drugs also tend to have less interest in their environment, have fewer emotional responses to stimuli, and have a depression of complex behaviors. Learned responses (but not instinctual responses) of avoidance to certain stimuli (e.g., audio reprimand, visual fear stimulus) are reduced with the use of phenothiazine tranquilizers. This is one reason why phenothiazines are used: to control learned fear responses such as those associated with thunderstorms, firecrackers, or other stimuli the animal has learned to fear.

However, because phenothiazines do not suppress instinctual responses, treatment can sometimes result in uncovering of underlying inappropriate behaviors. For example, phenothiazines are generally not recommended for use in suppressing aggressive behavior problems. Some aggressive animals may have learned adaptive behaviors that have reduced their displayed natural aggression to fit into the social order in a human household or to avoid receiving negative reinforcement (punishment). If a phenothiazine tranquilizer is used to attempt to "tranquilize" the displayed level of aggression, the animal's learned response to control aggressive tendencies may be lessened, allowing the instinctual aggressive behavior to reemerge. The animal actually may become more aggressive and startle more readily in response to stimuli or situations. Thus, as with all drugs, an understanding of the limitations of the phenothiazines for behavior-modification therapy is important.

ANTIDEPRESSANT DRUGS

Three classes of antidepressant drugs used in human beings have also found use in veterinary medicine: the *tricyclic antidepressants* (TCAs), the *selective serotonin reuptake inhibitors* (SSRIs), and the *monoamine oxidase inhibitors* (MAOIs). The TCAs are named for their chemical structure, and the latter two drug groups are named for the mechanisms by which they work.

Tricyclic antidepressants used in veterinary medicine include amitriptyline (Elavil [human product]) and clomipramine (Clomicalm [veterinary product], Anafranil [human product]). Both drugs work by decreasing the reuptake of serotonin from the synaptic cleft (the space in the synapse between two communicating neurons), which allows the neurotransmitter to accumulate and prolongs its activity. In addition to serotonin, amitriptyline also blocks reuptake of norepinephrine.

Amitriptyline and clomipramine have both been used to treat generalized anxiety and separation anxiety behaviors in dogs and cats. Amitriptyline has been used to decrease inappropriate spraying and excessive grooming in cats as well as excessive feather plucking in birds. Clomipramine has been approved and marketed for veterinary use as Clomicalm and is indicated for treatment of obsessive-compulsive disorders in dogs.

Obsessive-compulsive disorders are defined as behaviors that are repeated over and over again in the same way and appear to serve no real purpose. Because identification of a true obsessive-compulsive disorder is sometimes difficult to identify in animals (other than repeated licking, chewing, or grooming), a more common use for clomipramine is for treatment of separation anxiety and aggressive behaviors.

TCAs drugs do not blunt the overall normal behavioral responses to environmental stimuli to the same degree that phenothiazine tranquilizers do, but they do share some of the characteristics of the phenothiazines, including the possible increased risk for seizures from lowering of the threshold for initiation of seizure activity. As with all these antidepressants, TCAs should not be used with SSRIs or MAO inhibitors. Warnings and precautions of amitriptyline and clomipramine should be reviewed before using them in any patient because both drugs have several potentially adverse effects if used with certain other drugs or specific medical or disease conditions.

SSRIs used in veterinary medicine include the human drugs fluoxetine, fluvoxamine, paroxetine, and sertraline. Serotonin is a neurotransmitter identified as playing a significant role in determining mood and behavior. The SSRIs enhance the effect of the serotonin neurotransmitter by blocking its removal from the synaptic cleft. The serotonin remains for a longer period of time at its site of action, accumulates, and extends its effect. The SSRIs differ from the TCAs in that the SSRIs are more selective for blocking serotonin without significantly blocking the other neurotransmitters, such as norepinephrine.

The types of behaviors for which these drugs have been used are similar to the TCAs (obsessive-compulsive behaviors, anxiety, and aggression). The side effects of these drugs can be quite diverse. Some authors claim that SSRIs are safer than TCAs because SSRIs have less of a depressant effect on the heart than TCAs. Discontinuation of TCAs and SSRIs in veterinary patients relates more commonly to weak changes in behavior modification than to physiologic side effects. Still, a review of the potential side effects and adverse effects of these drugs must be done before the drug is administered.

The most commonly used MAOI in veterinary medicine is selegiline, also known as deprenyl. It is marketed as the veterinary product Anipryl for use in treating Cushing's disease and for canine cognitive dysfunction (old-dog senility). MAOIs increase the effect of dopamine by blocking the mechanism by which dopamine is taken up again by the mitochondria in the neurons. Unlike the phenothiazines, which block dopamine action and reduce its activity, MAOIs increase the amount of dopamine found in selected cells within the CNS and enhance the dopamine effect. Thus those behavioral problems related to a decrease of available dopamine in selected areas of the brain may be successfully treated with MAOIs. Because old-dog dementia, a senility-like syndrome, is thought to involve a decreased amount of dopamine in parts of the brain, selegiline has been advocated for improving cognitive function.

ANXIOLYTIC DRUGS

Anxiolytic drugs are tranquilizers belonging to the benzodiazepine group (e.g., diazepam, clonazepam, chlorazepate, lorazepam). As discussed in the anticonvulsant section, diazepam works by increasing stimulation of receptors for the neurotransmitter GABA. Because GABA is an inhibitory neurotransmitter, stimulation of these GABA receptors has a depressant effect on the CNS. However, the antianxiety effect of diazepam is thought to occur at a separate area of the brain from the CNS depression. At low doses of diazepam the animals become more relaxed and less excitable. The reduction in anxiety (nervousness in social interactions) does not occur until moderate-level doses of diazepam are used. At high doses the animals become quite sedated and ataxic and readily fall asleep.

Diazepam and the other members of this group are not used as frequently for behavior modification as some of the other drugs because of their nonspecific activity and their interference with the animal's ability to learn behavior modification. Because behavior modification through training is considered essential to successfully changing unwanted behavior patterns, the use of diazepam may compromise this process.

While diazepam and the benzodiazepines can be used to reduce general anxiety (without requiring behavior modification), they are not the best drugs to use in trying to reduce aggression in veterinary patients. If the pet's aggression is a direct response to anxiety, benzodiazepines may be useful in reducing the aggression. However, if the animal is currently less aggressive because anxiety or fear of punishment is holding that aggressive behavior in check, the use of benzodiazepines may remove that anxiety, allowing full expression of the underlying aggressive behavior.

OTHER BEHAVIOR-MODIFYING DRUGS

A wide variety of other medications have been used in an attempt to curb repetitive behavior, aggression, excessive vocalization or other anxiety behaviors, and self-destructive behavior. The list includes β blockers (see Chapter 5), antihistamines, anticonvulsants (phenytoin, phenobarbital), buspirone (a nonspecific anxiolytic human drug), and even progestin drugs. The range of these drugs reflects the complexity of the pharmaceutical side of behavior modification. Unfortunately, many of these drugs have significant side effects that either limit their use or require close monitoring of the animal to avoid significant clinical complications.

The point to remember is that no "magic bullet" exists for behavior therapy. Behavior modification requires training techniques, persistence on the part of the pet owner, and *possibly* medication to assist with the behavior-modification process. By understanding this point and being aware of the potential problems with using individual behavior-modifying drugs, the veterinary technician can help educate the client to have a realistic view of the capabilities and limitations of the behavior-modification process.

Box 9-1 Drug Categories and Names

ANTICONVULSANTS
Phenobarbital
Diazepam (Valium)
Potassium bromide
Others
  Primidone
  Phenytoin (Dilantin)
  Clonazepam (Klonopin)
  Lorazepam
  Clorazepate

BEHAVIOR-MODIFYING DRUGS
Antipsychotics (phenothiazine tranquilizers)
  Acepromazine
  Chlorpromazine

Haloperidol
Prochlorperazine
Antidepressants
  TCAs
    Amitriptyline (Elavil)
    Clomipramine (Clomicalm)
  SSRIs
  MAOIs
    Selegiline/deprenyl (Anipryl)
Anxiolytics
  Benzodiazepines
  Diazepam
  Clonazepam
  Chlorazepate
  Lorazepam

REFERENCES

1. Heldmann E, Holt D, Brockman DJ, et al: Use of propofol to manage seizure activity after surgical treatment of portosystemic shunts, *J Small Anim Pract* 40:590-592, 1999.

RECOMMENDED READING

Axlund TW: *Managing primary seizures (idiopathic epilepsy) in the dog.* In Proceedings of the Western Veterinary Conference, Las Vegas, NV, 2004.

Boothe DM: *Small animal clinical pharmacology and therapeutics*, Philadelphia, 2001, WB Saunders.

Luescher AU: *Compulsive disorders: treatment.* In Proceedings of the Western Veterinary Conference, Las Vegas, NV, 2004.

Maddison J, Page S, Church D: *Small animal clinical pharmacology*, Philadelphia, 2002, WB Saunders.

Mosby's drug consult, St. Louis, 2002, Mosby.

Neilson JC: *Compulsive disorders (around and around we go).* In Proceedings of the Western Veterinary Conference, Las Vegas, NV, 2003.

Plumb DC: *Veterinary drug handbook*, ed 5, Ames, IA, 2005, Blackwell.

Seibert LM: *Psychoactive drugs in behavioral medicine.* In Proceedings of the Western Veterinary Conference, Las Vegas, NV, 2003.

Self-Assessment

REVIEW QUESTIONS

Fill in the following blanks with the correct item from the Key Terms list.

1. _____ general term for a group of drugs that decreases the incidence or controls the onset of convulsions.

2. _____ seizures that manifest themselves as muscle movement.

3. _____ recurrent seizure activity (general term).

4. _____ measurement of mass of some drugs (e.g., phenobarbital).

5. _____ recurrent seizure activity of unknown origin.

6. _____ state of being in a seizure or term used to describe the condition of an animal having prolonged seizure activity.

7. _____ liver disease caused by a drug.

8. _____ another term for seizure (not convulsion).

9. _____ means "increased drinking."

10. _____ seizure that involves only localized muscle movement (e.g., one limb).

11. _____ his term meaning the metabolism of the drug has been sped up.

12. _____ means "increased appetite."

13. _____ seizure that produces convulsions that involve the whole body.

14. _____ behavior changes that occur before the actual seizure.

15. _____ part of the brain associated with controlling and generating emotions.

16. _____ mood-elevating drugs that include MAOIs, SSRIs, and TCAs.

17. _____ group of drugs that decreases fear responses.

18. _____ inhibitory neurotransmitter associated with the mechanism of action for diazepam and other benzodiazepine tranquilizers.

Fill in the following blanks with the correct drug name listed in Box 9-1.

19. _____ drug most commonly used and administered by the client for maintaining long-term control of seizure activity.

20. _____ drugs that work by blocking the removal of the serotonin neurotransmitter from the synapse.

21. _____ drug most commonly added to phenobarbital to enhance long-term control over persistent seizure activity.

22. _____ approved for use in dogs to control seizures; primary metabolite is phenobarbital; implicated in drug-induced hepatopathy.

23. _____ drug most commonly used for IV infusion control of status epilepticus.

24. _____ antipsychotic drugs that act by blocking dopamine stimulation of the limbic system.

25. _____ approved veterinary drug used to treat generalized anxiety and separation anxiety in dogs and cats; approved for obsessive-compulsive disorders in dogs.

26. _____ human anticonvulsant that is poorly absorbed and rapidly metabolized by dogs (Dilantin).

27. _____ veterinary-approved drug for use in treating Cushing's disease and canine cognitive dysfunction (old-dog senility).

28. Indicate whether the following statements are true or false.

    A. After a few weeks on phenobarbital to control seizures, the dose typically needs to be decreased to compensate for side effects that occur.

    B. Cats typically require a lower dose of phenobarbital than dogs do.

    C. The signs of polyuria and polydipsia in a dog on phenobarbital usually indicate potentially serious kidney disease.

    D. The preferred route for administration of diazepam in the dog is by mouth.

    E. Potassium bromide has an advantage as an anticonvulsant because it reaches equilibrium in the body (steady state) after only two or three doses.

    F. Phenothiazine tranquilizer drugs may cause inappropriate aggressive behaviors of animals to emerge.

    G. TCAs have an advantage over phenothiazine tranquilizers such as acepromazine because they do not suppress overall behavior as much as phenothiazines do.

    H. Increased presence of the dopamine neurotransmitter has been associated with a senility-like syndrome in dogs.

    I. Diazepam reduces anxiety by decreasing the amount of the neurotransmitter GABA.

    J. There is no simple "magic bullet" for behavior therapy.

APPLICATION QUESTIONS

1. You have a dog that ingested a type of rodenticide (rat poison) and has been in status epilepticus for almost 20 minutes. A bolus IV dose of diazepam has stopped the seizures, but the seizures are beginning again only 10 minutes after the diazepam was administered. What are the treatment options at this point?

2. Mrs. Jones' dog presented with a history of a generalized seizures lasting 3 minutes. This was the first incident of seizure activity for this dog. The dog was kept overnight for observation in the hospital and only had a small seizure the next morning that was readily controlled with a single IV bolus of diazepam. Because the dog was otherwise normal, the dog was released to Mrs. Jones the next day. In discussing long-term control of seizure activity, the veterinarian recommended phenobarbital instead of diazepam even though it was diazepam that controlled the seizures in the clinic. Why was this recommendation made?

3. A dog is presented to your veterinary hospital by an owner who has moved into the area. The dog has a history of idiopathic epileptic seizures of 9 months' duration that are fairly well controlled by the drug primidone. The veterinarian advises the owner to switch from primidone to phenobarbital. Why would the veterinarian recommend this when the primidone seems to be working adequately?

4. If the dog in question 3 was on 500 mg of primidone once daily, what would be a reasonable starting dose of phenobarbital to convert the dog from primidone to phenobarbital?

5. The drug order from the veterinarian is to give ½ grain of phenobarbital every 12 hours PO. Unfortunately, you have only one strength of phenobarbital tablet: 15 mg. What is the dose for this animal using the tablets you have in the pharmacy?

6. Mr. Smith comes in to get a refill on his dog's heartworm medication and mentions to you that his teacup poodle, who was diagnosed with idiopathic epilepsy last week and started on a low dose of phenobarbital, is pacing, acting anxious, panting, and not sleeping through the night as he used to. Normally phenobarbital tends to produce ataxia, sedation, wobbly gait, and lethargy for the first few days. Is this change in behavior likely from the drug even though it is the opposite of what is typically seen?

7. Mr. and Mrs. Johnson have a 6-year-old female spayed Pekinese with a history of intermittent seizure activity (seizure approximately every 10 days to 3 weeks). Because the owners both work, the seizures may have been more frequent or have occurred for a longer period. The last seizure was a generalized seizure that lasted 2 minutes. The veterinarian ruled out other possible seizure causes and prescribed ½ grain of phenobarbital to be given once daily PO to control the idiopathic epilepsy. The seizures appeared to be well controlled for 6 weeks and the clients were relieved and happy. Unfortunately, 2 days ago the dog started showing some of the preictal signs (aura) of seizure activity and today it had a generalized seizure. The clients have convinced themselves their pet has a brain tumor because the phenobarbital is no longer controlling the seizures. What is a more likely explanation for the breakthrough seizure activity? Also, calculate the animal's dosage of phenobarbital in milligrams.

8. In looking over the blood results for Mr. and Mrs. Johnson's dog in question 7, you see that the complete blood count and most of the blood chemistry profile results are within the reference range (within normal limits). However, ALP and ALT levels are higher than normal. You remember from your medical nursing and clinical pathology courses that an increase of these enzymes in the blood means that they are getting into the blood from the liver and can indicate injury to, or disease in, that organ. You also remember that anticonvulsant drugs can cause liver problems. Yet the veterinarian doesn't seem concerned about this! Should he be?

9. A 6-year-old female spayed terrier mix has been having breakthrough seizures in spite of the phenobarbital she has been prescribed. The veterinarian checked phenobarbital concentrations and found them to be 35 µg/mL for the peak concentration and 31 µg/mL for the trough concentration (therapeutic range is 20 to 40 µg/mL). He will start the dog on potassium bromide with the phenobarbital but tells the owner that it will take some time for the potassium bromide to reach its full effect and the dose will likely have to be adjusted. Why is this? And why not just give a loading dose to establish therapeutic concentrations more quickly?

10. Potassium bromide often causes vomiting. How can the incidence of vomiting be reduced?

11. Drugs that affect dopamine receptors in the brain almost always have side effects that seem to affect behaviors. Which drugs are more likely to be accompanied by behavioral changes: dopamine agonists or dopamine antagonists?

12. Why is the use of TCAs and phenothiazines a concern for dogs with a history of epileptic-type seizures?

13. Which would cause animals to become more tranquilized: a drug that blocks destruction of GABA or a drug that occupies a GABA receptor but has no intrinsic activity?

Antimicrobials

key terms

aerobic
anaerobic
antibiotic
antimicrobial
bactericidal
bacteriostatic
β-lactamase
β-lactam ring
cephalosporinase
chelate
cross-reactivity
cross-resistance
culture and sensitivity

crystalluria
dermatophyte
DNA gyrase
Fanconi's syndrome
fungicidal
hypersensitivity
keratoconjunctivitis sicca
leukopenia
minimum inhibitory
　concentration
myelosuppression
nephrotoxicosis
ototoxic

pathogens
penicillinase
pyogenic
residue
sensitive versus
　resistant
spectrum of activity
superinfection
suprainfection
susceptibility
thrombocytopenia

1. The different mechanisms by which antimicrobials kill or inhibit bacteria or other pathogens

2. The clinically significant adverse drug reactions of common antimicrobials and what the veterinary professional can do to limit their occurrence

3. The role bacterial resistance, drug absorption, distribution, location of bacteria, and drug elimination play in selection of antimicrobials

4. The drugs used to kill fungal agents, their advantages, disadvantages, and significant side effects

Antimicrobials are drugs that kill or inhibit the growth of microorganisms, or microbes, such as bacteria, protozoa, viruses, and fungi. The term *antibiotic* is often used interchangeably with the term *antimicrobial.* Technically an antibiotic is a substance produced by one microorganism that suppresses growth of another microorganism. The term antimicrobial applies to all drugs used to combat microorganisms, including antibiotics and chemically synthesized drugs. Today most antimicrobials, even antibiotics that were once manufactured with cultures of microorganisms, are chemically synthesized. Thus the distinction between antibiotic and antimicrobial is less important. Box 10-1, listing antimicrobials, can be found at the end of this chapter.

TYPES OF ANTIMICROBIALS

An antimicrobial can be classified according to the type of microorganism it fights (the drug's *spectrum of activity*) and whether it kills the microorganism or only prevents it from replicating and proliferating. The suffix *-cidal* denotes drugs that kill the microorganism (e.g., *bactericidal* and *fungicidal*). The suffix *-static* denotes drugs that inhibit replication but do not directly kill the microorganism (e.g., *bacteriostatic* and fungistatic). Drugs generally have the potential to both kill and inhibit *pathogens* (disease-causing organisms) with lower concentrations or short duration of treatment, resulting in a sublethal inhibiting effect, and higher concentrations or long durations of treatment, resulting in death of the pathogenic organisms.

Bacteriostatic drugs temporarily inhibit the growth of bacteria, but once the drug is removed the organism can begin to multiply again. Therefore drugs that only inhibit replication (*-static* drugs) depend more on a functional immune system to ultimately defeat the organism than *-cidal* drugs, which kill the pathogen outright. This is why people or animals with compromised immune systems (e.g., people with AIDS, cats with feline immunodeficiency virus infection, people or animals who receive chemotherapy) usually require drugs that are *-cidal* to treat infections.

The type of microorganism against which a drug is effective as well as its ability to kill the pathogenic organism are found the drug's description. Examples include the following:

Bactericidal	Kills bacteria
Bacteriostatic	Inhibits bacterial replication
Virucidal	Kills viruses
Protozoistatic	Inhibits protozoal replication
Fungicidal	Kills fungi

Disinfectants and antiseptics are also antimicrobials because they kill a variety of pathogens. Because they are generally applied to the surface of the body or on inanimate objects, they are discussed separately in Chapter 11.

GOALS OF ANTIMICROBIAL THERAPY

The goal of antimicrobial therapy is to kill or disable pathogens without killing the host. Unfortunately, many animals die each

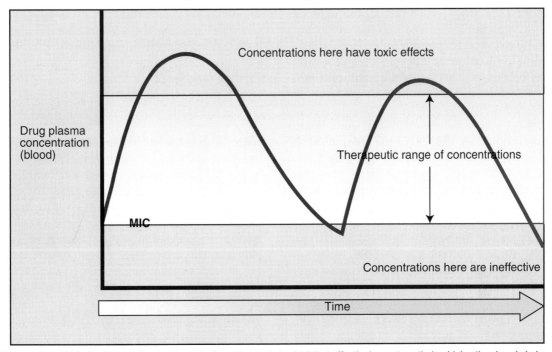

Figure 10-1 MIC is the lowest plasma concentration of an antimicrobial that effectively exerts antimicrobial action. Levels below this are ineffective, and levels exceeding the therapeutic range are toxic.

year because of side effects or inappropriate administration of antimicrobials. Successful administration of antimicrobials requires the following conditions:

- The microorganism must be susceptible to the antimicrobial drug.
- The antimicrobial must be able to reach the site of infection in high enough concentrations to kill or inhibit the microorganism.
- The animal must be able to tolerate high concentrations of the drug.

Factors such as client compliance, which includes ease of administration and convenient dosage interval and form, and cost also influence drug selection. However, the three conditions listed must be met before any other factors are considered.

The measurement of *susceptibility* of a bacterial strain to the effects of an antimicrobial is represented by the drug's *minimum inhibitory concentration* (MIC) against that bacterial strain. The MIC represents the lowest concentration of drug at which growth of the bacterium is inhibited (Figure 10-1). Bacteria and other pathogens typically have an MIC for almost all drugs. However, the concentrations required to kill or inhibit the bacteria may be so high that the host animal would suffer serious side effects or life-threatening toxicosis. Thus, if a bacterial strain has an MIC for an antimicrobial that is low enough to not produce significant side effects in the host animal, the bacteria is said to be *sensitive* to the drug. If the concentration required to kill or inhibit the pathogen is so high that significant side effects would occur in the host animal, the bacteria is said to be *resistant* to the drug.

For each bacterial strain, the MIC for antimicrobial drugs characteristically varies so that some antimicrobials are quite effective against some strains of bacteria but totally ineffective against other bacterial strains.

Similarly, a single bacterial strain may be highly susceptible to one antimicrobial but totally resistant to another antimicrobial. For example, a strain of *Staphylococcus* bacteria may be highly sensitive to the antibiotic gentamicin but quite resistant to penicillin. In this example, the *Staphylococcus* strain would have a relatively low MIC for gentamicin compared with the MIC for penicillin. A different species of bacteria such as *Pseudomonas,* however, might be fairly resistant to gentamicin; thus gentamicin would have a much higher MIC for *Pseudomonas* bacteria than *Staphylococcus* bacteria.

Because of the variability of different bacterial strains, obtaining a sample from the infection site, culturing (growing) the bacteria present in the infected area, and determining to which antimicrobials the particular bacterial strain is sensitive are recommended actions. This is commonly referred to as doing a *culture and sensitivity.*

Even if a culture and sensitivity indicates that the bacteria at the infection site are susceptible (sensitive) to a particular antimicrobial, unless the antimicrobials can reach the infection site in concentrations high enough to exceed that drug's MIC for the pathogen, the antimicrobial will be ineffective. In other words, the antimicrobial must be able to be absorbed from the administration site and distributed to the site of infection in sufficient quantity to produce concentrations in excess of the MIC. For example, if an animal had pneumonia (a bacterial infection in the lungs) and the culture and sensitivity testing indicated that the antibiotic neomycin would be effective against those bacteria, neomycin would seem to be the drug of choice. However, neomycin given by mouth is very poorly absorbed from the intestinal tract and never reaches sufficient concentrations in the lungs to affect the bacteria. Thus the drug's ability to reach the target tissue is as important as the sensitivity of the bacteria to that drug. A similar example was described in Chapter 3 regarding the inability

of penicillins to penetrate the blood-brain barrier, thus making them ineffective against a bacterial infection within the brain.

RESISTANCE OF MICROORGANISMS TO ANTIMICROBIAL THERAPY

Bacteria and other microorganisms have developed the ability to survive in the presence of antimicrobial drugs designed to kill them. This is referred to as resistance to the particular drug. Bacteria may be resistant to certain drugs because of genetic changes that were inherited from previous generations of bacteria, or they may acquire resistance as a result of spontaneous mutations of chromosomes or acquisition of an additional piece of DNA called an R plasmid (R = resistance).

The changes conferred by chromosomes or plasmids provide bacteria with a mechanism to defeat the effect of antimicrobials that would normally destroy or inactivate the bacteria. One of the most common examples is the ability of bacteria to produce enzymes that render antibiotics (such as penicillins and cephalosporins) useless. Other conferred changes may prevent a drug from attaching to a site on the bacterium where it is intended to work. Bacteria may also develop alternative metabolic pathways that circumvent an antimicrobial's ability to kill the bacteria.

Inappropriate use of antimicrobials does not necessarily cause bacteria to become resistant; however, it may allow a resistant population of bacteria to propagate more readily than other bacteria in the environment (Figure 10-2). For example, assume that in a population of millions of bacteria, a single bacterium spontaneously becomes resistant through expression of a chromosomal mutation. The antibiotic MIC required to kill this mutated bacterium is now 10 µg/mL, whereas the MIC for the rest of the bacterial population is only 1 µg/mL. If the standard dose of antibiotic used against these bacteria normally achieves concentrations of

CLINICAL APPLICATION
Time-Dependent versus Concentration-Dependent Effects

Even if barriers to drug distribution for a given infection are known and a drug can be selected that achieves drug concentrations in excess of the MIC, other variables with the MIC can reduce the effectiveness of an antimicrobial. For example, bacteriostatic drugs such as sulfonamides, tetracycline, and lincosamides inhibit the reproduction of susceptible bacteria when these drugs are present at the infection site at concentrations above the MIC. However, the MIC is typically lower than the concentration required for the drug to kill bacteria outright. If the bacteria are inhibited by the bacteriostatic drug, killing the bacteria ultimately depends on the animal's immune system. Therefore, to be most effective, bacteriostatic drugs should be administered so that drug concentrations at the infection site are maintained above the MIC to inhibit proliferation of the bacteria while the immune system destroys the infection. These drugs are said to be "time of contact" dependent to be effective.

This time-dependent characteristic may also extend to some of the bactericidal drugs. For example, the β-lactam drugs kill bacteria by preventing proper formation of the bacterial cell wall during replication. Because this interference only occurs at the point when the bacteria are dividing, penicillins or cephalosporins must be present at the site in concentrations that exceed the MIC at the time of bacterial cellular division. And because replication of bacteria is a continually ongoing process, theoretically the β-lactam drugs should be present at the infection site all the time. However, the immune system still plays a significant role in bacterial death; therefore some authors recommend 100% contact time for patients with a compromised immune system and 50% or greater contact time for those animals that have a working immune system.[1] The point to remember is that significantly increasing the peak concentration of penicillins or cephalosporins above the MIC does not, by itself, necessarily increase the effectiveness of these antimicrobials.

In contrast to the time-dependent bactericidal agents, concentration-dependent bactericidal agents must either achieve a peak drug concentration far exceeding the MIC or maintain a high level of concentration for a longer period of time to be maximally effective. For example, for gentamicin or amikacin to be truly effective, the peak drug concentration desired at the site of infection is at concentrations eight to 10 times the MIC for the bacteria even if this peak concentration only occurs over a relatively short period. Because of their postantibiotic effect, aminoglycosides achieving a single high peak concentration followed by lower concentrations over the remainder of the 24-hour dosing interval still retain maximal bactericidal effect while minimizing the risk for kidney damage.[2] Once-daily doses for gentamicin (dogs, 10-14 mg/kg; cats, 5-8 mg/kg) and amikacin (dogs, 15-30 mg/kg; cats, 10-15 mg/kg) have largely replaced the q8h and q12h dosage regimens for aminoglycosides for these reasons.[3]

The fluoroquinolones (e.g., enrofloxacin, marbofloxacin) have been shown in human beings to be most effective when, like aminoglycosides, they achieve peak concentrations eight to 10 times the MIC.[4] However, studies have also shown that having the total concentration of drug over time exceed the MIC is also a strong predictor for therapeutic success. From a practical point of view, this means the drug concentrations of quinolones should not only exceed the MIC, they should exceed them significantly as either a single high peak concentration or as a slightly lower peak stretched out over a more prolonged period but still well above the MIC.

What should be learned from this situation: When giving medications, following the dose regimen exactly is critical. The concentrations needed to be achieved at the infection site or the amount of time the drug exists at the infection site varies from drug to drug and is reflected in the drug's dosage regimen. Failure to follow the dose exactly may mean that the time-dependent or concentration-dependent characteristic of the drug is not achieved and the bacteria is allowed to survive (Table 10-1).

Abstracted from Bill RL: Insights into effective antimicrobial therapy and avoiding therapeutic failures in dogs and cats, *Vet Med* (in press).

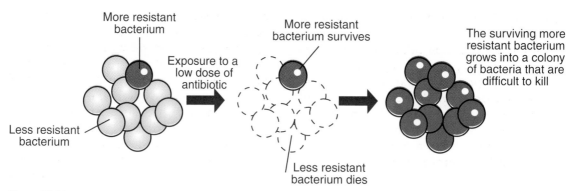

Figure 10-2 Mechanism by which small doses of an antimicrobial can lead to development of resistant strains of bacteria.

10 µg/mL or greater at the infection site, this is not a problem because both the mutated bacteria and the rest of the population will be killed. However, if the drug is incorrectly dosed at a low dose, administered improperly, or the dose used does not account for physiologic changes, the resulting concentrations achieved at the infection site may be less than 10 µg/mL. If concentrations were only 7 mg/mL, the bacteria in the general population would be killed but the more resistant bacteria would survive and replicate, producing more of the resistant strain of bacteria. Thus the next time the same antibiotic is used against these bacteria, it will be more difficult to kill them because this population has an MIC 10 times that of the original strain. To reduce the risk of allowing resistant strains to emerge, veterinary professionals must emphasize to clients or animal owners the need to use all of the prescribed medication at the stated dose.

Unfortunately, just using antimicrobials appropriately does not guarantee the prevention of resistant bacteria. In the preceding example the mutational change in the bacterium could have produced resistance requiring an MIC of 1000 µg/mL rather than only 10 µg/mL. Once a bacterium is resistant, the resistant characteristics and mechanism are passed on genetically to daughter cells. In the case of resistance conferred by R plasmids, the plasmid itself can be transferred to multiple bacteria by a process called transduction. With transduction the plasmids may confer bacterial resistance against multiple antimicrobial agents at one time, resulting in a bacterial colony that is resistant to several antimicrobials.

Veterinary professionals have an obligation to reduce development of microbial resistance to protect the health of the animal and general public. This can be accomplished by

TABLE **10-1** Time Dependent Versus Concentration Dependent

BACTERIOSTATIC DRUGS: MAINTAIN CONCENTRATIONS CONSTANTLY ABOVE THE MIC (TIME DEPENDENT)	BACTERICIDAL DRUGS: MAINTAIN CONCENTRATIONS CONSTANTLY ABOVE THE MIC (TIME DEPENDENT)	BACTERICIDAL DRUGS: MAINTAIN CONCENTRATIONS HIGH ABOVE THE MIC BUT NOT NECESSARILY CONSTANTLY (CONCENTRATION DEPENDENT)
Chloramphenicol*	Cephalosporins	Aminoglycosides
Lincosamide/clindamycin*	Penicillin family	Fluoroquinolones
Erythromycin (macrolides)		
Sulfonamide		
Tetracycline, oxytetracycline		

*Can be bactericidal for susceptible bacteria.

following simple principles of antimicrobial administration:

- Administer the appropriate dose at appropriate intervals, for the appropriate time, and in the appropriate manner.
- Educate clients regarding the importance of following the instructions for dispensed medication, including use of the medication until the supply is expended even if the animal's condition has improved after a few days.

CONCERN OVER ANTIMICROBIAL RESIDUES

A *residue* is the presence of a drug, chemical, or its metabolites in animal tissues or food products, resulting from either administration of that drug or chemical to an animal or contamination of food products. Antimicrobial residues in food animals are of growing concern. As discussed in Chapter 3, use of drugs in animals intended for food must be withdrawn a specific number of days before the animal is slaughtered or the food products are sold by the producer to allow enough time for the drug to be excreted from the body. Ensuring that no drug residue exists is important because most antimicrobial residues in food products are not degraded by cooking or pasteurization.

Exposure to low levels of antimicrobials in food can cause two effects in human beings: an allergic reaction (*hypersensitivity*) to the antimicrobial or selection for resistant bacteria in the intestinal tract, as described above. For example, a penicillin-sensitive person who consumes meat that contains penicillin residues might have an allergic reaction.

Another problem might occur as the result of a farm family consuming meat from livestock they slaughtered on their farm if the meat contained drug residues. For example, if an animal was on an antibiotic and the farmer decided to slaughter the animal for consumption rather than continue to feed and maintain the animal until the drug withdrawal time had elapsed, the family would consume the drug over several days or weeks, killing off the most susceptible (sensitive) bacteria and leaving only the more resistant bacteria in their intestinal tracts to grow and proliferate. This situation occurred in a family that contracted severe intestinal disease caused by overgrowth of pathogenic (disease-causing) bacteria after the beneficial bacteria in the intestinal tract were killed off by low-dose exposure to antibiotics.

Because of the public's concern over drug residues and the responsibility that veterinarians and veterinary technicians have in maintaining food safety, veterinary professionals must take the time to educate food animal producers on the appropriate use of antimicrobials and withdrawal times, label all dispensed medications with clear instructions for proper administration and withdrawal times, and be strong advocates for adhering to mandated withdrawal and residue avoidance regulations.

MECHANISMS OF ANTIMICROBIAL ACTION

Antimicrobials work by different mechanisms to kill or inhibit bacteria and other microorganisms. Antimicrobials generally exert their effects at five sites in microorganisms: the cell wall, the cell membrane, ribosomes, critical enzymes or metabolites, and nucleic acids.

Antimicrobials can interfere with formation of the bacterial cell wall. Normally the bacterial protoplasm draws water into the bacterium by osmosis, producing a tendency for the bacterial cell to swell. The intact bacterial cell wall keeps the bacterium from bursting, in much the same way that placing a balloon in a rigid container during inflation confines the balloon and prevents it from overinflating and bursting. Antimicrobials that interfere with bacterial cell wall formation usually affect it while the wall is forming during bacterial division. Once the bacterial cell wall is constructed, it is not readily affected by antimicrobial drugs. Thus drugs that target the bacterial cell wall are most effective against actively dividing bacterial colonies. Penicillin

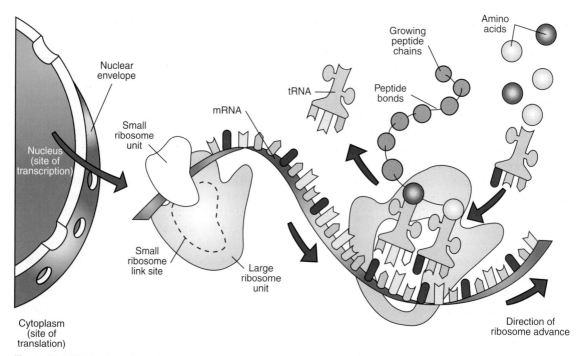

Figure 10-3 Mechanism of protein synthesis by a cell.

and cephalosporins are antimicrobials that act by disruption of new wall formation.

Antimicrobials can damage the bacterial cell membrane by making the microorganism leaky, which would allow either antimicrobials to more readily enter the bacterium or vital cytoplasmic components to leave. Unlike drugs that act on the bacterial cell wall, antimicrobials that affect the cell membrane can exert their effect on dividing or static (nondividing) bacteria.

Antimicrobials can inhibit protein synthesis in pathogenic microorganisms such as bacteria and fungi. Bacteria, just like mammalian cells, manufacture essential proteins from the amino acids in their cytoplasm (Figure 10-3). A strand of messenger RNA (m-RNA) carries a copy of the genetic code, or formula, for producing essential proteins by the cell. This strand m-RNA combines with a specialized organelle ("little organ") called the ribosome. Transfer RNA (t-RNA) molecules carry different amino acids to the ribosome, where they are attached

together in a sequence determined by the m-RNA's copied genetic blueprint. The properly linked amino acids produce a functional protein molecule. Some antimicrobials enter the bacterium, combine with the ribosome, and thereby disrupt normal protein production by interfering with the m-RNA or the ability of the t-RNA to get the amino acids to the ribosome. Without these essential proteins, the cell either stops dividing or dies. In some cases, the lack of essential proteins results in the leakiness of the cell membrane described above. Some antimicrobials that act by combining with ribosomes include lincosamides, macrolides, tetracyclines, and aminoglycosides.

Antimicrobials can interfere with critical enzymes needed by pathogenic bacteria to carry out their normal metabolic functions. Alternatively, antimicrobials can also bind with key intermediate compounds the bacteria need to function, essentially rendering these compounds worthless to the bacteria.

Either mechanism results in a bacterium that is unable to function properly. Sulfonamide antibiotics work primarily by this mechanism.

Finally, antimicrobials can impair production of bacterial nucleic acids (RNA and DNA). When antimicrobials damage or alter the function of nucleic acids in a pathogenic microorganism such as a bacterium or fungus, the cell usually cannot divide and may be unable to produce critical proteins needed by the cell. One of the concerns with antimicrobials that attack DNA is if the antimicrobial might also attack the mammalian DNA of the host animal or person. Even minor alterations of mammalian DNA can result in mutations that can, on rare occasions, help the organism (for example, the mutations that allow some bacteria to become resistant to an antimicrobial drug), but most mutations result in a disadvantage to the organism, resulting in decreased functioning, inability to reproduce, fetal abnormalities, or death. For that reason, antimicrobials that work by attacking DNA are scrutinized closely for any potential effect on mammalian DNA. Some antifungal drugs work in this manner and have the capability to produce fetal abnormalities in pregnant animals receiving the drug. However, newer antibiotics such as the quinolones (enrofloxacin, orbifloxacin, marbofloxacin, ciprofloxacin) work at sites on the pathogen's nucleic acid that are not found in mammalian cells, making these drugs much safer.

CLASSES OF ANTIMICROBIALS

Every year new antimicrobials are added to the veterinarian's roster of treatments to use against bacteria or other pathogens. Veterinary professionals have an obligation to be familiar with the most recent advances in veterinary medicine. Sometimes, however, keeping track of all the new drugs, including new antimicrobials, can seem overwhelming. However, most new drugs are often just modifications or improvements over drugs that are already available. Therefore understanding the basics of how

each general class of antimicrobial works, the overall spectra of activity, and the mechanisms behind the key side effects helps incorporate the new drug into working knowledge by simply aligning it within its family of antimicrobials.

PENICILLINS

Penicillins are among the most commonly used antibiotics in veterinary medicine and can usually be recognized by their *-cillin* suffix in the drug name. The most frequently used penicillins in veterinary medicine include the natural penicillin penicillin-G; the broad-spectrum aminopenicillins, which include ampicillin, amoxicillin, and hetacillin; the *penicillinase*-resistant penicillins cloxacillin, dicloxacillin, and oxacillin; and the extended-spectrum penicillins, including carbenicillin, ticarcillin, and piperacillin. Several other penicillins are used in human medicine but rarely in veterinary medicine because of cost and lack of Food and Drug Administration approval for use in animals.

Penicillins are generally effective against most gram-positive bacteria and a lesser number of gram-negative bacteria. Penicillins identified as broad-spectrum or extended-spectrum are more effective against a wider range of bacteria than the natural penicillins or penicillinase-resistant penicillins.

Penicillins are bactericidal and work primarily by interfering with development of the bacterial cell wall, making the bacterium more prone to lysis from osmotic imbalances. Penicillin drugs block bacterial enzymes that are essential for assembly of the bacterial cell wall. Several different enzymes are involved in bacterial cell wall assembly, and different penicillin antibiotics may affect different enzymes, which partially explains the reason one type of penicillin might be effective against a bacterial population and another is less effective. Because these cell wall assembly enzymes are needed by the bacterium only during cell division when a new cell wall is being produced, penicillins are only effective against an actively dividing colony of bacteria.

Thus if a bacteriostatic antimicrobial is used in conjunction with penicillin, the bacteriostatic effect prevents division of the bacteria and growth of the colony, decreasing the effectiveness of the penicillin. This is the origin of the myth that no bactericidal antimicrobial should be used simultaneously with a bacteriostatic antimicrobial. A more accurate statement would be that bacteriostatic antimicrobials should not be used, or used judiciously, at the same time as bactericidal drugs that require active bacterial growth and division. Other bactericidal drugs that disrupt protein synthesis or block essential enzymes can destroy bacteria regardless of whether bacterial colony growth has been inhibited by a concurrently administered bacteriostatic drug.

Penicillin Pharmacokinetics

Penicillins are generally well absorbed from injection sites and the gastrointestinal (GI) tract. However, penicillin G should not be given by mouth because it is inactivated by gastric acid; it can only be used as an injectable. Penicillins are generally well distributed to most tissues in the body; however, because penicillin molecules are hydrophilic at body pH, they typically will not reach therapeutic concentrations in the globe of the eye, the brain, or the prostate gland because of the cellular barriers between the tissue and the blood supply. If an animal develops meningitis (inflammation of the meninges covering the brain) the inflammation makes the blood-barrier more permeable to penicillin molecules, allowing them to enter the central nervous system (CNS). Unfortunately, even under these conditions penicillins usually do not reach significant therapeutic concentrations within the CNS.

Most penicillins are excreted largely unchanged by the kidney. Not only are penicillins filtered by passive diffusion, they are also actively transported (secreted) by the renal tubules into the forming urine. Because penicillins are actively secreted into the urine intact, the penicillin can attain much higher concentrations in the urine than in the blood, resulting in concentrations in the urinary tract that usually exceed the MIC for many bacteria found in the kidneys, bladder (where they cause bacterial cystitis), or genitourinary tract.

Penicillin Group Spectra of Activity

Each penicillin group has a slightly different bacterial spectrum. Some strains of bacteria, such as *Pseudomonas,* are highly resistant to penicillin's bactericidal effect, whereas other bacteria are quite susceptible. Therefore knowledge of each penicillin's antibacterial spectrum is important when the veterinary professional selects the most appropriate drug for treating a bacterial infection. Generally, if a strain of bacteria becomes resistant to one type of penicillin, such as amoxicillin, it is also resistant to most other penicillins. This phenomenon is known as *cross-resistance.*

Some bacteria, especially *Staphylococci,* acquire resistance to many penicillins by producing an enzyme that attacks a particular part of the penicillin molecule called the *β-lactam ring,* rendering the penicillin ineffective. These bacterial enzymes are called *β-lactamases* (β lactamase) or penicillinases if the enzyme specifically attacks penicillins.

One group of penicillins is not affected by bacterial β-lactamase enzymes. These β-lactamase–resistant penicillins include oxacillin, dicloxacillin, cloxacillin, and a few expensive products used in human medicine. These penicillins are often used in treatment of bovine mastitis or other infections in which a prevalence of β-lactamase–producing *Staphylococci* is likely to be found. A disadvantage of these penicillins is their overall spectrum of activity against many bacterial strains is far less than the spectra of the more common penicillins. Thus β-lactamase–resistant penicillins are used selectively for infections in which β-lactamase is likely to be produced by the bacteria.

Penicillin compounds normally inactivated by β-lactamase can sometimes be chemically combined with another compound to produce a modified, or potentiated, penicillin that is resistant to the β-lactamase enzyme. Clavulanic acid (potassium clavulanate) and sulbactam are added to penicillin drugs such as amoxicillin to produce a potentiated compound that renders bacterial β-lactamase enzymes inactive. For example, clavulanic acid is included with amoxicillin in the product Clavamox and its human equivalent, Augmentin. Clavulanic acid is a natural product of a *Streptomyces* species that inactivates the β-lactamase produced by other bacteria. When combined with a penicillin, it helps protect the penicillin's β-lactam ring from inactivation by these bacterial enzymes. These potentiated drugs are usually packaged individually in foil because the clavulanate readily absorbs moisture from the air, resulting in the tablets quickly decomposing if stored freely in a bottle.

Many gram-negative bacterial species are resistant to penicillin's bactericidal effect except at the high concentrations that occur in the urinary tract because of active transport of penicillin molecules into the urine. Some bacterial species, such as *Pseudomonas* found in otitis externa (outer ear infections in dogs) or necrotic tissue, are resistant to penicillin because the drug molecules cannot reach the cell wall components because of the presence of an impenetrable outer membrane, or capsule. Although general guidelines for which bacteria are likely to be sensitive or resistant to penicillins (or any antimicrobial) exist, the only way to determine for certain is to perform culture and sensitivity testing on the specific bacteria found in the infection.

Precautions for Use of Penicillins

When compared with many other antibiotics, penicillins are quite safe drugs primarily because they affect cell walls, and mammalian cells do not have cell walls. Hypersensitivity reactions (allergic reactions) are the most common adverse reaction to penicillins. Manifestations of hypersensitivity range from a mild skin rash to life-threatening anaphylactic shock. Anaphylactic reactions are more common with injectable penicillin products than with oral products and require aggressive emergency treatment, including administration of epinephrine and corticosteroids. Less-severe drug reactions include skin rashes (urticaria or hives), swelling of the face, swelling of lymph nodes, hematologic changes (eosinophilia, neutropenia), and fever. If an animal exhibits hypersensitivity to one type of penicillin, it is likely to react adversely to other penicillin drugs *(cross-reactivity)*. The veterinarian must be made aware of any possible adverse reaction to penicillin administration. Such reactions must be clearly marked on the animal's record to prevent future exposures and possibly fatal anaphylactic reactions.

When given orally, penicillins may destroy beneficial bacteria residing in the lumen of the intestinal tract, allowing more pathogenic (disease-causing) bacteria, which are generally more penicillin resistant, to proliferate. This condition, called *superinfection* or *suprainfection*, can produce severe diarrhea that can result in death in some species such as guinea pigs, ferrets, hamsters, and rabbits. Other species in which penicillins must be used with caution include snakes, birds, turtles, and chinchillas.

Because penicillins are readily available to food animal producers, the importance of observing withdrawal times for penicillins and all other antimicrobials should be emphasized. Because selected penicillins are used to treat or control mastitis in cattle, dairy milk is frequently tested for the presence of penicillins. A dairy producer that contributes drug-contaminated milk to a bulk storage tank of milk from multiple farms can end up "buying" the entire tank because the contamination renders the milk unacceptable for human consumption. Therefore the veterinary professional has the obligation to the public to educate and inform food animal producers regarding the appropriate withdrawal times and milk-discard times ("milk out" times) when penicillin products are used.

Considerations for Use of Specific Penicillins

Penicillin G is a natural penicillin that is usually administered by injection because it is largely inactivated by the acidic stomach environment if given orally. Penicillin G is available in three basic forms: an aqueous solution, which is penicillin complexed with potassium or sodium; a suspension form in which the penicillin G is combined with procaine; and a longer acting suspension form in which the penicillin G is combined with benzathine. Only the aqueous forms of penicillin G can be given intravenously. Sodium or potassium penicillin G can also be given subcutaneously and intramuscularly. The addition of procaine and benzathine to penicillin G delays absorption of the antibiotic from intramuscular or subcutaneous injection sites, extending the duration of drug activity. Procaine penicillin G usually provides adequate concentrations for 24 hours, and benzathine penicillins produce effective blood concentrations for 5 days. A disadvantage of the procaine and benzathine forms is that peak plasma concentrations may not be as high as those attained with the rapid absorption or sodium or potassium form of the drug (Figure 10-4).

Ampicillin and amoxicillin are aminopenicillins and have a more effective spectrum against gram-negative bacteria than penicillin G because of their ability to bind to sites on the gram-negative bacterial cell wall. Veterinary products are available in oral (capsules, coated tablets, and liquid suspension) and injectable forms. Oral amoxicillin is less affected than ampicillin by the presence of food in the GI tract; however, if possible the pet should be given the aminopenicillins on an empty stomach (if the animal can tolerate it). Although amoxicillin by itself is susceptible to destruction by β-lactamase, it is also available in combination with clavulanic acid (Clavamox, Augmentin), which protects the aminopenicillin against bacterial β-lactamase destruction.

Cloxacillin, dicloxacillin, and oxacillin have the distinction of being naturally resistant to β-lactamase. As previously mentioned, their overall spectrum of antibacterial activity is slightly less than that of the natural penicillins and the aminopenicillins. These penicillins are most commonly used to treat staphylococcal osteomyelitis (bone infections), staphylococcal pyoderma (skin infections), and staphylococcal mastitis (available as intramammary teat infusion syringes).

CEPHALOSPORINS

Cephalosporins are β-lactam antimicrobials that have a bacterial cell wall disruption mechanism of action similar to that of the penicillins. The *ceph-* or *cef-* prefix in the drug name identifies most members of this group, with *cef-* generally being used on the more recently discovered cephalosporins. Cephalosporins are classified by generations according to when they were first developed. First-generation cephalosporins are primarily effective against gram-positive bacteria such as *Streptococcus* and *Staphylococcus*. They are less effective against gram-negative bacteria than the second- or third-generation cephalosporins. Because cephalosporins are more resistant to bacterial β-lactamase than most penicillins, they are more effective against *Staphylococcus* species of bacteria than are penicillin drugs.

Although second-generation cephalosporins were more effective against more gram-negative bacteria than the first-generation drugs, they are generally less effective against gram-positive species than the older drugs. The same is true for third-generation cephalosporins. Thus each generation of drug has gained some advantage over the previous generation but has lost some advantages as well. These are general guidelines for the three generations of cephalosporins. Veterinary professionals should know the specific spectrum of each drug before using it for a bacterial infection.

Many different cephalosporin drugs are available. In addition to veterinary cephalosporin drugs, human cephalosporin drugs are

A

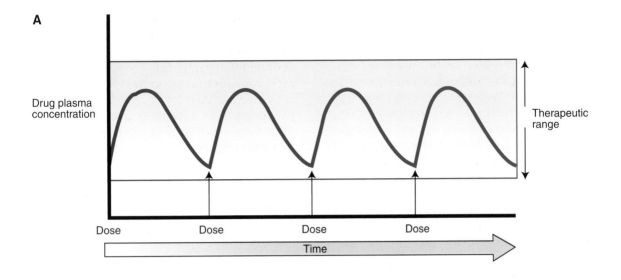

Drug plasma concentration

Therapeutic range

Dose   Dose   Dose   Dose

Time

B

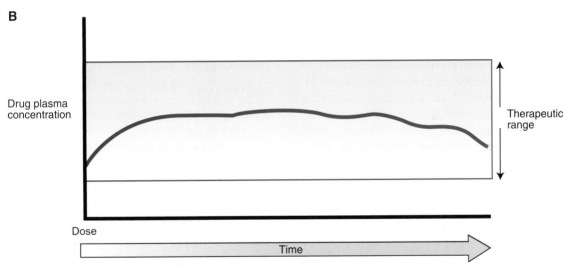

Drug plasma concentration

Therapeutic range

Dose

Time

Figure 10-4 Fluctuation of plasma drug concentrations produced by standard parenteral formulations and extended-absorption formulations of penicillin. **A**, Penicillin concentrations after parenteral administration. **B**, Penicillin concentrations when combined with procaine or benzathine.

also used; however, many of the more recent human drugs are too expensive to be used as the drug of first choice in most animal infections. Veterinary products include cefadroxil (first-generation, Cefa-Tabs, Cefa-Drops),

cephapirin (first-generation, Cefa-Lak and Cefa-Dri intramammary infusions), ceftiofur (third-generation, Naxcel and Excenel), and cefpodoxime (third-generation, Simplicef). Human products used in veterinary medicine include cephalothin (first-generation, Keflin), cephalexin (first-generation, Keflex), cefoxitin (second-generation, Mefoxin), and cefotaxime (third-generation, Claforan). Almost all third-generation cephalosporins, with the exception of cefpodoxime (Simplicef), are injectable, which is potentially a disadvantage if the drug is to be dispensed at the owner's home. Cefpodoxime is a third-generation, veterinary-approved cephalosporin that is capable of being administered orally.

Mechanism of Action

Cephalosporins are β-lactam antibiotics with bactericidal mechanisms similar to those of penicillins. The cephalosporins bind to, and inhibit, enzyme(s) responsible for the formation of bacterial cell walls, resulting in loss of the cell wall integrity. The loss of rigidity prevents the cell wall from maintaining the bacterium's osmotic balance and causes the bacterium to lyse easily with osmotic changes. Because more than one enzyme is involved in bacterial cell wall formation, the difference in spectra of activity for cephalosporins can be partially explained by the different affinities (attraction or ability to bind to) each cephalosporin has for the different cell wall–forming enzymes. Like penicillins, cephalosporins are most effective against rapidly dividing bacterial colonies. Because cephalosporin molecules have a β-lactam ring, they are susceptible to β-lactamase enzymes produced by bacteria but less so than the penicillins. Some β-lactamase enzymes may render cephalosporins ineffective without adversely affecting penicillin drugs. These bacterial β-lactamases are sometimes referred to as *cephalosporinases.*

Like penicillins, cephalosporins do not readily pass through the blood-brain barrier and therefore are not the drug of choice to treat bacterial infections of the CNS. β-lactam antibiotics generally pass through the placental membranes of pregnant females to enter fetal tissues and can also pass into the animal's milk after systemic administration.

Like penicillins, the concentrations of cephalosporins in urine can be high because most of the drug is excreted by filtration and active secretion into the renal tubules.

Precautions for Use of Cephalosporins

Cephalosporins, like penicillins, are considered safe antimicrobials because mammalian cells do not have cell walls. Also similar to penicillins is the potential for hypersensitivity reactions. However, the incidence of hypersensitivity reactions to cephalosporins is much lower than that of penicillins. Hypersensitivity reactions can cause fever, rashes, eosinophilia, and anaphylaxis. Superinfection caused by overgrowth of pathogenic bacteria may be associated with oral administration of first-generation cephalosporins. In addition, orally administered cephalosporins may cause anorexia, vomiting, and diarrhea. Because cephalosporins are most effective against a population of bacteria that is rapidly dividing, simultaneous use of bacteriostatic antibiotics may reduce the efficacy of cephalosporins.

AMINOGLYCOSIDES

Aminoglycosides are a powerful group of antimicrobials used in veterinary medicine to combat a variety of serious bacterial infections. Aminoglycosides used in veterinary medicine include gentamicin, amikacin, neomycin, streptomycin, kanamycin, tobramycin, and netilmicin. With the exception of amikacin, aminoglycosides can be identified by the *-micin* or *-mycin* suffix in the chemical or nonproprietary name. Note that many trade or proprietary names (not chemical or nonproprietary) of tetracyclines also use the *-mycin* suffix; drugs with these trade names should not be confused with aminoglycosides.

Mechanism of Action

Aminoglycosides are bactericidal through their action on the bacteria's ribosomal production of essential proteins. Because the ribosome is located within the bacterial cytoplasm, aminoglycosides must be transported through the bacterial cell membrane to exert their effects. Aminoglycosides are actively transported into the bacterium by an oxygen-dependent mechanism. For this reason, aminoglycosides are highly effective against many oxygen-dependent *(aerobic)* bacteria but are ineffective against most *anaerobic* (do not require oxygen) bacteria or against those bacteria that can survive in an anaerobic environment (so-called facultative anaerobic bacteria). The use of cell wall–inhibiting antibiotics such as penicillins enhances the ability of aminoglycosides to enter, and subsequently kill, the bacterial cell.

Once taken up by the aerobic bacterium, the aminoglycoside combines with the ribosome and prevents normal synthesis of protein from amino acids. The effect on the ribosomes is bactericidal.

Although the half-life of aminoglycosides is typically short (2 to 5 hours), the drug produces a postantibiotic effect that extends the killing activity of the drug beyond when plasma concentrations have dropped below the therapeutic range. Contemporary thinking is that once-daily dosing of aminoglycosides is equally effective and much safer than the older approved twice-daily and three times daily dosing regimens.

Although some cross-resistance occurs between members of the aminoglycoside family, it is not as common as with the penicillins. For example, some strains of *Pseudomonas* bacteria are resistant to gentamicin but sensitive to amikacin. Bacterial resistance is attributable to destructive enzymes produced by the bacteria or inability of the aminoglycoside to cross the cell wall or cell membrane.

Pharmacokinetics of Aminoglycosides

Aminoglycosides are hydrophilic at most physiologic pH levels and therefore are usually administered parenterally (by injection) because absorption across the GI tract wall after oral administration would be limited. The few aminoglycosides used orally are intended to remain in the intestinal tract and are not absorbed to any significant extent. Neonates, animals with intestinal hypomotility (slow gut movement), and animals with hemorrhagic or necrotic intestinal disease absorb greater amounts of aminoglycosides administered orally and thus are potentially at greater risk of systemic side effects.

Although aminoglycosides are not well absorbed across intact skin, they are well absorbed through denuded or abraded skin or when used to irrigate surgical sites. Thus applying a bandage soaked in aminoglycoside to a degloving injury (where the skin is traumatically removed from the paw) may result in a significant amount of drug being absorbed. When the drug is infused into the uterus or bladder to treat infection, most of it remains at the site and little is absorbed through the membrane surfaces.

When administered and absorbed parenterally, aminoglycosides remain mostly in the extracellular fluid. Because of this, the volume of distribution for aminoglycosides is significantly larger in neonates and young animals than in equivalent-sized adult animals because bodies of young animals generally contain a larger ratio of extracellular water to fat. For example, if 50 mg of amikacin were administered to a 10-lb puppy and 50 mg to a 10-lb adult dog, the puppy (which has a greater percentage of its body composed of water) would likely have lower drug concentrations in its body because the drug would be diluted in a proportionally larger volume of extracellular fluid.

The hydrophilic aminoglycoside molecules do not penetrate the blood-brain barrier of the brain or the globe of the eye to any significant degree. Because they are found in high concentrations in the bronchial secretions, aminoglycosides are often used to treat cases of pneumonia in which part of the infection is located within the lumen of the bronchioles.

In contrast to their inability to move into the brain or eye, aminoglycosides accumulate

CLINICAL APPLICATION
Topical Application Induces Renal Failure

A 4-year-old cat had a large draining abscess over the lumbar region from an attack by a dog 4 weeks previously. *Pseudomonas* susceptible to gentamicin was cultured from the wound. The wound was lavaged with a gentamicin solution twice within 24 hours. The cat was anesthetized and the wound cleaned. The cat recovered uneventfully from anesthesia. Gentamicin was administered SQ at 2.2 mg/kg q12h. Three days later the cat showed signs of elevated blood urea nitrogen (BUN) and creatinine, both signs of decreased renal function. The urine specific gravity, which is a measure of the degree of concentration of the urine, was 1.008. In an animal that is somewhat dehydrated, the urine specific gravity should reflect a more concentrated urine (for example, greater than 1.035), which indicates the body's attempts to conserve water and not lose so much in the urine. Because the kidneys are responsible for diluting or concentrating the urine under the control of antidiuretic hormone and aldosterone, the failure of the kidneys to concentrate urine appropriately suggested renal failure. The urine sediment contained red blood cells, white blood cells, and granular casts.

Because gentamicin *nephrotoxicosis* was suspected, the gentamicin was stopped and intravenous fluids begun at a rate of 6 mL/kg per hour. Ampicillin was used in place of the gentamicin. Unfortunately, the signs of renal toxicosis continued to worsen. The BUN and creatinine levels continued to climb even though IV fluid administration should have decreased these parameters. In spite of the fluids, diuretics (furosemide), and dopamine (designed to increased blood flow to the kidney), the urine output decreased. At the owner's request the cat was euthanized.

Necropsy showed severe necrosis of the proximal convoluted tubule of the kidney, one of the major sites where gentamicin and other aminoglycosides are taken up from the plasma by active transport. Serum samples previously obtained from the cat 7 to 8 hours after the second flushing of the wound with gentamicin showed a gentamicin concentration of 58.07 µg/mL. This would have been before the SQ administration of the drug. Serum samples that had been taken at 80 and 96 hours after the wound flushing showed concentrations of 10.43 µg/mL and 13.13 µg/mL, respectively. The serum sample at 96 hours was 24 hours after the last SQ dose of gentamicin had been administered.

The veterinarian used 2.0 µg/mL as the required trough (low point) concentration below which concentrations must drop to reduce the risk for nephrotoxicosis. The combination of gentamicin flushed directly into the wound (10 mL of gentamicin had been infused into the wound sites) and subsequent SQ administration of the gentamicin at a dose that would normally be well tolerated by a cat prevented the plasma concentrations from decreasing below 2.0 µg/mL. Thus conditions were ideal for aminoglycoside nephrotoxicosis and, in this case, the nephrotoxicosis was not reversible and the animal was euthanized.

What should be learned from this situation: Although aminoglycosides cannot cross intact skin or intact intestinal tract very readily, a break in the barrier (in this case flushing the wound directly with the drug) can allow the hydrophilic molecules to be absorbed quite well, achieving significant concentrations in the plasma. The only way that nephrotoxicosis can be prevented with aminoglycosides is to allow the plasma concentrations to drop low enough to allow the intracellular drug to passively diffuse out of the cell. The persistent plasma concentrations greater than 2 µg/mL because of the drug in the wound site and injected SQ did not allow the plasma concentrations to drop low enough for back-diffusion of gentamicin from the kidney cells to the plasma to occur. The end result was permanent damage to the kidneys. Thus veterinary technicians and veterinarians must remember that topically applied aminoglycosides should be considered the same as SQ administered drugs if the skin barrier is broken.

Taken from case report in Mealey KL, et al: *JAVMA* 204(12), June 15, 1994.

within the cells of kidneys and the inner ear by pinocytosis, an active transport process. This accumulation is thought to contribute to the nephrotoxicity and ototoxicity produced by large or frequent doses of aminoglycosides.

As mentioned in Chapter 3, the placenta does not pose a significant barrier to most drugs; therefore aminoglycosides cross the placenta readily and can produce nephrotoxicity and ototoxicity in a pregnant animal and its developing fetus.

Aminoglycosides are eliminated almost exclusively by glomerular filtration in the kidneys. Because the molecules are hydrophilic, minimal drug resorption occurs in the loop of Henle and most of the drug is excreted in the urine. This efficient elimination helps explain the short half-life of aminoglycosides (usually 2 to 5 hours depending on the species) in animals with normal renal function. Because these drugs are almost exclusively eliminated by the kidneys, any decrease in renal function from old age, dehydration, shock, or kidney disease can slow elimination and increase half-life, prolong high plasma drug concentrations, and increase the risk of nephrotoxicity or ototoxicity. Conversely, anything that increases renal perfusion could potentially increase the elimination of the aminoglycosides and shorten the half-life. When interpreting the measured plasma concentrations of an aminoglycoside drug and its elimination half-life, the presence of IV fluid therapy or factors that cause temporary decreased renal perfusion will artificially skew the half-life and observed concentrations, making a simple recommendation for dosage change based on the concentrations more difficult.

Precautions for Use of Aminoglycosides

Aminoglycosides are potentially nephrotoxic (toxic to the kidney) and *ototoxic* (toxic to the inner ear) even at normal doses. Therefore anyone who administers these drugs or monitors their effects in an animal should be aware of the way these drugs act in the body.

As previously mentioned, cells of the inner ear and kidney actively take up aminoglycosides, which causes the drug to accumulate within the cells and produce a toxic effect. Only by lowering the concentration of drug outside the cell can the amount of drug being taken up in the cells be reduced. Also, the accumulated drug within the cell can only leave those cells by passive diffusion from within the cell back into the plasma. Because aminoglycosides are hydrophilic and do not readily pass through cell membranes by passive diffusion, any diffusion requires a steep concentration gradient from inside the cell (where high concentrations are found) to the plasma (where lower concentrations are found). The only way to lower the drug concentrations outside the cell is to extend the dose interval (time between doses) so that the plasma concentration drops quite low. Failure to allow the plasma concentrations to drop low enough would mean a greater concentration of drug within the renal or otic cells and a more significant risk for nephrotoxicosis and ototoxicosis.

Thus, if the drug were to be given by continuous IV infusion over a 24-hour period, no trough plasma concentration would exist and thus no significant concentration gradient for drug molecules to diffuse out of the cells. The same would be true for q6h or q8h dose intervals. Toxicosis is related more to the lack of low concentrations than the presence of high concentrations.

When aminoglycosides are used in animals with reduced renal function, the same dose as normal is used but the interval between injections is increased to compensate for the decreased ability to eliminate the drug. When the dosage interval is extended, plasma concentrations of aminoglycoside are given more time than normal to decrease enough to prevent toxicity (Figure 10-5). The degree of renal dysfunction and measurements of plasma drug concentrations dictate the degree to which the dosage interval must be increased and whether a dosage increase is also needed.

A

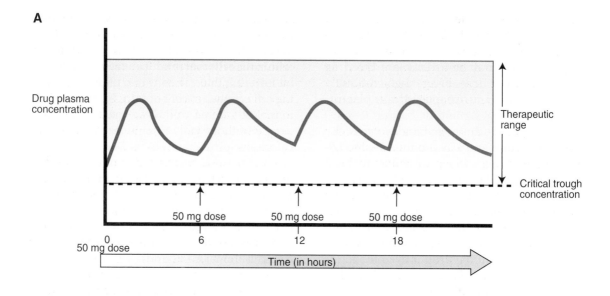

B

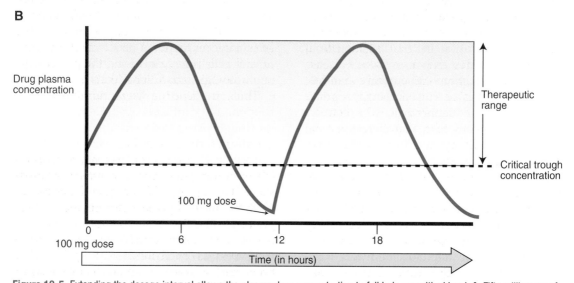

Figure 10-5 Extending the dosage interval allows the plasma drug concentration to fall below a critical level. **A**, Fifty milligrams of aminoglycoside given q6h: trough concentration does not decrease low enough to prevent nephrotoxicity. **B**, Same daily dose with 100 mg of aminoglycoside given q12h: trough concentration is low enough to decrease risk of nephrotoxicity.

If aminoglycosides are to be used in patients with marginal kidney function, renal function must be closely monitored with BUN, serum creatinine, urine sediment, and urine specific gravity measurements. An early sign of aminoglycoside nephrotoxicity is the appearance of casts or increased protein in the urine. In the absence of aminoglycoside plasma concentration measurements, daily urinalyses of high-risk patients for the presence of casts and protein may provide early indications of impending nephrotoxicity. By the time elevated

BUN and creatinine levels are detected on a blood chemistry panel, 70% to 75% of the kidney function has already been compromised. Nephrotoxicity may be reversible if the drug is withdrawn or the dosage is significantly altered before extensive renal tubular necrosis has occurred.

Aminoglycoside use resulting in ototoxicity can cause deafness in treated animals. Although deafness is not a serious disability in most domestic animals, it can pose a significant problem in certain animals. Dogs trained to assist hearing-impaired people require a considerable investment of time, expense, and emotion, all of which would be lost if a dog became deaf as a result of inappropriate aminoglycoside administration. Because ototoxicity also often affects balance (the vestibular system of the inner ear), service and working dogs can be rendered completely ineffective if unable to maintain their balance. Cats are apparently highly sensitive to the vestibular toxic effects of aminoglycosides and may show circling, fall over, or display repetitive rapid eye movements (nystagmus) as a result of inappropriate aminoglycoside administration. The benefits of aminoglycoside administration must be weighed carefully against the potential risks in these types of animals.

Neomycin appears to have the greatest potential for inducing nephrotoxicity in animals and people if it is systemically absorbed. However, it is not used as an injectable and is poorly absorbed from the intestinal tract, thus limiting its nephrotoxic risk under normal circumstances. Nephrotoxicity from gentamicin use has been reported in many species, including exotic animals, wildlife, and birds.

Although aminoglycosides are quite effective against many bacteria, cellular debris (such as pus) can render them ineffective. Cellular debris is composed of ruptured cells and cell contents, including the nucleic acids of ribosomes. As previously stated, aminoglycosides attach to the nucleic acids of ribosomes in bacteria to produce their bactericidal effect. If an aminoglycoside enters an infection site that contains a significant amount of cellular debris, the drug tends to bind to the nucleic acids in the cellular debris; therefore less drug is absorbed into the bacteria. Thus *pyogenic* (pus-producing) infections, such as abscesses or topical infections with necrotic tissue, must be cleaned or flushed thoroughly to remove cellular debris before applying aminoglycosides.

As previously mentioned, aminoglycosides require oxygen to be taken up by the bacteria. Therefore anaerobic conditions such as abscesses, deep puncture wounds, deep cavities in the mouth or gums, and the colon would be areas in which an otherwise excellent antibiotic would be rendered essentially ineffective.

Because aminoglycosides are such important drugs when used appropriately, and because aminoglycosides also have the potential to produce very serious side effects or be inactivated when used inappropriately, the veterinary professional must carefully consider the dosage regimen and the physiologic or pathologic conditions that exist in the patient at the time the drug is administered.

QUINOLONES

Quinolones, or fluoroquinolones, are a group of bactericidal antimicrobials that are continually expanding in human and veterinary medicine. The majority of fluoroquinolones can be identified by their *-floxacin* suffix in the nonproprietary name. The first quinolone introduced to veterinary medicine in North America in the late 1980s was enrofloxacin (Baytril). Since that time marbofloxacin (Zeniquin), orbifloxacin (Orbax), and difloxacin (Dicural) have been approved as veterinary drugs. Ciprofloxacin, a human drug that gained public attention with the emergence of the bioterrorism threat of anthrax, and sarafloxacin (Saraflox) are two other quinolones cited in veterinary literature. An older quinolone, nalidixic acid, and another human fluoroquinolone, norfloxacin, are not used in veterinary medicine to any significant extent.

CLINICAL APPLICATION
Nephrotoxicosis in a Horse

A 7-year-old Appaloosa mare was presented with a history of 2-week duration of fever, depression, cough, and serous nasal discharge that was nonresponsive to antibiotics and phenylbutazone. IV gentamicin was administered at a dose of 2 g q8h for 3 days without resolution. Ten grams of oxytetracycline was also administered intravenously. A blood chemistry profile showed an increase in BUN and creatinine levels, reflecting decreased renal function. The urine specific gravity was 1.014 in spite of the animal's dehydration, suggesting an inability of the kidneys to concentrate urine. A diagnosis of acute renal failure was made based on the clinical signs.

Therapy was initiated with high-volume IV fluids and furosemide (a diuretic). In spite of the correction of hydration status and maintenance of IV fluids the BUN and creatinine levels increased further. After an additional 6 days of IV fluids the BUN and creatinine levels began to go back down. An additional 14 days elapsed before renal parameters returned to normal. Four months later the horse was examined and found to be healthy with normal renal parameters.

What should be learned from this: The dose of gentamicin was higher than recommended and the drug was administered three times daily. The three times daily dosage regimen did not provide enough time for the plasma concentrations to drop low enough to allow backdiffusion of gentamicin from the kidney cells to the plasma. Thus the active transport of gentamicin into the renal cells resulted in damage to the kidney cells, producing the increased BUN and creatinine levels and the inability of the kidney to concentrate the urine. Fortunately, the drug was discontinued and IV fluids instituted before permanent renal damage occurred. Over the span of several days of supportive therapy the kidneys were able to return to an acceptable level of function.

The veterinary professional must select a dosage regimen of aminoglycosides that minimizes the risk for nephrotoxicosis. If nephrotoxicosis occurs, the drug needs to be stopped immediately and supportive treatment instituted. If an animal is at risk for nephrotoxicosis but the aminoglycoside is the only effective antibiotic available, the dosage interval between drug doses needs to be extended to allow enough time for plasma concentrations to drop low enough to allow diffusion of the drug out of the cell. Because of the postantibiotic effect and the equivalent effectiveness of once-daily and twice-daily dosages, three times daily dosage regimens are seldom used anymore.

Abstracted from case report in Bartol JM, et al: *Compend Contin Educ* September, 2000.

Enrofloxacin, marbofloxacin, and orbifloxacin are all approved for use in the dog and cat, and difloxacin is approved for use in dogs. Sarafloxacin was the first quinolone approved for use in food animals (poultry only); however, the Food and Drug Administration has withdrawn its approval for this drug. Considerable discussion and debate about the safe use of fluoroquinolones in livestock are ongoing.

Mechanism of Action

In bacteria the DNA molecule must be tightly coiled to be properly stored within the bacterial cell. The enzyme *DNA gyrase* (also called topoisomerase II) facilitates this supercoiling process. Quinolone antimicrobials interfere with DNA gyrase, preventing bacterial DNA supercoiling and subsequently disrupting DNA function; this rapidly kills the bacterium. Quinolones do not disrupt the mammalian cell function because the bacterial and mammalian DNA gyrases are different; hence quinolones are considered safe drugs to use.

The fluoroquinolones are effective against common gram-negative and gram-positive bacteria found in skin, respiratory, and urinary infections, including β-lactamase–producing *Staphylococcus, Pseudomonas, Klebsiella, Escherichia coli,* and *Salmonella* species. Enrofloxacin's activity against *Pseudomonas* is considered to be superior to gentamicin and on par with some of the more powerful aminoglycosides. In spite of this impressive spectrum of activity, veterinary-approved quinolones are not consistently effective against common gram-positive *Streptococcus* species. Therefore quinolones are not recommended for use in streptococcal infections. Quinolones are generally ineffective against most anaerobic bacteria.

Pharmacokinetics of Quinolones

Some variability in the absorption of oral quinolone products occurs across species. Quinolones are more efficiently absorbed from the intestinal tract of dogs and cats than from adult horses. Although young calves can adequately absorb orally administered enrofloxacin, bioavailability is less than 20% after oral administration in mature ruminants. Unlike some penicillins, enrofloxacin absorption after oral administration is not significantly affected by food; food only slightly delays the onset of absorption.

Most modern quinolones are highly lipophilic and accumulate in high concentrations in the kidneys, liver, lungs, bone, joint fluid, aqueous humor of the eyeball, and respiratory tissues. Concentrations of quinolones in the urine typically exceed plasma concentrations (some sources say they exceed concentrations by several hundred times); thus they are present at concentrations that far exceed the MIC for susceptible organisms in the urinary tract. Thus quinolones are often used to treat severe infections of the skin (pyoderma), respiratory tract, and urinary tract.

Because quinolones are able to accumulate in the prostate (an organ few antimicrobials are able to penetrate in significant concentrations) at concentrations two to three times that of plasma, it is one of the few antimicrobials that effectively treats prostate infections.

Each quinolone has a slightly different route of elimination. Enrofloxacin is mostly eliminated by the kidney; however, up to one fourth of the enrofloxacin is also metabolized to ciprofloxacin, which in turn is metabolized to inactive metabolites. Difloxacin is almost exclusively metabolized by the liver to inactive metabolites. Marbofloxacin and orbifloxacin are eliminated by a combination of liver and renal routes.

Precautions for Use of Quinolones

Although quinolones are considered very safe drugs, they can adversely affect developing joint cartilage. During periods of rapid growth in dogs, quinolones may cause bubblelike lesions in the joint cartilage. Because this cartilage is the weight-bearing surfaces in joints, concern exists about the potential for degeneration and arthritic changes as the animal grows older. Although these reported bubblelike changes occurred after administration of five times the normal dose, the manufacturer states that enrofloxacin is contraindicated in small- and medium-sized dogs between the ages of 2 and 8 months. The veterinary professional must remember that large-breed dogs have periods of rapid cartilage and bone development that extend well beyond 8 months; therefore use of quinolones is contraindicated for up to 12 months in large breeds and 18 months in giant breeds. Although enrofloxacin has been used in horses (extra-label use) and studies have not been done to look for similar cartilage changes in this species, avoiding this drug in young horses would be prudent because of the potential of cartilage damage.

Apparently quinolone absorption can be significantly reduced if administered orally with antacids or sucralfate (ulcer treatment medication). In human beings the absorption of orally administered quinolone can be reduced by up to 90% with concurrent administration of sucralfate. As a general rule of thumb, concurrent use of quinolones with any drug with two or three positive charges (divalent or trivalent cations) or with sucralfate should be avoided completely, or their administration separated from each other by at least 4 hours.

Some evidence supports the warning against using quinolones in animals that are prone to seizures. In instances described as rare or infrequent, quinolones have precipitated seizure activity in animals predisposed to seizures. Therefore the benefits of quinolone use should be weighed against the possibility of producing seizures before using either of these antibiotics in epileptic animals.

Although the initial 1997 dose of enrofloxacin for cats was labeled at 5 to 20 mg/kg once daily or divided twice daily, dosages of greater than 20 mg/kg in cats were discovered to potentially cause mild to severe changes in the retina, in some cases resulting in blindness. In 2000 the manufacturer issued a notice to veterinarians that the dose for cats would be reduced from a range of 5 to 20 mg/kg to a single dose of 5 mg/kg. Although this phenomenon has not been noticed for other fluoroquinolones, considering all quinolones as having the potential to produce this effect and to not exceed the label dose for the drug would be prudent.

Bacterial resistance to enrofloxacin was predicted to be slow in developing because of the mechanism of action of the quinolones. However, within a few months of release of the drug resistance to enrofloxacin was already being identified in some *Staphylococcus* and *Pseudomonas* species. As a general rule, antibiotics with a narrow spectrum of activity targeted specifically toward the bacteria causing the infection should be used. Indiscriminate use of quinolones for routine infections in which other older drugs could be equally effective could lead to development of bacterial resistance against this group of drugs. Thus quinolones should be reserved for more severe infections. This is an example of how newer drugs should not be automatically chosen over older, still effective antibiotics because of the risk for development of bacterial resistance to the newer drug.

The development of resistance to quinolones in human bacteria has prompted a ban on the extra-label use of quinolones in any food-producing animal, including the quinolones that were to be approved for use in poultry medicine. The use of enrofloxacin or other quinolones in other livestock is therefore illegal. With the concern over the impact of drug residues in human food, quinolones will not likely be approved on a large scale for livestock use in the near future. Therefore the veterinary technician needs to understand and be able to explain the science behind the decision not to use drugs such as enrofloxacin in livestock.

TETRACYCLINES

Tetracyclines are a group of bacteriostatic antimicrobials that have been used in veterinary medicine for many years, especially in food animal production. Many microorganisms are resistant to most of the older tetracyclines, forcing veterinarians to use other antimicrobials. Although overall use of tetracyclines has decreased in the past 10 years, tetracyclines are the drugs most commonly used for rickettsial diseases (Rocky Mountain spotted fever in human beings; ehrlichiosis and salmon poisoning in dogs; hemobartonellosis in dogs and cats), *Mycoplasma* pneumonia, chlamydial infections (especially those manifested as ocular disease in cats), psittacosis in birds, and borreliosis (Lyme disease). Tetracyclines have also been prescribed, with variable results, to help control tear staining (epiphora) on dogs' faces.

Tetracycline drugs can usually be recognized in the written form by the -*cycline* suffix of the nonproprietary name. The tetracycline family of drugs should be thought of as being composed of two general classes of drugs. The older tetracyclines include the drugs tetracycline and oxytetracycline, which are hydrophilic drugs with similar spectra of antibacterial activity and actions in the body. The second class of tetracyclines includes the newer and more lipophilic doxycycline and minocycline, which are being used more frequently in animals (extra-label use) because of their longer half-life, broader spectrum of antibacterial action, and better penetration of tissues than the older tetracyclines.

Mechanism of Action

Tetracyclines as a class bind to bacterial ribosomes and prevent transfer RNA from linking to the ribosome, thereby disrupting protein synthesis. In contrast to the aminoglycosides, which also bind to ribosomes and disrupt protein synthesis in a slightly different way, tetracyclines inhibit bacterial cellular function and division but do not cause immediate bacterial destruction. Because tetracyclines are usually bacteriostatic, they depend on a functional immune system to help them overcome a microbial invasion. Tetracyclines do not bind to the ribosomes of mammalian cells as readily as they do with bacterial ribosomes; therefore at normal dosages mammalian cells are not significantly affected by tetracyclines. However, at higher dosages protein synthesis in mammalian cells may be affected.

Pharmacokinetics of Tetracyclines

The two groups of tetracyclines vary in lipophilic/hydrophilic nature and hence they have different abilities to be absorbed from the GI tract and distributed to tissues with barriers. Generally, doxycycline and minocycline are more lipophilic and therefore orally absorbed much better than oxytetracycline or tetracycline. In addition, tetracycline and oxytetracycline are readily chelated (bound to and precipitated out of solution) by mineral ions with divalent cations (ions with two positive charges) such as calcium (Ca^{++}), magnesium (Mg^{++}), iron (Fe^{++}), and copper (Cu^{++}). If oxytetracycline or tetracycline is administered by mouth with a meal that includes dairy products, such as milk or cheese, or other foods high in divalent cations or trivalent cations (three positive charges), much of the drug is chelated in the gut and not absorbed. In addition to milk and cheese, other common items that can *chelate* tetracyclines include iron supplements, oral antacids (Mg^{++}), and antidiarrheal products that contain kaolin, pectin (Kaopectate), or bismuth subsalicylate (Pepto-Bismol). In contrast to oxytetracycline or tetracycline,

doxycycline's absorption is only reduced by approximately 20% in the presence of most of these products, which is not clinically significant in most cases.

Oxytetracycline is the most commonly used injectable tetracycline because of its good absorption from IM injection sites. In contrast to oxytetracycline, tetracycline is erratically absorbed from IM injection sites and therefore produces more reliable concentrations when administered by mouth. Oxytetracycline injectable is also commonly marketed in a longer acting form as LA-200, which is administered with a longer dose interval of 2 or 3 days.

Once absorbed into the systemic circulation, tetracyclines are distributed to most tissues and can reach significant concentrations in saliva and bronchial secretions. Because tetracycline and oxytetracycline are hydrophilic, they do not achieve significant concentrations in the CNS or penetrate mammalian cells to reach intracellular pathologic organisms. The more lipophilic doxycycline and minocycline more readily cross the blood-brain barrier and penetrate both the globe of the eye and the prostate gland better than oxytetracycline or tetracycline. Doxycycline is preferred over tetracycline and oxytetracycline for treatment of CNS signs associated with borreliosis (Lyme disease) in people.

Tetracyclines and oxytetracycline are excreted by filtration through the kidneys and to a lesser extent by the liver. Because renal elimination is an important excretion pathway for these two drugs, any change in kidney function such as renal disease or decreased renal perfusion may allow accumulation of drug in the body unless the dose is decreased. These two drugs are also excreted by the liver into the intestine, where they may be chelated by intestinal contents and excreted with the feces. Any tetracycline or oxytetracycline not chelated may be resorbed back into the body, a process known as enterohepatic circulation (movement from the intestine to the liver and back). Unlike the renal excretion of oxytetracycline and tetracycline, doxycycline is largely excreted into the intestine. Because it does not depend on glomerular filtration for elimination, the dose of doxycycline does not necessarily have to be reduced in animals with impaired kidney function.

Precautions for Use of Tetracyclines

The major problems with tetracyclines relate to their binding with calcium and other divalent cations. Tetracycline and oxytetracycline are chelated with the minerals of developing tooth enamel and dentin, imparting a yellow, mottled discoloration if given while teeth are developing. Therefore the veterinary professional should be careful not to administer tetracycline during the first few weeks of an animal's life while the adult teeth are being developed. Although doxycycline can cause the same effect, it is less likely to cause the discoloration than the more water-soluble oxytetracycline or tetracycline. In addition to tooth enamel, tetracyclines combine with the calcium in bones and at high doses may slow bone development in young animals.

As with other broad-spectrum antimicrobials, orally administered tetracyclines can produce superinfections from overgrowth of pathogenic bacteria in the gut. In ruminants, high oral doses can kill off significant numbers of normal ruminal flora, resulting in ruminoreticular stasis (rumen inactivity). In dogs, even if superinfections do not occur, diarrhea, vomiting, and anorexia are common usually from the direct irritation of the GI mucosa by orally administered tetracyclines. Cats tolerate tetracyclines even less and may show fever, depression, or abdominal pain. Because doxycycline absorption is not adversely affected to any significant degree by the presence of food in the intestines, food may be given with doxycycline to decrease some of these GI side effects.

IV injections of relatively small doses of doxycycline in horses have resulted in cardiac arrhythmias, collapse, and death. These signs have been observed in other species receiving rapid IV injections of normal doses, but horses appear to be especially susceptible to these effects. The proposed mechanism for this reaction may be chelation of calcium, which reduces the calcium needed for proper cardiac muscle function. Other theories relate to the vehicle (liquid) in which the drug is dissolved. Until further research is done, IV administration of doxycycline is not recommended in horses.

Because tetracycline drugs are bacteriostatic, they may interfere with the efficacy of penicillins and cephalosporins, which require an actively dividing bacterial population to exert their antibacterial action.

Expired tetracycline and oxytetracycline can decompose to form a nephrotoxic compound. This compound damages the cells of the kidney's proximal convoluted tubule, resulting in *Fanconi's syndrome*, a condition in which resorption of glucose from the glomerular filtrate is impaired, resulting in glucosuria (glucose in the urine). Unlike diabetes mellitus, where glucosuria is associated with high blood glucose concentrations, in Fanconi's syndrome glucose concentrations are normal.

SULFONAMIDES AND POTENTIATED SULFONAMIDES

Sulfonamides (sulfa drugs) were the first antimicrobials used on a widespread basis in human and veterinary medicine. Because they have been in use for many years, many strains of bacteria have become resistant to them. To increase the efficacy of sulfonamides and convert them from bacteriostatic to bactericidal drugs, they are sometimes combined with other compounds such as trimethoprim and ormetoprim to potentiate (increase) their antibacterial effects.

Some of the more common sulfonamides used in veterinary medicine include sulfadimethoxine (combined with ormetoprim in the veterinary drug Primor), sulfadiazine (combined with trimethoprim in the veterinary drug Tribrissen), sulfamethoxazole (combined with trimethoprim in the human drug Septra), sulfachlorpyridazine (used in livestock and poultry), and sulfasalazine (Azulfidine, used for its antiinflammatory effect in inflammatory bowel disease). Other sulfonamides are used to a limited extent in veterinary medicine as a result of the prevalence of resistant bacteria and the availability of cost-effective alternatives.

Sulfonamides are sometimes described as enteric or systemic sulfas. The site of action for an enteric sulfa such as sulfasalazine is within the intestinal tract, and therefore the drug is designed to not be absorbed into the body to any great extent. Systemic sulfas are absorbed from the intestinal tract with the intent to treat systemic infections within the body.

Mechanism of Action

To survive, bacteria must synthesize folic acid from raw materials and then use the folic acid in protein and nucleic acid metabolism. Sulfonamides inactivate a key enzyme involved in synthesis of folic acid, and the potentiating compounds trimethoprim and ormetoprim interfere with a separate enzyme in this metabolic pathway. Separately, sulfas and trimethoprim and ormetoprim are bacteriostatic, but when combined into potentiated sulfas they attack this essential metabolic pathway at two different locations and the drug becomes bactericidal.

Potentiated sulfas used in veterinary medicine have a fairly broad spectrum of antibacterial activity, including many gram-positive organisms such as streptococci, staphylococci, and *Nocardia*. Unfortunately, the true ability of a sulfonamide to be effective is limited by the wide prevalence of resistance among bacterial species. In spite of their limitations, sulfonamides are still among the drugs of choice for treatment of some protozoal infections, including *Coccidia* and *Toxoplasma* organisms. *Chlamydia* is usually susceptible to sulfonamides also.

Unlike other sulfonamides, sulfasalazine is not commonly used for its antimicrobial effect;

rather, it is used for its antiinflammatory effect on the colon. When sulfasalazine is given orally, less than one third of the drug is absorbed. The remainder stays in the bowel lumen, where it passes into the colon and is transformed by colonic bacteria into another sulfonamide (sulfapyridine) and an aspirinlike antiinflammatory drug (aminosalicylic acid). As discussed in Chapter 4, the salicylate inhibits prostaglandin formation, decreasing inflammation and hypersecretion associated with inflammatory bowel disease.

Pharmacokinetics of Sulfonamides

With the exception of the enteric sulfonamide sulfasalazine, sulfonamides and their potentiated forms are well absorbed from the GI tract of monogastric (single-stomach) animals. In ruminants the trimethoprim component of potentiated sulfas may be trapped in the rumen after oral administration and degraded to some degree, thereby reducing the amount of trimethoprim absorbed. Generally, sulfonamides exist in a nonionized lipophilic form at body pH and therefore are well distributed throughout the body, including in the pleural fluid, peritoneal fluid, synovial fluid, and ocular fluid. Concentrations in these fluids, including the cerebrospinal fluid during meningitis, can achieve 50% to 80% of the plasma concentration. Like the quinolones, most sulfonamides readily traverse the blood-prostate barrier and enter the prostate gland. Sulfonamides cross the placenta and have the potential to attain concentrations that are therapeutic or toxic to the fetus. Sulfonamides can also pass into the milk of nursing females.

Sulfa drugs vary in the degree to which they are excreted intact in the urine or metabolized by the liver before being excreted by the kidneys. Several sulfonamides are both filtered by the glomerulus and actively secreted into the renal tubules, achieving significant concentrations in the urine. This is one of the reasons sulfonamides are used for urinary tract infections.

In the potentiated compounds, the sulfonamide component and the potentiating compound (trimethoprim, ormetoprim) usually have different half-lives of elimination and different patterns of distribution. Trimethoprim is fairly quickly eliminated from the plasma; however, it may remain within some tissues for a longer time than its short half-life indicates. The pharmacokinetics of ormetoprim in domestic animals has not been well described. Clinically these pharmacokinetic differences are important because the sulfonamides and their potentiating compounds by themselves are bacteriostatic. Only if both compounds penetrate the infection site together, producing concentrations above the MIC for the bacterial species involved, is the bactericidal effect achieved. This may be the reason some clinicians administer trimethoprim-sulfonamide products twice daily, although once-daily use is recommended.

Precautions for Use of Sulfonamides

One of the more common reactions to sulfonamides in dogs is decreased tear production, resulting in *keratoconjunctivitis sicca* (KCS, or "dry eye"). Dogs with sulfonamide-induced KCS will suddenly begin to accumulate mucoid or crusty matter around the eye, show signs of ocular discomfort by rubbing the face or pawing at the eyes, and develop a dull corneal surface. A veterinarian should examine dogs with these signs immediately to determine if tear production is reduced. In the past many cases of sulfonamide-induced KCS could not be reversed. A cyclosporine ophthalmic ointment (Optimune) is now available that will restore production of near-normal levels of tears. However, affected dogs must be treated with cyclosporine for the rest of their lives.

Other reactions associated with sulfonamides include skin reactions, which are manifested as pruritus (itching), swelling of the face, and hives; hypersensitivity reactions in large-breed dogs; and liver dysfunction. Doberman pinschers are cited by some authors as being more susceptible to hypersensitivity (allergic) reactions.

Thrombocytopenia (decreased platelets), *leukopenia* (decreased white blood cells), and anemia have been reported in dogs and cats on sulfonamides. The mechanism of action for these toxic side effects is not well understood. Animals who are on high doses or prolonged duration of therapy with sulfonamide appear to be more susceptible to these effects, but they can apparently also occur at most dosages and relatively short duration of therapy.

Some sulfonamides or their metabolites may precipitate in the kidney if insufficient fluid volume is present (dehydration) or if the urine becomes acidic. The resulting *crystalluria* (crystals in the urine) can damage the renal tubules. The older sulfonamides and sulfadiazine are more prone to precipitation (crystallization) than the newer compounds. Because an alkaline pH keeps sulfonamides from precipitating as readily, and because herbivores generally have alkaline urine, crystallization is not as much a concern in herbivores as in carnivores, with their more acidic urine. Precipitation and crystallization can be prevented by water intake that is sufficient to maintain urine production and by preventing overdosing of sulfonamides. Therefore owners with pets on sulfonamides need to be advised to ensure that their pet has adequate water at all times (e.g., outdoor pen watering system is working or watering pan does not get overturned by the pet).

Because most sulfonamides are metabolized by the liver to some extent, many manufacturers advise caution in using these drugs in animals with hepatic disease. The kidneys are also important for elimination of metabolized and intact sulfonamides, so similar precautions should be observed in animals with reduced kidney function.

Salivation with oral administration of sulfonamide drugs in cats is common and profuse if the tablet is broken while administering the drug. The veterinary technician should work with the client to show how best to administer

CLINICAL APPLICATION
Skin Eruptions in Dogs on Sulfonamides

Case 1: A 5-year-old male miniature schnauzer was treated with oral trimethoprim-sulfamethoxazole at a dose of 24 mg/kg b.i.d. Eight days into treatment he developed pustules over most of the trunk. The trimethoprim-sulfa was discontinued and cephalexin (cephalosporin antibiotic) 25 mg/kg t.i.d. and prednisone 0.5 mg/kg b.i.d. were begun. No significant improvement occurred after 1 week. At this point the dog had a fever of 104.4° F and many ulcerative lesions on the neck, chest, axillary (armpit), and inguinal (groin) areas, covering an estimated 35% of the dog's body. Crusts and alopecia (hair loss) were evident on most other areas of the body. Skin scrapings were negative for parasites and skin fungus (*dermatophytes*). Bloodwork (complete blood count, blood chemistry profile) showed mild changes consistent with inflammation and the use of corticosteroids (increased serum alkaline phosphatase level). Biopsy suggested lesions consistent with a drug-induced condition (erythema multiforme).

The dog was treated with IV fluids to compensate for fluids lost from the open lesions and chlorhexidine (Nolvasan) whirlpool baths b.i.d. to reduce bacterial infection in the skin. The fever came down, no further lesions appeared, and existing lesions began to improve within 3 days of starting whirlpool baths. The dog was discharged 7 days after initiation of therapy with instructions to continue the chlorhexidine baths for an additional week. Most skin lesions were healed 2 weeks after the dog went home.

Case 2: A 10-year-old castrated male golden retriever with a long-term skin problem was put on trimethoprim-sulfamethoxazole at an oral dose of 22 mg/kg b.i.d. to combat the *Staphylococcus* bacteria cultured from the skin. The skin responded well initially; however, 12 days after starting the sulfa drug the dog stopped eating, developed a fever (105.8° F), and developed itchy skins lesions all over the body. Skin biopsies were taken and submitted for histopathology. Based on the history a tentative diagnosis of drug eruption (skin lesions from drug administration) was made. The trimethoprim-sulfamethoxazole was stopped and 0.2 mg/kg of oral prednisolone given b.i.d. for 4 days. Oral cephalexin (Keflex) was given at 23 mg/kg t.i.d. for 3 weeks. Eight days after stopping the sulfonamide no new lesions had formed and existing lesions were covered with crusts (healing).

Case 3: A 7-year-old castrated male mix-breed dog with a 3-year history of recurrent episodes of skin inflammation with infection was presented to the referral hospital after treatment with trimethoprim-sulfamethoxazole failed to improve the skin condition as it had in the past. The skin in the axillary areas was without hair (alopecia) and roughened. Reddened papules of an inch and a half to 3 inches were present on the trunk and abdomen. Skin scrapings and fungal cultures were negative. Biopsies were taken. Based on biopsy and clinical appearance, a tentative diagnosis of drug eruption was made.

The potentiated sulfonamide was stopped and the dog bathed with a 3% benzoyl peroxide shampoo every 5 day for 3 weeks. After 1 week most of the lesions had resolved.

What should be learned from these cases: Veterinary technicians must be aware of the dermal manifestation of drug eruption (skin reactions to drugs) so that if a client calls and mentions a change in the skin condition after starting the antibiotic, the veterinary technician will report this information accurately to the veterinarian for follow-up to determine if a drug reaction has occurred. Failure to properly report this information or to dismiss it as "normal" for a dog or cat with "bad skin" could result in the dermatitis becoming progressively worse and potentially endangering the animal's life from opportunistic pathogens that thrive on severely damaged skin.

Abstracted from case report in Medleau L, et al: *J Am Anim Hosp Assoc* May/June 1990.

the drug without the tablet becoming lodged in the back of the throat or mouth or broken by the cat chewing on the tablet.

Unlike the systemically absorbed sulfonamides, the enteric sulfa sulfasalazine potentially poses a risk to cats because they cannot metabolize absorbed salicylates as well as dogs. As mentioned previously, sulfasalazine is metabolized by GI bacteria to sulfapyridine and aminosalicylic acid. If the salicylate compound is absorbed in sufficient amounts to overwhelm the cat's ability to metabolize the drug, it can produce toxicity. Therefore sulfasalazine must be used cautiously in cats and animals with aspirin (salicylate) hypersensitivity.

Regardless of which sulfonamide is used, veterinary professionals should know the signs of an adverse reaction to sulfonamides and advise animal owners of possible side effects to prevent the serious complications caused by an adverse reaction.

OTHER ANTIMICROBIALS USED IN VETERINARY MEDICINE

LINCOSAMIDES

Lincosamide antibiotics include lincomycin, clindamycin (Antirobe), and pirlimycin (Pirsue). These drugs are bacterial protein inhibitors and can be bacteriostatic or bactericidal, depending on the concentrations attained at the infection site. The lincosamides are generally effective against many gram-positive aerobic cocci. Clindamycin has good efficacy against many anaerobic bacteria, which makes it an effective drug for use in deep pyodermas (skin infections), abscesses, dental infections, bite wounds, and osteomyelitis caused by *Staphylococcus aureus*. Pirlimycin (Pirsue) is a drug approved for use as an intramammary infusion for mastitis treatment in lactating cattle.

Because lincosamides are generally metabolized in the liver and then excreted in the urine or bile, severe liver or renal disease can prolong the half-life of elimination and necessitate reducing the dose to prevent toxicity.

Pirlimycin is an intramammary infusion drug used in cattle; therefore withdrawal times for milk and tissue residues are important. Current recommendations for milk withdrawal are 36 hours and for tissue residues (for slaughter purposes) are 28 days after the last treatment.

Lincomycin is approved for use in a variety of species, including dogs, cats, swine, and poultry, but clindamycin is only approved for use in dogs. Lincosamides in general are contraindicated for use in rabbits, hamsters, guinea pigs, horses, and ruminants because they can cause serious GI effects in these species, resulting in death. Even in approved species, vomiting, diarrhea, and bloody diarrhea may occur from overgrowth of pathogenic bacteria caused by killing of competing anaerobic bacteria in the intestinal tract. Lincosamides can pass into the milk of lactating animals, which may cause nursing puppies and kittens to develop diarrhea.

Simultaneous use of kaolin antidiarrheal preparations such as Kaopectate and lincomycin can reduce absorption of the lincosamide up to 90%. If the two compounds must be used in an animal, they should be given 2 hours apart, preferably with the lincomycin being given 2 hours before the antidiarrheal drug. Absorption of clindamycin is not affected as greatly by concurrent administration of kaolin.

MACROLIDES

The macrolide antibiotics include erythromycin, the human drug azithromycin (Zithromax), tilmicosin (Micotil), and tylosin (Tylan). Although tylosin is approved for use in dogs and cats, its primary use is in livestock. In contrast, tilmicosin is approved for treatment of respiratory disease only in cattle. These drugs are bacteriostatic and work by inhibiting bacterial protein synthesis. They share similar spectra of antibacterial activity and bacterial cross-resistance. Because the spectrum of activity is similar to penicillin, the macrolides are often used as penicillin substitutes in animals or people allergic to penicillin.

Although macrolides are well distributed to most body tissues (including the prostate gland), they do not penetrate the CNS or cerebrospinal fluid very well. Macrolide antibiotics are primarily excreted unchanged in the bile, with a small portion (less than 5% for erythromycin and slightly more for tylosin) being eliminated by the kidney.

Erythromycin is similar in molecular structure to motilin, a compound found in the intestinal tract that stimulates intestinal motility. Thus, in human beings and veterinary patients, intestinal cramping, abdominal pain, and diarrhea may occur while on erythromycin. Suprainfection from overgrowth of bacteria is also a concern with erythromycin and azithromycin. Human beings put on this drug are often advised by their physicians to eat yogurt to resupply the intestinal tract with beneficial bacteria. Bacterial overgrowth is likely a significant contributor to the severe diarrhea sometimes seen in horses and foals put on erythromycin for respiratory disease.

Although erythromycin is indicated for treatment of selected infections in foals (*Rhodococcus equi* bacterial infections), oral use of erythromycin in adult horses is controversial because it may produce fatal diarrhea. For a similar reason, use of oral erythromycin in ruminants and oral tylosin in horses is contraindicated. Even though oral erythromycin should not be used in ruminants, injectable erythromycin is often effective against stubborn respiratory infections in ruminants.

Azithromycin has a slightly broader spectrum of activity than erythromycin and accumulates in significant concentrations in the respiratory tract. Because azithromycin is also effective against *Mycoplasma* organisms, a bacterial strain found in pneumonia and feline respiratory disease, this drug has been increasingly used in human and veterinary medicine for persistent respiratory diseases.

Tilmicosin (Micotil) is a macrolide approved for SQ administration for treatment of bovine respiratory diseases. The drug concentrates well in lung tissues and is especially effective against the organisms that cause bovine respiratory disease complex. The drug is highly irritating if given intramuscularly and can cause death if given intravenously. Horses, swine, primates, and human beings are much more sensitive to the toxic effects of tilmicosin, which include tachycardia (rapid heart rate) and potentially fatal arrhythmias.

Deaths in livestock handlers from accidental injection of Micotil have been reported in the toxicology, agricultural, and livestock literature. In a case described in a publication from the National Ag Safety Database, a cattleman accidentally injected himself with Micotil after being knocked down by a charging cow. In this case, the cattleman died 1 hour after injection from cardiac arrest. In another case reported in the *Journal of Toxicology*, the subject was attempting to inject a steer when he accidentally injected himself in the forearm.[5] Clinical signs did not appear for 5 hours, at which point severe chest pains occurred. In this case the injected individual survived.

Because tilmicosin can be dangerous to human beings, veterinary professionals must be especially careful to prevent accidental injection into human beings by not carrying uncapped syringes loaded with the drug, carrying no more of the drug than needed for one animal (do not use multidose syringes or put multiple doses in one syringe), and taking precautions to prevent contact of the drug with the eyes. A physician should be contacted immediately in cases of accidental human injection or contact with the eyes.

METRONIDAZOLE

Metronidazole (Flagyl) is a bactericidal antimicrobial that is also effective against protozoa that cause intestinal disease, such as *Giardia* (giardiasis), *Entamoeba histolytica* (amebiasis), *Trichomonas* (trichomoniasis), and *Balantidium coli* (balantidiasis). Although no approved veterinary form of metronidazole exists, human formulations are used for treatment of protozoal infections of the large bowel in dogs and cats and enteric bacterial infections caused by anaerobic bacteria in horses, dogs, and cats. Because metronidazole has been used successfully in common domestic species, it is also being used to treat anaerobic infections in avian and reptilian species. Resistance to metronidazole by *Giardia* and some bacteria is beginning to be noticed and reported in the veterinary scientific literature.

The exact mechanism of action of metronidazole is not known, but it may be metabolized to a form that can disrupt synthesis of DNA and nucleic acids. This change in form can only occur under conditions of low oxygen; therefore metronidazole is only effective against anaerobic bacteria and has minimal effectiveness against aerobic bacteria. For that reason, metronidazole is often selected for use in the lumen of the intestinal tract or for soft tissue infections that form anaerobic conditions (e.g., deep puncture wounds).

As mentioned in Chapter 4, metronidazole has been reported to produce some neurologic side effects, including loss of balance, head tilt, nystagmus (rapid, repeated horizontal, vertical, or circular eye movement), disorientation, and even tremors and seizures. These effects are observed more frequently in animals receiving an overdose; however, they have also been observed in animals treated with recommended doses for long periods of time.

CHLORAMPHENICOL AND FLORFENICOL

Chloramphenicol is an antimicrobial that is bacteriostatic at low concentrations but may become bactericidal at higher dosages. It works by binding to ribosomes in sensitive bacteria and disrupting bacterial protein synthesis. However, chloramphenicol can also disrupt mitochondrial function in bone marrow cells of mammals and has produced fatal aplastic anemia in human beings. For this reason, chloramphenicol use in food animals is completely banned.

In the past chloramphenicol has been used to treat small animals because of its ability to penetrate tissues and fluids, including the prostate gland, globe of the eye, and CNS fluids, and its effectiveness against rickettsiae. Because some new antimicrobials have greater antibacterial activity and fewer side effects, chloramphenicol is less commonly used in small animal practice.

In dogs, most of a chloramphenicol dose is metabolized by glucuronide conjugation, and very little drug is excreted unchanged into the urine. Because cats poorly metabolize chloramphenicol in the liver, more of the drug is excreted intact by the kidneys. Therefore adequate renal function is a more important consideration for chloramphenicol use in cats than in dogs. The reduced metabolism and slower rate of elimination in cats are the reasons that chloramphenicol doses for cats are significantly lower than those for dogs. Neonates (especially neonatal kittens) can easily develop chloramphenicol toxicosis because of their poor hepatic function. In addition, chloramphenicol can be passed in the milk of lactating animals and subsequently ingested by the nursing offspring. Therefore lactating animals should not be given chloramphenicol.

Chloramphenicol can inhibit hepatic biotransformation of drugs such as phenobarbital, pentobarbital, and primidone. Concurrent use of any of these anticonvulsant or barbiturate drugs with chloramphenicol necessitates a reduction in their dose to prevent accumulation within the body.

Chloramphenicol is bacteriostatic at most dosages used in veterinary medicine; therefore it interferes with the bactericidal effects of penicillins, which require an actively growing bacterial population to exert their effect. Chloramphenicol binds to the same site on the ribosome as tylosin, erythromycin, lincomycin, and clindamycin and may reduce the efficacy of these drugs if used simultaneously. However, the clinical effect of this antagonism has not been established in veterinary patients.

As mentioned, chloramphenicol can disrupt division of mammalian bone marrow cells, resulting in suppression of bone marrow cell formation *(myelosuppression)* and subsequent nonregenerative anemia, lymphopenia, and neutropenia. Therefore when handing chloramphenicol powder in capsules or tablets or while mixing the powder into a suspension, veterinary technicians must avoid repeated contact with or inhalation of the powder. Precautions include washing hands after handling capsules or tablets, avoiding inhalation of chloramphenicol powder, and using care when breaking chloramphenicol tablets or opening capsules.

Florfenicol (Nufluor) is a newer antibiotic related to chloramphenicol but with some significant differences that enable this drug to be safely used in cattle for bovine respiratory diseases such as shipping fever or pneumonia. Like chloramphenicol, florfenicol is bacteriostatic, disrupts protein synthesis at the bacterial ribosomes, and penetrates tissues fairly well. Unlike chloramphenicol, florfenicol is approved for use in cattle and, according to the manufacturer's literature, lacks the chemical component that makes chloramphenicol toxic to human bone marrow. Florfenicol is only approved for IM injection administered as 2 injections 48 hours apart. The drug has a 28-day withdrawal time. Because insufficient data are available regarding florfenicol's effect on bovine reproduction, pregnancy, and lactation, the drug should not be used in cattle of breeding age. The veterinary technician should thoroughly read the drug information on this and any new drug before use.

RIFAMPIN

Rifampin is a bactericidal or bacteriostatic antimicrobial belonging to the class of antimicrobials known as rifamycins. It is primarily used with or without erythromycin for treatment of *Corynebacterium equi* (Rhodococcus) infections in young foals, *Staphylococcus* infections, and some fungal agents (*Histoplasma, Aspergillus, Blastomyces*) when used in conjunction with the antifungal agent amphotericin B. Some

sources debate the clinical effectiveness of rifampin against these fungal agents in spite of the synergy caused by amphotericin's ability to enhance penetration of rifampin into the fungal organisms.

Rifampin suppresses formation of the RNA chain by inhibiting an RNA polymerase needed for RNA synthesis. Like quinolones, rifampin only affects bacterial RNA polymerase and does not disrupt the function of mammalian RNA polymerases.

Rifampin is a potent inducer, or accelerator, of hepatic microsomal enzyme function responsible for metabolism of some other drugs. Rifampin accelerates metabolism of those drugs, with subsequent shortened half-lives and lower plasma concentrations. Some of these drugs include heart medications such as propranolol and quinidine, the antibiotic chloramphenicol, benzodiazepine tranquilizers such as diazepam and zolazepam (found in Telazol), barbiturates such as phenobarbital and pentobarbital, and corticosteroids such as prednisone and dexamethasone.

Rifampin imparts a reddish-orange color to urine, tears, sweat, and saliva. Owners of animals being treated with rifampin should be informed of this change so they are not unduly alarmed.

MISCELLANEOUS ANTIBIOTICS

Bacitracin is an antibiotic that works similarly to penicillins and cephalosporins in that it inhibits the formation of bacterial cell walls. Bacitracin has the potential to produce nephrotoxicity; therefore its use is confined to topical antibiotic preparations or ocular (ophthalmic) preparations, sometimes in conjunction with neomycin (an aminoglycoside) or polymyxin B (an antibiotic effective against *Pseudomonas* bacteria).

The nitrofurans are a group of antimicrobials that includes nitrofurantoin (Furadantin). Nitrofurantoin is eliminated by the kidneys so rapidly that it usually does not attain therapeutically significant concentrations in tissues.

However, because approximately half of the drug administered is filtered unchanged through the glomerulus and actively secreted into the renal tubule, it is used to treat infections of the lower urinary tract (in the bladder and urethra) in dogs, cats, and occasionally horses. Because of the drug's cost and potential for GI and systemic toxicity, it is limited to use for urinary tract infections that are not susceptible to other antibiotics.

ANTIFUNGALS

This group of antimicrobial drugs was developed to be effective against many of the fungal organisms that cause superficial mycoses (fungal skin infections), such as ringworm, and the deep or systemic mycoses (fungal infections within the body) such as histoplasmosis, blastomycosis, cryptococcosis, coccidioidomycosis, candidiasis, sporotrichosis, and aspergillosis. The number of antifungal agents is likely to continue to expand because of the need for these agents for immunocompromised human patients who are typically susceptible to fungal pathogens. Because most antifungal drugs have potentially severe side effects, veterinary technicians must be aware of the correct procedures for safe handling, administration, storage, and disposal of antifungals.

AMPHOTERICIN B

Amphotericin B is effective against most of the deep mycoses listed above. Amphotericin is administered parenterally (primarily intravenously, but doses exist for SQ administration) for treatment of deep or systemic mycotic infections because it is poorly absorbed from the GI tract. Once amphotericin B reaches the fungal elements, it binds and damages a specific molecule (ergosterol) on the fungal cell membrane, causing damage and allowing critical cellular components to leak from the fungal cell. This effect can be fungicidal or fungistatic, depending on the concentration of drug achieved at the fungal infection site. One advantage of amphotericin B over the imidazole antifungal agents is the rapid onset of fungicidal activity (hours) compared with the imidazoles (days).

Amphotericin B binds to circulating lipidproteins (lipoproteins) like cholesterol and then to cholesterol in cell membranes. It distributes and concentrates well in kidney, liver, spleen, and lung tissue but does not accumulate as well in bone, body fluids (pleural fluid, pericardial fluid, peritoneal fluid, joint fluid), or the CNS. The metabolism of amphotericin B is complex and not well understood.

Amphotericin can cause several serious side effects, including nephrotoxicosis, fever, anorexia, and nausea. Of these, nephrotoxicosis (kidney toxicity) is the most common and most significant. Most canine patients (some studies say more than 80%) show some degree of nephrotoxicosis after amphotericin B administration. Nephrotoxicosis occurs because of the strong vasoconstrictive effects amphotericin has on the renal blood supply (results in poor circulation, tissue anoxia, and kidney cell death) and its direct toxic effect on the renal tubules (primarily the distal convoluted tubule). Renal function (including BUN, creatinine, and urinalysis) should be closely monitored before and during treatment with amphotericin B so the degree of renal damage can be evaluated. Renal damage is dose related; therefore more renal damage occurs with high doses or prolonged dosing of amphotericin.

Although some sources state that the nephrotoxic effect of amphotericin can be blunted by administration of IV fluids (to maintain renal blood flow), damage to the kidney may be to some degree irreversible. If, however, the irreversible damage is limited the animal can still have decent renal function after conclusion of the amphotericin treatment.

AZOLES: THE IMIDAZOLE DERIVATIVES

Azole antifungal agents, also called imidazole derivatives, are composed of two groups (imidazoles, which contain two nitrogen atoms, and triazoles, which contain three) and include several compounds such as ketoconazole, itraconazole, fluconazole, miconazole, and clotrimazole. Of these drugs, ketoconazole is the prototype imidazole. Ketoconazole, itraconazole, and fluconazole are typically administered orally, whereas miconazole and clotrimazole are administered topically.

Nearly all deep or systemic mycoses in animals today are treated with these drugs or with amphotericin B. Because imidazole derivatives have fewer side effects than amphotericin B, they are often used as the first drug of choice for the treatment of most deep fungal agents except the ones that are rapidly growing where the quicker onset of amphotericin would be preferred.

The imidazole derivatives interfere with the fungal agent's ergosterol synthesis, resulting in damage to the fungal cell membrane function and subsequent fungal cell membrane leakage. This effect usually takes 5 to 10 days of treatment before it becomes fungicidal; hence the delay in onset of activity. Although the azoles do not produce nephrotoxicosis as does amphotericin, they do have their own adverse reactions that must be monitored in patients receiving these drugs. GI side effects are the most common adverse reaction with the imidazole derivatives, with ketoconazole probably being the least tolerated of the azoles. Vomiting is more commonly associated with higher doses of the azoles, occurs more commonly in cats than dogs, and can be reduced by splitting the daily dose into small individual doses given more frequently.

Hepatotoxicity is a potentially serious side effect more commonly reported with ketoconazole use than the other imidazole derivatives. It is more of a risk in patients with existing liver impairment but is rarely seen in normal animals during the first few weeks of therapy. Selected liver enzymes (e.g., alanine aminotransferase) will normally go up in many animals without indicating liver failure. As long as this is the only liver enzyme that has significant change and the animal is otherwise without liver failure signs, the treatment protocol for the azole antifungal agent probably does not need to be changed.

Ketoconazole should be used with caution in breeding dogs because ketoconazole decreases steroid production in dogs and thus may reduce concentrations of testosterone and glucocorticoids (cortisol). Dogs given large doses of ketoconazole may require supplementation with corticosteroid drugs to compensate for reduced production of endogenous glucocorticoids (adrenal gland insufficiency). Testosterone and cortisol levels rebound after ketoconazole is withdrawn. Interestingly, cats appear to be more resistant to this effect than dogs.

Clotrimazole and miconazole are recommended for use with topical yeast infections, superficial dermatophytes and, in the case of clotrimazole, for use as an intranasal infusion to treat nasal aspergillosis.

GRISEOFULVIN

Although it has been replaced by itraconazole to some extent, griseofulvin is a fungistatic drug used primarily to treat infections from *Trichophyton* and *Microsporum* species of dermatophytes ("skin plants") found superficially on dogs, cats, and horses. These fungi usually infect the skin, hair, nails, and claws, causing the condition known as ringworm. Griseofulvin is available as an oral powder (for horses) or as tablets. To be absorbed from the GI tract, the particles of griseofulvin must be very small. Therefore griseofulvin products are produced in microsize and ultramicrosize formulations. Because the ultramicrosize formulation is smaller, it is better absorbed than the microsize formulation. Because these two formulations are absorbed to different extents (different bioavailability) the dosage must be adjusted when switching from one formulation to the other.

Griseofulvin is metabolized by the liver and conjugated with glucuronide. Cats are slow to conjugate any drugs with glucuronide, so they eliminate griseofulvin slowly. The slow rate of elimination predisposes cats to accumulate a toxic level of the drug. For this reason, doses of griseofulvin for cats are lower than for dogs.

Griseofulvin is reportedly teratogenic in cats, producing cleft palates and other skeletal, skull, and nervous system defects in kittens of queens treated during gestation. Therefore griseofulvin is contraindicated for use in pregnant animals.

More common side effects of orally administered griseofulvin are anorexia, vomiting, and diarrhea. Although more severe effects such as anemia and leukopenia have been reported, these are rare at normal dosages. Griseofulvin should be used with caution in cats and especially in kittens because of the increased sensitivity of these animals to this drug.

Box 10-1 Antimicrobial Drug Categories and Names

PENICILLINS

Natural penicillins
  Penicillin G
Aminopenicillins
  Ampicillin
  Amoxicillin
Penicillinase-resistant
  Cloxacillin
  Dicloxacillin
  Oxacillin
Extended-spectrum
  Carbenicillin
  Ticarcillin
  Piperacillin
Penicillin adjuncts
  Clavulanic acid
  Sulbactam
  Benzathine
  Procaine

CEPHALOSPORINS

First-generation
  Cefadroxil (Cefa-Tabs, Cefa-Drops)
  Cephapirin (Cefa-Lak, Cefa-Dri)
  Cephalexin (Keflex)
  Cephalothin (Keflin)
Second-generation
  Cefoxitin (Mefoxin)
Third-generation
  Ceftiofur (Naxcel, Excenel)
  Cefpodoxime (Simplicef)
  Cefotaxime (Claforan)

AMINOGLYCOSIDES

Amikacin
Gentamicin
Kanamycin
Neomycin
Streptomycin
Tobramycin

QUINOLONES (FLUOROQUINOLONES)

Enrofloxacin (Baytril)
Marbofloxacin (Zeniquin)
Orbifloxacin (Orbax)
Difloxacin (Dicural)
Ciprofloxacin

TETRACYCLINES

Tetracycline
Oxytetracycline (LA-200)
Doxycycline
Minocycline

SULFONAMIDES

Sulfadiazine (Tribrissen)
Sulfadimethoxine (Primor)
Sulfamethoxazole (Septra)
Sulfachlorpyridazine
Sulfasalazine (Azulfidine)

SULFONAMIDE-POTENTIATING COMPOUNDS

Trimethoprim
Ormetoprim

OTHER ANTIMICROBIALS

Lincosamides
  Lincomycin
  Clindamycin (Antirobe)
  Pirlimycin (Pirsue)
Macrolides
  Erythromycin
  Tylosin (Tylan)
  Tilmicosin (Micotil)
  Azithromycin (Zithromax)
Metronidazole (Flagyl)
Chloramphenicol
Florfenicol

Box 10-1 Antimicrobial Drug Categories and Names—cont'd

Rifampin	Ketoconazole
Bacitracin	Itraconazole
	Fluconazole
ANTIFUNGALS	Miconazole
Amphotericin B	Clotrimazole
Azoles: imidazole derivatives	Griseofulvin (Fulvicin)

REFERENCES

1. Aucoin DP: *Rational approach to antimicrobial selection.* In Proceedings of the Atlantic Coast Veterinary Conference, Atlantic City, NJ, 2002.
2. Freeman CD, Nicolau DP, Belliveau PP, et al: Once-daily dosing of aminoglycosides: review and recommendations for clinical practice, *J Antimicrob Chemotherapeutics* 39:677, 1997.
3. Papich MG: *Strategies for using antibiotics in animals.* In Proceedings of WSAVA 2002 Congress, Granada, Spain, 2002.
4. Andes D, Craig W: Animal model pharmacokinetics and pharmacodynamics: a critical review, *Int J Antimicrob Agents* 19:261-267, 2002.
5. Von Essen S, Spencer J, Hass B, et al: Unintentional human exposure to tilmicosin, *J Toxicol* 41(3):229-233, 2003.

RECOMMENDED READING

Bertone JJ: *Rational antibiotic choices.* In Proceedings of the Western Veterinary Conference, Las Vegas, NV, 2003.
Bill RL: *Twenty ways to avoid complications from antimicrobial therapy.* In Proceedings of the American Veterinary Medical Association Annual Meeting, Philadelphia, July 2004.
Boothe DM: *Small animal clinical pharmacology and therapeutics*, Philadelphia, 2001, WB Saunders.
Booth DM: Fluorinated quinolones. In Bonagura JD, editor: *Kirk's current veterinary therapy XIII*, Philadelphia, 2000, WB Saunders.
Collins BR: *Antimicrobial drug use in rabbits, rodents, and other small mammals.* In Proceedings of the Miles Antimicrobial Therapy in Caged Birds and Exotic Pets Symposium, Orlando, FL, January 1995.
Dow S: *More effective use of antibiotics.* In Proceedings of the North American Veterinary Conference, Orlando, FL, January 2002.
Maddison J, Page S, Church D: *Small animal clinical pharmacology*, Philadelphia, 2002, WB Saunders.
Mosby's drug consult, St. Louis, 2002, Mosby.
Plumb DC: *Veterinary drug handbook*, ed 5, Ames, IA, 2005, Blackwell.
Morely PS, Dargatz DA, Lappin MR, et al: *Veterinarians and antimicrobial drug use.* In Proceedings of the American College of Veterinary Internal Medicine, Charlotte, NC, 2003.
Papich MG, Taboada J: *Making the best first choice antibiotic selections.* In Proceedings of the North American Veterinary Conference, Orlando, FL, January 2005.
Taboda J: Systemic mycoses. In Ettinger SJ, Feldman EC, editors: *Textbook of veterinary internal medicine*, ed 5, Philadelphia, 2000, WB Saunders.

Self-Assessment

Fill in the following blanks with the correct item from the Key Terms list.

1. _____ drug concentration at the lower end of the therapeutic range for the antibiotic; the concentration of drug at which bacteria are inhibited.

2. _____ means "decrease in number of platelets."

3. _____ disease-causing agents.

4. _____ range of bacteria that can be killed by a particular antimicrobial.

5. _____ means "kills bacteria."

6. _____ traces of leftover drug in the tissue long after the antimicrobial drug has been stopped.

7. _____ chemical structure found in penicillins and cephalosporins; can be the site of action for some bacterial enzymes.

8. _____ having an allergic reaction to a drug.

9. _____ process by which one compound binds to another compound, causing the compounds to precipitate out of solution; occurs with tetracyclines and calcium.

10. _____ means "toxic to the kidney"; occurs with aminoglycosides.

11. _____ presence of crystals, typically precipitated drug molecules, in the urine.

12. _____ means "skin plant"; refers to fungal agents such as ringworm.

13. _____ term meaning bone marrow production of blood cells has been depressed or stopped; occurs with drugs such as chloramphenicol.

14. _____ enzyme inhibited by quinolones and prevents the nuclear material inside the bacteria from being condensed so the bacteria can divide.

15. _____ drug-induced condition that results in glucosuria without hyperglycemia; associated most often with tetracyclines.

16. _____ means "keeps bacteria from growing or multiplying."

17. _____ means "decreased number of white blood cells."

18. _____ term indicating bacteria that can be inhibited or killed by a particular drug.

19. _____ condition that occurs when an antibiotic given by mouth kills off beneficial bacteria in the GI tract and allows pathogenic bacteria to proliferate.

20. _____ means "toxic to the ear"; occurs with aminoglycosides.

21. _____ condition called "dry eye" because of the decreased function of the tear glands; can result from the use of sulfonamide antibiotics.

22. _____ process by which bacteria are isolated and their susceptibility to different antimicrobial drugs determined.

23. _____ microbes that grow under conditions of little or no oxygen.

24. _____ means "produces pus."

25. _____ translates to "against life" and refers to drugs that kill pathogens; today applies mostly to antibacterial drugs.

26. _____ the resistance of bacteria to several related antimicrobial drugs.

27. _____ enzyme produced by bacteria (especially *Staphylococci*) that can disable penicillins and cephalosporins.

28. _____ bacteria that cannot be killed by a particular drug.

29. _____ microbes that require oxygen to grow.

Identify the correct drug for each description from the drugs listed in Box 10-1.

30. _____ group of antimicrobials that can be rendered ineffective by the presence of pus; nucleic acid in the debris of ruptured cells can bind to the drugs and prevent them from reaching the bacteria.

31. _____ group of tetracyclines that is able to penetrate the CNS through the blood-brain barrier; has a longer half-life than the other tetracyclines and a slightly broader spectrum of activity.

32. _____ group of antimicrobials that works by inactivating key enzymes involved in the bacteria's synthesis of folic acid, which the bacteria needs to function.

33. _____ amino-type members of this group; greater spectrum of activity than the natural members of the group.

34. _____ first of the quinolones to be approved for use in the United States; indicated for use with cats and dogs; do not use above 5 mg/kg in cats to decrease the risk for blindness.

35. _____ β-lactam antibiotics that are naturally resistant against penicillinase.

36. _____ expired drugs that can decompose to form a nephrotoxic compound that damages the proximal convoluted tubule of the kidney, which prevents reabsorption of sugar from the urine and results in glucosuria; also called Fanconi's syndrome.

37. _____ group of antibiotics known for being very safe with the exception of hypersensitivity reactions that many animals seem to have with drugs of this group; hypersensitivity reactions can be life-threatening compared with the reactions seen with sulfonamide antibiotics.

38. _____ antifungal used for deep mycoses; causes damage to the kidneys of the animal almost every time.

39. _____ these antimicrobials are readily chelated with calcium and magnesium; do not use orally in nursing animals or allow animals to drink milk or eat dairy products while taking these drugs by mouth.

40. _____ added to penicillin G to slow absorption and extend therapeutic concentrations for up to 3 days.

41. _____ use of this drug in any animal intended for food is grounds for losing the license to practice veterinary medicine; can cause aplastic anemia in human beings.

42. _____ group of β-lactam antimicrobials classified by generations.

43. _____ group of antimicrobials taken up with an active transport process that is oxygen dependent; ineffective against anaerobes.

44. _____ group of drugs that works by binding to DNA gyrase and preventing the bacteria from replicating.

45. _____ members of the penicillin group that have the greatest range of activity against bacteria.

46. _____ drugs that can cause adult teeth to turn yellow if they were present in the body when the enamel was being laid down on the developing adult teeth.

47. _____ ototoxic and nephrotoxic.

48. _____ group of antimicrobials indicated for use in prostatic infections because they can penetrate the blood-prostate barrier and accumulate within the prostate at concentrations higher than the surrounding plasma or blood.

49. _____ antimicrobials that work by interfering with the development of the bacterial cell wall.

50. _____ sulfonamide drug used for its antiinflammatory characteristics in the colon; metabolized in the colon to aminosalicylic acid, an antiinflammatory drug.

51. _____ group of antimicrobials contraindicated in dogs who are in rapid growth phases because of the possibility of forming small, bubblelike lesions in the joint cartilage.

52. _____ like penicillins and cephalosporins, this drug group also causes hypersensitivity reactions, mostly of the skin (e.g., pruritus, swelling of the face, hives).

53. _____ bacteriostatic antimicrobials; used most commonly for rickettsial diseases such as Rocky Mountain spotted fever or Lyme disease; has two classes of drugs: one group is lipophilic and the other is hydrophilic.

54. _____ early signs of toxicosis from this antimicrobial group are the presence of casts and increased protein in the urine.

55. _____ used to treat superficial fungal infections (ringworm); teratogenic in cats and can produce cleft palates or other skeletal deformities.

56. _____ most potentially nephrotoxic aminoglycoside.

57. _____ water-soluble tetracyclines; used in livestock to a great degree.

58. _____ two groups of antibiotics only effective against bacteria that are rapidly dividing.

59. _____ IV injection of relatively small doses of this drug in horses has resulted in arrhythmias, collapse, and death.

60. _____ added to sulfonamide antibiotics to increase their killing power.

61. _____ added to penicillin G to slow its absorption and extend its action over 5 days.

62. _____ group of antimicrobials associated with KCS.

63. _____ natural member of this group; β-lactam; do not give orally.

64. _____ lincosamide drug that works well against anaerobic bacteria and therefore is used to treat deep pyoderma, abscesses, and dental infections.

65. _____ macrolide antibiotic similar in its chemical structure to a compound called motilin; cause abdominal cramping, pain, and diarrhea.

66. _____ macrolide antibiotic that has produced deaths in people who have accidentally or intentionally injected themselves.

67. _____ bactericidal antimicrobial effective against intestinal protozoa such as *Giardia*; can cause neurologic side effects even at normal doses.

68. _____ drug with excellent ability to penetrate tissues; does not cause aplastic anemia as does the other member of its group.

69. _____ added with neomycin and polymyxin B to make a widely used antibiotic cream or ointment.

70. _____ added to amoxicillin to make amoxicillin resistant to the bacteria's β-lactamase enzyme.

71. _____ group of antifungals that is the treatment of choice for deep mycoses; fewer side effects than amphotericin B.

72. _____ group of otherwise safe antimicrobials capable of causing superinfections in guinea pigs, ferrets, hamsters, and rabbits; should be used with caution in snakes, birds, turtles, and chinchillas.

73. Indicate whether the following statements are true or false.

    A. Cloxacillin has a broader spectrum of activity than ampicillin.

    B. If an animal has a reaction to penicillin G, amoxicillin should be safe to give because its formula is different enough from the formula of penicillin G.

    C. Generally, first- and second-generation cephalosporins are more effective against gram-negative bacteria than the first-generation drugs.

D. With aminoglycosides, the total daily dose should be divided among four doses (q.i.d.) instead of given once daily (s.i.d.).

E. Aminoglycosides readily penetrate cellular barriers.

F. Aminoglycosides are almost exclusively eliminated by the kidneys.

G. In aminoglycoside toxicosis, the BUN and serum creatinine concentrations go up before casts and protein begin to appear in the urine.

H. If an animal develops diarrhea while on oral tetracycline, antacids, kaolin, or Pepto-Bismol are acceptable treatments.

I. For susceptible bacteria in the liver or lungs, a systemic sulfonamide is preferred over an enteric sulfonamide.

J. Amphotericin B begins to kill fungal organisms much quicker than ketoconazole or itraconazole.

K. When changing the griseofulvin dose form from microsized to ultramicrosized, the dose would probably have to increase.

APPLICATION QUESTIONS

1. Why are penicillins, even those with a broad spectrum of activity, not used to treat bacterial infections of the brain or the eye?

2. An owner calls the hospital early this morning and tells you that her dog, who was in yesterday to have a tooth removed and a dental cleaning of the rest of its teeth, is lethargic, has a temperature of 102.5° F, and is swollen around the face (eyes are almost swelled shut). You relay this information to the veterinarian and he says to bring the dog in right away because his symptoms might be related to the antibiotic injection given yesterday. How so?

3. You have a cat in the hospital with a viral disease that impairs its immune system. It also has a secondary bacterial infection. As the veterinarian is discussing the treatment options with you, she mentions that she needs to select a -cidal antimicrobial for the bacterial infection. Why?

4. Griseofulvin and enrofloxacin are both antimicrobials that work by affecting the pathogen's nucleic acid. Griseofulvin has the potential to produce birth defects in mammals because of its mechanism of action. But enrofloxacin and the other quinolones do not produce birth defects even though they affect the bacterial DNA. Why is enrofloxacin not a threat to mammalian DNA and a cause of potential birth defects as griseofulvin is?

5. Even though a dog's culture and sensitivity come back showing both amoxicillin and sulfadiazine are effective against the bacteria causing the lung infection, the veterinarian does not want to use the drugs together. "They would tend to work against each other," she says. What does she mean by this?

6. You notice that the veterinarian often chooses either a penicillin or potentiated sulfonamide antibiotic for initial therapy for canine bacterial bladder infections. Why these two drugs? What makes them particularly useful for bacterial cystitis?

Chapter 1

Disinfectants and Antiseptics

key terms

antiseptics	germicides	scrubs
bactericidal	halogens	solutions
biofilm	microbicidal	spore form
coagulum	microbiostatic	sporicidal
cytotoxic	naked virus	sterilizers
disinfectants	nosocomial infections	tinctures
enveloped virus	protozoacidal	vegetative form
fungicidal	sanitizers	virucidal

objectives

After studying this chapter, the veterinary technician should be able to define or describe:

1. The scientific and nonscientific terminology used to describe the characteristics of disinfecting agents

2. The different mechanisms by which disinfectants and antiseptics kill or inhibit bacteria or other pathogens

3. The clinically significant adverse reactions of commonly used disinfectants and antiseptics, and what the veterinary professional can do to keep these from occurring

4. The roles bacterial resistance, presence of organic material, and other factors play in the selection of disinfecting agents

Disinfection is the destruction of pathogenic microorganisms. Disinfection is important in maintaining the health of all animals whether on a farm, in a veterinary hospital, in a research facility, or in a breeding colony. However, disinfection is often taken for granted. With literally hundreds of disinfecting products available to the veterinary professional and the general public, sorting through all the options and selecting a disinfecting agent that is most applicable to the needs of a particular clinical situation can be overwhelming. Thus disinfecting agents are often chosen because of a practice's long-term use or an appealing price or sales pitch. This haphazard method of selecting disinfecting agents can lead to contamination of clean or sterile areas and subsequent spread of pathogenic microorganisms. The role of the veterinary technician should be to understand the limitations of all disinfecting agents used in their facility and know when these limitations are likely to be encountered during use.

Disinfection of hospital equipment and premises is especially important because of the natural selection for resistant strains that occurs when populations of microorganisms are exposed to low concentrations of antimicrobial chemicals (see Chapter 10). *Nosocomial infections,* which are infections acquired during a period of hospitalization, are especially difficult to control because of the resistance of the organisms involved. Common sites of nosocomial infections are the urinary tract (associated with urinary catheters), respiratory tract (associated with endotracheal tubes), surgical sites, wounds, and intravenous (IV) catheter insertion sites. Improper use of disinfecting agents can cause an otherwise healthy animal to acquire an infection during its stay in the veterinary hospital. With the increased incidence of highly resistant bacteria (so-called "super bugs"), proper disinfection takes on an increasingly important role in prevention and treatment of infections in veterinary patients. Box 11-1, listing disinfecting agents, can be found at the end of this chapter.

TERMINOLOGY DESCRIBING DISINFECTING AGENTS

The terminology used to describe disinfecting agents can be confusing. In addition to the scientific terms, many vague terms are frequently used by the general public. The veterinary technician must understand the terms used to describe *disinfectants* to make rational decisions about the appropriate use of the proper agent.

Antiseptics are chemical agents that kill or prevent the growth of microorganisms on living tissues. Disinfectants are chemical agents that kill or prevent growth of microorganisms on inanimate objects such as surgical equipment, floors, and tabletops. Disinfectants typically are more potentially toxic to veterinary patients, staff, or clients because they are intended for use on non-living tissue. In some cases, a disinfectant may be a more concentrated form of an antiseptic. Therefore the distinction between the two terms may be blurred. However, if the veterinary technician applies the general rule of antiseptic = living tissues and disinfectant = inanimate objects, this delineation usually applies.

Some disinfectants are listed as high-, intermediate-, and low-level disinfectants. This designation generally refers to the ability of the disinfectant to kill the tougher pathogens (e.g., high-level disinfectants are more likely to kill bacterial spores and *naked viruses*). Antiseptics and disinfectants may also be described as *sanitizers* or *sterilizers*. The difference refers to the degree of microbial destruction achieved. Sanitizers are chemical agents that reduce the number of microorganisms to a "safe" level without eliminating all microorganisms. Sterilizers are chemicals or other agents that destroy all microorganisms.

Many household cleaning products are advertised as *germicides*. A germicide is any chemical agent that kills microorganisms. Because microorganisms include viruses, bacteria, protozoa, and fungi, the term germicide is nonspecific and should not be used by veterinary professionals.

TABLE **11-1** Relative Efficacy of Disinfectants and Antiseptics

	ALCOHOL	IODINE IODOPHOR	CHLORINE	CHLORHEXIDINE	QUATERNARY AMMONIUM COMPOUNDS	GLUTARALDEHYDE
Bactericidal	++	+++	++	+++	++	+++
Lipid enveloped virucidal	++	++	+++	++	+	+++
Nonenveloped virucidal	–	+	+++	+	–	++
Sporicidal	–	+	+	–	–	++
Effective in presence of soap	++	+++	++	+	–	++
Effective in hard water	+*	++	++	+	–	++
Effective in presence of organic material	–	–	–	+++	–	++

Ratings are relative indicators. Effectiveness depends on concentration of compound used. The more plus signs, the greater the efficacy. A minus sign means the compound is not effective.
*Do not dilute in water; they do not mix well and will render the alcohol much less effective.

The veterinary professional should know against which organisms the antiseptic or disinfectant is effective (Table 11-1). *Bactericidal* chemicals kill bacteria, *virucidal* chemicals kill viruses, *fungicidal* chemicals kill fungi, *protozoacidal* chemicals kill protozoa, and *sporicidal* chemicals kill microbial spores.

Unlike some antimicrobials, disinfectants need to be *microbicidal* rather than *microbiostatic* because inanimate objects do not have an immune system, and disinfectants must therefore completely eliminate all microorganisms on their own.

Whether the pathogen can form a spore is also important in selecting the disinfectant. Bacteria and fungi can exist in two forms: an actively growing *vegetative form* or a more static *spore form*. Bacterial spores are designed to be able to survive in a dormant state for years to decades so that under appropriate growing conditions they can switch to the vegetative form and begin multiplying again. For example, *Clostridium tetani*, the bacterial agent of tetanus, and *Bacillus anthracis*, the bacterial agent of anthrax, have been shown to exist as spores buried in the ground for decades only to be reactivated on exposure to appropriate conditions of temperature, moisture, and aerobic or anaerobic environment. Because these spores are capable of surviving extreme environmental conditions for years,

they are also resistant to the majority of disinfectants. Therefore, the possibility of the spores carried into the veterinary hospital environment or contaminating surgical procedures in the field means that sporicidal disinfection plays an important role in proper veterinary care.

Some bacteria, such as the *Pseudomonas* species, are highly resistant to disinfection and antiseptics because of their ability to produce a *biofilm*. In these situations, implants or catheters that are contaminated with *Pseudomonas* may be covered with a glycocalyx material (a "slime") that prevents the disinfecting agent from penetrating to reach the bacteria. This is of great concern with external fixation devices (pins and clamps) used to immobilize broken bones. If a bone implant (e.g., pin, plate) becomes infected with a biofilm-producing bacteria, the implant usually has to be removed. For these high-risk situations, high-level disinfectants are required to reduce the chances of contamination.

APPROPRIATE USE OF DISINFECTING AGENTS

Because the use of disinfecting agents is often assumed to require little more than common sense, the basic tenets of proper disinfection are often ignored. The results are inadequate reduction of populations of pathogenic microorganisms and the potential for the spread of disease.

Following are the characteristics of the ideal disinfecting agent:

- Broad-spectrum antimicrobial activity. A single disinfectant that could destroy all viruses, bacteria, and other pathogens would be ideal. Realistically, the chemicals used in most disinfectants often leave certain groups of pathogens untouched. Therefore the veterinary professional should know the various disinfectants' spectra of antimicrobial activity to select the appropriate one for use against the microorganisms most likely to be inhabiting the site of application.

- Nonirritating and nontoxic to animal and human tissue. Many disinfecting agents are irritating or toxic, especially those with a broad spectrum of antimicrobial activity. Several disinfecting agents can cause toxicity if accidentally ingested, and some are dangerous if too much is applied to the skin or mucous membranes. Even approved antiseptics can be *cytotoxic* (cell killing) if applied in inappropriate concentrations or to open wounds. Veterinary technicians should be aware of the potential dangers that disinfectants pose to themselves and animals under their care.

- Easily applied to inanimate objects and without causing corrosion or stains. Concentrated hydrochloric acid could certainly destroy the microorganisms on the surface of a surgery table. However, the corrosive action of the acid would damage the table surface and create minute crevices in which contaminants and microorganisms could accumulate. Also, some antiseptic or disinfecting agents contain dyes that stain porous or easily marked surfaces.

- Stable and not easily inactivated. Most disinfecting agents take several seconds or minutes to reduce the population of microorganisms to safe levels. If during that time the agent is in contact with cellular debris, blood, or other organic materials, it may be inactivated by these contaminants and therefore cannot sufficiently reduce the number of microorganisms. The same is true for some surgical antiseptics when they make contact with soap residue left over from the scrubbing of the skin before application of the antiseptic. Ideally, a disinfecting agent should not lose its potency or effectiveness while in storage for an extended time.

- Inexpensive. Because disinfecting agents are used to such a great extent in veterinary medicine, these agents must be economical and affordable. Although this is an important consideration in selecting a disinfectant, it should not be the most important criterion.

The ideal disinfectant or antiseptic has yet to be discovered. Each disinfecting agent currently in use in veterinary medicine lacks one or more of the ideal characteristics listed. However, by being aware of the deficiencies of any given disinfectant and matching its strengths with the given task, technicians can select the appropriate agent.

SELECTING AN APPROPRIATE DISINFECTING AGENT

Three factors should be considered before selecting a particular disinfectant for a given application:

- The type of microorganism the agent must eliminate (bacteria, viruses, fungi, or vegetative or spore forms)
- The environment in which the disinfectant will be used (living tissue versus inanimate object or presence or absence of dirt or debris)
- The characteristics of the disinfectant (corrosiveness, cost, and antimicrobial spectrum)

Technicians should know whether the pathogens of greatest concern in a given situation are viruses, bacteria, fungi, protozoa, or a combination. Technicians should also consider whether spores, especially bacterial spores, are likely to be encountered. If a virus is likely to be present, technicians should know the general susceptibility of that virus to disinfecting agents. Some

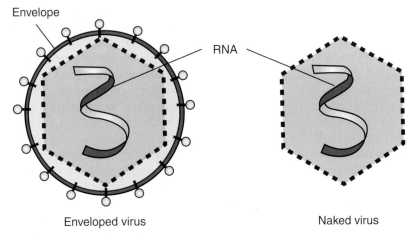

Figure 11-1 Enveloped and nonenveloped (naked) virus particles.

viruses, such as feline infectious peritonitis virus, feline leukemia virus, and canine distemper virus, are surrounded by a lipid envelope. This envelope is fairly easily destroyed by many disinfectants, rendering the virus harmless and unable to infect cells. Thus *enveloped viruses* are much easier to kill with disinfecting agents than unenveloped (naked) viruses such as feline distemper virus or parvoviruses (Figure 11-1). Knowledge of a microorganism's inherent resistance or susceptibility to disinfecting agents is an important consideration in the selection of an appropriate disinfectant.

The environment in which the disinfecting agent is used influences its efficacy. Some otherwise excellent agents may be inactivated by dirt or organic material such as pus, blood, and cellular debris, necessitating a thorough cleaning of the site before application of the agent. The presence of organic material in small crevices of a hospital surface (surgical table, counter top, even surgical instruments) can provide a barrier to even the strongest disinfectant. Certain instruments, such as endoscopes, are notoriously difficult to clean completely and may retain pathogens in microscopic cracks and crevices. If a recurrence of infections occurs in a hospital environment, the presence of organic material reservoirs usually plays a major role in the cause.

Thorough cleansing of the site or surface is always prudent; however, technicians should know which disinfectants function poorly if cleansing is not properly performed. Some disinfectants are inactivated by soap or heavily mineralized ("hard") water. In these situations, special attention must be paid to thorough rinsing and preparation of the site after initial cleansing. Without knowledge of these special limitations, the veterinary technician could select a disinfectant of little value in a particular circumstance.

Antiseptics applied to living tissue must be properly diluted and thoroughly rinsed after they have produced their beneficial effect. Failure to do so may result in an unacceptable level of absorption of the antiseptic and the subsequent appearance of toxic signs. The same is true for disinfectants used on surfaces or instruments that are then placed in contact with the animal. For example, failing to rinse disinfected endotracheal tubes properly has been reported to result in local tissue reaction and even systemic toxicosis.

As illustrated by the above examples, the limitations and precautions of the products clearly require the veterinary technician to take the time to become familiar with the needs of their particular veterinary environment so that patient care is not compromised and money is not wasted on an agent that will be ineffective.

TYPES OF DISINFECTING AGENTS

ALCOHOLS

Ethyl alcohol and isopropyl alcohol are among the most common antiseptics applied to skin. Alcohol's main mechanism of action is denaturing (altering) either the pathogen's surface proteins or essential metabolic proteins needed by the pathogen to survive. *Solutions of 70% alcohol are most commonly used to disinfect surgical sites, injection sites, and rectal thermometers.* Advantages of alcohol include its low cost, general lack of toxicity when applied topically, and bactericidal activity against gram-positive and gram-negative bacteria. However, technicians should be aware that alcohol is ineffective against bacterial spores. In addition, alcohol must be applied in sufficient quantities and remain in contact with the site for several seconds to be effective against bacteria (several minutes for fungi). Therefore a cursory swipe with an alcohol-soaked swab on an animal's skin, especially if the skin is encrusted with dirt or feces, does little to disinfect an injection site.

Only enveloped viruses are susceptible to the virucidal effects of alcohol. Because alcohol does not penetrate dirt or feces, technicians should be aware of the potential for transmission of enteric (intestinal) viruses such as parvovirus if fecal debris is not adequately removed from a rectal thermometer or fecal loop.

Unlike some other antiseptics, alcohol should not be applied to open wounds because it causes pain and may also facilitate survival of pathogens. Open wounds usually contain a serum exudate that is rich in protein. Alcohol denatures the structure of this protein, causing it to form a superficial barrier, or *coagulum* (Figure 11-2). This coagulum may seal in or protect underlying bacteria, thereby preventing topical disinfectants from reaching the organisms. The infection could then spread to underlying tissues.

Repeated application of alcohol to intact skin, whether as an antiseptic or a vehicle for other compounds, removes some of the skin's lipid component, resulting in drying. Animals may develop dry skin, pruritus (itchiness), or flaky skin after repeated alcohol application.

Because alcohols are not as effective at cleaning sites or dissolving and removing organic material, alcohols are generally effective only if dirt and organic material are removed from the skin before application. Alcohol should

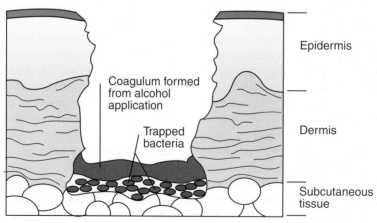

Coagulum formed from alcohol application

Trapped bacteria

Epidermis

Dermis

Subcutaneous tissue

Figure 11-2 Application of alcohol to an open wound can create a coagulum, trapping bacteria beneath it.

be selected as an antiseptic only if (1) the site is clean, (2) the microorganisms present are susceptible to alcohol, and (3) the alcohol is applied in enough quantity to keep the area moist for a sufficient time. Failure to follow these guidelines results in incomplete disinfection and contamination by microorganisms.

CHLORINE COMPOUNDS

Chlorine compounds belong to a larger group of compounds known as *halogens*. Chlorine kills the vegetative forms of bacteria, algae, and fungi by denaturing proteins and chemically reacting with essential enzyme systems needed by the pathogen. In addition to these agents, chlorine also kills both enveloped and unenveloped viruses. Therefore chlorine is one of the few disinfectants effective against parvovirus. As with most other disinfectants, chlorine is not effective against bacterial spores.

Chlorine disinfectants are most commonly available as sodium hypochlorite (Clorox). It is inexpensive and easily obtained. As might be expected, contact with high concentrations of chlorine compounds can cause bleaching and deterioration in fabric. Chlorine is also corrosive to most metals except high-quality stainless steel. Repeated chlorine application can result in pitted or damaged metal tabletops, which can then provide reservoirs for debris accumulation and proliferation of pathogens. The pungent vapor of chlorine compounds can irritate the eyes and other exposed mucous membranes if the compounds are used in a poorly ventilated area. Failure to rinse a chlorine-disinfected surface on which an animal subsequently rests can easily result in skin irritation.

Although chlorine is the most commonly used disinfectant for fighting enteric viruses such as parvovirus, when in contact with organic material such as feces, blood, and pus, the free chlorine combines with the organic material, significantly reducing the availability of chlorine to react with the pathogen. Therefore any site for chlorine disinfection should be thoroughly cleaned before application of chlorine compounds. In addition, the chlorine solution should remain in contact with the site for several minutes to ensure destruction of pathogens.

Color-fast bleaches do not contain sodium hypochlorite but instead contain concentrated hydrogen peroxide. Despite its effervescent foaming when applied to a wound, hydrogen peroxide has minimal bactericidal activity and is considered to be potentially cytotoxic. Therefore common bleach and color-fast bleaches should not be confused as being similar products.

IODINE COMPOUNDS AND IODOPHORS

Iodine compounds and iodophors are most commonly used as topical antiseptics before surgical procedures or for disinfection of tissue. Iodine compounds are also classified as halogens. An iodophor is a combination of molecular iodine and a carrier molecule that releases the iodine over time, prolonging the antimicrobial activity. The most common iodophor is iodine complexed with polyvinyl pyrrolidine, a combination more commonly known as povidone-iodine.

When combined with a detergent, iodophors are often referred to as surgical *scrubs*. Surgical scrubs are designed to clean dirty surgical sites while providing some low-level disinfection. In contrast to the scrubs, iodophor solutions and products classified as iodine solutions or *tinctures* do not contain detergent and therefore do not have any particular ability to remove organic material and debris. Aqueous solutions, which contain iodine dissolved in water, and tincture of iodine, which is iodine in an alcohol solution, both have higher concentrations of free iodine available for microbicidal activity than the iodophor (povidone-iodine) form. However, both preparations are considered potentially more irritating and cytotoxic.

Iodine and higher concentrations of iodophors are bactericidal, virucidal, protozoacidal, and fungicidal. For example, these topical agents are quite effective against the dermatophytes that cause ringworm. Iodine is potentially effective against bacterial spores if the iodine solution remains moist and in contact with the site for more than 15 minutes. Iodophors are considered less effective because of the relatively lower concentration of available iodine at any given moment. Overall, iodine can be inactivated by organic material, especially blood, but it is not inactivated by organic material quite as readily as chlorines are.

Although concentrated iodine solutions or tinctures can be irritating to tissue, iodophor compounds are generally not irritating when properly used. However, proper use means that the technician must distinguish between an iodophor scrub and an iodophor solution when applying an iodophor. In circumstances where the iodine is needed inside the body (e.g., in an abscess site), presence of the scrub soap is not appropriate and a solution without detergent must be used. Conversely, the detergent in surgical scrubs plays an important role in cleansing the skin before surgery. Neither form should be used in the peritoneal cavity, and high concentrations of iodine should be avoided on denuded skin because of the potential for significant irritation and systemic absorption. Because some iodine and iodophor preparations exist in concentrated forms, technicians should always check the container label to see whether dilution of the product is required before applying it to living tissue. Although less corrosive to inanimate surfaces than chlorine compounds, higher concentrations of iodine compounds can also be corrosive to metal if left in contact for an extended period.

CHLORHEXIDINE

Chlorhexidine, a member of a class of antiseptics known as biguanides, is one of the most commonly used disinfectant and antiseptic compounds in veterinary medicine. Chlorhexidine is used for a variety of purposes, including cleaning cages, treating teat infections in cattle, and maintaining oral hygiene in companion animals. Its wide range of uses is likely related to its low tissue irritation and its virucidal, bactericidal (both gram-positive and gram-negative), and fungicidal properties. Some authors, however, state that the virucidal and fungicidal activities of chlorhexidine are limited.

Chlorhexidine remains more active in the presence of organic material, including blood, than the halogen compounds (chlorine and iodine), but thorough cleansing of the application site is still recommended for it to achieve maximal effectiveness. Chlorhexidine may be inactivated by anionic detergents, but less so by nonionic soaps. Detergents and soaps are typically identified on the side of their containers if they are anionic, cationic, or nonionic products. Regardless of the type of soap or detergent used to clean a surface, thorough rinsing is always a good policy before application of chlorhexidine. Hard water (mineralized water) and saline solutions may cause precipitation; however, the precipitation does not appear to significantly reduce the antimicrobial activity.

Chlorhexidine binds to the outer surface of the skin and appears to have some residual activity for up to 24 hours if left in contact with the site. Additionally, chlorhexidine also binds to the surface of the oral mucous membranes and the teeth; hence it has been marketed as an oral antiseptic to be used in conjunction with dental procedures.

The veterinary technician should be careful when applying chlorhexidine to open wounds because many concentrations of chlorhexidine are toxic to fibroblasts (one of the important cells involved with the healing process). When applied to intact skin, chlorhexidine has minimal tissue irritation.

Some discussion still exists regarding the potential ototoxicity of chlorhexidine after instillation of chlorhexidine into the middle ear. Therefore aggressive use of chlorhexidine may warrant some caution. Some brands of chlorhexidine warn against using the compound on cats and kittens, whereas others do not have such a warning. Because both ototoxic and adverse effects in kittens have been identified with chlorhexidine, the veterinary technician should be aware of these potential side effects even if they are not commonly observed.

GLUTARALDEHYDE

Glutaraldehyde is a chemical sterilizer with a wide spectrum of activity against bacteria, viruses, fungi, and bacterial spores. It is generally not inactivated by organic debris and is effective in the presence of hard water. However, its effectiveness can be influenced by the pH of the environment in which it is placed. For example, glutaraldehyde is sporicidal at an alkaline pH (above 8) but generally not at an acidic pH.

Glutaraldehyde has become more commonly used because of its ability to kill bacteria that normally protect themselves by generating biofilm. Because of its effectiveness, glutaraldehyde is used to sterilize equipment that cannot be heat sterilized (e.g., endoscopic equipment). Glutaraldehyde is chemically related to formaldehyde, the noxious smelling preservative most often associated with older preserved animal or tissue specimens. Glutaraldehyde shares some of the tissue irritation and corrosion characteristics of formaldehyde; therefore the technician should take precautions when using this compound (e.g., safety goggles and a well-ventilated working area). Any equipment disinfected with glutaraldehyde must be thoroughly rinsed before use in or on living tissue.

QUATERNARY AMMONIUM COMPOUNDS

Quaternary ammonium compounds, or "quats," are used in veterinary medicine to disinfect the surfaces of inanimate objects. One quaternary ammonium compound used in veterinary medicine is benzalkonium chloride. Quaternary ammonium compounds are effective against gram-positive bacteria, but they are ineffective against bacterial spores and have poor efficacy against fungi and gram-negative bacteria. Although quaternary ammonium compounds can destroy enveloped viruses,

they are ineffective against unenveloped viruses such as parvovirus. They act rapidly at the site of application and normally are not irritating to the skin or corrosive to metals.

Quaternary ammonium compounds readily bind to organic materials, rendering them less effective against many pathogenic microorganisms within or under such debris. Thus thorough cleansing of a site before application of a quaternary ammonium compound is essential for adequate reduction of microbial populations. Because quaternary ammonium compounds are inactivated by detergents and soaps, the cleaned application site must be rinsed to remove all soap or detergent residue before the disinfectant is applied. Finally, hard water reduces the antimicrobial activity of quaternary ammonium compounds. Therefore proper cleansing, rinsing, and drying the site before application of the quaternary ammonium compound are essential to maintain its effectiveness.

Although quaternary ammonium compounds are generally low in toxicity and nonirritating to skin, prolonged contact may irritate epithelial surfaces. Use of these compounds in aviaries or other avian confinement operations without proper rinsing has resulted in damage to the mouth, toes, eyes, and respiratory tract of birds kept in these confines. A similar situation could occur in dogs and cats if a highly concentrated industrial quaternary ammonium compound is applied but not adequately rinsed from the corners of cages or horizontal surfaces with poor drainage.

OTHER DISINFECTING AGENTS

A veterinary technician may come across many other disinfecting agents in veterinary practice or research. The ones listed in this text constitute the majority of compounds routinely used. However, the veterinary technician must understand the benefits and drawbacks of any disinfecting or antiseptic agent used in the veterinary facility to avoid contamination of surgical sites, instruments, or hospital equipment. The following agents are occasionally used or are used less now than they were previously. Because they still are used, and sometimes used inappropriately, the veterinary technician should be aware of them.

Peroxides are sometimes used to debride (remove) dead, injured, or necrotic tissue and kill bacteria. Hydrogen peroxide is weakly bactericidal and may do more good by debriding devitalized ("without life") tissue to make the environment less receptive to pathogen growth. Although the foaming action of oxidizing agents in wounds is dramatic, these compounds are not virucidal and may actually damage tissue that is healthy or marginally viable. For that reason, hydrogen peroxide has fallen out of favor as an antiseptic. Note that although hydrogen peroxide as a liquid antiseptic is largely ineffective, as a disinfectant used in special sterilizers it is classified as a high-level disinfectant effective against many microorganisms, including spores. Peroxide sterilization may have a role as a potential replacement for the more toxic ethylene oxide gas sterilization method.

A product was introduced in 2003 to the United States veterinary market that was composed of the peroxide compound potassium peroxymonosulfate mixed with a surfactant, organic acids, and buffers. The manufacturer claims that it is virucidal—including against nonenveloped viruses—bactericidal, and fungicidal even in the presence of organic material and hard water. The powder formulation (Trifectant, EVSCO Pharmaceuticals, Buena, N.J.) is said to have no environmental residue problems and has low toxicity if applied topically or swallowed. Additional information is available from the manufacturer.

Phenols are a part of a larger group of related compounds found in mouthwashes, surface disinfectants, and many household disinfectants such as Lysol, pine oil, and similar cleansers. Phenol compounds are quite effective against gram-positive bacteria but generally ineffective against gram-negative bacteria, viruses, fungi, and spores. Phenols are not as easily inactivated by organic material as detergents, quaternary ammonium compounds, and chlorine solutions. However, because phenols are more toxic if taken into the body and because they have a slower onset of action than povidone-iodine or chlorhexidine, they are not commonly used as antiseptics for preparing surgical sites.

Although most household phenols are generally safe if used on inanimate surfaces, prolonged contact with concentrated solutions may damage the skin. For example, bird perches disinfected with phenols may cause lesions on the feet of birds. Dermal ulceration has been reported in reptiles kept in cages that are consistently disinfected with phenols. Dogs may develop skin lesions when runs are cleaned with phenols and not adequately rinsed. Ingestion of phenols can result in severe liver damage.

Hexachlorophene is a phenol surgical scrub that has largely been phased out because of its suspected neurotoxicity (damage to the nervous system) and teratogenic effects (birth defects) in human health care professionals who came in contact with high concentrations on a regular basis. Do not confuse hexachlorophene with chlorhexidine; chlorhexidine is not a phenol compound.

Ethylenediamine tetraacetic acid and Tris buffer are two products that can be compounded and used together to irrigate ear infections or wounds or fistulas infected with *Pseudomonas*. They are considered effective against a fairly narrow spectrum of gram-negative bacteria and *Staphylococcus aureus*.

Acetic acid is sometimes used as a 0.25% solution to kill *Pseudomonas* organisms as well as a variety of other gram-positive and gram-negative bacteria. Vinegar solution is primarily acetic acid and is sometimes recommended for yeast infections in otitis externa (ear inflammation caused by bacterial or yeast infections). Because better products are available that have greater efficacy and less tissue irritation, acetic acid is not often recommended today for use in veterinary medicine.

Box 11-1 Drug Categories and Names

Alcohols	Quaternary ammonium compounds
Chlorine compounds	Peroxides and oxidants
Iodine and iodophors	Phenols (hexachlorophene)
Chlorhexidine (biguanides)	Ethylenediamine tetraacetic acid and Tris buffer
Glutaraldehyde	Acetic acid

RECOMMENDED READING

Boothe HW: Disinfectants, antiseptics, and related germicides. In Boothe DM, editor: *Small animal clinical pharmacology and therapeutics,* Philadelphia, 2001, WB Saunders.

Clem MF: Sterilization and antiseptics. In Auer JA, editor: *Equine surgery,* Philadelphia, 1992, WB Saunders.

Dwyer RM: Environmental disinfection to control equine infectious diseases, *Vet Clin North Am Equine Pract* 20:531-542, 2004.

Greene CE: Environmental factors in infectious disease. In Greene CE, editor: *Infectious diseases of the dog and cat,* ed 2, Philadelphia, 1998, WB Saunders.

Justine AJ: *Role of technicians: nosocomial infections.* In Proceedings of the Northeast Veterinary Conference, North Grafton, MA, 2004.

Lemarie RJ, Hosgood G: Antiseptics and disinfectants in small animal practice, *Compendium of Continuing Education* 17:1339, 1995.

Lozier SM: Topical wound therapy. In Harari J, editor: *Surgical complications and wound healing in small animal practice,* Philadelphia, 1993, WB Saunders.

Phillips MA, Vasseur PB, Gregory CR: Chlorhexidine diacetate versus povidone-iodine for preoperative preparation of the skin, *J Am Anim Hosp Assoc* 27:105, 1991.

Rochar MC, Mann FA, Berg JN: Evaluation of a one-step surgical preparation technique in dogs, *J Am Vet Med Assoc* 203:392, 1993.

Smith BP: *Design and implementation of comprehensive infection control programs.* In Proceedings of ACVIM Forum, Minneapolis, MN, 2004.

Swaim SF, Riddel KP, Geiger DL: Evaluation of surgical scrub and antiseptic solutions for surgical preparation of canine paws, *J Am Vet Med Assoc* 198:1941, 1991.

Self-Assessment

REVIEW QUESTIONS

Fill in the following blanks with the correct item from the Key Terms list.

1. _____ chemical agents that kill or prevent growth of pathogens on living tissues.

2. _____ antiseptics or disinfectants that reduce the number of microorganisms to a "safe" level.

3. _____ chemical agents that kill or prevent growth on inanimate objects.

4. _____ means "kills microbial spores."

5. _____ infection acquired during a period of hospitalization.

6. _____ means "kills protozoa."

7. _____ glycocalyx coating over surgical implants that prevents antiseptics from reaching the bacteria.

8. _____ means "kills viruses."

9. _____ antiseptics or disinfectants that destroy all microorganisms.

10. _____ means that something is capable of killing cells.

11. _____ type of virus that is difficult to kill with most antiseptics.

12. _____ means "kills fungi."

13. _____ antiseptic combined with a soap.

14. _____ antiseptic (such as iodine) dissolved in an alcohol solution.

15. _____ means "kills bacteria."

Fill in the following blanks with the correct drug described in Box 11-1.

16. _____ one of the most commonly used antiseptic/disinfectants in veterinary medicine; precipitates in hard water; should only be diluted with distilled water; can delay healing by inhibiting fibroblasts.

17. _____ type of disinfectant commonly found in hand soaps, mouthwash, and Lysol; members of this group have been reported to be neurotoxic and teratogenic in human beings with prolonged contact.

18. _____ common antiseptic found in most surgical scrubs; is inactivated by organic material but not to the extent of the chlorine compounds; exists also as a tincture and as solutions used as antiseptics.

19. _____ effective against naked viruses (parvovirus); potent odor; corrosive.

20. _____ virucidal against enveloped viruses, but not naked viruses such as parvovirus; is inactivated by soaps; benzalkonium chloride is example.

21. _____ must remain in contact with site for several minutes to produce bactericidal effect; not effective against parvovirus; forms a coagulum on top of oozing wounds that can trap bacteria; inexpensive.

22. _____ active antiseptic ingredient is combined with a carrier such as polyvinyl pyrrolidine that releases it over time.

23. _____ sodium hypochlorite is the ingredient found in most household versions.

24. _____ disinfectant used to sterilize equipment that cannot be heat sterilized because of its effectiveness against bacteria that produce biofilm.

25. Indicate below whether the following statements are true or false.

   A. Color-fast bleaches have chlorine as their active ingredient.

   B. A microbiostatic agent is appropriate to disinfect the surgery table because they tend to be less corrosive than microbicidal agents.

   C. The vegetative form of bacteria is more susceptible to disinfectants and antiseptics than the spore form of bacteria.

   D. Generally applying an antiseptic to a surgery site before cleaning the site of dirt and debris is better so the bacteria in the debris can be killed before cleaning.

   E. Swabbing an injection site and then administering the injection does not provide sufficient antisepsis.

   F. Phenols are components of common household cleansers such as Lysol. Therefore soaking a bird perch in a phenol compound or disinfecting a reptile cage with spray-on phenol disinfectant should be effective in controlling bacterial growth on these objects.

   G. Hexachlorophene and chlorhexidine are similar compounds.

   H. Ounce per ounce, iodophors tend to have less irritation and last longer than free iodine compounds, but they do not achieve as high a concentration of iodine at the disinfecting as iodine compounds in the free form.

APPLICATION QUESTIONS

1. You are reading the insert of a new disinfectant and you see a statement that identifies the disinfectant as a cytotoxic agent. This sounds good because that means it will kill more things, and that is what you want in a disinfectant. Or is it?

2. The standard procedure in your veterinary clinic is to use alcohol to clean a rectal thermometer used on dogs with parvovirus as a means of disinfection. Critique this method of disinfection.

3. Chlorine disinfection of a parvovirus-contaminated metal surface (such as an examination table or stainless steel cage) needs time but should not be used for too long. What is the truth behind this statement?

4. A chlorine residue is left on a concrete or nonmetal surface where a parvovirus-infected animal is being housed. Will the residue destroy parvovirus that lands on it?

5. Can color-fast bleaches be used to control parvovirus?

6. Many antiseptics and disinfectants come packaged in concentrated solutions that have to be diluted. Why is distilled water or nonionized water better than regular tap water for diluting some disinfecting compounds?

7. Rinsing soap from a site of antisepsis is also important before application of the antiseptic agent. Why?

8. Why is chlorhexidine supposed to be good for skin, oral, and dental procedures?

Antiparasitics

outline

key terms

acetylcholine
acetylcholinesterase
adulticide
anthelmintic
anticestodal
antinematodal
antiprotozoal
antitrematodal
cestocides
coccidiostats
delayed neurotoxicity
ectoparasites
emboli
endectocides

endoparasites
γ-aminobutyric acid
glutamate
hemoptysis
insect development
   inhibitors
insect growth regulators
infective third-stage larvae
insecticides
intima (arterial)
juvenile hormone mimics
macrocyclic ring
microfilaremia
microfilaricide

monoamine oxidase
muscarinic receptors
mydriasis
nicotinic receptors
ovicidal
P-glycoprotein
proglottids
pruritus
selective toxicity
SLUDDE
synergist
taeniacides
vermicide
vermifuge

1. The terminology used to describe antiparasitics

2. The mechanisms by which commonly used antiparasitics work

3. Precautions that apply to specific antiparasitics

Drugs and chemicals for use against intestinal parasites, fleas, ticks, heartworms, and other parasites constitute the widest array of products available to veterinary professionals and the general public. Not only are prescription medications available, but many of these compounds are also found as nonprescription products in drugstores, grocery stores, and general retail stores. Thus the veterinary professional needs to keep abreast of all the new products brought out and marketed to the veterinarian and be aware of the wide assortment of questions and issues that come from the direct-to-consumer marketing that many drug companies have used. Box 12-1, listing antiparasitic drugs, can be found at the end of this chapter.

The veterinary professional needs to understand that many products have similar ingredients or combinations of ingredients have similar mechanisms of action, and in some cases may simply be modifications of existing products with which the veterinary professional is already familiar. Part of the process of comprehending the seemingly endless number of proprietary antiparasitic product trade names is to be familiar with the shorter list of nonproprietary names of compounds. Second, understanding which compounds, as may be hinted by the similarity of their nonproprietary names, have similar characteristics is also important (e.g., ivermectin and selamectin, or fenbendazole and oxibendazole).

IMPORTANCE OF THE VETERINARY TECHNICIAN'S ROLE

Parasites can be found in almost any environment regardless of how clean that environment may appear to the untrained eye. Internal and external parasites produce disease in the animals they infect and may have the potential to infect human beings (e.g., ascarid larvae migrate through human body organs if the eggs are accidentally ingested) or to transmit diseases to human beings (e.g., Lyme disease is transmitted to human beings by the tick). For that reason, the veterinary technician plays an important role in educating and protecting the general public from inadvertent exposure to diseases caused or carried by common parasites found in and on veterinary patients.

The veterinarian professional can also help clients sort out the information they hear about what is best for their pets or livestock business. Aggressive marketing groups have learned that by directly "educating" the general public about what they should ask their veterinarian to do, they put pressure on veterinarians to purchase their particular antiparasitic product for sale to their clients who "demand" it. In addition to the direct-to-consumer marketing, the advent of mail-order availability of veterinary products more typically dispensed under a veterinarian's direction bypasses the veterinarian and one of the key safeguards against inappropriate antiparasitic use. For example, pet owners who are immunocompromised from being chemotherapy patients, AIDS patients, transplant recipients, and so forth can be highly susceptible to zoonotic transmission of parasites. If they purchase an antiparasitic product that does not completely remove the pet's parasite or is unable to break the parasite life cycle by itself, they are putting themselves at risk for exposure to the parasite because of a false belief that they have eliminated the problem.

Given the current environment and availability of veterinary products, aggressively educating clients to prevent unfortunate outcomes from the inappropriate use of these drugs becomes increasingly important for veterinary professionals. The veterinary technician is often delegated, or falls into, the role of primary educator in these situations. Therefore today's veterinary technician really needs to have a solid understanding of antiparasitic products.

Because of the quickly changing market and product development of antiparasitic drugs, the information in this text reflects contemporary veterinary practice as of 2005. To remain up to date with current principles of veterinary antiparasitic practice, the veterinary professional must constantly review journal articles and informational brochures that describe and assess the effectiveness of antiparasitic products. Indeed, between the time this text has been written and when it is published, additional veterinary products will have been brought to market. Therefore the most important information to be extracted from this text is the basic concepts behind the drugs, how they work, and how they can be safely applied. This foundation information will provide veterinary professionals with a knowledge base from which they can assess the multitude of new products released every year.

PRINCIPLES
OF ANTIPARASITIC USE

Decisions about purchasing flea sprays, deworming medications, and other antiparasitic drugs for the veterinary practice are often based on an aggressive marketing pitch, attractive incentive offers, or comfort with a product that has always worked in the past. Unfortunately, this can sometimes result in additional expense to the practice and the animal owner for a product that may only be minimally better or as equally effective as another compound. Therefore, when selecting an appropriate antiparasitic compound for use, the following characteristics of the *ideal parasiticide* should be considered:

- *Selective toxicity:* The chemical should be highly toxic to the parasite but should have little effect on the host's tissue and the person applying or administering the product.
- *Does not induce resistance in the target parasite:* With repeated exposure to the same parasiticide, many external and internal parasites can develop resistance to certain products. The ideal compound would not favor development of resistance and thus would avoid evolutionary selection for a "superparasite" that is incapable of being killed by common antiparasitics.
- *Economical*: An economical yet effective product is most desirable for treatment of parasitism. Economics is one of the most critical factors in selection of a parasitic control agent in livestock production. Economics plays a comparatively smaller role in equine or small animal parasite control.
- *Effective against all parasite stages with one application:* Ideally, internal antiparasitic drugs should kill all the adult parasites as well as any migrating larvae or immature forms with a single treatment. Likewise, external antiparasitics should be effective with one treatment and convenient to reapply because fleas, flies, lice, and mites usually cannot be totally eradicated from the environment, and reinfestation is likely to occur. Because of the life cycle of the parasite, a single application of an antiparasitic drug is often not effective by itself, even though such a single-use application would be ideal.

Other desirable characteristics include a fragrant odor or lack of offensive odor (external antiparasitics) and environmental safety. No single product incorporates all these ideal features, although over the years products have become generally safer for the animal owner, the animal, and the environment. Still veterinary professionals should understand the specific needs of the animal and client, the environment in which the product will be used, and the characteristics of the antiparasitic product to make a rational, economical, and safe recommendation.

As a general rule, internal and external antiparasitic agents should be used with caution in old, young, debilitated, or pregnant animals. Certain antiparasitics may also be risky to use in selected groups of animals. For example, collies are considered a high-risk group for ivermectin. Because of the idiosyncrasies of each antiparasitic drug, the veterinary professional should become very familiar with the particular high-risk groups for all antiparasitic compounds used in a particular practice.

Just as the best antibiotic is not effective unless it reaches the infection site, parasiticides are only effective when most of the drug reaches the location of the parasite. If the parasite is free living within the lumen of the intestinal tract, an orally administered antiparasitic need not be absorbed systemically to be effective. In contrast, if the intestinal parasite's life cycle includes a stage of arrested development (slowed metabolism) or larvae migration is throughout the body, a single dose of a drug that kills only the adult worms within the intestinal tract will not eliminate the problem. In this example larvae of the adult intestinal parasite would eventually migrate back to the intestinal tract and mature to new adult worms, causing a recurrence of the clinical signs. Therefore the veterinary professional must understand the features of the parasite's life cycle and where the parasiticide acts on that life cycle. One of the major reasons for failure of antiparasitic treatment is misunderstanding the limitations of the activity of the antiparasitic compound against various stages of the parasite's life cycle.

Because many of today's antiparasitic drugs require either specific locations for application or specific intervals between doses to be safe and fully effective, client education is essential for successful antiparasitic treatment of internal or external parasites. For example, failure of a client to give a medication at the prescribed time may allow parasites to pass through a critically vulnerable phase of the life cycle without the parasiticide being present, thus resulting in failure to eliminate the parasite. Failure to properly educate a client about removal of animal feces containing parasite eggs may result in an increased risk for reinfection from intestinal parasites from the contaminated environment.

Today's veterinary clients are savvier about their animal's health; therefore explaining the reasoning behind the instructions given the clients to perform certain control procedures is often necessary. An appropriate, clear explanation for the reasons behind the control measure is more likely to ensure client compliance with the instructions and thus increase the odds of breaking the parasite life cycle and controlling the parasitic infection.

INTERNAL ANTIPARASITICS

Although many discussions about parasites break them down into internal or external parasites, many drugs today are capable of killing both. These types of drugs are called *endectocides,* so named for their ability to kill some *endoparasites* (internally living parasites) and some *ectoparasites* (externally living parasites). This section discusses drugs used to kill or control parasites that reside primarily inside the body; however, some of the drugs will also be discussed in the external antiparasitic section.

A walk down any drugstore or supermarket pet product aisle reveals that products for treating intestinal worms in dogs and cats constitute a multimillion dollar industry. This is also true of the antiparasitic products available for livestock and horses at feed stores, farming implement stores, and tack shops. For that reason, veterinary professionals are often asked questions concerning safe use of these nonprescription or over the counter (OTC) products. As previously emphasized, properly educating clients about antiparasitics not necessarily sold by a veterinary practice is also part of the veterinary professional's responsibility to the animal's health.

TERMINOLOGY USED TO DESCRIBE INTERNAL ANTIPARASITICS

Various terms are used to describe internal antiparasitics. Veterinary technicians should be familiar with these terms to better understand the effects and limitations of a particular product. *Anthelmintic* is a general term used to describe compounds that kill various types of helminth internal parasites or worms. A *vermicide* is an anthelmintic that kills the worm, as opposed to a *vermifuge*, which only paralyzes the worm and often results in passage of live worms in the stool.

Antinematodal compounds are anthelmintics used to treat infections of nematodes, or roundworms. Nematodes include hookworms, ascarids, whipworms, strongyles, and almost any worm that is circular or round when it is looked at in cross-section (as opposed to tapeworms, which are sometimes called flatworms because of their flatter cross-section appearance). Unfortunately, because one antinematodal drug does not kill every type of roundworm, the veterinary technician must be familiar with the spectrum of antiparasitic activity for each of the products they dispense.

Anticestodal compounds or *cestocides* treat infections of cestodes, which are tapeworms or segmented flatworms. Anticestodals are sometimes referred to as *taeniacides,* an older term that takes its name from the *Taenia* species of tapeworm. Again, a particular cesticidal drug may not be effective against all species of tapeworms commonly encountered in veterinary practice. Therefore the veterinary technician should carefully read the package insert to determine the drug's spectrum of anticestodal activity.

Antitrematodal compounds treat infections of trematodes, which are flukes or unsegmented flatworms, including *Paragonimus, Fasciola,* and *Dicrocoelium* parasites. *Antiprotozoal* compounds treat infections of protozoa, which are single-celled organisms such as *Coccidia, Giardia,* and *Toxoplasma. Coccidiostats* are antiprotozoal drugs that specifically inhibit the growth of coccidia. Many antibiotics also have antiprotozoal properties (e.g., sulfonamides, quinolones).

Many of the parasiticides today have a broad spectrum of activity. Drugs that are antinematodal may also be anticestodal and have additional effectiveness against external parasites. Thus the classification of drugs as antinematodal versus anticestodal, or internal parasiticide versus external parasiticide has blurred the past few years. As previously mentioned, endectocides are effective against internal and external parasites. Thus many of these products mentioned in one category (antinematodal, anticestodal, internal parasiticide, external parasiticide) will be mentioned in multiple sections.

ANTINEMATODALS

AVERMECTINS AND MILBEMYCIN GROUP (THE MACROLIDES)

Thanks to the 1976 discovery that a *Streptomyces* bacterium growing near a golf course in Japan possessed a broad range of parasiticide and insecticide properties, a group of new, safer compounds with broad spectra of activity has become available to the veterinarian. This group includes the avermectins (ivermectin, selamectin, doramectin, and eprinomectin) and the milbemycins (milbemycin oxime and moxidectin). Interestingly, the milbemycins had been discovered and were being used against agricultural pest insects for at least 3 years before the avermectins were discovered in Japan. It was only when it was discovered that the structurally similar avermectins had excellent activity against a wide variety of internal parasites that the milbemycins were then developed for use as anthelmintics. Thus, even though they were discovered first, milbemycin did not hit the veterinary market until well after the first avermectins, specifically the ivermectin products, were already well established as internal parasiticides.

To keep the multitude of compounds and their uses straight, the veterinary professional must remember that ivermectin (Heartgard, Ivomec, Eqvalan), selamectin (Revolution), milbemycin (Interceptor, Sentinel), moxidectin (ProHeart, Cydectin for cattle, Quest for horses), doramectin (Dectomax for use in livestock), and eprinomectin (Eprinex for use in cattle) are all structurally similar and have similar mechanisms of action. The *macrocyclic ring* found in each of these compounds gives rise to the collective name for the group as the macrolides or macrocyclic lactones. Thus, when hearing these various terms (macrolides, avermectins, or milbemycins) remember they are all the same familiar set of commonly used veterinary products.

The mechanism of action for all these compounds is primarily through stimulation of a receptor site for the neurotransmitter *glutamate.* Glutamate is an inhibitory neurotransmitter that increases the flow of chloride ions into the neuron. When the glutamate receptor on a chloride channel is stimulated, the chloride influx into the cell changes the neuron's charge away from its depolarization threshold (membrane charge at which the whole neuron fires), making it harder for the neuron to depolarize when stimulated to do so. In parasites, glutamate receptors also mediate a similar inhibiting effect on the parasite's muscles. The net effect of this mechanism is to make the neurons unable to depolarize and the muscles unable to contract, causing paralysis and the subsequent death of the parasite. In some cases, the paralysis of the worm's muscles necessary for feeding results in the worm starving to death. The absence of these glutamate receptors in tapeworms and flukes explains why the macrolides are largely ineffective against most members of these parasite classes.

It was previously thought the receptor of the inhibitory neurotransmitter *γ-aminobutyric acid* (GABA, which is involved with the effect of some tranquilizers like diazepam) played the main role in the macrolide's inhibitory effect in parasites. However, subsequent research published has shown that although an enhanced GABA-mediated inhibitory effect results from these drugs, glutamate is the primary receptor involved with the majority of the drug effect on parasites. The increased GABA receptor effect is still thought to be involved in the toxic effects observed in mammals (e.g., ivermectin toxicosis in collies).

In spite of their broad spectrum of activity against both internal and external parasites, the macrolides are still considered to be among the safest compounds to use in mammals. As previously mentioned, tapeworms and flukes are not readily killed by macrolides because they do not have the glutamate receptors. However, mammals do have glutamate receptors and should theoretically be sensitive to the same paralytic effects of macrolides. The mammalian glutamate receptors in mammals are located within the central nervous system (CNS), safely behind the blood-brain barrier mentioned in Chapter 3. Part of the blood-brain barrier's protective function is the presence of a special protein *(P-glycoprotein)* whose function appears to be to move drugs from the blood-brain barrier cells back into the blood. The net effect of P-glycoprotein, therefore, is to prevent some drugs in the blood from reaching the brain tissue. Animals that are highly sensitive to the effects of macrolides such as ivermectin have been shown to have lower quantities of this P-glycoprotein present, thus increasing the ability of the macrolide parasiticides to penetrate the blood-brain barrier and reach glutamate receptors within the CNS. Certain lines of collies and collie-like breeds appear to be more sensitive to macrolides. However, occasionally individual animals of noncollie breeds may also show sensitivity to drugs such as ivermectin, milbemycin, or other macrolide compounds. Toxicosis can occur in any mammal if sufficient doses of the macrolide are given and the P-glycoprotein mechanism is overwhelmed.

IVERMECTIN

Ivermectin was the first macrolide to be available for use in veterinary medicine. Its wide spectrum of activity includes everything from heartworms and intestinal parasites to external parasites. In addition veterinarians have used the drug for many extra-label (not approved) applications. It was, and still is, quite common to see ivermectin listed in the veterinary literature as an experimental or extra-label treatment for internal and external parasites in a wide variety of exotic animals, wildlife, avian species, and nonconventional household pets (e.g., hedgehogs, snakes, other reptiles). Many dosages also exist for use of ivermectin in dogs and cats to treat extra-label parasites such as demodectic mange, ear mites, microfilariae of the heartworm, and a wide variety of less frequently seen internal parasites. As long as the drug is not used in animals intended for use as human food, and as long as the veterinarian applies the Food and Drug Administration (FDA) guidelines for use of the drug in an extra-label manner, these uses are mostly considered prudent and acceptable.

Ivermectin is now being incorporated with other anthelmintics to produce parasiticides with a wider spectrum of activity. For example, Heartgard-Plus is a combination of ivermectin, for prevention of heartworm disease, and pyrantel pamoate, an effective drug for control of intestinal ascarids (roundworms). Many more combination drugs are expected to be seen in the future. By understanding what each drug in the combination does separately, the veterinary technician can more easily understand the spectrum and potential side effects of these combination drugs.

Ivermectin toxicosis in collies and other dogs has been widely documented in the veterinary literature. The sensitivity to ivermectin and other macrolides appears to be caused by a genetically transmitted, autosomal recessive trait. When this genetic trait manifests itself, it is apparently from a genetic deficiency of the P-glycoprotein mechanism in the blood-brain barrier, resulting in a lessened ability to keep the avermectins from passing from the blood into the CNS. Although beagles exposed to a single dose of 2 mg/kg of ivermectin typically do not show adverse reactions, doses as low as 0.1 mg/kg have produced toxicosis in collies, with a dose of 0.2 mg/kg producing death. Cats do not appear to be especially sensitive to ivermectin.

Because all avermectins act as inhibitory compounds (they inhibit the neuron or muscle and keep it from depolarizing) animals with ivermectin toxicosis show signs associated with CNS depression. Typically signs begin with sedation progressing to ataxia (wobbly, "drunken" gait) and, if sufficient exposure has occurred, to stupor and coma. *Mydriasis* (pupil dilation) and apparently loss of menace reflex (moving the hand toward the eye to check for reflex avoidance) suggest either blindness or inability of the pupils to respond to light. Vomiting and salivation are also frequently observed in the early stages. Even though the manufacturer of the ivermectin-based Heartgard warns that collie-related breeds should be observed for signs of ivermectin toxicosis for 8 hours after administration of the monthly heartworm preventative, the dose used with this product is well below that which should cause ivermectin toxicosis even

CLINICAL APPLICATION
Ivermectin Toxicosis in Two Australian Shepherds

A 10-month-old male Australian shepherd presented to a veterinary hospital 24 hours after having received 4000 µg of a cattle ivermectin preparation. The dog was reluctant to move, was salivating profusely, had slowed respiration and heart rate, and had a subnormal temperature. On neurologic exam the dog was poorly responsive to stimuli and had head bobbing, facial muscle twitches, and pinpoint, nonresponsive pupils. Reflexes in the limbs were normal to exaggerated. Complete blood count and serum biochemistry profiles were within reference ranges. Based on the history of exposure and clinical signs consistent with CNS depression, including depression of brainstem control centers (respiratory, cardiovascular, temperature), a presumptive diagnosis of ivermectin toxicosis was made.

The dog was treated with supportive care. Intravenous (IV) fluids were given to maintain hydration, ophthalmic ointment was applied to both eyes to prevent drying of the cornea and corneal ulceration formation, supplemental heat was provided to maintain the body temperature, and the dog was turned over every 4 hours to prevent decubital ulcers (pressure sores, or bed sores, on the skin). Glycopyrrolate (an anticholinergic drug) was given to help reverse the low heart rate by reducing the parasympathetic nervous system effect on the heart. Glycopyrrolate was chosen over atropine because atropine penetrates the brain and could produce unwanted side effects in the CNS, whereas glycopyrrolate does not appreciably penetrate the blood-brain barrier.

Unlike drugs that are excreted by the body through the kidney, ivermectin is metabolized and excreted by the liver. Therefore the administration of IV fluids to increase the urine production (diuresis) was not instituted because it would not facilitate the removal of the hepatically eliminated ivermectin.

Over the next 10 days the dog slowly increased motor control. Because the dog was unable to feed itself, a gastrostomy (*gastro*, meaning stomach; *stoma*, meaning hole) tube was placed through the stomach and body wall so food gruel could be placed into the stomach by the tube. By day 8 the dog could stand if helped. Vision returned on day 10. On day 11 the dog was able to walk with a wobbly gait (ataxia) and was sent home with its owners.

The owners reported behavior changes after the dog went home. He became aggressive toward a companion cat, would try to nip the owners, and snapped at objects near his head. These behavior changes had disappeared by the time the dog was returned to the veterinary hospital on day 19 to have the gastrostomy tube removed. At day 19 the dog was clinically normal without any residual neurologic or physical signs.

A 3-year-old, female Australian shepherd also showed similar clinical signs after being fed 7600 µg of an equine ivermectin preparation. In this case the respiratory depression was more profound and, in addition to the other supportive measures, the dog had to be maintained on ventilator-assisted oxygen (positive-pressure ventilation) to keep blood oxygen concentrations within acceptable limits. This dog was on a ventilator until day 11 after ingestion, and eventually recovered 21 days after administration of the ivermectin.

What should be learned from these cases: In both of these cases, the dogs showed signs shortly after being given 167 µg/kg and 340 µg/kg of ivermectin. Small animal heartworm preventative medication typically has approximately 6 µg/kg (0.006 mg/kg) ivermectin. Therefore it would take ingestion or administration of a significant volume of small animal products to achieve the doses administered to these two animals. However, because the ivermectin preparations that were ingested were labeled for use on livestock and horses and thus had relatively high concentrations of the drug, ingestion of only a small volume of product produced severe toxicosis.

The second lesson from this case report is that other breeds besides collies are susceptible to the side effects of ivermectin. Collie-like breeds (e.g., Shetland sheepdogs, Australian shepherds) appear to have the potential to be equally as sensitive to ivermectin (and presumably all macrolide parasiticides) as collies themselves.

Adapted from Hadrick MK, Bunch SE, Kornegay JM: Ivermectin toxicosis in two Australian shepherds, *J Am Vet Med Assoc* 206:1147-1150, 1995.

in the collie breed. Therefore, when toxic cases are reported, they are usually associated with administration of ivermectin in an extra-label manner, usually with a concentrated large animal or equine product.

Finally, the third lesson is that ivermectin has no antidote. The only way an animal with ivermectin toxicosis can survive is if aggressive treatment is used to maintain the body systems: IV fluid to maintain arterial blood pressure, supplemental oxygen for the depressed respiratory system, and additional heat to counteract hypothermia. Remember that decubital ulcers (pressure sores, or bed sores) can become infected with bacteria such as *Pseudomonas,* ultimately resulting in septicemia (bacteria or bacterial toxins in the blood) and death.

The best treatment for ivermectin toxicosis is prevention of it in the first place. The veterinary technician should always educate the client on how to properly dispose of unused ivermectin livestock medications and explain the potential risk to other animals if accidentally ingested or administered.

SELAMECTIN

Selamectin (Revolution) entered the veterinary market after ivermectin and milbemycin oxime. It was targeted as a broad-spectrum endectocide approved for use against several internal and external parasites. Unlike ivermectin, which is available primarily as oral or injectable forms, selamectin was approved as a topical application for control of fleas, ear mites, and prevention of heartworm disease in both dogs and cats. Later, selamectin was also approved for treatment of sarcoptic mange and tick control in dogs and for the treatment and control of intestinal hookworms and roundworms in the cat. Because the drug manufacturer must invest significant time and resources into providing the data and testing to get each indication (use) of the drug approved by the FDA, it is easy to see why the approved range of uses for a

parasiticide is typically much smaller than the range for which it is actually used in an extra-label manner by practicing veterinarians. It also helps explain why a product may be released initially with a limited number of approved uses, and then over time the parasiticide manufacturer announces additional FDA-approved indications.

Just as new indications or uses for a drug are posted by the drug company after the drug has been released into the market, new cautions or warnings may also be released as a result of adverse reactions reported from the thousands of veterinarians and animal owners who are dispensing or using the drug on animals in the field or the real world. For example, in the summer of 2002 the parent company of Revolution announced changes in the label to emphasize the need for caution when using the drug in "sick, debilitated, or underweight animals." In this case the company moved this precautionary statement to a warning level (more significant than a caution) by changing the phrasing from "use with caution" to "do not use..." In addition, they also raised the minimum age of use in cats from 6 weeks to 8 weeks and added a comment that side effects ranging from itching to fever and rarely seizure or death have been reported. These changes illustrate once again how the veterinary professional must keep abreast of new information to adjust treatment protocols to ensure safe use of parasiticides.

LIVESTOCK MACROLIDES: DORAMECTIN AND EPRINOMECTIN

Doramectin (Dectomax) is available as both an injectable and topical "pour-on" approved for use in cattle and swine, whereas eprinomectin (Eprinex) is approved for use as a topical application in cattle. Both products are approved for use against a variety of internal parasite worms, as well as grubs, lice, and mange. Although doramectin is reported to be free of toxic signs in cattle at 25 times the recommended dose, the manufacturer states that use of doramectin in other species may result in severe adverse reactions, including death in dogs. Both drugs have specific indications and restrictions for their use even within cattle species (e.g., restricted use in lactating cattle of a certain age or veal calves). Therefore the veterinary professional should know, and comply with, the restrictions applied to the drugs and should communicate to the livestock producer the importance of compliance with these restrictions to prevent drug residues.

MILBEMYCIN OXIME

As previously stated, milbemycin (Interceptor, Sentinel) compounds (milbemycin oxime and moxidectin) are macrolide compounds chemically similar to the avermectins previously described. Milbemycin was originally used against agricultural insects (mites) and was only looked at for its antinematodal activity after the antinematodal activity of avermectins became known.

Although dosages exist for milbemycin use in everything from heartworm preventative in cats to treatment of demodectic and sarcoptic mange, the FDA-approved uses for milbemycin are for heartworm prevention for dogs and cats (Interceptor), as a treatment/control for hookworms and roundworms, and as a treatment of ear mites (Milbe-Mite), an indication that reflects its original use against agricultural mites. Milbemycin has shown some promise in treatment of demodectic mange resistant to other mange medications. Milbemycin oxime works by the same mechanism as the avermectins and appears to have a similar pattern of sensitivity reactions in macrolide-sensitive collies. Because milbemycin's principal use is as a heartworm preventative, it will be discussed in greater detail in that section.

MOXIDECTIN

Moxidectin (Cydectin, Quest, ProHeart), like other members of this group, has a wide range of potential uses. The list of parasites for which moxidectin is indicated in cattle (as a pour-on) and horses (as an oral gel) includes intestinal parasites, mites, cattle grubs, horse stomach bots, lice, flies, and nematodes living in other parts of the body. Moxidectin is available as an OTC equine product and therefore has been widely used by the lay public for a spectrum of parasites well beyond the approved label uses. Still, very few reports of moxidectin toxicity in horses have been reported. One clinical case report described three foals that had been administered moxidectin doses far exceeding the recommended dose. Clinical signs were consistent with overdose signs seen with ivermectin: CNS depression that progressed to coma. Moxidectin is not approved for use in horses younger than 4 months. Two of the three foals in this moxidectin toxicity case report were less than 2 weeks old, with the third foal being a 4-month-old miniature horse foal.[1]

In dogs, moxidectin was used as an injectable 6-month heartworm preventative and a treatment for hookworms (ProHeart). As of September 2004 the manufacturer had voluntarily recalled the product due to FDA concerns over reported adverse drug reactions.

BENZIMIDAZOLES

Like the macrolides, benzimidazoles are a rather large collection of antiparasitic drugs developed in the 1960s from the prototype compound thiabendazole. This drug was used in both human beings and animals, especially livestock, for treatment of a wide variety of nematodal infections. Because of the greater spectrum of activity of newer anthelmintics and endectacides, this group has decreased in popularity for veterinary use. However, the relatively low cost of the drugs still makes them attractive for livestock operations.

All the benzimidazoles act by attacking special proteins in the cells (β-tubulin) that are responsible for helping the cell divide. Fortunately, because mammalian β-tubulin is different from the parasite's β-tubulin, mammalian cells are not significantly affected by the toxic

CLINICAL APPLICATION
Respiratory Failure Attributable to Moxidectin Intoxication in a Dog

A 5-month-old male collie presented after it had ingested an unknown quantity of Quest Gel, a moxidectin deworming agent for horses. The owner had administered the deworming agent to some horses and the dog likely ate some of the Quest Gel that had ended up in the horse feed (undigested horse feed was found in the stool of the dog 2 days after it was admitted to the hospital).

The onset of signs began 2 hours after exposure and progressed rapidly from lethargy to 4-limb ataxia to seizure activity. The dog was seizing at the time of admission to the hospital. Diazepam infusion controlled the seizure activity; however, subsequent examination showed that the mucus membranes had become cyanotic after seizure activity had been controlled. The dog was intubated and given 100% oxygen. The gums returned to a more normal pink color within 5 to 10 minutes after starting the oxygen.

The neurologic examination indicated a state of coma with a lack of all myotatic reflex responses (e.g., patellar reflex), flexor reflexes (e.g., pinching toe and no limb withdrawal seen), and perineal reflex (pinching anal area and no twitching of external anal sphincter noticed). Pupillary light reflexes were weak but present. Glucocorticoid drugs (dexamethasone, prednisone sodium succinate) were administered and the dog was placed on a portable ventilator with 100% oxygen for transport to a veterinary referral center 4 hours away.

Treatment at the referral hospital focused on maintaining breathing with positive pressure ventilation, administration of active charcoal and other drugs to decrease absorption of any remaining moxidectin in the GI tract, changing the animal's position to prevent pulmonary edema and decubital ulcers, and passive range of motion exercises (physical therapy). Feeding by a nasogastric tube was begun on day 2 after admission to the referral hospital.

Neurologic function slowly returned over 6 days. During this time the dog developed clinical signs consistent with aspiration pneumonia; bacterial culture and cytology of endotracheal lavage fluid indicated the presence of bacteria. Treatment with amikacin helped keep this potentially life-threatening complication in check.

Ten days after admission to the referral hospital, the dog was sent home although it was still lethargic. Two weeks after discharge the neurologic examination and thoracic radiographs (for aspiration pneumonia signs) were considered normal.

What should be learned from this situation: The concentration of moxidectin and other avermectins is very high in equine products. In this case, the concentration of moxidectin in Quest Gel is 20,000 µg/mL. In one study, a single dose of moxidectin at 90 µg/kg in collies (270 µg in a 66-lb. collie) produced mild ataxia, lethargy, and salivation in one of six dogs. In contrast, beagles given 1130 µg/kg every day for a year did not show any of these signs. This pattern of sensitivity in collies should come as no surprise given the similarities in chemistry and mechanisms between ivermectin and moxidectin.

Because a single milliliter of avermectin horse products has the potential to produce severe toxicosis in collie-related breeds, this case reemphasizes the need to carefully ensure that equine deworming medications are safely disposed of. The resulting toxicosis from avermectin products requires extensive supportive care for periods up to 5 weeks depending on the dosage ingested. Thus, for the wide array of avermectin products, a moment of extra precaution in safely disposing the medication can literally save days or weeks of intensive medical care.

From Beal MW, Poppenga RH, Birdsall WJ, et al: Respiratory failure attributable to moxidectin intoxication in a dog, *J Am Vet Med Assoc* 215:1813-1817, 1999.

effects of the benzimidazoles. Because of the action of benzimidazole on the parasite's cells, it usually takes 3 to 5 days of exposure to the drug to have the optimal killing effect on the parasite. Therefore most dosage regimens of benzimidazoles require the pet owner or livestock producer to administer the drug on consecutive days. The β-tubulin mechanism of action is generally safe for mammalian cells for the reasons stated previously; however, rapidly dividing mammalian cells (which are very dependent on properly functioning tubulin to make the microtubules that aid cellular division) may be affected by higher doses of benzimidazoles. It has been suggested that there is the potential for teratogenic effects (birth defects) in some benzimidazoles. Some of the benzimidazoles were known to have hepatotoxic effects; however, most of those compounds have been replaced by other parasiticides.

There are several drugs in this class and they can usually be recognized by the -*azole* suffix of the chemical name. In addition to the prototype thiabendazole, other benzimidazoles include fenbendazole (Panacur, Safe-Guard), oxibendazole (Anthelcide EQ), albendazole, (Valbazen), and oxfendazole (Benzelmin). Most of these products are formulated as pastes and solutions for use in control of equine intestinal parasites. Most also have applications in cattle, other food animals, and companion animals. Characteristics that distinguish one benzimidazole from another are noted below.

Thiabendazole has a wide range of activity against ascarids and strongyles. The drug is safe when used at recommended dosages and rarely causes significant side effects, although dying parasites may produce some signs associated with an inflammatory reaction to the dead parasite. In addition to its antiparasitic activity, thiabendazole is unique in that it also has some antiinflammatory and antifungal activity. For this reason thiabendazole is sometimes added to otic (ear) medications (e.g., Tresaderm Otic) and topical products.

Oxibendazole has long been used as an equine dewormer. While oxibendazole is apparently safe for use in horses, this drug when used in combination with diethylcarbamazine as a daily heartworm preventative had caused liver dysfunction (periportal hepatitis) in dogs. This combination of oxibendazole and diethylcarbamazine is no longer manufactured in the United States. Oxibendazole is still used against nematode species found in the horse.

Fenbendazole (Panacur for dogs, horses, and livestock, Safe-Guard for livestock) has a wide spectrum of activity against nematodes and a variety of other parasites. Fenbendazole is effective against a limited number of species of tapeworms, but should not be used as a general cestocide unless the particular species of tapeworm has been identified. Vomiting is occasionally noted in dogs given this medication, but the liver problems associated with some of the other benzimidazoles have not been reported with fenbendazole. In the dog, the drug must be given for 3 consecutive days for maximal efficacy in killing the more common intestinal parasites, but it must be given for 10 to 14 days for other parasites such as the lungworm or liver fluke. Dosages exist for treating cats and "pocket pets" (e.g., mice, gerbils) with fenbendazole. Likewise, livestock and horses require several consecutive days of treatment with fenbendazole to break the parasite life cycle.

Albendazole (Valbazen) is known to have a spectrum of activity that includes nematodes, trematodes (flukes), cestodes, and protozoa. It is one of the benzimidazoles that is thought to have the potential for teratogenic effects, and it has been linked to bone marrow suppression because of its effect on rapidly dividing cells. Therefore, although albendazole is still used in livestock, it should not be used in pregnant animals because of the potential for teratogenic effects. Like most of the benzimidazoles, ivermectin and modern anticestodals have largely supplanted the need for albendazole in companion animals.

Oxfendazole (Benzelmin) is a benzimidazole approved for use as a suspension or paste in horses. Like the other benzimidazoles, it is very effective against a wide variety of nematodes and has potential for use in livestock, even though the products are not approved for use in species other than the horse.

PYRANTEL

Pyrantel anthelmintics (Strongid, Nemex) are highly effective antinematodals and considered very safe. They are marketed as pyrantel pamoate and a more water-soluble salt, pyrantel tartrate. Although pyrantel products are labeled for use against common nematodes in dogs and horses, dosages exist in the veterinary literature for many species treated by veterinarians. Pyrantel mimics the action of the neurotransmitter *acetylcholine* on nicotinic acetylcholine receptors, causing initial stimulation and then paralysis of this class of acetylcholine receptors on muscles, thus killing the parasite by paralysis.

The pleasant taste of liquid pyrantel pamoate facilitates giving the oral suspension to animals by the veterinary professional or the client. Because of its safety and pleasant flavor, a large number of OTC pyrantel products are also available to the general public in a wide variety of retail stores. For this reason, many pet owners will choose to "worm" their pet with these products. Because this drug is effective against ascarids (roundworms) and hookworms, but has no activity against tapeworms, clients may not understand why their pet has tapeworms when they have "dewormed" the dog at home with pyrantel purchased OTC.

Because the drug particles of pyrantel quickly settle to the bottom of the bottle in the oral suspensions, these suspensions should be thoroughly shaken and mixed before administration to ensure accurate dosing of the medication. Failure to thoroughly mix the suspension before each dose can result in underdosing when using the diluted concentrations at the top of the bottle, or overdosing when using the higher concentrations found at the bottom of the bottle.

Pyrantel pamoate has been incorporated into a number of veterinary products to extend their spectra of activity. Heartgard-Plus combines the heartworm preventive ivermectin with pyrantel, Drontal combines the anticestodal praziquantel with pyrantel, and Drontal-Plus combines the antinematodal activity of pyrantel and the benzimidazole febantel with the anticestodal activity of praziquantel.

PIPERAZINES

Piperazine is a vermicide found in most of the "once a month" deworming medications sold in grocery stores and pet shops. Piperazine is very safe but has a very narrow spectrum of activity and is only effective against ascarids. Like pyrantel, when pet owners use piperazine products to deworm their pet, they may believe there is no reason to submit their pet's fecal sample to check for parasite eggs. The veterinary technician should inform the client that piperazines do not kill hookworms, tapeworms, whipworms, or protozoa (coccidia) that commonly infect dogs and cats. Unlike pyrantel, which kills both ascarids (roundworms) and hookworms, piperazine does not kill hookworms, and severe hookworm infestations can kill a young puppy due to blood loss. Thus, the false sense of security a puppy owner might get from using a piperazine product is even more dangerous than when they use an OTC pyrantel product.

Piperazine works by paralyzing the parasite's nervous system at the neuromuscular junction. For this reason, the drug is considered a vermifuge because it does not directly kill the worms. The flaccid paralysis of the ascarid adult worm means that the parasites can then no longer swim upstream against the normal peristaltic waves of the intestinal tract and may appear as a wriggling mass of live roundworms passed with the stool. If the worm is only partially paralyzed and is not passed out with the normal movement of feces, the ascarid may survive the dose of piperazine and go on to reinfect the animal.

ORGANOPHOSPHATES

Organophosphates are a class of compounds that were originally developed to be used as nerve gas in warfare, which attests to the potential these compounds have to kill their mammalian hosts as well as the parasites. Organophosphates act by binding to the *acetylcholinesterase* enzyme that normally breaks down and terminates the action of the neurotransmitter acetylcholine. With the enzyme bound, acetylcholine continues to stimulate the receptor, causing overstimulation of the nervous system and, for those receptors on the neuromuscular junction, eventually blockade of the receptor at the neuromuscular junction and subsequent paralysis of the muscle.

Most of the antiparasitic organophosphates were used as external parasite compounds for fleas and flies. The use of these as internal antiparasitics is almost nonexistent because of their risk for toxicity in the patient and the development of safer antiparasitics equally effective against the same spectrum of parasites.

More information concerning the mechanism of action and toxicity of organophosphates is included in the section on external antiparasitics.

ANTICESTODALS

Anticestodes and cestocides are drugs that are designed to destroy tapeworms. Modern cestocides have the ability to destroy tapeworms, including the head, with minimal effects on the host animal. The two major drugs, praziquantel and epsiprantel, both work by similar mechanisms. Both drugs cause increased permeability of calcium with subsequent loss of intracellular calcium, resulting in paralysis of the parasite. In addition, the protective covering of the tapeworm becomes permeable, resulting in leakage of essential nutrients and unveiling antigens against which the host's body can produce antibodies to help kill the parasite.

PRAZIQUANTEL

Praziquantel is marketed in injectable and tablet forms for use in dogs and cats (Droncit) and in other products that combine praziquantel with other antiparasitics (e.g., Drontal = praziquantel + pyrantel pamoate). The advantages of praziquantel are its efficacy with a single dose and its activity against a wide range of anticestodes, including *Echinococcus* species.

Unlike some of the older anticestodal drugs (taeniacides), praziquantel reduces the tapeworm's resistance to digestion by the host's intestinal tract. After praziquantel administration, the entire worm disintegrates, including the head buried in the bowel wall. Therefore owners usually do not see tapeworm segments (*proglottids*) passing in the feces after administration of praziquantel because the worm disintegrates.

Although a single dose of praziquantel is effective, elimination of the tapeworm *Dipylidium caninum* requires elimination of fleas from the host and the immediate environment because fleas are involved in that tapeworm's life cycle. Failure to prevent flea infestation is likely to result in reinfection.

While praziquantel is effective against the adult tapeworms, it is not *ovicidal* (capable of destroying the tapeworm eggs). Therefore after administration of the drug and the death of the parasite, microscopic tapeworm eggs may pass in the feces for a period of time. Because accidental ingestion of tapeworm eggs by human beings poses a potential public health hazard, the veterinary professional should instruct the pet owner to follow proper hygiene procedures (washing hands) after cleaning a cat litter box or disposing of feces that might be contaminated with tapeworm eggs.

Vomiting is an occasional side effect of praziquantel use in dogs and cats. The injectable form of praziquantel has a slightly greater incidence of vomiting than the oral. Pain at the injection site, ataxia, drowsiness, and weakness have been reported in cats and dogs after receiving the injectable form.

EPSIPRANTEL

Epsiprantel (Cestex) is an oral anticestodal effective against *Taenia* and *Dipylidium* tapeworms. The manufacturer does not list it as being effective against *Echinococcus* species, a species of tapeworm that can infect wild carnivores and has been associated with a fatal liver disease in human beings when the tapeworm eggs are accidentally ingested. Unlike praziquantel, epsiprantel is not absorbed to any significant degree from the GI tract. This lack of absorption minimizes the risk of systemic side effects. Like praziquantel, epsiprantel causes digestion of the entire tapeworm within the bowel, so there is little evidence of the tapeworm in the stool. Epsiprantel does not come in an injectable form.

ANTIPARASITICS USED IN HEARTWORM TREATMENT

Heartworms are helminths that produce clinical disease in both the dog and the cat. Because this disease is commonly encountered in veterinary medicine in most parts of North America and because its treatment is more complex than other internal parasites, it is discussed separately from the other internal parasitic worms.

Heartworm disease is the set of clinical signs caused by infestation of *Dirofilaria immitis* adult worms in the heart and pulmonary arteries. The adult worms cause disease by their physical presence, which obstructs blood flow through the right ventricle. Heartworms also cause the inner lining of the pulmonary arteries (the *intima*) to proliferate and thicken, increasing resistance to blood flow. Because of these effects, heartworm disease can result in an inability of the heart to adequately pump blood to the lungs, resulting in failure of the right side of the heart (right-sided congestive heart failure), and, in severe cases, death. Unfortunately, treatment of heartworm disease can result in side effects or adverse reactions that also have the potential to cause death. Because both the disease and the treatment are potentially life threatening, the veterinary professional should be very familiar with the current literature and recommendations produced by veterinary parasitologists and the American Heartworm Society. The Recommended Reading list at the end of this chapter has some sources of information on heartworm infection.

To effectively eliminate heartworm from the mammalian host, multiple drugs affecting different stages of the life cycle of *Dirofilaria* must be used. An *adulticide* is a drug used to kill mature (adult) heartworms that live in the right chambers of the heart. Female adult heartworms produce microscopic young (larvae) called microfilariae, which circulate in the bloodstream of infected dogs and are taken up by mosquitoes when they feed on an infected dog's blood. *Microfilaricides* are drugs used to kill the circulating microfilariae produced by the adult heartworms. After the microfilariae have been ingested by a mosquito, they undergo changes to become *infective third-stage larvae* (L3). These infective larvae migrate to the head and mouth parts of the mosquito, through which they enter another dog's body the next time the mosquito feeds. The injected infective larvae migrate through the dog's body and eventually reach the right ventricle, where they mature to adult worms. Heartworm preventatives are drugs given to kill these infective larvae so they are not allowed to mature to adults and produce heartworm disease. Generally, adulticides (at the dose used to kill adult heartworms) are not effective against microfilariae or the infective L3 larvae. Hence more than one drug is needed to effectively eliminate all stages of the heartworm from an infected dog.

HEARTWORM ADULTICIDES

For many years the only drug approved for treatment of adult heartworms was thiacetarsemide sodium (Caparsolate). In 1996, melarsomine dihydrochloride (Immiticide) was approved as an adulticide and has since become the only approved adulticide available.

Melarsomine is an organic arsenical adulticide that is administered as a deep IM injection given twice every 24 hours. The manufacturer of Immiticide is quite specific about the location into which the drug should be injected. The drug should only be injected into the epaxial muscles, which are located dorsally on either side of the spinal column. Specifically, the drug should be injected into the epaxial muscles between the third and fifth lumbar vertebrae, 1 to 2 inches lateral to the dorsal spinous process, which marks the center of the spinal column. Dogs that weigh less than 10 kg (22 lb.) should be injected with a 23-gauge, 1-inch needle, and larger dogs with a 22-gauge, 1.5-inch needle. The longer needles are required to place the drug deep within the belly of the epaxial muscles. The small-gauge needle (small gauge = narrow needle diameter) helps prevent drug leakage from the injection site.

Although fewer side effects occur with melarsomine than the older thiacetarsemide, several side effects, some of them potentially serious, have been reported since its introduction. Swelling and pain at the injection site are frequently reported. It is important to ensure that the entire drug is injected into the site before withdrawing the needle to avoid additional pain and swelling at the injection site.

Gagging, coughing, lethargy, and pulmonary congestion have been reported with melarsomine use; however, some of these effects may be caused by the killing of the adult heartworms, resulting in fragments of worms floating into the pulmonary arterial system until they lodge in small lung arterioles (thromboembolism), where they cause localized inflammation.

Melarsomine is contraindicated in animals with class 4 heartworm disease, in which large numbers of heartworms are found in the right ventricle and the right atrium and the venae cavae. Animals with this caval syndrome usually require surgical removal of the adult heartworms. Class 3 heartworm disease, which is characterized by fatigue, dyspnea, severe right heart changes on radiographs, and right heart failure, can be treated with melarsomine in a modified dosage regimen, which involves giving 1 dose of melarsomine, resting the animal for 1 month, and then giving the regular set of 2 injections.

Levamisole is a drug that at one time was advocated as an inexpensive alternative adulticide to thiacetarsemide when canine heartworm disease was first recognized in the United States. Although levamisole did kill adult heartworms to some extent, the inconsistent number of worms killed and the side effects (primarily CNS related) make it much less useful for this purpose than melarsomine. However, because levamisole is inexpensive and available, veterinary technicians may occasionally hear of an animal (typically an economic hardship case) being treated with this drug to reduce (but not eliminate) adult heartworms and clear microfilariae from the blood.

Some of the macrolide antiparasitics (e.g., ivermectin, selamectin) have been shown to reduce the number of adult worms when given over several months. It is presumed that exposure to these drugs over prolonged periods reduces the life span of the adult heartworm. Although this therapy will only reduce the adult worm load and not eliminate it, it is an alternative for owners who choose not to put their pet through the full adulticide treatment or for animals that might not be able to tolerate the adulticide drugs.

In the weeks after adulticide treatment with melarsomine, the dead adult heartworms degenerate, forming *emboli* that can travel from the heart to the lungs by the pulmonary arteries, eventually lodging in the smallest arterioles in the lung where they initiate an inflammatory reaction. Pulmonary inflammation from worm emboli will appear as coughing, fever, and sometimes the presence of blood in the productive cough *(hemoptysis)*. These signs typically appear between 1 and 2 weeks after the adulticide therapy, but they can appear any time in the 4 to 6 weeks after adulticide therapy. Therefore, during this postadulticide period, the animal must be prevented from exercising or becoming excessively excited because of the potential for increased blood flow through the heart and lungs, an increased turbulence and breaking up of dead worms, and increased bombardment of emboli in the lungs.

If signs of emboli-induced pulmonary inflammation appear, glucocorticoids are indicated to combat the inflammatory signs. It has been suggested that the simultaneous administration of glucocorticoids with adulticide therapy may increase the ability of the adult heartworm to survive. Although melarsomine's adulticidal effectiveness does not appear to be adversely affected by glucocorticoids, there is the suggestion that the removal of worm emboli trapped in the small pulmonary arterioles may be prolonged because of the glucocorticoid's effect. However, for situations in which acute, life-threatening pulmonary edema is occurring secondary to obstructive worm emboli in the lungs, the need to control or attenuate the inflammation with glucocorticoids takes a much higher priority than concern about a slowed removal of the emboli.

Aspirin has been recommended in the past to reduce inflammation associated with pulmonary emboli and decrease some of the platelet effects that contribute to the thickening of the pulmonary blood vessels. However, aspirin would be contraindicated for those animals coughing up blood secondary to the inflammatory effects of worm emboli in the lungs because of its inhibition of platelet functions and the subsequent reduction in the ability of the body to form small platelet clots. In fact, some veterinary cardiologists do not recommend aspirin use at all in heartworm-positive animals because of the potential for hemorrhage secondary to damaged pulmonary vasculature from the heartworm disease. Therefore aspirin use in helping prevent or reduce clinical signs associated with heartworm disease or postadulticide inflammatory reactions is considered more controversial than it used to be.

Note that cats are not treated with adulticide drugs because of the high risk for death from inflammatory lung disease caused by the dead adult heartworms. Cats typically have fewer adult heartworms than dogs, and the life span of the adult heartworm is shorter in the cat (2 to 3 years) than the dog. However, because the cat's heart and pulmonary arteries are much smaller than the dog's, it only takes a small number of adult heartworms to produce severe heartworm disease in cats. For these same reasons, emboli of decaying dead adult worms killed by an adulticide are more likely to obstruct the larger pulmonary vessels, producing a severe, and potentially fatal, pulmonary inflammatory reaction. Studies of melarsomine use in cats experimentally infected with heartworms also showed that the kill rate of the adult worms was significantly lower in cats than has been demonstrated in dogs. This lower kill rate and the risk of life-threatening worm emboli if the worms are killed are the basis for the current recommendation that melarsomine not be used to treat heartworm disease in cats.

MICROFILARICIDES

After the animal has been allowed 3 to 4 weeks to recover from adulticide treatment and embolic pulmonary inflammation, a microfilaricide can be administered to eliminate circulating heartworm microfilariae. It has become standard practice to use a single dose of diluted large-animal injectable ivermectin (1% Ivomec injectable or Eqvalan) by mouth as the microfilaricide of choice. Depending on the medium in which the ivermectin is dissolved, the product is diluted 1:10 either in water (Eqvalan) or propylene glycol (Ivomec) and then administered at the rate of 1 mL/20 kg of body weight. Administration of the undiluted drug can be done with a TB syringe; however, because the large-animal ivermectin dose formulations are very concentrated, the undiluted dose would be 0.1 mL for every 20 kg of body weight and an accurate dose would be difficult to measure.

Because milbemycin oxime (Interceptor) is also a macrolide, it has also been used as a microfilaricide at a dose of 0.5 mg/kg. Use of ivermectin or milbemycin as a microfilaricide is considered an extra-label use because neither drug is approved by the FDA for this purpose. Because of their similarities to ivermectin and milbemycin, selamectin has the potential to be microfilaricidal, although no microfilaricide dosage regimen has been established. According to the literature from the manufacturer of moxidectin, moxidectin "is not effective for microfilariae clearance."

Animals treated for *microfilaremia* (microfilariae in the blood) with ivermectin or milbemycin should be observed for a few hours for adverse effects. Occasionally a rapid kill of many microfilariae will produce a shocklike syndrome that can usually be treated with standard shock therapy (IV fluids, glucocorticoids, and supportive therapy). Dogs determined to have a high microfilariae count are sometimes given a reduced dose of ivermectin to reduce the number of microfilariae, allowed to recover for a few days, then given a standard dose to eliminate the remainder.

The blood should be examined microscopically for circulating microfilariae 3 weeks later, and a second dose of microfilaricide should be given if microfilariae are still present. Persistence of microfilariae after the second dose suggests the possibility of surviving adult heartworms. The second adulticide therapy should be given following the time table and guidelines published by the American Heartworm Society or similar protocols published in the veterinary literature.

PREVENTATIVES

After microfilariae have been cleared from the blood, the animal can begin receiving heartworm preventive to prevent reinfection caused by the infective larvae injected into the animal by the mosquito. Heartworm preventives are available in two basic forms: those given daily (diethylcarbamazine) and those given monthly or at longer intervals (macrolides).

Diethylcarbamazine (DEC) was a daily preventative medication capable of killing the infective larvae as they molt from one stage to the next and therefore is given daily during seasons when an animal could be bitten by a mosquito and for 2 months thereafter (some sources say 1 month after the first frost). The macrolide products ivermectin, milbemycin oxime, selamectin, and moxidectin have largely supplanted the use of DEC and as of this writing no veterinary-approved DEC products were available in the United States.

Many of the macrolide preventative drugs come in forms that have other anthelmintics added (e.g., pyrantel) to expand the spectrum of their approved uses. In addition, some of these products are now approved for use in cats as well as dogs. Because these products change constantly, it is important that the veterinary professional keep abreast of each new product, or each new approved use of the old product, to understand the mechanisms and potential side effects. As of this writing, the current products for heartworm prevention are shown in Table 12-1.

The dose of ivermectin (Heartgard) for prevention of heartworm infection (0.006 mg/kg) is much lower than the dose used for microfilaricidal activity (0.05 mg/kg). Thus the likelihood of a collie breed experiencing an adverse reaction to ivermectin used as a heartworm

TABLE **12-1** Current Products for Heartworm Prevention

DRUG	TRADE NAME(S)	ROUTE, DOSE INTERVAL	APPROVED FOR USE IN DOGS?	APPROVED FOR USE IN CATS?
Ivermectin	Heartgard and others	PO monthly	Yes	Yes (some products)
Milbemycin oxime	Interceptor	PO monthly	Yes	No (doses do exist)
Selamectin	Revolution	Topical monthly	Yes	Yes

preventive is minimal. Nevertheless the manufacturer recommends observing the animal for 8 hours after administration of the preventive dose of ivermectin. Heartgard-30 Plus includes the antinematodal drug pyrantel with ivermectin. The formulation of ivermectin approved as a preventive for use in cats (Heartgard for Cats) comes in chewable cubes that are packaged in two forms; one for use in cats less than 5 lb and one for cats greater than 5 lb. Like the canine Heartgard, the medication is administered once a month. It is recommended that the Heartgard be crumbled into food or given to the cat in small pieces to facilitate dissolution of the cube and absorption of the drug. Heartworm testing is recommended before the cat is started on Heartgard. Even if the test results are positive for the presence of adult heartworms, the drug can still be used to prevent further infection from mosquito-injected infective larvae. The drug appears to be safe in cats even at three times the recommended dose.

In addition to preventing heartworms, milbemycin oxime (Interceptor) also eliminates adult hookworms, ascarids (*Toxocara canis*), and whipworms. Like ivermectin, milbemycin oxime kills migrating microfilariae at any stage of development. At higher doses, milbemycin may also cause a mild shocklike syndrome in some dogs with significant numbers of circulating microfilariae. At normal doses, such reactions are infrequent. Studies in collies have shown the drug to be safe at up to 20 times the recommended dose. Milbemycin has also shown some promise in treatment of demodectic mange that is resistant to other treatments.

Selamectin (Revolution) is a heartworm preventative that uses the topical application as its route of administration. The drug is apparently safe to use around children who play with the pet and come into contact with the topically applied drug, but it is always a good general policy to avoid touching the area where the product has been applied until it completely dries. In addition to its heartworm prophylaxis, selamectin is approved for use against hookworms, roundworms, adult fleas, ear mites, ticks, and sarcoptic mange mites.

As more is understood about heartworm disease in both the dog and the cat, new products will be introduced. The information provided in this section will provide a foundation for understanding how new heartworm products work, how they are similar or different from established heartworm medications, and how the safety of the product compares to those products already existing.

ANTIPROTOZOALS

Protozoa are single cellular organisms that most frequently cause GI disease, but can also produce disease in almost every other organ system. Antiprotozoal drugs are most commonly used against coccidia, *Giardia*, and *Sarcocystis neurona*, the agent of equine protozoal myeloencephalitis (EPM). They include a wide range of products, including sulfonamide antimicrobials (e.g., sulfadimethoxine), metronidazole, benzimidazole anthelmintics (e.g., fenbendazole, albendazole), furazolidone (Furoxone), amprolium, and others. A relatively new product targeted toward the cause of EPM is ponazuril (Marquis). Control of protozoal infections requires treatment of existing infections and successful environmental control to prevent reinfection from fecally contaminated feed, grazing areas, and water supplies.

Amprolium is an antiprotozoal used in calves and the avian species. It is structurally similar to thiamin but does not possess thiamin's intrinsic vitamin activity. Thus when the parasite absorbs amprolium, competitive antagonism between amprolium and thiamin occurs and thiamin activity is inhibited. The parasite dies from thiamin deficiency. Use of amprolium in large doses for extended periods can also result in thiamin deficiency in the host animal.

For many years metronidazole (Flagyl) was the drug of choice against *Giardia.* It still is an excellent choice even with the risk of neurologic side effects sometimes seen with animals on metronidazole (see Chapter 10). Metronidazole also has antibacterial and antiinflammatory properties, thus making it a great drug for use in those situations where low-grade inflammatory bowel disease, either with or without *Giardia*, is the primary cause for chronic diarrhea.

Fenbendazole (Panacur) is a benzimidazole anthelmintic drug that is also a very effective and safe drug for use against *Giardia* and is therefore the drug of choice by some gastroenterologists for treating *Giardia* in pregnant animals and cats. Febantel, found in some combination drugs such as Drontal, is metabolized to fenbendazole and oxyfenbendazole and thus would be expected to have a similar efficacy against protozoa as fenbendazole. Albendazole is also a benzimidazole that is very effective against protozoa, including *Giardia*; however, it has been associated with loss of appetite, lethargy, and even suspected bone marrow depression resulting in leukopenia (low white cell count). Because of these side effects, albendazole is not favored as much as fenbendazole, febantel, or metronidazole for treatment of *Giardia.*

In 1999 a vaccination for *Giardia* was introduced. It was found to reduce the severity of infection in animals with active *Giardia* and reduce the shedding of cysts in the feces. The vaccine was approved for use in both dogs and cats; however, it is not likely to be considered a routine vaccine like rabies or distemper. Dogs or cats at higher risk for exposure to *Giardia* because of potential exposure to outside natural water sources of *Giardia* or close contact with many animals (e.g., show animals) may benefit from this vaccine as well as animals with chronic giardiasis that do not respond well to the drugs mentioned previously.

Ponazuril is an antiprotozoal drug introduced in 2001 as Marquis for the treatment of equine protozoal myeloencephalitis caused by *Sarcocystis neurona.* The drug is effective against several species of coccidia and although its mechanism of action is not known, it is believed to target metabolic functions or organelles not found in vertebrate cells. Several side effects ranging from loose stools, skin reactions, to a possible estrogen-like effect on the uterus were noted in trials for this drug.

EXTERNAL ANTIPARASITICS

External antiparasitics are used to control flies, grubs, and lice on livestock, flies (bots and maggots) on horses, and fleas, ticks, and mange mites on companion animals. In addition to decreasing skin disease in companion animals or increasing weight gain in livestock by controlling these external parasites, an additional benefit is the control of diseases that are spread to human beings by arthropod vectors such as Lyme disease, bubonic plague, and Rocky Mountain spotted fever. Because the targets for these external antiparasitics are members of the six-legged insect family, they are more commonly grouped together under the lay term *insecticides* even though they are effective against eight-legged creatures such as spiders (arachnids).

Insecticides and external antiparasitics are available in many formulations. For example, flea products have been marketed as flea collars, powders, dips, aerosol sprays, pump sprays, baths, foggers, foams, pour-ons, drop-ons, and even roll-ons. Most of these formulations are designed to appeal to the convenience of application for the companion animal owner, or in some cases they are marketed in a novel delivery system designed to set the product apart from its competitors. In contrast to the individual animal application in companion animals, insecticides and external antiparasitics for livestock are designed for ease of application to large groups of animals; hence they may be incorporated into rubbing bars and dust bags that deliver a dusting of the chemical that kills or repels insects. Other formulations for livestock include pour-on products that are absorbed through the skin, sprays, dips, impregnated ear tags from which insecticide diffuses into the body, and feed additives. Whereas products for companion animals are designed to be applied in a carefully controlled manner and dose for each animal, products formulated for food animals can easily be overdosed or underdosed depending on the length of time or amount of chemical with which the animal comes in contact.

By far the most common application of external parasiticides is for control or elimination of fleas in the dog and cat. Many of the modern flea products are targeted at specific stages of the flea life cycle, as opposed to the entire life cycle. Therefore, the veterinary technician must understand the flea life cycle and the limitations of each flea product to properly educate the client and prevent the client from having inappropriate expectations for one product solving all of his or her pet's flea problems.

The generic flea's life cycle can be summarized as follows. The female flea feeds on the pet's blood and produces thousands of eggs in a normal lifetime. These eggs fall off the pet and within a few days will hatch larvae in the pet's environment. Flea larvae then create a pupa (a cocoon) in which they can remain for months. When the environmental conditions are right, the young adult flea will emerge from the cocoon and seek the pet or the pet owner on which to feed and continue the life cycle. Because some flea products only stop one component of the flea life cycle (e.g., just the egg or just the adult) failure to kill the other stages of the life cycle simultaneously will allow adult fleas to continue to plague the pet (in the case of compounds that kill larvae or affect eggs) or will only temporarily eliminate the flea problem until the eggs hatch or the new adults emerge from the pupa. As stated previously, the veterinary technician must thoroughly understand this life cycle and how the individual drugs affect it to provide appropriate advice for the client (Figure 12-1).

ORGANOPHOSPHATES AND CARBAMATES

Although organophosphates and carbamates (carbaryl, methylcarbamate) are used much less often as veterinary antiparasite compounds as they used to be, some products are still available. In addition, cases of organophosphate or carbamate toxicity from non–animal related sources still occur in veterinary medicine. Therefore the discussion of these particular insecticides focuses more on their toxic effects.

Organophosphates and carbamates, which are two chemically different types of insecticides, are usually grouped together because of their similar mechanisms of action, effects on insects, and toxic effects. Unlike the old chlorinated hydrocarbon compounds like DDT and lindane, organophosphates and carbamates decompose readily in the environment and do not pose a significant threat to wildlife. Although limited in use for animal applications, they have several agricultural applications, including use on crops, on garden plants to control aphids and other pests, in the soil to control lawn grubs, and on nursery trees.

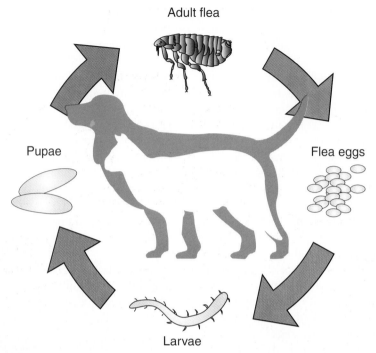

Adult flea

Pupae

Flea eggs

Larvae

Figure 12-1 Flea life cycle.

Organophosphates and carbamates are general names for this broad class of insecticides. Manufacturers modify the basic organophosphate molecule to produce new products and may not state specifically that the product is an organophosphate or carbamate product. However, a tip-off that a product contains organophosphates or carbamates can be found in a container's warning label to physicians stating that the product "contains a cholinesterase inhibitor" and should be treated as such in cases of accidental contact or ingestion.

Organophosphates and carbamates work in similar ways. As shown in Figure 12-2, they bind to acetylcholinesterase, which is the enzyme that normally breaks down the neurotransmitter acetylcholine to terminate its action at the receptor site. With the acetylcholinesterase inhibited, acetylcholine neurotransmitter released by the axon continues to stimulate receptor sites. It is important

to realize that there are two classes of acetylcholine receptors, *muscarinic receptors* and *nicotinic receptors,* and that stimulation of each class of receptor results in different clinical signs.

In spite of governmental recalls and tighter use restrictions on many organophosphate products and carbamates, toxicity cases from exposure to these insecticides are still seen by veterinary practices. Depending on the type of organophosphate or carbamate product and the dose administered to the animal, clinical signs of toxicity can manifest either as muscarinic receptor signs, nicotinic receptor signs, or a blending of both. For that reason it is important for the veterinary professional to recognize these signs and understand how each set is a potential threat to the animal's life.

Stimulation of muscarinic receptors produces the classic signs of toxicity related to parasympathetic nervous system stimulation.

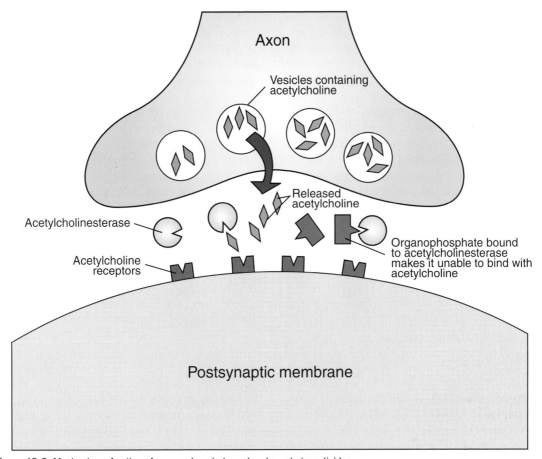

Figure 12-2 Mechanism of action of organophosphate and carbamate insecticides.

Because the parasympathetic nervous system normally stimulates the GI tract motility and secretions and antagonizes the sympathetic nervous system effects in the heart, bronchioles, and pupil, muscarinic receptor signs of organophosphate toxicosis can be remembered by the acronym *SLUDDE:* **s**alivation, **l**acrimation (tearing), **u**rination, **d**efecation, **d**yspnea (difficult breathing because of bronchoconstriction and increased respiratory secretions), and **e**mesis. Bradycardia is also consistent with overstimulation of the parasympathetic nervous system. Signs of CNS muscarinic receptor stimulation include seizures caused by CNS stimulation. One of the most characteristic muscarinic signs of organophosphate or carbamate toxicity is miosis (pinpoint pupils). Miosis may not be present with toxicity caused by every organophosphate because certain organophosphates produce this sign more than others. When miosis does appear with other SLUDDE signs, it is highly suggestive of organophosphate or carbamate toxicity.

Some organophosphate and carbamate products may produce clinical signs associated predominantly with the nicotinic receptor stimulation. The nicotinic receptors that produce the clinical signs of toxicity are those located at the neuromuscular junction where nerve axons contact skeletal muscles. Instead of GI or respiratory signs, stimulation of the nicotinic receptor initially produces muscle tremors that progress in severity until the nicotinic receptors that stimulate the muscle to contract lock up and block transmission of axonal depolarization waves to the voluntary or skeletal muscles. Thus, toxicity signs associated with nicotinic receptor stimulation appear initially as tremors, progressing to shaking, and then to ataxia and paralysis. Because the diaphragm is a skeletal muscle, the diaphragm and the intercostal muscles that help lift the rib cage during inspiration can also be paralyzed, contributing to the respiratory failure. Pupils in these animals may be dilated (especially in cats).

Treatment of acute organophosphate toxicity consists of removing any insecticide remaining on or in the animal, and blocking the parasympathetic effects. Atropine is the drug of choice for reversing clinical signs of toxicity because it is a muscarinic receptor antagonist (blocker) that decreases the effect of the excessive acetylcholine at the muscarinic receptor site. Because the greatest risk to the animal's life is hypoxia caused by the combination of bronchoconstriction and excessive airway secretions, atropine at 10 times the typical preanesthetic dose is often the first drug of choice for reversing the more life-threatening signs associated with toxicosis. Atropine does not block nicotinic receptor sites except at very high doses, so nicotinic signs of toxicosis may not significantly improve from atropine administration at recommended organophosphate antidote doses. Glycopyrrolate is also a muscarinic receptor blocker and will relieve the SLUDDE signs. One difference between atropine and glycopyrrolate is that atropine more readily penetrates the blood-brain barrier than glycopyrrolate; therefore it would be more effective at reversing muscarinic signs associated with the CNS. Atropine and glycopyrrolate are both drugs found in almost every veterinary practice for use as part of a preanesthetic regimen. However, an additional drug, pralidoxime, can be obtained from a local human

hospital, pharmacy, or emergency department that reverses organophosphate toxicosis by separating the organophosphate from the acetylcholinesterase molecule, thereby freeing the enzyme molecule to work again.

A *delayed neurotoxicity* syndrome has been reported in people, cats, dogs, and some livestock that have recovered from an acute toxicity from certain organophosphates. This syndrome usually occurs 1 or 2 weeks after short-term exposure to large doses of some organophosphates. The animal becomes ataxic in the hind legs, may buckle over, and may have difficulty maintaining posture. This state may progress to complete paralysis of the hind limbs. Apparently metabolism of certain organophosphates produces a metabolite that is toxic to the myelin sheath covering the nerves. This damage may result in death of the neuron and impaired function of the muscles innervated by that neuron. The effect has been likened to "chemical transection" of the nerve. Affected cattle may show weakness, depression, droopy ears, and bloat. Fortunately, this syndrome is fairly rare. Because no antidote or reversal agent is available for this syndrome, treatment is supportive and symptomatic; in livestock affected animals are usually culled from the herd.

PYRETHRINS AND PYRETHROIDS

Pyrethrins and pyrethroids constitute the largest group of OTC insecticides marketed for use against external parasites and common household insect pests such as flies and mosquitoes. Unlike organophosphate and carbamate insecticides, pyrethrins and pyrethroids have a large therapeutic index, meaning that the dose that is effective (kills the parasite) is much smaller than the dose that produces toxicosis in the animal host.

Pyrethrins are natural insecticides derived from chrysanthemum flowers. They produce a quick "knockdown" effect, as evidenced by the way flies drop or fleas fall from an animal sprayed with pyrethrins. However, the killing activity of pyrethrins is not as marked as the stunning effect, and the immobilized flies or fleas may recover after several minutes. For that reason, the basic pyrethrin molecule has been modified to enhance the insecticidal effect. These pyrethrinlike insecticides are called pyrethroids. Most pyrethroids can be recognized by the *-thrin* suffix such as resmethrin, allethrin, permethrin, tetramethrin, deltamethrin, and cyfluthrin. One of the exceptions to this rule is fenvalerate, a common pyrethroid ingredient in insecticidal applications.

Pyrethrin and pyrethroids both work by locking open the sodium channels that allow sodium ions to move into the neuron to initiate depolarization of the nerve. By increasing the influx of sodium into the nerve, pyrethrin compounds overstimulate the nervous system of the parasite. Pyrethrin and pyrethroids are classified as type 1 or type 2 compounds based on whether this overstimulation of the nervous system results in increased nervous system activity (seizures) or in paralysis from the receptors locking up from overstimulation. Unfortunately, pyrethrin and pyrethroid toxicity can also occur in mammals (especially cats), and affected animals often show similar signs of nervous system stimulation.

Pyrethrins and pyrethroids for the most part have very selective toxicity, meaning that they require a very small dose to be toxic to insects in contrast to a much larger dose necessary to produce adverse effects in animals. Although pyrethrins are very safe for mammals, fish unfortunately readily absorb pyrethrin insecticides through their skin and can easily become poisoned and die. Therefore pyrethrin and pyrethroid use around streams, lakes, decorative ponds, fish farms, and aquaculture establishments must be carefully controlled. Fortunately, pyrethrins and pyrethroids degrade in the environment fairly quickly.

Synergists are compounds added to the pyrethrin products to enhance their insecticidal effect. The synergist most commonly used with pyrethrins is piperonyl butoxide. This synergist is generally safe, but it has been reported to cause neurotoxicity signs in cats licking their treated hair coat. Because pyrethroids usually have sufficient insecticidal activity by themselves, they are not often combined with a synergist. However, some pyrethrin and pyrethroid flea products now include *insect growth regulators,* which are compounds that retard or stop the development of fleas without directly killing the flea.

Veterinary technicians should be aware of features of certain pyrethroids. Resmethrin is degraded by ultraviolet light and has been reported to leave an odor like stale urine. Permethrin and fenvalerate adhere to synthetic fibers such as those found in nylon or synthetic carpets, which causes these insecticides to lose their residual activity. Permethrin and deltamethrin have been used in flea and tick collars and other antiparasitic products because of their effectiveness in killing and repelling ticks as well as fleas. This combination of flea and tick killing activity is appealing to the public because of their increased awareness of tick-borne diseases such as Lyme disease (borreliosis) and Rocky Mountain spotted fever. It is important to recognize that the manufacturers of permethrin products, or products that contain combinations of permethrin and other compounds (e.g., imidacloprid and permethrin in Advantx), state that such products should not be used in cats and contact between cats and permethrin should be avoided.

Because so many pyrethrin, pyrethroid, and combination products exist in the veterinary and public market, the veterinary professional should carefully review the precautions, species or age limitations, and specific application instructions to fully understand how to safely use or prescribe these products.

AMITRAZ

Amitraz, a diamide insecticide, was one of the first effective agents available for treatment of demodectic mange in dogs. The amitraz formulation for demodectic mange in dogs comes in a liquid form to be used as a dip or sponge-on bath (e.g., Mitaban). Gloves should be worn during application of this product to decrease contact with the skin of the person administering the dip or bath as the potential for intoxication from topical exposure is possible. With the normal dipping procedure, animals may show CNS depression manifested by clinical signs of sedation and incoordination for 24 to 72 hours after treatment. Some depression of the body's thermoregulatory mechanism may cause dogs damp from their dip to become hypothermic (low body temperature). Therefore after a dip the animal should be placed in a well-padded cage so it does not lose body heat to the metal of the cage. *Pruritus* (itching) often occurs for several days after treatment and is thought to be caused by death of the mites and the body's subsequent reaction to the mite body as a foreign protein.

Amitraz is not effective in killing fleas; however, it can kill and repel ticks. Preventic is an amitraz tick collar for dogs. Preventic Plus is an amitraz tick collar that also contains an insect growth regulator for fleas called pyriproxyfen (Nylar). Amitraz can be highly toxic if ingested by animals or people. Therefore veterinary technicians should caution pet owners that amitraz collars should not be handled by children or be available where children or pets can find, play with, or chew on them. It is also very important that the discarded segments of collars trimmed off to make it fit better on the pet be promptly disposed of so they are not accidentally picked up by children or animals.

It is not entirely clear by what mechanism amitraz kills ticks or mites; however, it is known that amitraz is an α_2 receptor agonist similar to sedative/tranquilizer drugs like xylazine (Rompun) and detomidine (Dormosedan). The α_2 receptor in the brain decreases the release of norepinephrine from axons and thus decreases the excitatory effect on the brain, bringing about sedation. The sedative side effects observed with amitraz are consistent with this α_2 receptor activity.

Amitraz is also known to inhibit *monoamine oxidase* (MAO), an important enzyme involved in the normal recycling or reclaiming of the norepinephrine neurotransmitter. Because many behavior-modifying drugs are MAO inhibitors (MAOI), the manufacturers of amitraz products strongly recommend not using amitraz on animals that are being treated with MAOIs, tricyclic antidepressants, or serotonin-reuptake inhibitors. Because of the increased use of psychotropic drugs for behavior modification in veterinary medicine, the potential for this interaction is much more likely to occur than might have been the case just a few years ago.

If a dog loses its amitraz collar and begins to appear depressed or sedated, the owner should suspect amitraz toxicity from ingestion and get the dog to a veterinarian as soon as possible. Death from ingestion of amitraz collars has been reported in both the veterinary and human medical literature. Fortunately, because amitraz is an α_2 agonist, the α_2 antagonist drugs yohimbine (Yobine), tolazoline (Priscoline, Tolazine), and atipamezole (Antisedan) can be used to reverse many of the toxic effects caused by excessive sedation. Because the half-life for the reversal agents is very short compared with the half-life for amitraz, multiple dosages of the α_2 antagonists are going to have to be administered to maintain the reversal effect.

MACROLIDES

Although most of the macrolides likely have effects on mites and other insects, two macrolide products are specifically targeted toward external parasites. Milbemycin oxime was discussed as an internal parasiticide and as a heartworm preventative. Its original use was as an agent against agricultural mites. Milbemycin was approved in 2002 for use as an otic preparation against ear mites (*Otodectes cynotis*) in the cat (MilbeMite). Preliminary studies on adverse effects and toxicity indicate a low risk for toxicosis from this product when applied to the ear in accordance with the manufacturer's directions.

Selamectin (Revolution) is approved for use against fleas in dogs and cats, sarcoptic mange mites in dogs, ears mites in dogs and cats, and for tick control in dogs. As mentioned in the section on internal parasites, it is a topical product ("spot on") applied once a month to the back of the dog or cat. It is directly insecticidal, as opposed to blocking the life cycle or inhibiting development of a life cycle stage. Topical application is deemed safe when used according to the manufacturer's recommendations.

Several extra-label dosages exist for ivermectin and some of the other macrolides, especially for exotics or wildlife species. Although the use of macrolides in an extra-label manner may be routine in some practices, it still warrants caution and intensive client education about the potential side effects of the product in that species. In many cases, little information is published regarding potential complications. Therefore the veterinary professional is always obligated to inform the client that the medication being used is not approved for that species or for that particular use and procure the client's permission to use the product in the prescribed manner. This does not ensure against litigation if an animal dies or is injured because of the extra-label use of this or any compound, but it does facilitate the communication and partnership between the veterinarian and the client, especially if something does not go as planned.

IMIDACLOPRID

Imidacloprid (Advantage, K9 Advantx) is a chloronicotinyl nitroguanidine insecticide used topically to kill adult fleas and exists in formulations approved for dogs and cats. Like the organophosphates, carbamates, and pyrethroids, imidacloprid is an insect neurotoxin. Imidacloprid acts in a similar manner to the nicotinic effects of organophosphate toxicosis by combining with the parasite's nicotinic acetylcholine receptor, stimulating it initially, then causing it to lock up, effectively blocking any further neurotransmission by this receptor.

Advantage contains only imidacloprid for fleas, whereas K9 Advantx also contains permethrin, a pyrethroid compound that acts as a tick and mosquito parasiticide and repellent. Because of the cat's decreased ability to metabolize permethrin and suspected adverse reactions by cats to this compound, the manufacturer states that K9 Advantx must not be used on cats. The manufacturer goes on to advise caution in households where cats live with dogs treated with K9 Advantx, especially if the cat has close contact with the dog or grooms the dog.

Imidacloprid is applied to the back of the neck in cats or between the shoulder blades in dogs (and over the rump area of large dogs). The drug is disseminated across the skin by the animal's movement. Imidacloprid is poorly absorbed through the skin and kills adult fleas on contact. The manufacturer claims 4 weeks of residual activity in cats, with a slightly longer residual effect in dogs. Because the insect's nicotinic acetylcholine receptor has a different structure than mammalian receptors, imidacloprid does not combine with the host animal's nicotinic receptors and therefore the drug has a significant margin of safety. Toxicity to fish is also stated by the manufacturer to be low.

FIPRONIL

Fipronil (Frontline, Top Spot) is a neurotoxic insecticide that blocks the GABA receptor, resulting in decreased chloride moving into the nerve cell. In so doing, fipronil removes the inhibitory effect of chloride influx on the neuron function, resulting in overstimulation of the neuron, hyperexcitability of the nervous system, and subsequent death. The safety of fipronil is attributable to the differences in affinity (its ability of the drug to bind) of fipronil to the structure of insect GABA receptors compared with the structure of mammalian GABA receptors. Because the fipronil molecule does not bind readily to mammalian GABA receptors, and hence does not stimulate the GABA receptor, the drug is relatively safe to use in mammals. Unfortunately, fipronil is highly toxic to some types of fish and therefore must be used with caution to prevent accidental contamination around aquariums or pools of fish.

Frontline is marketed as a spray product and as a concentrated topically applied liquid (Frontline Top Spot) for use in dogs and cats. The topical liquid product is applied on the back between the shoulder blades and works its way over the rest of the body surface by the animal's movements. Fipronil is stored in the sebaceous glands associated with the hair follicles; apparently this site acts as a depot of the compound that is then exuded back onto the skin surface. The residual effect of fipronil in efficacy trials indicated a residual insecticidal effect of at least 30 days, even if the animal is bathed. Thus Frontline is being marketed as a once-a-month spray and topical liquid.

The binding of fipronil to the dermis, hair follicles, and sebaceous glands makes toxicity from licking unlikely. A disadvantage of fipronil in its present spray formulation is that, like many sprays, the active ingredient is dissolved in an alcohol base. Alcohol dries the skin, causes salivation if the site is licked while wet, and often has an unpleasant odor because of the volatility. An advantage of the topical drop application over the spray is that cats are often intolerant of sprays and would have to be physically restrained long enough to ensure proper dose application. Clients and veterinary professionals should wear gloves when applying this product to prevent exposure to the drug.

NITENPYRAM

Nitenpyram (Capstar) is an oral tablet used in dogs and cats to kill adult fleas. Nitenpyram claims to be faster in onset of flea-killing activity than fipronil or imidacloprid, although the clinical significance of this difference may be minimal. Nitenpyram is a nicotinelike compound that combines with a nicotinic type of acetylcholine receptor mentioned with the organophosphate compounds. Nitenpyram initially stimulates the nicotinic acetylcholine receptor, causing increased nervous system activity (increased flea movement and seizures) followed by the receptor locking up (receptor blockade), resulting in the receptor no longer being able to stimulate the muscle and subsequently producing paralysis and ultimately death of the flea. Unlike organophosphates, which can produce a similar nicotinic receptor blockade in both insects and mammals, nitenpyram is designed to have greater affinity (attraction) for insect nicotinic receptors than mammalian nicotinic receptors because of subtle differences between mammal and insect nicotinic receptor structure. It is this preferential affinity for the insect's receptor that confers the safety of nitenpyram in mammals.

Nitenpyram is effective only against the adult flea. Therefore, if it is used as the only flea product, it will need to be used as long as viable flea eggs and pupa exist and continue to hatch. Because nitenpyram has a short half-life, it can be safely given on a daily basis without concerns for accumulation of drug. The manufacturer recommends using Capstar with an insect growth regulator or *insect development inhibitor* such as lufenuron (Program), the combination of which would strike at more than one part of the flea life cycle and more effectively reduce the flea population. As of this writing, Capstar was being marketed with Program and Sentinel products as a flea management system.

The manufacturer warns that flea-infested pets treated with nitenpyram will actually increase their scratching for a short period after administration of the drug because the initial nicotinic receptor stimulation that produces increased nervous system and muscle activity produces seizurelike activity of the flea and hence the urge by the animal to itch. The veterinary technician should notify the owner of this temporary but common side effect, explain why this effect is occurring, and reassure the owner that it is not a drug reaction to the nitenpyram.

INSECT GROWTH REGULATORS, INSECT DEVELOPMENT INHIBITORS, AND JUVENILE HORMONE MIMICS

Insect growth regulators (IGRs), insect development inhibitors (IDIs), and *juvenile hormone mimics* (JHMs) are compounds that affect immature stages of insects and prevent maturation to adults. IGR is the term often applied to any compound, regardless of mechanism, that interferes with insect development; IDIs and JHMs are types of insect growth regulators.

Lufenuron (Program) is an IDI available as a tablet and chewable tablet for dogs and cats and as a 6-month injectable for use in cats. Lufenuron is combined with milbemycin oxime in an oral tablet heartworm preventative/flea controller product called Sentinel.

Lufenuron is absorbed and distributes throughout an animal's tissue fluids. When the adult flea bites and feeds on the animal, the lufenuron is taken into the adult flea and affects egg development. Lufenuron interferes with the deposition of chitin into the flea egg and the exoskeleton of the larvae within the egg. Chitin accounts for the "crunch" noticed when an insect is crushed and is a key structural component of the exoskeleton. Thus the larvae may die because of the poor construction of the egg, or the larvae may be unable to hatch out of the egg because of a lack of an effective egg tooth, which is also composed of chitin. Larvae that do hatch out of the eggs because of lower exposure

to lufenuron will be smaller and less likely to survive because of poor chitin deposition in their exoskeleton. Although chitin deposition occurs in adult fleas, the concentration of lufenuron achieved in adult fleas is insufficient to significantly affect chitin formation. Therefore, lufenuron is not effective against adult fleas. Because lufenuron targets chitin and because mammals do not have chitin in their bodies, lufenuron is considered a very safe compound.

To enhance absorption of orally administered lufenuron, the medication should be given with a meal. When absorbed into the mammal's body, lufenuron is distributed to all tissues, including fat, where it is taken up and retained. This constitutes a depot of lufenuron that will slowly move back into circulation and be redistributed to tissues over a period of 1 month. This explains why Program tablets are administered once a month and the Program 6 Month injectable can provide extended protection for half of a year.

The manufacturer of Program 6 Month injectable notes that localized tissue reactions have occurred with this drug. Vomiting and listlessness have also been reported. Program 6 Month injectable is not to be used in dogs because of a severe local reaction that occurs in dogs that is not observed in cats. It is also interesting to note that the tablet doses of lufenuron are higher than the equivalent doses used in dogs (in contrast to many other drugs). In this case, lufenuron is less efficiently absorbed from the intestinal tract in cats than it is in dogs (lower bioavailability in cats), necessitating a higher dose in cats to achieve equivalent drug concentrations found in dogs.

Because lufenuron affects eggs laid by adult fleas, there is a lag time of up to 2 weeks between when lufenuron treatment is started and when significant changes in flea reproduction are noted. Thus, for lufenuron to be effective to a client's satisfaction, it is highly recommended that a flea adulticide be used simultaneously to reduce the pet's aggravation from flea bites.

It is interesting to note that the enzyme system needed for chitin deposition and disrupted by lufenuron is also needed by some fungal agents for normal function. Thus lufenuron is being investigated for its potential use as an agent for treatment of superficial skin fungal infections (e.g., ringworm).

Methoprene and fenoxycarb were some of the first IGRs incorporated into topically applied insecticidal products and flea collars. While generally regarded as safe, the manufacturer of fenoxycarb voluntarily withdrew this product from the market in 1996 because of concerns over the results of government testing involving the use of high doses of the drug. Methoprene, however, is still used in veterinary products as an insect growth regulator.

Whether incorporated into a flea collar or applied topically, these compounds distribute over the animal's skin and thus work by direct contact with the flea. Adult female fleas absorb the drug and incorporate the IGR into the flea eggs. The drug-impregnated eggs hatch, but the larvae do not mature to adult fleas. Although methoprene would also be effective if it came into contact with the immature larval stages of fleas in the environment, flea pupae in carpets are probably protected from methoprene because of the carpet fiber length and methoprene's propensity to adhere to fibers.

It is important to reemphasize that these IGRs do not have any adulticidal activity (do not kill mature fleas). Therefore these products are typically used as one component of a flea-control program along with environmental control of fleas and judicious application of an adulticide to kill mature fleas on an animal.

Pyriproxyfen (Nylar) is a JHM with a mechanism of action thought to be similar to, but perhaps more potent than, that of methoprene. Nylar is marketed for control of fleas in the environment but may also be formulated in a product for use on the animal. Early research suggests that pyriproxyfen may have some activity against adult fleas, but the effect is not immediate.

INSECT REPELLENTS

Insect repellents are used to repel insects and keep them off animals. Repellent formulations include fly sprays, ear tags, and products applied to the tips of dogs' ears. Some of these products are insecticides as well as repellents. In horses and cattle, repellents prevent flies from laying eggs on the skin, reducing bot and warble infestations. In outdoor dogs, especially those with upright ears such as German shepherds and Doberman pinschers, flies sometimes continually bite the ear tips, producing oozing wounds and encrustations of black, scabby material (ear tip fly strike). Application of a repellent to the ears of these dogs reduces fly strike.

Some pyrethrins and pyrethroids, such as permethrin, have natural repellent properties. Butoxypolypropylene glycol (Butox PPG) is a repellent that has been incorporated into flea and tick spray products for use in dogs and cats. It is also used in equine fly repellents because it provides a shine that is of cosmetic value in show animals. Butoxypolypropylene glycol can cause dermal irritation if a harness or collar is applied over the area while the haircoat is still wet with spray.

Diethyltoluamide (DEET) is a common ingredient in repellent products formulated for use in people. It also was used with fenvalerate in the product Blockade (manufactured by Hartz), which was withdrawn from the market for several months because of reports that it caused death in several treated cats and dogs. Signs of toxicosis from this product include excitation, tremors, seizures, ataxia, and vomiting. People who use DEET in pure (100%) formulations have reported numbness of the lips or tingling associated with repeated use or application of large amounts.

Box 12-1 Drug Categories and Names

INTERNAL PARASITE DRUGS

Antinematodals
 Avermectins and milbemycins
  Ivermectin (Heartgard, Ivomec, Eqvalan)
  Selamectin (Revolution)
  Doramectin (Dectomax)
  Eprinomectin (Eprinex)
  Milbemycin oxime (Interceptor, Sentinel)
  Moxidectin (Cydectin, Quest, ProHeart)
 Benzimidazoles
  Thiabendazole
  Fenbendazole (Panacur, Safe-Guard)
  Oxibendazole (Anthelcide EQ)
  Albendazole (Valbazen)
  Oxfendazole (Benzelmin)
 Pyrantel pamoate and pyrantel tartrate
 Piperazines
 Organophosphates

ANTICESTODALS

Praziquantel
Epsiprantel

HEARTWORM MEDICATIONS

Melarsomine (Immiticide)
Levamisole
Ivermectin (Heartgard)
Milbemycin oxime (Interceptor)

Selamectin (Revolution)
Diethylcarbamazine (DEC)

ANTIPROTOZOALS

Amprolium
Metronidazole
Fenbendazole (Panacur)
Ponazuril (Marquis)

EXTERNAL PARASITE DRUGS

Organophosphates and carbamates
 Antidotes
  Atropine
  Glycopyrrolate
  Pralidoxime (2-PAM)
Pyrethrins and pyrethroids
Piperonyl butoxide
Amitraz
Macrolides
 Avermectin
 Milbemycins
Imidacloprid (Advantage, Advantx)
Fipronil (Frontline, Top Spot)
Nitenpyram (Capstar)
Lufenuron (Program, Sentinel)
Methoprene
Pyriproxyfen (Nylar)
Diethyltoluamide (DEET; repellent)

REFERENCES

1. Johnson PJ, Mrad DR, Schwartz AJ, et al: Presumed moxidectin toxicosis in three foals, *JAVMA* 214: 678-680, 1999.

RECOMMENDED READING

Heartworm Infection

Atkins CD: *Feline heartworm disease: what's different.* In Proceedings of the Waltham/OSU Symposium, Small Animal Cardiology, Columbus, OH, 2002.

Boothe DM: *Treatment of heartworms in dogs and cats.* In Proceedings of the North American Veterinary Conference, Orlando, FL, January 2003.

Dillon R: *Heartworm adulticides: rapid kill vs slow kill— the complications.* In Proceedings of the Western Veterinary Conference, Las Vegas, NV, 2003.

Hutchens DE, Paul AJ: Moxidectin: spectrum of activity and uses in an equine anthelmintic program, *Compendium for Continuing Education,* April 2000.

Snyder PS, Levy JK: *Heartworms in cats, the rest of the story.* In Proceedings of the North American Veterinary Conference, Orlando, FL, January 2003.

Tanner PA, Keister DM, Dunavent BB: *Clinical pathology changes in dogs with severe heartworm disease following treatment with immiticide,* Proceedings of the American Association of Veterinary Parasitologists, Abstract 75, Auburn, AL, March 1995.

Internal Parasites

Boothe DM: *Small animal clinical pharmacology and therapeutics,* Philadelphia, 2001, WB Saunders.

Furr M, et al: Efficacy of ponazuril 14% oral paste as a treatment for equine protozoal myeloencephalitis, *Veterinary Therapeutics* 2:215-231, 2001.

Lech PJ: Ponazuril, *Compendium for Continuing Education,* June 2002.

Leib MS: Giardia *infection in dogs and cats.* Proceedings of the Purdue University Fall Conference for Veterinary Technicians and Veterinarians, West Lafayette, IN, September 2001.

Tams TR: *How I treat Giardia.* In Proceedings of the North American Veterinary Conference, Orlando, FL, January 2003.

Thompson RCA, Robertson ID: *Gastrointestinal parasites of dogs and cats: current issues.* In Proceedings of the Bayer Zoonosis Symposium, Orlando, FL, 2003.

External Parasites

Foil CS: *Flea control update.* In Proceedings of Western Veterinary Conference, Las Vegas, NV, 2003.

Kwochka KW: *Canine and feline demodicosis treatment options.* In Proceedings of the Western Veterinary Conference, Las Vegas, NV, 2004.

Miller WH Jr, Scott DW, Cayatte SM, et al: Clinical efficacy of increased dosages of milbemycin oxime for treatment of generalized demodicosis in adult dogs, *J Am Vet Med Assoc* 207:1581-1584, 1995.

Self-Assessment

REVIEW QUESTIONS

Fill in the following blanks with the correct item from the Key Terms list.

1. _____ inhibitory neurotransmitter involved with the effects of diazepam tranquilizers; originally thought to account for the majority of ivermectin's clinical signs until glutamate was discovered to be the primary neurotransmitter that accounts for ivermectin effects.

2. _____ tapeworm segments.

3. _____ type of cholinergic receptors that, when stimulated, produce muscle tremors and eventually paralysis.

4. _____ compounds that specifically inhibit coccidia protozoa.

5. _____ means "dilated pupils."

6. _____ term used to describe compounds that kill flukes.

7. _____ means that the drug expels the worms while they are still alive.

8. _____ condition that occurs after recovery from acute organophosphate toxicosis.

9. _____ type of cholinergic receptors that, when stimulated, produce the classic SLUDDE signs of organophosphate toxicosis.

10. _____ anthelmintics that kill both internal and external parasites.

11. _____ neurotransmitter associated with parasympathetic effects.

12. _____ general term used to describe compounds that kill a wide range of internal parasites.

13. _____ molecule responsible for moving drugs like ivermectin from the CNS into the blood; part of the blood-brain barrier functional mechanism.

14. _____ term used to describe compounds that kill worms that are round in cross-section.

15. _____ inhibitory neurotransmitter thought now to account for the effects of ivermectin.

16. _____ refers to something that floats along in the blood vessel until it lodges and causes obstruction (e.g., degenerating heartworm pieces obstructing pulmonary arteries).

17. _____ type of drug that kills heartworm adult worms.

18. _____ term used to described compounds that kill protozoa.

19. _____ parasites that live on the outside of the animal's body (e.g., fleas, ticks).

20. _____ means "coughing up blood."

21. _____ means "kills parasite eggs."

22. _____ enzyme that destroys acetylcholine to terminate acetylcholine's action.

23. _____ means "itching."

24. _____ term used to describe compounds that kill tapeworms.

25. _____ compounds that kill the young produced by adult heartworms.

26. _____ means that an insecticide is much more poisonous to the parasite than it is to the host animal.

27. Although it is preferable to remember the nonproprietary name for most drugs, many of the antiparasitic drugs are commonly referred to only by their trade names. Thus for this group of drugs, the veterinary technician should know which trade names correspond to which nonproprietary drug names. For each of the following trade names, identify the active ingredient.

   A. Advantage

   B. Program

   C. Immiticide

   D. Revolution

   E. Interceptor

   F. Heartgard

   G. Sentinel

   H. Panacur

   I. Strongid, Nemex

   J. Droncit

   K. Frontline, Top Spot

   L. Capstar

Identify the correct drug for each description from the list in Box 12-1.

28. _____ one of the safest groups of the external insecticides; characterized by its quick knock down; made from chrysanthemum.

29. _____ group of internal and external antiparasitic drugs that works primarily by stimulation of the inhibitory neurotransmitter glutamate's receptors.

30. _____ originally developed for demodicosis; extremely toxic if ingested; α_2 agonist.

31. _____ toxicosis from this endectocide results in CNS depression and is exhibited by ataxia, depression, blindness, and coma; toxicosis may last for several days.

32. _____ safe roundworm medication found in grocery stores; once-a-month OTC dewormer; no effect on worms other than ascarids; vermifuge.

33. _____ topically administered endectocide; used to control fleas and ticks, ear mites, sarcoptic mange, and as a heartworm preventative for dogs and cats; avermectin-type drug.

34. _____ antiprotozoal used primarily in calves and avian species; similar in structure to thiamin and therefore acts by causing a thiamin deficiency.

35. _____ arsenical adulticide against *Dirofilaria*; requires a deep IM injection.

36. _____ drugs blocked from getting to the brain by P-glycoprotein.

37. _____ group of insecticides that works by blocking acetylcholinesterase.

38. _____ milbemycin type of antiparasitic approved for use in cattle and horses; was the active ingredient in the 6-month heartworm preventative ProHeart.

39. _____ prototype drug for the benzimidazoles; attacks β-tubulin in the parasite cells; has antiinflammatory and antifungal activity so is used in some ear medications.

40. _____ antiprotozoal drug developed to be effective against the agent that causes EPM.

41. _____ microfilaricide most commonly used (not milbemycin).

42. _____ benzimidazole anthelmintic; approved for use in dogs, horses, and livestock; must be given for 3 consecutive days in the dog to be effective; includes the trade name livestock medication Safe-Guard.

43. _____ antinematodal; considered very safe; effective against hookworms as well as ascarids; pleasant-tasting liquid suspension administered PO; often combined with other anthelmintics like praziquantel or ivermectin.

44. _____ toxic signs include SLUDDE signs or muscle tremors progressing to paralysis.

45. _____ single-treatment tapeworm medication; effective against many different species of tapeworms, including *Echinococcus*.

46. _____ heartworm preventative avermectin approved for use in cats and dogs once a month as an oral medication; was the first canine heartworm preventative.

47. _____ orally administered macrolide heartworm preventative but not an avermectin; also approved to control hookworm, ascarid, and whipworm infections.

48. _____ topically applied flea insecticide; put between the shoulder blades; wide margin of safety; blocks nicotinic cholinergic receptor site for acetylcholine.

49. _____ flea tablet; inhibits chitin formation in larvae and egg; is an IDI.

50. _____ daily administered oral heartworm preventative medication; has largely been replaced by the monthly use of avermectins and milbemycins.

51. _____ macrolide heartworm preventative for use in cats and dogs that is similar in structure and mechanism of action as the avermectins; also approved to treat ear mites in cats.

52. _____ antibacterial drug that is also antiprotozoal, especially against *Giardia*; has neurologic side effects at high doses.

53. _____ injectable and pour-on avermectin-type drug approved for use in cattle and swine to treat several internal parasites, grubs, lice, and mange; has been reported to have caused severe adverse reactions in other species, including fatalities in dogs.

54. _____ insecticides associated with SLUDDE signs.

55. _____ added to pyrethrins to increase their killing activity; a synergist drug.

56. _____ topically applied insecticide; removes the inhibitory effect of GABA on the nervous system, causing overstimulation of the insect and death; is very safe because the receptor site for this drug in insects is very different from the receptor site in mammals; can be toxic to some fish.

57. _____ antidote for organophosphate or carbamate toxicosis; readily available in most veterinary practices; blocks acetylcholine receptor.

58. _____ oral tablet flea adulticide; rapid death of the fleas; nicotine type compound, so stimulates muscle movement of the fleas initially then paralyzes them; animals may have a transient period of increased itching after administration because of seizurelike activity of the fleas as they die.

59. _____ JHM for fleas; larvae do not mature to adults; adulticide activity is minimal; similar to methoprene.

60. _____ insect repellent often used in human repellent products; can cause neurologic side effects.

61. Indicate below whether the following statements are true or false.

   A. Heartworm disease can be acquired from a blood transfusion taken from a heartworm-positive dog that has circulating microfilaria.

   B. Cats should be treated for adult heartworms with melarsomine.

   C. The "L" in SLUDDE stands for "locomotion."

   D. Glutamate is an excitatory neurotransmitter.

   E. Live ascarid worms may be expelled after administration of piperazine.

62. What dog breed is more susceptible to ivermectin toxicosis?

APPLICATION QUESTIONS

1. You have a dog that presented to the hospital after ingestion of diazinon, an organophosphate insecticide commonly found in lawn applications for grubs. What is the readily available first drug of choice for treatment of this toxicosis? Does this drug have

an advantage or disadvantage over glycopyrrolate? What other less-available drug is also used? What are the differences in their mechanisms of action?

2. A client calls and is somewhat angry because the veterinarian gave his dog an injection of a wormer and he is not seeing any worms come out as he does with the store-bought medicine for worms. You look on the record and see the medication given was praziquantel. What do you tell this pet owner?

3. An owner, whose dog was successfully treated for heartworms with melarsomine 2 weeks ago, calls and is quite frustrated at having to keep the dog inside or on leash-only exercise. "He seems fine and is very energetic. Can he be allowed to run in the fenced-in backyard?" What should you say?

4. A client asks you a question about the heartworm preventative you have been instructed to dispense to her. "My parents always had to give a daily heartworm preventative and their veterinarian always said it was really bad to give it if the dog already had heartworms. Do we have the same risk if the dog has heartworms and we put him on this once-a-month heartworm preventative?"

5. Pyrethrins and pyrethroids are safe insecticides commonly found in premise sprays and foggers. A pet store owner wants to fog his store with a pyrethrin product to get rid of the spiders and other bugs that inhabit the various nooks and crannies. Are there any problems with pyrethrin use in this situation?

6. What should clients be advised about any amitraz-type of flea or tick collars?

7. Why should amitraz mange, flea, or tick products not be used on animals that are also being treated with medication for behavioral problems?

8. Why is it that IDIs, IGRs, and JHMs such as lufenuron, methoprene, or pyriproxyfen are incomplete solutions to flea problems? Why do they not provide the pet with immediate relief from fleas?

Antiinflammatory Drugs

outline

key terms

Addison's disease

adrenocorticotropic hormone

aldosterone

alopecia

arachidonic acid pathway

atrophy

autoimmune reactions

B-lymphocytes

catabolic effects

cell-mediated immunity

cortex (of endocrine gland)

corticotropin-releasing factor

Cushing's syndrome

cyclooxygenase

eicosanoids

eosinopenia

glucocorticoids

gluconeogenesis

glycogenesis

humoral immunity

hyperadrenocorticism

hypersensitivity reaction

hypoadrenocorticism

iatrogenic

leukotrienes

lipoxygenase

lymphopenia

mineralocorticoids

monocytopenia

neutrophilia

phospholipase

phospholipid

propionic acid

prostaglandins

renal papillary necrosis

thromboxanes

T-lymphocytes

objectives

After studying this chapter, the veterinary technician should be able to define or describe:

1. The terminology used to describe antiinflammatory drugs

2. The mechanism by which inflammation occurs

3. The mechanisms by which glucocorticoids and NSAIDs work

4. How glucocorticoids and NSAIDs differ in their effects and side effects

5. Precautions that apply to glucocorticoids, nonsteroidal antiinflammatory drugs, and cyclooxygenase-2 inhibitor drugs

Inflammation is a protective mechanism that increases the blood supply to a traumatized or infected area, increases migration of leukocytes (white blood cells) into the area, and increases the activity of phagocytes (cells that engulf and destroy foreign material and microorganisms). If this protective mechanism is activated inappropriately or if its activity goes beyond what is beneficial (such as with arthritis, severe allergic reactions, or autoimmune disease), drugs are necessary to prevent excessive tissue damage.

Drugs that relieve pain or discomfort by blocking or reducing the inflammatory process are called antiinflammatories. Two general classes of antiinflammatories exist: steroidal antiinflammatory drugs (corticosteroids) and nonsteroidal antiinflammatory drugs (NSAIDs). These drugs all have the common effect of relieving pain indirectly by decreasing inflammation in the local tissue. Because these drugs have not traditionally decreased the perception of pain at the level of the central nervous system like the opioids, antiinflammatories were not considered to be true analgesics (pain-killing drugs). However, some of the antiinflammatory drugs appear to be able to produce a reduction in pain that has a quicker onset and greater activity than can be explained by a reduction in inflammation alone. Therefore some antiinflammatory drugs are now considered to have analgesic properties. This is just one example of how the area of antiinflammatory drugs is rapidly changing in veterinary therapeutics and will require the veterinary professional to be vigilant in keeping up with how these drugs apply to contemporary veterinary practice. (Box 13-1 listing drug categories and names can be found at the end of this chapter.)

INFLAMMATION PATHWAY

After an insult or injury such as trauma, burns, or infection, tissues respond by producing several substances collectively called *eicosanoids* that produce the classic signs of inflammation and also initiate the steps of the healing process.

Many of these substances also stimulate pain receptors in the injured tissue or increase the sensitization of pain receptors that, when stimulated, send their impulses to the spinal cord and brain, resulting in the animal perceiving pain at the site of the inflammation. See Chapter 8 for a description of the pain pathway. If the production of eicosanoids is reduced or inhibited, the inflammatory process would be diminished and stimulation or reaction of the pain receptors could be decreased, reducing the perceived pain at the site of injury.

ARACHIDONIC ACID PATHWAY

Any time cells are traumatized, a well-described series of steps occurs in a sequence similar to knocking over the first domino in a line of dominos. This sequence is called the *arachidonic acid pathway.* The sequence starts with trauma to a cell membrane, which causes the *phospholipid* molecules that comprise the cellular membrane to be converted into arachidonic acid by the enzyme *phospholipase.* The arachidonic acid is then acted on by either *cyclooxygenase* enzymes (COX) to produce eicosanoids called *prostaglandins* and *thromboxanes,* or by the enzyme *lipoxygenase,* which produces another group of inflammatory mediators called *leukotrienes.* The prostaglandins, thromboxanes, and leukotrienes diffuse out of the cell to initiate a very wide variety of physiologic reactions (the next steps in the sequence) that are associated with the inflammatory response.

Corticosteroids, especially the *glucocorticoids,* reduce inflammation by blocking the action of phospholipase and hence stabilize the cell's phospholipid membranes. This blocks the early portion of the pathway shown in Figure 13-1, reducing production of most inflammatory mediators. NSAIDs have no significant effect on phospholipase but inhibit cyclooxygenase and, to varying degrees, lipoxygenase, reducing production of prostaglandins, thromboxane, and leukotrienes. Glucocorticoids also depress cyclooxygenase, thus potentially inhibiting the arachidonic acid pathway at two different sites.

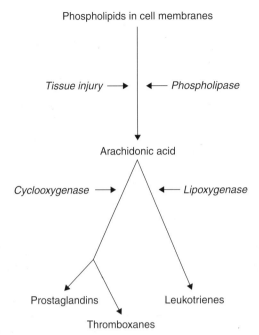

Phospholipids in cell membranes

Tissue injury ⟶   ⟵ *Phospholipase*

Arachidonic acid

Cyclooxygenase ⟶   ⟵ *Lipoxygenase*

Prostaglandins   Leukotrienes

Thromboxanes

Figure 13-1 The arachidonic acid cascade for production of inflammatory mediators.

When these inflammatory mediators are decreased by corticosteroids or NSAIDs, this decreases the production of several other compounds, including histamine, kinins, substance P, and superoxide radicals, which contribute to the redness, swelling, heat, and pain associated with inflammation.

CORTICOSTEROIDS

The term corticosteroids (technically called adrenocorticosteroids) refers to a group of hormones produced by the *cortex* (the outer layer) of the adrenal gland. There are two groups of corticosteroids: *mineralocorticoids* and glucocorticoids. Although both groups of hormones are produced by the same gland, they have very different effects on the body.

Mineralocorticoids, as the name implies, affect the minerals in the body, such as sodium, potassium, and other electrolytes. Mineralocorticoids are involved with water and electrolyte

balance in the body but have little or no antiinflammatory effect. *Aldosterone* is the mineralocorticoid hormone of medical significance in animals with adrenocortical insufficiency. A low functioning adrenal gland cortex (*hypoadrenocorticism* or *Addison's disease*) results in a potentially fatal hyperkalemia (increased blood potassium) and hyponatremia (decreased blood sodium) because of a lack of aldosterone production. Mineralocorticoid drugs like desoxycorticosterone pivalate (Percorten-V) are used to treat animals with Addison's disease signs.

In contrast, glucocorticoids produce an antiinflammatory effect by inhibiting phospholipase, and to a lesser degree cyclooxygenase, thus decreasing the production of prostaglandins and leukotrienes involved with inflammation. The glucocorticoids also appear to inhibit the production of other mediators that are involved in toxic and immune-mediated cellular damage, which helps explain corticosteroid's role in controlling allergic reactions. Corticosteroids also reduce production of cell factors that cause increased vascular permeability of the capillaries and in so doing help maintain the integrity of the capillaries and reduce some of the mechanisms by which swelling occurs in injured tissues.

Every corticosteroid drug has both mineralocorticoid (sodium retention) and glucocorticoid (antiinflammatory, glycogen deposition) effects to some degree. Therefore corticosteroids are generally classified as a glucocorticoid or a mineralocorticoid depending on which effect predominates. Because this chapter concerns antiinflammatory effects, glucocorticoid drugs are the focus.

GLUCOCORTICOIDS

When veterinarians use the terms cortisone, corticosteroids, or just steroids, they are usually referring in a loose way to glucocorticoid drugs. Glucocorticoids are natural hormones normally produced by the adrenal cortex in

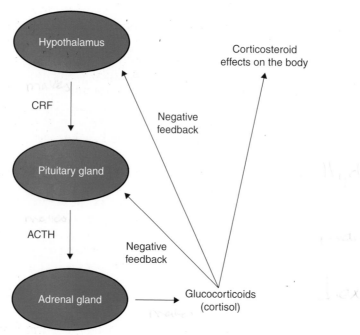

Figure 13-2 Regulation of glucocorticoid production.

response to release of *adrenocorticotropic hormone* (ACTH) by the anterior pituitary gland. The release of ACTH from the anterior pituitary is in turn controlled by *corticotropin-releasing factor (CRF)* from the hypothalamus. The production of hydrocortisone (cortisol) and cortisone by the adrenal gland provides the needed systemic effect on the body and simultaneously stimulates the negative feedback needed to curtail release of CRF and ACTH. Thus the CRF-ACTH-cortisol negative feedback loop (Figure 13-2) is similar to the self-regulating mechanisms described for other hormones in Chapter 7.

Exogenous glucocorticoids are administered as drugs used to reduce inflammation (e.g., prednisone, prednisolone, methylprednisolone) and have the same negative-feedback effect on the hypothalamus and pituitary gland as the endogenous (internally produced) cortisol. This negative feedback from exogenous corticosteroid drugs can result in potentially severe side effects through suppression of the adrenal gland if glucocorticoids are used inappropriately.

TYPES OF GLUCOCORTICOID DRUGS

Glucocorticoids are classified according to their duration of biologic activity (antiinflammatory effect, changes in glucose metabolism or storage). A glucocorticoid that exerts an antiinflammatory effect for less than 12 hours is considered to be a short-acting glucocorticoid. Hydrocortisone is a short-acting glucocorticoid and a common ingredient in topical medications. Hydrocortisone is very similar to the natural cortisol hormone. Cortisone is another common short-acting glucocorticoid often cited as being the same as hydrocortisone (e.g., cortisone products), but it is chemically different and must be converted by the liver to hydrocortisone before it becomes active. Cortisone is not used in veterinary medicine to any appreciable amount even though hydrocortisone is found in a wide variety of topical veterinary preparations.

Many of the glucocorticoids used systemically in veterinary medicine are classified as intermediate-acting glucocorticoids and exert their biologic activity for 12 to 36 hours. These drugs include the "preds" (prednisone, prednisolone, methylprednisolone, and isoflupredone) and triamcinolone. Although prednisolone and prednisone are often considered to be interchangeable, they are slightly different in that prednisone must be converted by the liver to prednisolone to exert its maximal effect. Because of their duration of activity, these drugs are ideally suited for alternate-day dosing for conditions related to allergic or inflammatory disease.

The long-acting glucocorticoids, such as dexamethasone, betamethasone, and flumethasone (the methasones) exert their biologic activity for more than 48 hours. This longer duration means there is greater beneficial effect on cells and tissues; however, it also means that suppression of CRF and ACTH occurs for a longer period, with potential side effects resulting from this effect.

FORMULATIONS OF GLUCOCORTICOIDS

It is not unusual to see that one glucocorticoid drug comes in many different forms. For example, dexamethasone is available as dexamethasone, dexamethasone acetate, and dexamethasone sodium phosphate. What is the difference in these drug forms?

Glucocorticoid drugs are generally available in three injectable forms: aqueous solutions, alcohol solutions, and suspensions. The type of formulation determines the drug's route of administration and often its clinical use. Glucocorticoids in aqueous (water) solution are usually combined with a salt such as sodium phosphate or sodium succinate to make them soluble (dissolvable) in water. Therefore dexamethasone sodium phosphate and prednisolone sodium succinate (Solu-Delta-Cortef) are aqueous solutions of glucocorticoids. The advantage of the aqueous forms is that they can be given in large doses intravenously with less risk of an adverse reaction than alcohol solutions or suspensions (suspensions should never be given intravenously). The aqueous forms of glucocorticoids are often used in emergency situations such as with shock or CNS trauma because they can be delivered intravenously in large amounts and have a fairly rapid onset of activity.

Unlike glucocorticoids in aqueous solutions, glucocorticoid molecules dissolved in alcohol do not need to be attached to a salt to dissolve. Thus if the label of a vial of dexamethasone specifies the active ingredient as dexamethasone without mention of sodium phosphate salt, it is likely an alcohol solution form of the glucocorticoid drug.

Suspensions of glucocorticoids contain the drug particles floating, but not dissolved, in the liquid vehicle. Hence, suspensions are characterized by their need to resuspend the drug by shaking the vial before use; their opaque appearance after shaking and resuspension of the drug; and the terms acetate, diacetate, pivalate, acetonide, or valerate appended to the glucocorticoid drug name. Because glucocorticoids in suspension exist as relatively large crystals, the crystals injected subcutaneously must be dissolved before the drug can be absorbed from the injection site. Because the crystals in the injected suspension dissolve over several days, they release small amounts of glucocorticoid each day and provide prolonged duration of activity. The acetate form of glucocorticoid suspensions is very lipid soluble and therefore used in topical ophthalmic medications.

Suspensions of glucocorticoids must be stored within a certain temperature range. Extremes of hot or cold temperatures (e.g., being left in the practice truck on a hot day or a very cold night) can cause the crystals to change size or shape, resulting in a change in the ability of the crystal to dissolve, an alteration in the length of absorption, and pain, irritation, or inflammation at the site of injection (if the crystals are larger than normal).

EFFECTS OF GLUCOCORTICOIDS

Because glucocorticoids affect many different types of cells in the body, they produce a wide variety of effects and side effects. Glucocorticoids decrease inflammation by blocking the phospholipase and cyclooxygenase enzymes that would form prostaglandins and other eicosanoids and attract other inflammatory cells to the site of tissue damage. In addition, glucocorticoids also prevent release of lytic enzymes within cells that would cause the cells to self-destruct. By preventing cell death, glucocorticoids also help maintain the integrity of the capillaries and reduce leakage of fluids from systemic circulation, which, in turn, decreases swelling in the injured area. In addition to decreasing many of the signs of inflammation, glucocorticoids also inhibit fibroblasts that normally help close wounds and produce scar tissue. Although decreasing fibroblast activity can delay healing of wounds, decreasing excessive scar formation can prevent later damage or loss of tissue/organ function caused by contraction of scar tissue.

Glucocorticoids are often used to decrease the overreaction of the immune system associated with *autoimmune reactions* such as lupus or autoimmune hemolytic anemia, or *hypersensitivity reactions* such as allergic reactions. Unfortunately, this same immunosuppression by the glucocorticoids can prevent parts of the immune system from being as effective in fighting some invading organisms. At most therapeutic doses, glucocorticoids suppress one type of lymphocyte called the *T-lymphocytes.* T-lymphocytes are associated with the *cell-mediated immunity* in which cells like macrophages are attracted to, and engulf, foreign materials or selected disease-causing organisms. Because the primary defense against fungal agents (e.g., histoplasmosis, blastomycosis, aspergillosis) is by cell-mediated immunity (versus *humoral immunity,* which is the production of antibodies by *B-lymphocytes*), the use of glucocorticoids can increase the risk for severe infections from fungal agents and certain other types of invaders. Generally, at normal therapeutic doses of glucocorticoids, humoral immunity and antibody formation to antigens, a process required for vaccinations to confer immunity, is not significantly depressed. This is important to remember because of the large number of dogs that are on glucocorticoids for allergy-related skin inflammation and whose owners want them vaccinated while the animal is still on doses of prednisone or prednisolone. At higher than normal doses of glucocorticoids some suppression of humoral immunity as well as cell-mediated immunity may occur.

Use of glucocorticoids dramatically alters the leukogram (the number of different white blood cells in the complete blood count); therefore, a history of recent use of glucocorticoids may affect how the shift in white blood cells is interpreted by the veterinarian. Glucocorticoids cause lymphocytes, eosinophils, and monocytes to become sequestered (taken up, or stored) within the lungs, spleen, and other organs, thereby decreasing the number of cells observed in systemic circulation (*lymphopenia, monocytopenia, eosinopenia*).

In contrast, glucocorticoids increase the number of platelets and neutrophils in circulation, giving rise to *neutrophilia.* The neutrophilia is initially caused by the mobilization of neutrophils that are "parked" along the blood vessel wall (the "marginated pool" of neutrophils). Thus, on a complete blood count (CBC) it appears that more neutrophils have suddenly appeared in the blood when it may be more of a reflection of neutrophils simply rejoining the circulation instead of lingering along the vessel wall. Longer term neutrophilia is also due to increased production of the neutrophils by the bone marrow and a reduced removal from the circulation.

The combination of neutrophilia, lymphopenia, and monocytopenia is considered characteristic of glucocorticoid drug administration or stress (in which endogenous corticosteroids are released). While this combination of cells constitutes the classic "stress leukogram" on the CBC, it's important to remember that different animal species will vary in the extent to which monocytopenia or eosinopenia is observed; therefore interpretation of the stress leukogram will also vary according to species.

Although the short-term lymphopenia seen with the stress leukogram is mostly caused by sequestration of the lymphocytes in tissues outside the blood, glucocorticoids are capable of destroying malignant lymphocytes associated with lymphosarcoma, a fairly common cancer of lymphatic tissue (e.g., lymph nodes, lymph tissue in the gastrointestinal [GI] tract) in dogs, cats, and cattle. Because lymphocytes are the primary cell that proliferates in lymphosarcoma, glucocorticoids are part of the treatment protocol for this cancer.

In the GI tract, glucocorticoids increase gastric acid secretion and decrease mucus production, predisposing the patient to hyperacidity and gastric ulceration. The use of glucocorticoids with NSAIDs may significantly increase the risk of GI ulceration.

Corticosteroids are said to be catabolic because they enhance catabolism (breakdown) of protein in the body as part of their mechanism to provide amino acids for *gluconeogenesis* and subsequent elevation in glucose needed by the body to handle stress. With the breakdown of proteins over time, these *catabolic effects* can be observed clinically as muscle wasting (*atrophy*), thinning of the skin, loss of hair (*alopecia*), and decreased bone density. The "pot-bellied" appearance of dogs after long term glucocorticoid treatment is primarily due to catabolism of abdominal muscles, the subsequent loss of abdominal muscle tone, and an inability to tuck up the abdominal viscera.

Some forms of ophthalmic medications contain glucocorticoids that are used to relieve inflammation in the eye. These preparations are absolutely contraindicated if corneal ulceration is present. If glucocorticoids are used in the presence of a corneal ulcer, the catabolic effect of corticosteroids can catabolize protein that forms the middle layers of the cornea, resulting in a deepening ulcer. Because glucocorticoids suppress fibroblast activity that normally heals injuries, this effect will also slow corneal ulcer healing. The combination of catabolism and delayed healing can result in a breakdown of the corneal stroma to the point that the cornea ruptures.

There is an additional risk of ophthalmic corticosteroid use, especially in horses, because of the suppression of the cell-mediated immunity. Common fungal agents found in barn and stall environments may be found in the normal eye without producing clinical disease. However, because cell-mediated immunity is the primary defense against fungal infections, the suppression of this aspect of immunity in conjunction with a relatively minor injury to the eye (e.g., corneal scratch) may allow a fungal agent to establish a clinical infection in the eye. Because many ophthalmic preparations exist in forms with and without glucocorticoids, the veterinary technician should always double-check to be certain that the packaged preparation is exactly what has been prescribed.

As discussed in Chapter 7, exogenous glucocorticoids can induce premature parturition or abortion in cattle and mares. After 20 days of gestation, bitches may abort 2 to 5 days after receiving large doses of glucocorticoids.

As the *gluco-* part of the name implies, glucocorticoids also have effect on glucose metabolism in the body. Specifically, glucocorticoids increase the conversion of amino acids to glucose (gluconeogenesis), increase deposition of glucose in the liver as glycogen (*glycogenesis*), and decrease the ability of glucose to move from the blood into the cells, resulting in an elevation of glucose in the blood. Because glucocorticoids increase blood glucose concentrations, animals with diabetes mellitus who are given high doses of glucocorticoids, or who are put on glucocorticoid drugs for an extended period, may require an increase in their dose of insulin to compensate. Generally, if a glucocorticoid drug is used for only a short period, little or no change in the insulin dose is clinically required.

DISEASE CAUSED BY GLUCOCORTICOID USE

Overproduction of glucocorticoids by the tumors of the adrenal cortex or other pathologic conditions results in a condition called *hyperadrenocorticism,* or *Cushing's syndrome.* Underproduction of glucocorticoids by the adrenal cortex results in a condition called hypoadrenocorticism, or Addison's disease.

A state of hyperadrenocorticism can also be produced by overuse of exogenous glucocorticoid drugs, such as might occur with long-term administration of large glucocorticoid doses to control an allergic skin problem in dogs. When a disease is caused by a treatment by the veterinarian (or physician), the disease has the word *iatrogenic* attached to it. Thus iatrogenic Cushing's would occur in an animal showing hair loss, thinning skin, and pot-bellied appearance because of the glucocorticoid drugs prescribed by the veterinarian.

In addition to the alopecia, muscle atrophy, and pot-bellied appearance of the Cushingoid patient, the hyperadrenocorticism would also cause slow healing of wounds and the triad of signs: polyuria, polydipsia, and polyphagia. Although the increased water consumption, urination, and appetite become apparent soon after the animal begins receiving glucocorticoids, the signs of alopecia and atrophy do not become apparent until the animal has been treated with glucocorticoids for weeks.

It would seem to be common sense that if an animal begins to show signs of iatrogenic hyperadrenocorticism after being treated with glucocorticoids for several weeks, the veterinarian would want to stop the drug immediately. However, stopping the drug cold turkey can potentially result in a severe swing from hyperadrenocorticism to hypoadrenocorticism. The presence of high levels of natural cortisol in the blood normally provides the negative feedback to the hypothalamus and pituitary that shuts down production and release of CRF and ACTH, respectively. Essentially, the exogenous glucocorticoid drug is providing the same beneficial effects that the natural cortisol would and has the same negative feedback effect on the hypothalamus and pituitary. When glucocorticoid drugs are used for an extended period, the lack of CRF and ACTH secretion means that the adrenal cortex is not stimulated to produce cortisol. Like any other tissue in the body, if the adrenal cortex is not stimulated it begins to atrophy. With atrophy the capacity of the adrenal gland to produce natural cortisol is significantly diminished.

If glucocorticoid drug administration is suddenly stopped after weeks of daily use, the levels of corticosteroid drug in the blood will decline and the hypothalamus and pituitary will be stimulated to release CRF and ACTH again. Unfortunately, when the ACTH stimulates the adrenal cortex to produce cortisol to replace the decreasing glucocorticoid drug, the adrenal gland is unable to respond to a sufficient level. The net effect is a drop in glucocorticoid/cortisol blood levels, resulting in an Addisonian crisis. Animals with an Addisonian crisis show signs of weakness, lethargy, vomiting, and/or diarrhea. In severe cases the animal will die. Therefore an animal on corticosteroid drugs for an extended period must be tapered off the drug over days to weeks for the atrophied adrenal gland to have time to regenerate its functional capacity.

SAFE USE OF GLUCOCORTICOIDS

As previously described, glucocorticoids have the potential to produce a wide variety of undesirable side effects in addition to their beneficial effects. The following are guidelines for safe use of these potent drugs:

- If another antiinflammatory drug, such as an NSAID, can accomplish the same result, use it rather than a glucocorticoid (as long as no contraindications exist for NSAID use).

- Avoid continuous use of glucocorticoids because of the suppression of the adrenal cortex and its subsequent atrophy. To decrease the risk of adrenal suppression, it is preferable to use an intermediate-acting glucocorticoid such as prednisolone instead of the long-acting glucocorticoids for those animals requiring systemic administration of glucocorticoid (versus topical administration) for an extended period.
- Use the smallest dose of glucocorticoids that provides a clinical response, and reduce the dose as the clinical condition improves. Aim to reduce the dose to an alternate-day dosing (every 2 days) to decrease continuous suppression of the hypothalamus and pituitary.
- If an animal has been receiving glucocorticoids for an extended period, the dose should be gradually reduced to allow the adrenal cortex to regain its ability to function normally.

Most of these precautions pertain to dogs. Cats seem to be more resistant to development of Cushing's syndrome and are relatively tolerant of long-term use of glucocorticoids.

NONSTEROIDAL ANTIINFLAMMATORY DRUGS (NSAIDs)

Nonsteroidal antiinflammatory drugs (NSAIDs) are drugs that decrease inflammation like the corticosteroids but do not contain the molecular steroid ring structure and do not have many of the side effects of the glucocorticoid drugs. NSAIDs are among the most rapidly expanding group of drugs used by veterinarians. Many of the veterinary drugs have come from the human medicine side as a result of human beings being more sensitive to the side effects of glucocorticoids and needing NSAIDs to control chronic inflammation.

Most NSAIDs work by blocking the activity of cyclooxygenase enzymes and thus inhibiting the production of prostaglandins. Although most NSAIDs are not thought to block formation of the leukotriene group of eicosanoids, some NSAIDs such as ketoprofen, ibuprofen, and tepoxalin (Zubrin) inhibit lipoxygenase and decrease their production. Even though NSAIDs probably have a wide range of cellular effects, generally most of the antiinflammatory activity is focused on cyclooxygenase inhibition. In the 1990s research showed that cyclooxygenase existed in two forms. Cyclooxygenase-1 (COX-1) existed in the kidney, stomach, and other organs of the body, where it produced prostaglandins that were involved in the normal, physiologic regulation of the organ's functions. For example, COX-1 plays a very important role in causing the secretion of stomach-protective mucus, maintaining blood supply to the stomach, and decreasing acid production. COX-1 was also found to play a very important role in the kidney where COX-1 prostaglandins counteracted vasoconstriction and allowed vasodilation of the renal blood supply. In contrast, COX-2 is an enzyme that produces the prostaglandins associated with the clinical signs of inflammation. Thus, from a simplistic view COX-1 could be said to be the "good guy" and COX-2 the "bad guy." NSAIDs that selectively inhibit COX-2 without significantly inhibiting COX-1 would theoretically be able to decrease inflammation without decreasing production of the normal helpful prostaglandins in the kidneys and stomach. This has been the advantage cited by the manufacturers of the newer NSAIDs used in veterinary medicine since the mid-1990s.

Of course the real story of COX-1 and COX-2 is not as simple as this. For example, it has been found in mice that COX-2 actually helps play some role in the healing of gastric ulcers in mice. And COX-1 produces some prostaglandins that actually enhance the inflammatory reaction. In addition, most of the drugs with selective COX-2 inhibition lose some or all of that selectivity as the dose increases, meaning that they eventually inhibit as much COX-1 enzyme as they do COX-2. Still, COX-2 selective inhibitor

NSAIDs do have some advantage over non-selective COX inhibitors as far as fewer side effects on the stomach and kidney at normal doses.

COX-2 selective inhibitor drugs approved for use in veterinary medicine include carprofen (Rimadyl), etodolac (EtoGesic), deracoxib (Deramaxx), and meloxicam (Metacam). Tepoxalin (Zubrin) is a nonspecific COX inhibitor that also inhibits lipoxygenase. These drugs are discussed in greater detail below.

NSAIDs AS ANALGESICS

Older NSAIDs reduce discomfort and pain primarily by decreasing inflammation with a secondary effect of decreased stimulation of pain receptors. Generally, they had very little true analgesic effect, meaning they did not work at the CNS to decrease the perception of pain. However, newer NSAIDs appear to have an additional analgesic effect that cannot be explained by antiinflammatory activity alone. Therefore, some NSAIDs are now approved for use in preventing or diminishing postoperative surgical pain. Even though analgesic properties are attributed to some NSAIDs, they are not very strong analgesics by themselves and are not very effective by themselves in relieving severe visceral pain (pain associated with organs, such as the intestine in equine colic) or severe somatic pain (pain associated with the body surface, such as burns or severe abrasions).

NSAIDs may play an increasing role in what is being referred to as preemptive analgesia, which refers to the use of drugs before surgery or traumatic tissue manipulation to reduce the amount of pain perceived by the patient. As mentioned in Chapter 8 the spinal cord has the ability to modulate or alter the amount of pain messages that actually reach the brain. Normally the spinal cord impulses of pain are somewhat dampened by naturally occurring opioids and by nerve pathways that decrease the ability of the pain-transmitting neurons in the spinal cord to depolarize.

When pain occurs in the body, the repeated pain signals sent to the spinal cord cause these same pain-transmitting neurons to depolarize much more readily. Hence, under painful conditions the spinal cord not only transmits the signals from the pain receptors, but the neurons in the spinal cord will actually increase the number of pain impulses being sent to the brain. Thus if NSAIDs can be used before a surgery to decrease the build-up of inflammatory prostaglandins at the injury site, the pain receptors at that site will not be stimulated as readily, the number of pain impulses reaching the spinal cord will be diminished, the spinal cord's pain-transmitting neurons will not depolarize as readily, and the number of pain messages reaching the brain (perception of pain) will be diminished. So even though the NSAIDs are not considered true analgesics, used in this manner they do decrease the perception of pain by the patient.

NSAID PRECAUTIONS AND SIDE EFFECTS

All NSAIDs are tightly bound to plasma proteins circulating in the blood. Under conditions of hypoalbuminemia (low blood albumin concentrations), there is less protein available to bind the NSAID drug molecules, resulting in more NSAID molecules being in the free form and readily able to distribute from blood to the tissues. The end result of this increased distribution of the drug may be higher concentrations of NSAIDs in the tissues and enhanced beneficial effects and detrimental side effects. This effect of protein binding was described in Chapter 3. The same situation may occur if there is a normal amount of plasma albumin, but another drug displaces the NSAID molecules from the protein, resulting in more NSAID molecules free to distribute to the tissues.

There is some debate as to how clinically significant this displacement or the effect of hypoalbuminemia can be. Some experts claim that the risk for toxic side effects is significantly increased under these conditions while others say that increased elimination of the free drug molecules compensates for the increased availability of the NSAID molecules. It is generally agreed that adverse effects due to hypoproteinemia or displacement of NSAIDs from the bound protein are much more likely to occur with NSAIDs that are greater than 90% protein bound. For an NSAID that is 90% highly protein bound, a reduction in binding of only 5% increases the amount of free drug from 10% to 15% (a 50% increase in free drug available to go to the tissue and produce an effect). Contrast this with an NSAID that is only 50% protein bound. That same 5% reduction in protein binding would only result in a 10% change of freely available drug molecules. Regardless, it is still prudent to carefully monitor any animal that is taking NSAIDs while experiencing hypoalbuminemia or simultaneously taking another drug that may displace the NSAID molecules from their carrier protein.

The most common side effects of NSAIDs occur in the GI tract. PgE and PgI_2 are two types of prostaglandins that normally decrease the volume, acidity, and pepsin content of gastric secretions released during normal digestion. As discussed in the chapter on GI drugs, these "good" prostaglandins also stimulate secretion of sodium bicarbonate to neutralize the acidic stomach contents entering the intestine. They also increase perfusion of the gastric mucosa, stimulate gastric and enteric mucus production, and stimulate turnover and repair of the GI epithelial cells. Thus prostaglandins play an important role in maintaining the health of the GI tract by protecting the lining from the harsh environment of the stomach lumen and by facilitating healing should an injury to the stomach lining occur. Because nonselective COX inhibitor NSAIDs block production of all prostaglandins, including the good prostaglandins, the net effect can be a reduced ability to withstand the acidic stomach contents, gastritis (inflammation of the stomach) and, if the superficial cells of the stomach lining are eroded away, GI ulcers. This effect is similar to that caused by glucocorticoids.

It would make sense that this injury and inflammation of the stomach lining would result in affected animals having anorexia, diarrhea, ulcerations of the stomach or duodenum, and evidence of digested blood in the stool. Animals who receive an NSAID overdose or who are on nonselective NSAIDs for an extended period are most at risk for these problems. If ulcerations occur, sucralfate, histamine 2 (H2) blockers (e.g., cimetidine or ranitidine), and omeprazole are used to treat the open ulcer and reduce the acidity of the stomach (see Chapter 4). In addition, misoprostol, a drug similar in composition and effect to prostaglandin E, is sometimes used to counteract the antiprostaglandin effect of NSAIDs on the GI tract. It is important to remember that these treatments will not prevent ulcer formation in animals receiving high doses of NSAIDs. These drugs are discussed to a greater degree in Chapter 4.

NSAIDs also block beneficial prostaglandins that help regulate the renal blood supply. Under conditions of hypotension (decrease of arterial blood pressure in the body) the body normally causes vasoconstriction of the renal arterioles in an attempt to channel blood to the essential organs (e.g., brain). Although this reflex is beneficial for the overall body if used for a short period, a severe decrease in blood flow to the kidney (or any tissue or organ) can result in the cells not obtaining enough blood and hence dying from a lack of oxygen carried in the blood (tissue hypoxia). To prevent a marked decrease in blood flow to the kidney under conditions of hypotension, prostaglandin E_2 is released by the kidney. This prostaglandin dilates the renal arterioles and allows continued perfusion of kidney cells despite the decreased blood pressure and reduced overall renal perfusion.

If these hypotensive conditions and the vasoconstriction of the renal vasculature occur while an animal is being treated with NSAIDs, the protective vasodilating prostaglandins will not be released, the kidney will be unable to offset the stimulus for renal vasoconstriction, blood flow to the kidney will be markedly reduced, and parts of the kidney may die from ischemia (lack of oxygen availability). The renal papillae are the projections of the renal collecting ducts that dump urine into the collecting cavity (renal pelvis) within the kidney. These papillae have relatively sparse blood supply and hence are very susceptible to the decreased renal blood flow. Thus under these conditions of poor perfusion the renal papillae die from the tissue ischemia, producing the condition *renal papillary necrosis.*

Interestingly, COX-2, the enzyme that normally produces prostaglandins associated with inflammation, also produces prostaglandins in the kidney that are needed for normal renal function. Thus the COX-2 selective-inhibition NSAIDs are not significantly safer for prevention of renal problems than the older non-selective NSAIDs.

In addition to renal papillary necrosis associated with NSAID use in hypotensive animals, it has been suggested that at higher doses some NSAIDs may be directly toxic to the renal tubules and can be truly nephrotoxic.

With the increasing use of NSAIDs, especially the COX-2 selective NSAIDs, veterinarians have become aware of the hepatotoxicity (liver toxicity) of NSAIDs. All NSAIDs (both selective and non-selective COX inhibitors) have the potential to produce hepatotoxicity. The effect is thought to be idiosyncratic, meaning that factors that predispose an animal to the hepatotoxicity are unknown and the occurrence of the problem unpredictable. It occurs with a low frequency and is not thought to be associated with preexisting liver problems. Thus the presence of elevated liver enzymes on a blood chemistry profile is not a contraindication to use NSAIDs.

There appears to be some species differences in the ability to tolerate NSAIDs. As a general rule, the incidence of GI side effects is reported much more frequently in dogs than horses. Whether this is from the overall use of NSAIDs is not known; however, older NSAIDs such as phenylbutazone have been used for many years in horses with relatively few reported GI side effects at normal doses. Dogs given some of these traditional equine NSAIDs typically show signs of gastritis and digested blood in the stool within a few days of starting these drugs. Cats are generally considered to be poorly tolerant of NSAIDs, mostly from their reduced ability to eliminate the drug and hence their increased risk for accumulation and toxicity. Aspirin has been used safely in cats when the dose used is small and the dose interval (time between doses) is extended to every 2 days to allow for the feline's slowed metabolism of these drugs.

SPECIFIC NSAIDs

COX-2 inhibitors constitute the newest group of NSAIDs in veterinary medicine. Carprofen (Rimadyl) was the first COX-2 selective inhibitor drug released for use in veterinary medicine in the United States. Other COX-2 selective inhibitors include etodolac (EtoGesic), deracoxib (Deramaxx) released in 2002, meloxicam (Metacam) released in 2003, and firocoxib (Previcox) released in 2005.

The basis for the theoretical benefit of these drugs was previously described as well as some of the limitations of this benefit. It is important to remember that GI side effects will occur with this class of drugs and that veterinary professionals should not become complacent about the risk for gastritis and ulceration in animals on these drugs. In addition, the idiosyncratic reaction producing the hepatopathy is always a potential serious side effect. The interaction of COX-2 inhibitors and hypotension can still produce renal papillary necrosis; thus avoiding dehydration or any other cause of decreased arterial blood pressure is important.

CLINICAL APPLICATION
Are These COX-2 Inhibitors Like Vioxx and Celebrex?

The veterinarian is prescribing to Mr. and Mrs. Jones one of the COX-2 inhibitor NSAIDs for their German shepherd's arthritic hips. In the course of conversation, Mrs. Jones suddenly asks, "Isn't this the same kind of drug that Vioxx and Bextra are?" When the veterinarian starts to explain that they are similar drugs, Mr. Jones chimes in, "Won't this drug cause strokes and heart attacks in our dog? We don't want that drug!" Within minutes the Jones' have made up their minds. Their pet is not going to have any part of those "heart-killing" drugs.

What should be earned from this situation: Owners read the news and hear about problems with medications on the human side, which they will often transfer to concern over their pet's medications. In this case there are a number of points about this class of drugs that would help the veterinary professional reduce the owners' fears.

Vioxx and Bextra are two human COX-2 inhibitor NSAIDs that were taken off the market in September 2004 and April 2005, respectively, as a result of concerns with higher risks of adverse cardiovascular events (strokes and heart attacks).

Celebrex, as of summer 2005, is in this same class of human drugs and is still available.

The COX-2 selective veterinary products do not have a history of causing adverse cardiovascular effects.

Domestic animals do not develop narrowing of the arteries from plaque formation inside the arteries (atherosclerosis) like people do. These narrowed arteries restrict blood flow and help generate blood clots that give rise to strokes and heart attacks.

The dog and cat have different pharmacokinetics with the veterinary COX-2 inhibitory NSAIDs than their human counterparts. The drugs behave differently in veterinary patients than they do in human patients.

It is important to listen to the pet owners' concern and to educate them on the differences between human and veterinary drugs or the way human beings and veterinary patients respond to the same drug. Acknowledge their concern, but be able to answer their questions with current information. Stay informed!

One of the unintended problems arising from the oral COX-2 inhibitors is the flavoring of the chewable tablets. There have been several reports of dogs chewing apart dropped bottles of the flavored formulations of these drugs, ingesting large numbers of the flavorful tablets and causing an NSAID toxicosis. Clients should be informed that these chewable medications need to be stored safely away from the pet to avoid this overdose situation.

Tepoxalin (Zubrin) is a rapidly disintegrating tablet introduced in 2003 that seems to run counter to the increasing use of COX-2 inhibitor drugs. The ratio of inhibition of COX-1 to COX-2 is 30:1, meaning that COX-1 is inhibited 30 times more than COX-2. The drug is marketed as a dual-pathway NSAID because in addition to inhibiting the cyclooxygenase arm of the arachidonic pathway, tepoxalin also inhibits

lipoxygenase enzyme that produces leukotrienes. Leukotrienes are potentially potent components of the inflammatory process; therefore inhibition of this arm of the arachidonic acid pathway should contribute to inflammation control. The manufacturer counters the COX-1/COX-2 inhibition ratio by stating that the blocking of leukotrienes blocks some of the earliest steps in the formation of gastric inflammation and ulceration.

Tepoxalin is packaged in a blister pack to avoid any contact with moisture. The tablet rapidly disintegrates on contact with moisture and therefore care needs to be taken that the tablet does not come in contact with any moisture before being placed in the dog's mouth. Once placed the mouth needs to be held closed for about 4 seconds to allow for full disintegration of the tablet and swallowing. Because tepoxalin is better absorbed in the presence of food, the manufacturer recommends that treated animals should be fed either at the time of medication administration or within 1 to 2 hours after feeding.

Phenylbutazone is an older NSAID but is still one of the most commonly used NSAIDs in equine medicine. It has been used for years in horses for relief of musculoskeletal inflammation. Phenylbutazone decreases inflammation primarily by nonselectively inhibiting cyclooxygenase enzymes and decreasing prostaglandin formation.

As with most other NSAIDs, phenylbutazone is metabolized by the liver. The primary metabolite of phenylbutazone is oxyphenbutazone, which is also an active antiinflammatory agent. Phenylbutazone is highly protein bound (greater than 99% in horses), and the relative amount of free drug available for distribution to tissues varies considerably if the animal has low blood albumin levels (hypoalbuminemia) or the NSAID is displaced from the protein by other protein-bound drugs (that is, other NSAIDs, sulfonamides, or phenytoin).

It is important to be aware of the interactions of phenylbutazone with other medications the animal is taking. For example, phenylbutazone induces increased hepatic metabolism and other drugs metabolized with the same enzyme system (e.g., phenytoin, digitoxin). Similarly, other drugs such as barbiturates and corticosteroids that use the same hepatic microsomal enzymes for metabolism increase phenylbutazone metabolism, resulting in a shorter half-life and overall decreased concentrations attained in the body. Thus the effectiveness of phenylbutazone or other drugs may be altered by concurrent administration of several medications.

The adverse effects of phenylbutazone are similar to those of other NSAIDs: risk of GI ulceration; renal papillary necrosis if renal perfusion is decreased; and retention of water and sodium from decreased renal function. Two other adverse effects of phenylbutazone are bone marrow suppression resulting in neutropenia, thrombocytopenia, and anemia and tissue necrosis if the drug is injected intramuscularly or subcutaneously. Bone marrow suppression is more common in people and dogs than horses. Blood dyscrasias (abnormal blood cells) have been reported in dogs.

In horses, phenylbutazone should be given intravenously or by mouth. Accidental perivascular injection (outside the vein) can cause severe inflammation and tissue necrosis. Accidental injection of phenylbutazone into the carotid artery can cause marked CNS stimulation (that is, seizures and collapse). For these reasons, the veterinary professional must be careful to ensure that this drug is administered properly.

Aspirin (acetylsalicylic acid) is a fairly safe nonselective COX-inhibiting NSAID. Owners commonly give aspirin to their pets without advice from the veterinarian. Aspirin belongs to a larger group of compounds known as the salicylates, which include bismuth subsalicylate, found in antidiarrheal preparations such as Pepto-Bismol and, since its new formulation released in 2003, Kaopectate.

Aspirin decreases inflammation by blocking the cyclooxygenase pathway. Because thromboxane normally promotes platelet aggregation, thromboxane inhibition by aspirin is used to decrease platelet clumping. Daily aspirin doses are often given to reduce the likelihood of clot formation and subsequent blockage of coronary blood vessels in people at risk for heart attack.

Dogs with heartworm infection often have narrowed pulmonary vessels caused by proliferation of the endothelial lining of the vessel, an effect stimulated by thromboxanes. In the past aspirin was used to inhibit thromboxanes, reduce platelet clumping, and hence stop or reverse the thickening of the inner lining of the pulmonary blood vessels. However, some cardiologists now advise against using aspirin for this purpose because of the increased risk for hemorrhage due to poor platelet adhesion.

Cats with hypertrophic cardiomyopathy, a condition in which the heart muscle thickens, resulting in stiff ventricular walls and reduced

Saddle thrombosis

cardiac output, often have "turbulent" blood flow through the diseased heart. This turbulent flow causes platelets to clump and form clots. Because these clots usually form on the left side of the heart, they flow with the blood into the aorta and commonly lodge at the caudal bifurcation (forking) of the dorsal aorta, where it divides to pass into the hind legs. The resulting clot, often called a saddle thrombus, can markedly reduce blood flow to the hind legs, resulting in eventual loss of the use of the limbs. Aspirin is one of the drugs that have been advocated in these cats to reduce clot formation associated with hypertrophic cardiomyopathy.

Because of its short half-life and GI side effects in horses, aspirin is not used very often for inflammation control in horses. However, it has been used as part of the treatment protocol for uveitis (inflammation of the iris and ciliary body of the eye).

Like other NSAIDs, aspirin is metabolized by the liver. Aspirin is conjugated with (joined to) glycine and glucuronic acid by the liver enzyme glucuronyl transferase. Because cats have little of this enzyme, aspirin is metabolized much more slowly in cats than in other species. Aspirin has a half-life of 1.5 hours in people, approximately 8 hours in dogs, and 30 hours in cats. Thus as with many other drugs, the aspirin dosage for cats is lower than dosages in other species and usually consists of one "baby" aspirin (81 mg) every 2 or 3 days. If used prudently, aspirin is safe for cats.

Ibuprofen, ketoprofen, and naproxen are derivatives of *propionic acid* and share common modes of action and side effects. Like other NSAIDs, these drugs work by nonselective blocking of COX and subsequent decreased prostaglandin formation. These NSAIDs also block leukotriene formation and thus reduce inflammation associated with this other branch of the arachidonic cascade. Ketoprofen and naproxen are used in horses; however, the use of any of the propionic acid compounds in dogs has a high incidence of gastritis and ulcers. Few adverse reactions with these drugs have been reported in horses, although gastric mucosal damage and renal papillary necrosis are possible. In contrast, after 2 to 6 days of treatment, dogs consistently experience vomiting. Because of the fairly high incidence of side effects and the availability of safer NSAIDs, these propionate derivatives are not usually recommended for use in dogs.

All three drugs are available as OTC human medications. In addition to several generic brands, ibuprofen is marketed as Advil and Motrin, and naproxen is marketed as Aleve. Practicing veterinary technicians should recognize the brand names and understand the potential dangers when well-meaning owners indiscriminately give these drugs to their animals.

Flunixin meglumine (Banamine) is used primarily in equine medicine for treatment of colic. Although flunixin is a COX inhibitor and thus has an antiprostaglandin antiinflammatory effect, it also has an analgesic component that is more potent than that of other older NSAIDs such as phenylbutazone. In addition to analgesic and antiinflammatory effects, flunixin also blocks the effects of endotoxins (poisons produced by the liberation of toxins from the cell wall of gram-negative bacteria) associated with colic in horses. *horse*

In dogs, flunixin meglumine provides analgesia superior to that of aspirin or phenylbutazone. It has been used as an analgesic in dogs with hip dysplasia, arthritis, intervertebral disk disease, and anterior uveitis. However, dogs are very sensitive to the GI side effects of flunixin. Some clinicians recommend using flunixin for no longer than 3 days because of the risk of vomiting, hemorrhagic gastroenteritis, and pyloric ulceration. In contrast, horses are relatively resistant to side effects and can receive up to 5 times the recommended dose without major side effects. *arthritis dog*

Although flunixin has also been used in an extra-label manner in cattle, swine, and other species, the doses are based on anecdotal evidence rather than controlled clinical trials.

Meclofenamic acid (Arquel) has been available for use in equine medicine for over 25 years. It is most commonly administered as granules that are mixed in the feed, and accumulates in appreciable quantities in the joint fluid after oral administration. This drug has antiinflammatory and analgesic actions and is used in horses to treat lameness associated with joint inflammation. It has also been used to treat chronic joint degenerative diseases in dogs, such as hip dysplasia or chronic arthritis.

Like flunixin, meclofenamic acid is well tolerated in horses (up to 4 times the recommended dose) but can produce GI signs in dogs with long-term use. When dogs are being treated with meclofenamic acid, the owner should be advised to watch for anorexia, diarrhea, or changes in stool color (melena) that might indicate GI side effects.

Dimethyl sulfoxide (DMSO) is an excellent industrial solvent derived from wood pulp that is also used to dissolve drugs that do not readily dissolve in water. In addition, this compound also has an antiinflammatory mechanism different from other NSAIDs. DMSO is not an antiprostaglandin drug, but works by inactivating the destructive process caused by superoxide radicals (free oxygen radicals) that are a normal byproduct of the inflammatory process. These superoxide radicals produce hydroxyl radicals and hydrogen peroxide, which damage cells. DMSO traps or scavenges the hydroxyl radicals while the metabolite of DMSO traps oxygen radicals. The combined activity reduces the cellular damage produced by the inflammatory process.

DMSO is used topically and parenterally, primarily in horses. DMSO is also a component of some otic (ear) preparations used in dogs and cats (Synotic). DMSO is widely used in extra-label ways to treat a variety of conditions, including swelling from CNS trauma, mastitis, mammary swelling associated with nursing,

postoperative pain, burns, and other superficial trauma. However, the only approved uses are for acute injury associated with trauma or as an antiinflammatory in otic preparations.

DMSO is known for its ability to penetrate intact skin and has been used as a vehicle to carry dissolved drug into the body when applied topically. DMSO can also carry toxins or harmful substances when it enters an animal or penetrates the skin of the person applying it. The skin in the area of application should be thoroughly cleansed to avoid absorption of bacterial toxins or other chemicals such as oil, grease, and insecticides. DMSO is also available as an industrial-grade solvent. Although considerably less expensive than the medical-grade form, the industrial-grade should never be used on veterinary patients because of toxic impurities such as benzene that are found in many of these products. People applying DMSO should protect themselves by wearing high-quality rubber gloves during topical application.

The smell of DMSO is said to resemble garlic or raw oysters. This odor is evident during topical application, and the drug can sometimes be tasted after it is absorbed into the body. After DMSO is applied topically, erythema (redness), edema, and pruritus may develop at the application site. These reactions reflect release of histamine and other vasoactive amines from mast cells in the skin. Although the cutaneous reaction is usually mild, a more severe reaction may occur if the animal has mast cell tumors. DMSO causes these large aggregates of mast cells to release large amounts of histamine.

If given intravenously to horses, DMSO can cause hemolysis and passage of hemoglobin in the urine (hemoglobinuria). Severe hemolysis and release of hemoglobin can adversely affect the kidneys; therefore hemolysis should be minimized by using DMSO solutions with a concentration below 20% for IV administration.

In large doses, DMSO has produced defects in the offspring of hamsters and avian species. Although these effects have not been demonstrated in other species, the use of

DMSO in pregnant animals should be weighed against any benefits the drug may provide. A conservative approach would include use of another NSAID that has been documented as safe for use in pregnant animals.

CHONDROPROTECTIVE AGENTS

Within the past few years a number of products have entered the veterinary market that are designed to slow the process of arthritis in joints by supporting the health of the joint cartilage. These drugs are called chondroprotective agents because they protect the cartilage (*chondro*, meaning cartilage) from degradation and may actually promote repair of the cartilage.

POLYSULFATED GLYCOSAMINOGLYCANS (PSGAGs OR PGAGs)

The polysulfated glycosaminoglycans, or PSGAGs for short, mimic the components of the normal joint cartilage. These rather large and complex molecules in joint cartilage trap molecules of water and give cartilage its springy characteristic and ability to tolerate stressful shocks. In addition, PSGAG may inhibit or reduce activity of enzymes in the joint fluid that degrade cartilage. The addition of PSGAG in the drug form (Adequan injectable) increases the amount of these compounds within the joint cartilage. Uses of PSGAGs would be for injured joints (either from trauma or surgical intervention) or to decrease degeneration of joints because of conformation problems (e.g., hip dysplasia).

HYALURONIC ACID OR HYALURONATE SODIUM

Hyaluronic acid is an essential component of the synovial fluid, where it is assumed to increase the thickness or viscosity of the joint fluid and, in so doing, act as a lubricant for contact between cartilage surfaces. In addition, hyaluronic acid or hyaluronate sodium acts as an antiinflammatory compound through its suppression of production of prostaglandins and by scavenging free radicals that are destructive to the joint cartilage and tissue. The veterinary products (Legend, Hyalovet, and others) are injected either IV or into the joint space to relieve inflammation of the synovium (tissue surrounding the joint) of horses and, to a lesser extent, dogs.

GLUCOSAMINE AND CHONDROITIN SULFATE

Glucosamine and chondroitin sulfate are referred to as nutraceuticals because they are used like drugs but are actually natural products found in the body or used by the body for normal healthy function. Nutraceuticals are not regulated by any agency and their label, by law, cannot imply that the compound is to be used as a therapeutic agent. Glucosamine and chondroitin sulfate are actually precursors for PSGAG formation by the chondrocytes (cartilage-forming cells) and for the proteoglycans that are found in cartilage. Chondroitin sulfate binds with collagen fibers in the cartilage and supports the collagen strands. The presence of both chondroitin and glucosamine in the serum increases efficiency of the chondrocytes to repair cartilage, stimulates production of hyaluronic acid (glucosamine's action), and inhibits some of the destructive enzymes found in injured or diseased cartilage (chondroitin's action). The challenge with these products is the variability in the amount of active product since some products are extracts from living organisms (mussel, sea cucumber, sea algae, shark cartilage) and others are purified extracts (more expensive). Cosequin is perhaps the best known of the glucosamine/chondroitin sulfate nutraceuticals used in veterinary medicine.

OTHER DRUGS USED TO FIGHT INFLAMMATION

ACETAMINOPHEN

Acetaminophen is not an antiinflammatory drug. However, because of its analgesic and antipyretic (fever-reducing) properties, it is often grouped with NSAIDs. Unlike NSAIDs, acetaminophen (Tylenol) does not block prostaglandin formation associated with inflammation but reduces the perception of pain by a mechanism not clearly defined and decreases the effect of endogenous pyrogens (substances that increase fever).

Acetaminophen does not cause the GI upset, ulcers, or interference with platelet clumping associated with NSAIDs. However, the metabolites of acetaminophen can have other severe side effects, especially in cats. Acetaminophen is normally conjugated with glucuronic acid and sulfate for metabolism and elimination. A small portion of acetaminophen is also metabolized to a toxic metabolite. In most species this toxic metabolite is quickly conjugated with glutathione to form a nontoxic metabolite. Because of the relatively less effective glucuronide and sulfate conjugation in cats, more of the toxic metabolite tends to be produced. Unfortunately, the supply of glutathione needed by the liver to biotransform this toxic metabolite to a nontoxic metabolite is limited in the cat. Therefore the toxic metabolite accumulates in the liver and other tissues, producing cellular destruction. In addition to liver damage, the red blood cells are also severely affected. The hemoglobin in red blood cells is converted to methemoglobin, which is much less capable of efficient oxygen transport. Increased red blood cell hemolysis and Heinz bodies are evident on blood smears. Cats with methemoglobinemia have chocolate-colored mucous membranes and dark urine caused by methemoglobin in the blood and urine.

An acetaminophen dose of 50 mg/kg to 60 mg/kg can poison a cat. A single extra-strength acetaminophen tablet (500 mg) can kill an average-size cat. In dogs, a higher dose (above 150 mg/kg) is required before signs of hepatic necrosis, weight loss, and icterus (jaundice) become evident.

Treatment of acetaminophen toxicity focuses on providing the sulfhydryl groups of glutathione to convert the toxic metabolite to its nontoxic form. The drug most commonly used to treat acetaminophen toxicity is acetylcysteine (Mucomyst), a mucolytic agent used in treatment of respiratory infections.

ORGOTEIN

Orgotein (superoxide dismutase or SOD) exerts its antiinflammatory effect by inactivating superoxide radicals. This drug is marketed as a veterinary product and is used to prevent or reduce joint damage. Superoxide radicals associated with joint inflammation degrade hyaluronic acid, the main component in joint fluid that is responsible for joint fluid viscosity and lubrication of the joint. Orgotein works as an enzyme, superoxide dismutase, to convert superoxide radicals into oxygen and hydrogen peroxide, which are then converted to water and oxygen, thus preserving the integrity of hyaluronic acid. Orgotein is most commonly used to treat horses with joint and vertebral disease.

GOLD SALTS

Gold salts, such as aurothioglucose, are used in human medicine for treatment of rheumatoid arthritis. These compounds are apparently taken up by macrophages and possibly prevent release of lysosomal enzymes. Gold salts also decrease histamine release from mast cells and inhibit prostaglandin formation. In veterinary medicine, gold salts have been used to treat severe immune-mediated skin problems such as the various forms of pemphigus.

PIROXICAM

Piroxicam (Feldene), an NSAID formulated for use in people, is sometimes used in small animal medicine for certain types of tumors. Because of the gastric side effects and risk for renal papillary necrosis, and the availability of safer NSAIDs, this drug is not used often in veterinary medicine for its NSAID effects.

Box 13-1 Drug Categories and Names

CORTICOSTEROIDS (ADRENOCORTICOSTEROIDS)

GLUCOCORTICOIDS

Short-acting
 Hydrocortisone
 Cortisone
Intermediate-acting
 Prednisone
 Prednisolone
 Triamcinolone
 Methylprednisolone
 Isoflupredone
Long-acting
 Dexamethasone
 Betamethasone
 Flumethasone

NSAIDs

COX-2 inhibitors
 Carprofen (Rimadyl)
 Etodolac (EtoGesic)
 Deracoxib (Deramaxx)

Meloxicam (Metacam)
 Firocoxib (Previcox)
Tepoxalin (Zubrin)
Phenylbutazone
Aspirin (salicylates)
Propionic acid derivatives
 Ibuprofen (Advil, Motrin)
 Ketoprofen (Ketofen)
 Naproxen (Aleve)
Flunixin meglumine (Banamine)
Meclofenamic acid (Arquel)
Dimethyl sulfoxide (DMSO)
Chondroprotective agents
 Polysulfated glycosaminoglycans (PSGAGs)
 Hyaluronic acid
 Glucosamine
 Chondroitin sulfate (Cosequin)
Acetaminophen
Orgotein (superoxide dismutase)
Gold salts
Piroxicam

RECOMMENDED READING

Boothe DM: *Small animal clinical pharmacology and therapeutics*, Philadelphia, 2001, WB Saunders.

Brayton CF, Schwark W: Use and misuse of DMSO. In Bonagura JD, editor: *Kirk's current veterinary therapy XII*, Philadelphia, 1996, WB Saunders.

Hansen B: *Updated opinions on analgesic techniques.* In Proceedings of ACVIM, Charlotte, NC, 2003.

Hansen B: Acute pain management. *Vet Clin North Am Small Anim Pract* 30:899-916, 2000.

Mathews KA: *Pain management for the critically ill I & II.* In Proceedings of the Western Veterinary Conference, Las Vegas, NV, 2004.

Mosby's drug consult, St. Louis, 2002, Mosby.

Plumb DC: Veterinary drug handbook, ed 5, Ames, 2005, Blackwell.

Shaffran N: *NSAIDS: not just for osteoarthritis anymore!* In Proceedings of ACVIM, Minneapolis, MN, 2004.

Tranquilli WJ: *NSAIDs and perioperative pain management in dogs.* In Proceedings of the Atlantic Coast Veterinary Conference, Atlantic City, NJ, 2004.

Trepanier LA: *Drug interactions and differential toxicity of NSAIDs.* In Proceedings of ACVIM, Minneapolis, MN, 2004.

Self-Assessment

REVIEW QUESTIONS

Fill in the following blank with the correct item from the Key Terms list.

1. _____ group of adrenocorticosteroids associated with the antiinflammatory response.

2. _____ cyclooxygenase-produced eicosanoids cause platelets to adhere to each other and thus contribute to the clotting mechanism.

3. _____ means "loss of hair" and is a clinical sign of Cushing's disease.

4. _____ type of immunity provided by antibodies.

5. _____ combination of NSAID use plus arterial hypotension can produce this kidney condition that can result in kidney failure.

6. _____ lipoxygenase produces this eicosanoid.

7. _____ diseases caused by the body's own defense mechanisms turning against its own tissues; examples would be lupus or certain hemolytic anemias in which the red blood cells are attacked by the body.

8. _____ increase in neutrophils.

9. _____ effect meaning that tissue is being destroyed or broken down; seen with steroids such as corticosteroids.

10. _____ type of cell that produces antibodies against invading pathogens.

11. _____ refers to the outer part of the adrenal gland (or any gland or organ that has an outer layer).

12. _____ another name for hyperadrenocorticism.

13. _____ enzyme that produces prostaglandins and thromboxanes.

14. _____ the collective term for all the prostaglandins, leukotrienes, and thromboxanes produced by the arachidonic acid pathway.

15. _____ means "low numbers of eosinophils"; can be seen on the complete blood count when some species of animals are given corticosteroids.

16. _____ condition characterized by clinical signs consistent with insufficient amounts of glucocorticoids.

17. _____ the production of glycogen in the liver.

18. _____ hormone released from the hypothalamus that stimulates the pituitary to release ACTH.

19. _____ means "decreased monocytes" and occurs in some species with the use of glucocorticoid drugs.

20. _____ means "decreased size"; seen with the muscles and skin in animals with hyperadrenocorticism.

21. _____ means that the animal has an elevated level of either natural cortisol or exogenous corticosteroids (drugs).

22. _____ means the patient is exhibiting clinical signs consistent with low levels of corticosteroids.

23. _____ means disease or condition "caused by the veterinarian."

24. _____ hormone released by the adrenal gland; is a mineralocorticoid.

25. _____ arachidonic acid is acted on by COX and this enzyme to produce the eicosanoids.

26. _____ this group of adrenocorticosteroids affects mainly the electrolytes (sodium, potassium) and water balance in the body with little or no antiinflammatory effect.

27. _____ creation of glucose from amino acids (which come from catabolism of protein).

28. _____ a "decrease of lymphocytes in circulation."

29. _____ ibuprofen, ketoprofen, naproxen all belong to the same group of compounds characterized by this chemical structure.

30. _____ type of body defense mechanism characterized by cells that attack pathogens or foreign proteins (as opposed to the antibody response).

31. _____ thromboxanes and these inflammatory mediators are produced by cyclooxygenase.

32. _____ series of enzymes resulting in the production of eicosanoids after an injury.

33. _____ cells involved in cell-mediated immunity; do not produce antibodies.

34. _____ hormone released by the pituitary gland that stimulates the adrenal gland to produce corticosteroids.

Identify the correct drug for each description from the list in Table 13-1.

35. _____ NSAID that comes in a rapidly disintegrating tablet; not a selective COX-2 inhibitor; called a "dual-pathway NSAID because it also blocks lipoxygenase.

36. _____ chondroprotective agent that is a component of the joint synovial fluid; acts as a lubricant, and increases the viscosity of the fluid; may also suppress production of prostaglandins and scavenge free radicals.

37. _____ intermediate-acting glucocorticoid that is not a "pred."

38. _____ older NSAID commonly used in equine medicine for relief of inflammation associated with the musculoskeletal system; 99% protein bound; bone marrow suppression has been reported in dogs.

39. _____ first COX-2 selective inhibitor released for veterinary medical use in the United States.

40. _____ intermediate-acting corticosteroid; in the active form (does not have to be metabolized to become active).

41. _____ antiinflammatory that works differently from NSAIDs or glucocorticoids; scavenges superoxide radicals; stinks.

42. _____ short-acting glucocorticoid; applied topically.

43. _____ besides carprofen, the other three COX-2 selective inhibitors used in veterinary medicine.

44. _____ long-acting glucocorticoid that comes in aqueous solution, alcohol form, and suspension form.

45. _____ prototype drug for the salicylates; commonly available OTC drug; nonspecific for its COX activity (hits both COX-1 and COX-2); used to reduce the risk for spontaneous clot formation.

46. _____ derivatives of propionic acid; OTC drugs; high incidence of gastric ulcers when given by owner to pet dogs.

47. _____ NSAID used primarily in horses for relief from colic; has more analgesic effect than phenylbutazone; thought to provide some protection against endotoxins.

48. _____ chondroprotective agent that mimics the components of normal joint cartilage; traps water molecules and helps provide springy characteristic that allows the cartilage to tolerate impact; inhibits degrading enzymes in the joint fluid.

49. _____ intermediate-acting corticosteroid; must pass through liver to be converted to its active form, prednisolone.

50. _____ nutriceutical chondroprotective agents; precursors for PSGAGs; appear to increase the efficiency with which cartilage repairs itself.

51. _____ human OTC drug used to relieve discomfort from pain but is not an NSAID; very toxic to cats; rarely used in dogs.

52. Indicate whether the following statements are true or false.

   A. A long-acting glucocorticoid drug combined with acetate, diacetate, pivalate, or valerate would identify it as an aqueous solution.

   B. Vaccines should not be given to a dog that has been on prednisone for allergic skin reactions because the immune system will not be able to adequately respond.

   C. In hypoalbuminemic animals (low blood protein) the dose of NSAIDs may have to be increased to achieve the same effect on the tissues.

D. The two most common target organs for NSAID toxicity are the liver and the kidney.

E. NSAIDs should be able to provide enough analgesia to allow an animal with a broken leg to be positioned for a radiograph of the leg without using anesthesia.

53. Indicate which of the following are associated with glucocorticoid effects:

A. Increased retention of sodium.

B. Maintain integrity of capillaries.

C. Decreased fibroblast activity.

D. Decreased T-lymphocyte activity.

E. Decreased scar tissue formation.

F. Increased B-lymphocyte activity.

G. Lymphocytosis.

H. Increased eosinophils and monocytes.

I. Increased neutrophils.

J. Muscle wasting and atrophy.

54. What effect do NSAIDs have on the following: stomach and intestinal mucus production, production of sodium bicarbonate by the GI tract wall, and repair of the GI epithelial cells.

APPLICATION QUESTIONS

1. You have heard the veterinarian talk about being cautious about using glucocorticoids in animals that are diabetics. What is the connection between a lack of insulin and glucocorticoid effects?

2. If an animal has an adrenal cortex tumor that is producing glucocorticoids, what would the clinical condition be called? Would levels of natural cortisol be higher or lower than normal? What about CRF and ACTH levels?

3. An animal has been on dexamethasone tablets for 5 weeks to control severe allergies. He is showing signs of hyperadrenocorticism. If you were to check concentrations of ACTH, CRF, and natural cortisol, would they be higher or lower than normal? What would this clinical condition be called? Should the dexamethasone be stopped immediately to prevent worsening of clinical signs?

4. The veterinarian has just prescribed a COX-2 selective NSAID for Mrs. Jones' German shepherd with arthritic hips. Mrs. Jones is grumbling about the high cost of the medication and finally asks you why she cannot use aspirin because it is much cheaper. What is the medical reason for using the more expensive and newer COX-2 inhibitors over aspirin drugs?

5. The owner of an animal that is being discharged from the hospital after orthopedic surgery wants to know why there a drug is given for pain before the surgery. "That doesn't make any

sense," she says. "And according to the doctor, it was an aspirin-like drug! Who takes aspirin before having bone surgery?" What do you say to explain this?

6. What precautions should you take when working with DMSO?

7. A client is surprised to find out from you that acetaminophen (Tylenol) is so toxic to cats. "So, aspirin must be poisonous, too, since they are really the same thing, aren't they?" Answer her and explain why acetaminophen is so poisonous to cats.

8. What signs are seen with acetaminophen toxicosis in the cat? What is the treatment of choice?

Answers to Self-Assessment

Chapter 1

REVIEW QUESTIONS

1. elixir
2. emulsion
3. tincture
4. extract
5. gel cap or capsule
6. ointment or cream (not paste)
7. syrup
8. paste
9. sustained-release medication
10. enteric coated
11. generic drug
12. ampule
13. repository or depot drug
14. inert ingredients
15. indication
16. extra-label or off-label
17. side effect or adverse effect
18. Tylenol is the proprietary name (capitalized like a proper noun)
19. False. That would be a contraindication.
20. False. These are reversed. A dose is given one time.
21. True. They must follow the guidelines for their use, however.
22. True.

23. False. These are lozenges to be held in the mouth. Veterinary patients will not do this.
24. False. The ® symbol indicates a copyrighted logo or drug name.
25. True.

APPLICATION QUESTIONS

1. Today's veterinary technician cannot diagnose, do surgery, or prescribe treatment or medications, but the veterinary technician needs to understand how the drug works, its uses and contraindications, and the signs of adverse reactions to properly monitor in-hospital patients, to detect any possible adverse reactions early, and to educate clients or animal owners about the drug or if they have questions.

2. A generic drug is a drug manufactured by a company other than the original parent company. Generic drugs are less expensive because the generic drug company did not have to make the tremendous financial investment required to research, develop, test, and market the original drug. Generic drugs are required to have the same amount and type of active ingredient as the parent brand of drug. They are generally considered to be equivalent to the parent drug, although minor differences in the types of inert ingredients may affect the drug's performance in the body.

3. The enteric coating protects the medication from the acid in the stomach. Acid can denature or destroy some types of drugs; thus the generic coating allows the

drug to pass through the stomach to the less-acidic environment of the intestine, where it can dissolve and be absorbed.

4. SR is commonly put on the label of sustained-released oral medications. Sustained release means that the drug is dissolved or released over a longer period of time, thus supplying amounts of drug to be absorbed for a longer duration.

5. Suspension should never be given intravenously. Suspensions always need to be shaken (sometimes carefully, as in the case of insulin) to equally disperse the drug within the liquid medium before removal of the drug from the bottle or vial.

6. A repository drug is a depot drug. Both are designed to be absorbed over a long period after being injected into the body. Therefore the dosage interval should be longer between injections of a depot or repository drug than a nondepot drug.

7. An extract is derived from plant or animal parts. It is relatively cheaper to produce than chemically synthesizing the drug. However, some inconsistency in the amount of active ingredient occurs in some extracts.

8. The Food and Drug Administration. It is also advisable for the veterinarian to contact the technical support personnel at the drug company about any reaction he or she suspects is from the drug.

9. The veterinarian is saying to use the drug for disease X but if condition Y exists, the drug should not be used.

10. A. Not appropriate. A valid veterinarian/client/patient relationship has not been established because the veterinarian has not seen the animal.

   B. Not appropriate. If there is an FDA-approved drug form for the condition, that drug formulation is the only one that can be used.

   C. Not appropriate. No veterinarian/client/patient relationship is established for the other animals. Plus, the veterinarian has transferred the responsibility of diagnosis to the livestock producer.

   D. Maybe. Three weeks may or may not be long enough of a withdrawal time. The law requires a significantly extended withdrawal time for extra-label use drugs. A longer period would be preferable.

   E. Possibly appropriate if the drug is properly labeled and records are maintained. Goats and sheep are minor species and therefore it is not uncommon to use cattle medications in these species because there are very few, if any, medications specifically approved for use in these minor species.

   F. Good use of following the requirements for extra-label use. Make sure the label has the veterinarian's name and the active ingredient listed on it.

Chapter 2

REVIEW QUESTIONS

1. The strength (concentration) of the tablets is missing. There are 24 amoxicillin tablets (Amoxitab is a trade name) required, but we do not know if they are the 50 mg, 100 mg, 200 mg, or 400 mg size.

2. OTC

3. C-I. C-I is the highest level of potential abuse, and C-V is the group with the least amount of abuse potential.

4. cytotoxic

5. material safety data sheet

6. Occupational Health and Safety Administration

7. compounding

8. antineoplastic agents or drugs

9. household

10. mutagenic, which means capable of producing mutations

11. False. Two years is the typical recommended minimum.

12. False. Mixing two drugs in a syringe, bottle, or container is considered compounding because you are then administering these as a new combined drug with physical and pharmacologic interactions.

13. False. "Room temperature" is 59° to 86° F, whereas a refrigerator would keep drugs cool (46° to 59° F) to cold (not exceeding 46° F). "Warm" and "excessive heat" also describe specific ranges of temperature.

14. False. The Poison Prevention Packaging Act does not apply to veterinarians. However, there is an ethical obligation to warn pet owners of the risk of accidental ingestion of medication in containers that are not childproof and to emphasize keeping the medication out of reach of children.

15. True. The smaller the roman numeral, the more potential for abuse.

16. True. C-II drugs are the most potentially abusive drugs veterinarians are legally allowed to prescribe.

17. False. Although not a regulation, it is recommended that the log be kept in a bound notebook of sequentially numbered pages to reduce the risk of a page being removed and replaced by another page with adjusted inventory information to hide diversion of abuse substances.

18. A. 2000 mg

B. 0.05 g

C. 6.36 kg

D. 50.6 lb

E. 83,000,000 mg

F. 143 lb

G. 400 g

H. 1363.6 mg

I. 6818.2 g

J. 430 mg

K. 0.056 lb

L. 4181.8 mg

M. 0.025 L

N. 43 mL

O. 1500 mL

P. 0.8 L

Q. 55 mL

R. 0.00025 L

19. Convert 15 lb to kilograms. First: 15 lb × 1 kg/2.2 lb = 6.82 kg. Now determine how much drug is needed for this sized cat: 6.82 kg × 15 mg/kg = 102.3 mg of drug needed. Now determine how much physical drug you need to inject: 102.3 mg × 1mL/100 mg = 1.02 mL. Note that when multiplying the dose by the concentration in the bottle, the problem has to be set up so the "mg" in the numerator and denominator cancel each other out, leaving "mL" by itself on top. The 1.02 mL is rounded to the nearest 1/10 mL = 1.0 mL.

20. First convert the dog's weight to kilograms: 55 lb × 1 kg/2.2 lb = 25 kg. Now

determine how much drug a 25-kg dog will need: 25 kg × 0.08 mg/kg = 2 mg of drug needed. Now select the tablet size, keeping in mind that you do not want to break a tablet into anything smaller than one half of a tablet. If the 1-mg tablet size is used then we need: 2 mg × 1 tablet/ 1 mg = 2 tablets per dose. If a 5-mg tablet size is used, it comes out to 2 mg × 1 tablet/5 mg = 0.4 tablet per dose, rounded to 0.5 tablet per dose. This is not as accurate as using the two 1-mg tablets, but it is close enough if this drug is safe. Now determine how many tablets you will need for 5 days of treatment if the drug is to be given q6h (every 6 hours). For the two 1-mg tablet dose, you would need 2 tablets/dose × 4 doses/ day × 5 days = 2 × 4 × 5 = 40 tablets for the 5-day period. For the ½ tablet of the 5-mg strength tablets: 0.5 tablet/dose × 4 doses/ day × 5 days = 0.5 × 4 x 5 = 10 total for the 5-day period. Cost of the medication: 40 tablets (1-mg tablets) × $0.35/tablet = $14.00, or 10 tablets (5-mg size) × $0.35/tablet = $3.50.

21. 16-lb Chihuahua = 7.27 kg = dose range of 21.8 mg to 36.4 mg; use ½ of a 50-mg tablet. ½ tablet/dose × 1 dose/day × 180 days = 90 of the 50-mg tablets needed. 90 tablets at $0.03 per tablet = $2.70 for the 180 days. 27-lb terrier-X = 12.3 kg = dose range of 36.8 mg to 61.4 mg; use 1 whole 50-mg tablet per dose. 1 tablet/ dose × 1 dose/day × 180 days = 180 tablets. 180 tablets × $0.03 per tablet = $5.40 for the 180 days worth of medica-tion. 66-lb collie = 30 kg = dose range of 90 to 150 mg; use either 1 of the 100-mg tablets, 1½ of the 100-mg tablets, or ½ of the 200-mg tablets; costs would be, respectively, $9.00, $13.50, or $6.30.

22. 10% solution = 10 g/100 mL = 10,000 mg/ 100 mL = 100 mg/mL. 43% = 43 g/100 mL = 43,000 mg/100 mL = 430 mg/mL.

23. 7.5% solution = 7.5 g/100 mL = 7500 mg/ 100 mL = 75 mg/mL. If there is 75 mg/mL, you want to know how many are in 0.13 L or 130 mL. 130 mL × 75 mg/mL = 9750 mg in 130 mL of solution.

APPLICATION QUESTIONS

1. A valid veterinarian/client/patient relationship does not exist in this case. The veterinarian has not seen this animal, does not know what type of medication the animal is currently using for motion sickness, and does not know if there are any physical contraindications that would prevent the safe use of the drug in this animal.

2. A. Give 3 mg every 4 hours by mouth as needed

   B. Dispense 1 bottle; give 2 drops in both eyes two times daily

   C. Give 2 mL by the intraperitoneal route immediately

   D. Needs to have 3 L every day

   E. 15 mg intravenously three times daily

   F. 4.5 mL of the 5 mg/mL concentration 4 times daily

3. Technicians cannot legally order C-II drugs. Only a veterinarian with a current state license, state controlled substance permit, and DEA certification number can order C-II drugs.

4. This is not adequate. A thief can pick up and carry the box off. The storage compartment has to be made of a material of "substantial construction" that cannot be removed. A wooden cabinet, if locked and the key controlled by the veterinarian, may provide sufficient security as long as the cabinet cannot be easily broken into.

5. Generally, yes. The minimum requirement for DEA standards is 2 years. However, some states may require keeping the logs for longer than 2 years.

6. Surgical masks in one layer are porous enough to allow an aerosolized drug to pass through them. A single pair of latex surgical gloves may not be enough to prevent a drug from getting through.

7. If the veterinarian is selling "blue goo" to other practices with or without a label, this is drug manufacturing as opposed to compounding the product for a specific client and a specific animal. This would be considered illegal.

8. "Units" are just another way of measuring concentration of the drug (insulin in this case) in a solution. The U-100 preparation of insulin contains 100 U of insulin/mL. There are 10 mL in a vial, hence 100 U/mL × 10 mL = 1000 U of insulin in one vial. The dog requires 3.2 U per dose, thus the number of doses from this vial would be 1000 U × 1 dose/3.2 units = 312.5 doses = 312 doses (a half of a dose is of no value).

9. Meters squared (m^2) is another way of describing the animal instead of kilograms or pounds of body weight. Use meters squared in the same way as kilograms and pounds of body weight. 0.8 m^2 × 0.22 mg/m^2 = 0.176 mg. 0.176 mg × 1 mL/0.15 mg = 1.17 mL to be given at full strength. The veterinarian wants you to use 60% of the original dose. Therefore 60% = 0.60 and 60% of the dose would be 0.60 × 1.17 mL = 0.7 mL of drug. You can also calculate the reduction in dose by taking the calculated dose in mg (0.176 mg) and determining what 60% of that would be (0.1056 mg) and then determining the milliliters of elixir to be used: 0.1056 mg × 1 mL/0.15 mg = 0.7 mL.

10. The number of tablets per dose for this dog would be determined by dividing the 115 total tablets by 10 days and three times a day dosing: 115 divided by 10 = 11.5. 11.5 divided by 3 = 3.83333 tablets per dose. No client is going to be able to slice off 0.8333 of a tablet. The error came in determining total milligrams of drug needed for the whole 10 days. What needed to be done is determine the milligrams of drug needed for one dose, then convert that amount into the tablet dose. The milligram dose was 190.1, which translates into 3.8 of the 50-mg tablets per dose. Round that 3.8 tablets to 4 tablets per dose. Now determine how many tablets are needed per day (4 tablets per dose × 3 doses per day = 12 tablets) and how many are needed for 10 days (12 tablets per day × 10 days = 120 tablets total).

11. 8-lb dog = 3.636-kg dog. At a dose of 8 mg/kg, this dog needs a dose of 29.1 mg. Tablets are 15 mg in size so the dog gets 2 tablets per dose. Each tablet costs $0.13 ($130 divided by 1000 tablets) and the dog gets two tablets a day; therefore the cost per day of tablets is 2 × $0.13 = $0.26 per day. If the client has only $10, then we divide the $10 by the cost per day to determine how many days of medication the client can have. $10 × day/$0.26 = 38.4 days = 38 days (a partial day does not count).

Chapter 3

REVIEW QUESTIONS

1. first-pass effect
2. dose interval
3. absorption
4. ion trapping
5. passive diffusion

6. ionized or hydrophilic

7. facilitated diffusion (not active transport)

8. alkaline or basic drug

9. IM

10. maintenance dose

11. elimination or excretion

12. distribution

13. liver

14. metabolism or biotransformation

15. redistribution (distribution is going from blood to tissue)

16. enterohepatic circulation

17. steady state

18. intradermal

19. agonist

20. 240 mg q12h; 160 mg q8h; 80 mg q4h (6 × a day); 160 mg t.i.d.; 480 q24h; 120 mg q.i.d.

21. C is the correct answer. Choice A = 100 mg × 0.7 = 70 mg. Choice B = 150 mg × 0.5 = 75 mg. Choice C = 200 mg × 0.4 = 80 mg. Choice D = 250 mg × 0.2 = 50 mg.

22. Most superficial = intradermal (within the layers of the skin), then subcutaneous (below the skin), then intramuscular.

23. Into the abdominal or peritoneal cavity (IP = intraperitoneal)

24. A. passive diffusion through extracellular fluid between cells.

    B. phagocytosis or pinocytosis because it is a large molecule.

    C. active transport: able to accumulate drug in spite of the concentration gradient.

    D. facilitated diffusion: moves along a concentration gradient so no cellular

energy is being expended, and because it is hydrophilic it is not likely to passively diffuse through the lipid cellular membrane; thus it needs a carrier to get through the membrane.

25. Ionized molecules dissolve in water. Nonionized molecules pass through membranes.

26. pH of 3.

27. Acid drugs in acidic environments are more likely nonionized and therefore lipophilic.

28. pKa = 6. This drug becomes more ionized in more acidic environments and more nonionized in alkaline environments. That would make the drug an alkaline, or basic, drug.

29. A. ionized

    B. ionized

    C. nonionized

    D. nonionized

    E. ½ in ionized form and ½ in the nonionized form

    F. nonionized

    G. ionized

    H. ionized

    I. nonionized

30. This is SQ, so drug most in ionized (hydrophilic) state will most rapidly diffuse to capillary and enter systemic circulation (absorption). Fastest (#1) = basic drug pKa 9.4 (100 ionized molecules for every 1 nonionized). #2 = acid drug pKa 6.4 (10 ionized molecules for every 1 nonionized). #3 = acid drug pKa 8.4 (1 ionized molecule for every 10 nonionized molecules). #4 = basic drug pKa 5.4 (1 ionized molecule for every 100 nonionized molecules).

31. A. decrease dose: it takes longer for the drug concentrations to drop by ½.

B. increase dose: the drug is being converted to a metabolite (presumably an inactive metabolite) at a quicker rate.

C. decrease dose: less protein in the blood for binding means more drug molecules in the free form and available to distribute to tissues to produce a greater effect.

D. decrease dose: with the drug distributed to fewer tissues and hence less diluted by the volume of tissue fluid, the amounts of drug in the tissues will become more concentrated. Decrease dose to prevent concentration from exceeding therapeutic range.

32. A. Always look for two concentrations that are one half to one fourth of each other. In this problem there is 160 μg/mL at 1 hour after dose and 40 μg/mL at 5 hours after dose. 160 divided by 2 = 80 and 80 divided by 2 = 40. Thus the concentrations went through two half-lives to go from 160 to 40 μg/mL. How long did it take to drop from 160 to 40 μg/mL? 160 was at 1 hour after dose and 40 was at 5 hours after dose. The elapsed interval between these two samples was 5 – 1 = 4 hours. Thus if 4 hours = 2 half-lives, then 1 half-life must be 2 hours. Therefore no matter at what concentration we start on this dose curve, 2 hours later the concentration will be half of what it was.

B. If the half-life is 2 hours and the concentration at 2 hours after injection is shown as 100 μg/mL, then 2 hours later at 4 hours after injection the concentration will be one half. At 4 hours after injection the concentration will be 100 divided by 2 = 50 μg/mL.

C. 40 μg/mL at 5 hours after injection will be half again 2 hours later at 7 hours after injection. At 7 hours after injection the concentration will be 20 μg/mL.

D. The estimated peak concentration occurring immediately after the completion of the IV bolus push should theoretically be double (twice) what it is at 2 hours after injection because this drug has a 2-hour half-life. Thus, the peak concentration at 0 hr after injection is estimated at 100 μg/mL × 2 = 200 μg/mL.

E. Steady state = 5 × the half-life. 5 × 2 hours = 10 hours to reach steady state.

33. A. False. If metabolism has been induced, it has been sped up. The drug is being broken down quicker and therefore inactivated more rapidly. The dose needs to be increased. This is the explanation for why tolerance develops to drugs such as barbiturates, alcohol, and opioid/narcotics.

B. True.

C. True.

D. False. An antagonist is a drug molecule that occupies a receptor site without producing an effect. In so doing, the antagonist blocks the agonist from occupying the receptor site and therefore reverses the agonist's effect.

E. True. If Vd increases there is more volume of fluid into which the drug is dissolved and therefore the drug is more diluted.

34. Capillaries have openings called fenestrations through which drug molecules can enter. Drug molecules can leave through fenestrations to go from systemic circulation to tissues (distribution). The capillaries in the brain, prostate, and globe of the eye do not have fenestrations and therefore the only way a drug can get into these areas from systemic circulation is if the drug is in a lipophilic (nonionized) state.

APPLICATION QUESTIONS

1. PO means per os, so it is given by mouth. IV = intravenously, so it is placed within the veins. SQ = subcutaneously, so it goes in the tissue beneath the skin. IM goes into the deep belly of a muscle. Obviously the IV drug will reach its peak in the plasma first because all of the drug, if given as a bolus, is placed immediately into the blood (no absorption phase). IM, in muscle that is well perfused and usually moving, is almost as quick to reach its peak concentrations. SQ and PO will be much more variable in their onset of peak concentration because of the various factors that influence their absorption.

2. The veterinarian is correct in his or her statement. The value of 40 µg/mL within 2 hours sounds impressive, but if the bottom end of the therapeutic range is 50 µg/mL, the drug will still be in the subtherapeutic range after 2 hours. Or, if the toxic range for this drug starts at 30 µg/mL, at 2 hours this animal is going to be very ill. Without knowing what the therapeutic range is for this drug, this single concentration value is worthless.

3. The loading dose is a large dose given initially to establish concentrations within the therapeutic range (or at least close to it). Once therapeutic drug concentrations in the body are established, the smaller maintenance dose will keep the drug concentrations there. The advantage of using the loading dose is that therapeutic concentrations are established very quickly. If just a maintenance dose is used, it may take hours or even days for the drug to gradually accumulate to its steady state within the therapeutic range.

4. IV bolus administration results in very high initial concentrations within the plasma (blood) shortly after the bolus is administered. Unfortunately, if these high concentrations are above the therapeutic range, these high initial concentrations may result in the animal showing toxic signs until plasma concentrations decrease. For a drug like digoxin that has a narrow therapeutic index there is not much difference between plasma concentrations of drug that provide benefit and those plasma concentrations that cause toxicity. Thus it would be safer to use a route of administration that has less prominent swings in peaks, such as the PO or SQ route. Digoxin is usually used PO in veterinary medicine.

5. In this situation the drug is being administered as the same total daily dose amount (50 mg q6h = 200 mg and 100 mg q12h = 200 mg). But because more drug is being administered at one time with the 100 mg q12h dosage regimen, higher concentrations at the peak are going to be achieved. And because the 100 mg q12h regimen goes longer between doses, the concentrations are going to be allowed to drop for a longer period, resulting in trough concentrations lower than with the 50 mg q6h dosage regimen. Thus with the 100 mg q12h dosage regimen, the greater swings in concentrations from peak to trough may result in periods when the concentrations exceed the therapeutic range (toxicity) or drop below the therapeutic range (subtherapeutic).

6. An IV bolus or push means that the whole amount of the drug is being delivered within a few seconds. An IV infusion means that the drug is being dripped into the animal over minutes to hours. A major difference between these two is that the bolus will result in very high concentrations in the blood (plasma) until it gets a chance to distribute to the body. During that time it is possible that the high concentrations can result in toxic

signs. The IV infusion has no prominent peak concentration but shows slowing increasing concentrations over time.

7. Do not let the drug leak or get out of the vasculature (veins, arteries). Some drugs can be extremely irritating to tissues if deposited outside the vein. In some cases the tissue can die and slough off. If you administer a drug intravenously and it goes extravascularly, you should be able to notice a distension of the tissue surrounding the injection site. With irritating drugs there will also likely be a pain response from the animal. If you do not detect the extravascular administration, the next day you may find that the injection site is warm, sensitive, and swollen.

8. Aerosol drugs are meant to be administered by a nebulizer into the respiratory tract. The highest concentrations will be lining the inside lumen of the trachea, bronchi, and bronchioles in the respiratory tree. This is the goal with antibiotics administered by aerosol nebulization to combat bacterial infections brought into the lungs by air.

9. An intracarotid injection would send the concentrated drug directly to the brain. There are several drugs used in horses that will produce a violent reaction if inadvertently given in the carotid artery instead of the jugular vein.

10. Facilitated diffusion and active transport are processes that use special proteins located within the cell membrane to move drugs across the membrane. There are a finite (limited) number of these proteins present. Therefore, if all the available proteins are occupied with transporting drug molecules across the membrane, the transport process is operating at its maximal speed (its top speed limit). Passive diffusion, because it does not require special proteins to get across the membrane, is not limited to the maximal rate that a carrier system can operate.

11. SQ and IM administered drugs are placed into extracellular water (fluid) and therefore need to be hydrophilic drugs so they can readily dissolve and move away from the site of administration toward the capillaries between loosely packed cells by passive diffusion. There are no membranes for these drugs to penetrate when given by SQ or IM route of administration (the fenestrations in the capillaries allow drug molecules to enter the capillary without going through the capillary endothelial cell membranes). Unfortunately in the GI tract the cells lining the lumen of the gut are very tightly packed together so that there are no extracellular gaps; hydrophilic drugs cannot get through the GI cellular membranes and hence are poorly absorbed. Thus, while this horse might consume the drug in the appropriate dose, if the drug is mostly in the hydrophilic state in the lumen of the GI tract, it will not be absorbed.

12. Acid drugs in general become more lipophilic as they are placed in increasingly acidic environments. Alkaline drugs become more ionized in this same situation. And because the GI tract requires drugs to be in the lipophilic form to be absorbed, acidic drugs are more likely to be absorbed from the GI tract at a pH of 2 or 3.

13. Acid drugs in the lipophilic form in the stomach pH of 2 or 3 will enter a more alkaline environment of pH = 7.4 when they move through the cell membrane into the cell's cytoplasm. This more alkaline pH will result in more of the nonionized molecules becoming ionized (hydrophilic) and thus trapped within the confines of the cellular membrane.

14. Remember that reabsorption from the kidney tubules back into systemic circulation

is by passive diffusion and requires a drug molecule to move through the renal tubular cell membrane. Thus a lipophilic drug is reabsorbed from the renal tubules but a hydrophilic drug remains in the tubules and is excreted with the urine. Because this is a poison, the drug needs to be in the hydrophilic form so it will be excreted and not reenter the body to do more damage. This poison is an acid type compound. Any time the pH of its environment is more alkaline, an acid drug is going to become more ionized. Therefore a urinary alkalizer should be used to make the drug molecules more hydrophilic within the renal tubules and be less reabsorbed.

15. Enteric coatings are designed to protect the drug from the gastric acid environment. If a drug is broken down or inactivated by the extreme acidity of the stomach, the enteric coating might allow more active drug to make it to the duodenum where it can be absorbed.

16. Pylorospasm would slow the gastric emptying. If the drug was not inactivated in the stomach, the only difference would be a delayed onset of the drug's activity (assuming not much of the drug is absorbed from the stomach because it is a basic drug). If the drug is degraded by the acidic stomach environment, then both a delay of onset plus a reduced amount of intact drug present to be absorbed would occur.

17. If the intestinal transit time was shortened (things moving through quicker) a tablet might not have enough time to physically break down in size small enough to be absorbed before it is moved through the small intestine into the colon, which does not absorb drugs as readily as the small intestine.

18. Same concept that a highly hydrophilic compound will not be absorbed into the body from the GI tract and thus will not have an effect on the body overall. If injected or absorbed across mucous membranes or damaged skin, it can gain access to systemic circulation and cause its damage (or if a drug, its beneficial effect). Another reason why a PO drug might be ineffective is that even if it is absorbed across the gut wall, it might be taken out by the liver (first-pass effect) and not reach systemic circulation in significant concentrations.

19. In cold conditions the body protects itself from heat loss by causing vasoconstriction of blood vessels near the surface of the body. This vasoconstriction reduces perfusion of the superficial tissues and thus means a drug injected SQ has to diffuse a lot further to find an open capillary and be absorbed.

20. Fat is poorly perfused tissue. Therefore any drug injected into a fat pad will be very poorly absorbed (or have significantly delayed absorption) and will have a reduced effect upon the body.

21. Blood-brain barrier of tight-junctioned capillaries and glial cells means the drugs must be in the lipophilic form to get into the brain from the blood. To get around the blood-brain barrier, some drugs are injected directly into the cerebrospinal fluid surrounding the spinal cord. This fluid will then transport the injected drug into the brain.

22. Redistribution is the movement of drug from tissue A back into the blood and then to tissue B. In this case, the anesthetic thiopental is diffusing back into the blood from the brain and then into the fat tissue. As concentrations drop in the brain, the animal starts to breathe and may actually start to wake up.

23. Decreased. With fewer than normal numbers of protein molecules floating around

in the blood, there are fewer sites for the administered drug to be tied up. With more of the administered drug in the free form, and therefore capable of distributing to tissues, a normal dose will end up delivering higher concentrations of drug molecules to the tissues and possibly producing an overdose. The dose should be decreased.

24. Drug B has the greater distribution as reflected by the total volume of fluid in which it is dissolved. If drugs A and B are given in the same amounts, drug B would be more diluted and thus have lower concentrations (even though those concentrations are distributed to a larger number of organs or tissues).

25. Volume of distribution is usually called the apparent Vd because it is always an approximation based on what the concentration of drug is within the plasma only (we cannot easily go out and biopsy organs to find out what their drug concentrations are all the time!). In the case of digoxin, so much of the drug moves out of the plasma into the skeletal and cardiac muscle that concentrations within the plasma are very low. It would therefore appear from looking at plasma concentrations that digoxin is diluted in a very large volume of fluid. In fact, it is simply that the drug is being bound to sites outside of the plasma.

26. Lower concentrations. More fluid in the body to dilute the drug, thus lower concentrations.

27. An antagonist to the insecticide would probably be ineffective because the insecticide has combined with a receptor in such a way that an antagonist will not be able to readily replace it at the receptor site. This is in contrast to a competitive agonist/antagonist situation in which simply by giving more antagonist, the effect of the agonist can be reversed.

28. Butorphanol has intrinsic narcotic activity (sedation, relief of pain) when it combines with narcotic (opioid) receptors, but its sedation and pain relief effect is much weaker than that of hydromorphone. Therefore, if butorphanol replaces hydromorphone at the opioid receptors, the animal's degree of narcosis and analgesia (pain relief) will be decreased, but not totally eliminated. With the use of a true antagonist like naloxone that has little or no intrinsic activity, the narcosis and analgesia of hydromorphone would be completely reversed.

29. A chelator is an example of a non–receptor-mediated drug activity in which the effect for which the drug is intended does not require a cellular receptor. In this case, there is a direct chemical reaction between the chelator drug and ions that produces its effect.

30. Cats have a limited ability to conjugate glucuronide and other compounds with drugs, and thus drugs that depend on this process for normal metabolism will be metabolized at a slower rate. Young animals have immature livers that are not able to biotransform drugs as readily as older animals and therefore hepatically biotransformed drugs must be used with caution in very young animals. Because the kidney does not have to mature and because the cat's kidneys are just as efficient as any other species' kidneys, this same concern does not necessarily apply to drugs that are exclusively renally excreted.

31. Phenobarbital induces its own metabolism, meaning that the liver metabolism of phenobarbital speeds up. Because the phenobarbital is broken down quicker, the concentrations of drug in the body decrease more rapidly and thus less drug accumulates between dosages.

Thus an increase in drug dose will be necessary to compensate for the more rapid metabolism caused by induced phenobarbital metabolism.

32. Decreased blood flow to the kidney means less drug delivered to the kidney and subsequently less drug excreted by the kidney.

33. Penicillin is actively secreted into the renal tubule lumen and thus can achieve concentrations in the urine that may be much higher that those in the plasma. Thus the bacteria are killed in the urine by the higher concentrations attained through active secretion.

34. Enterohepatic circulation means that the poison is excreted by the liver, dumped into the intestine, and then reabsorbed back into the body where it can continue to cause damage. The activated charcoal, which is added to give the poison something to stick to in order to decrease its absorption, must be given as long as the poison is being excreted back into the intestinal tract. Otherwise the poison will have a much longer effect on the body.

35. Clearance is a measure of how quickly a drug is removed from the blood. Rapid clearance means rapid movement out of the blood and presumably from the body.

36. This question has to do with the time to reach steady state (5× half-life). Until steady state is achieved, the drug concentrations are climbing upward. A drug with a long half-life, such as phenobarbital, will not achieve steady-state concentrations for days as opposed to a drug like penicillin, which has a half-life of approximately 2 hours and thus would be at steady state by 10 hours after the first administration of the drug. Because phenobarbital is slowly increasing over days, it may be present in very low concentrations during the first few hours (or days) after the drug is begun and not have therapeutic concentrations. Therefore it might benefit from administration of a loading dose to establish therapeutic concentrations much faster.

37. Theoretically the withdrawal time should be shorter for drug A because its half-life is so rapid and that means the drug is leaving the blood at a faster rate (and it is assumed that it is leaving the body when it is leaving the blood). Several other factors may enter into the withdrawal time, such as how long it takes for the drug to leave the body tissues (not just the blood) or if lower concentrations of residues are required of one drug or the other in order for the meat or food products (eggs and milk) to be considered safe for human consumption.

Chapter 4

REVIEW QUESTIONS

1. gastric

2. enteric

3. colonic

4. acetylcholine

5. gastrin

6. parietal or oxyntic cells

7. emetic center

8. tenesmus

9. vagus nerve

10. sympathetic nervous system

11. parasympathetic nervous system

12. CRTZ, chemoreceptor trigger zone

13. gastritis

14. monogastric

15. sucralfate (Carafate)

16. bismuth

17. dimenhydrinate, diphenhydramine

18. DSS, dioctyl sodium succinate

19. metronidazole

20. apomorphine

21. xylazine

22. metoclopramide (Reglan)

23. loperamide, diphenoxylate

24. omeprazole

25. sulfasalazine (Azulfidine)

26. misoprostol ("prost" suggests a prostaglandin)

27. pancreatic enzyme supplements

28. bismuth subsalicylate (Pepto-Bismol, Kaopectate)

29. cimetidine (Tagamet), ranitidine (Zantac), famotidine (Pepcid)

30. acepromazine

31. The parasympathetic nervous system (rest and restore system) would do everything to increase digestion. Therefore, GI motility increases, GI secretions increase, and blood flow to the GI tract increases.

32. Phosphate.

33. Prostaglandins in the stomach help protect the stomach from acid and enhance the ability of the stomach to repair itself. Therefore stomach mucus will be increased, stomach acid production will be decreased, and blood flow and cell turnover will both be increased to assist in repair and health of the tissue.

34. A. No: corrosive substance

    B. Yes

    C. No: horses do not vomit

    D. No: dog is already vomiting

35. A. True.

    B. True.

    C. False. Prostaglandins would increase the sodium bicarbonate as a means of protecting the stomach lining by neutralizing stomach acid.

    D. False. When given intravenously or in the sulcus of the eye, the drug achieves high concentrations in the blood very quickly. This stimulates the CRTZ, which stimulates the emetic center and produces vomiting. With PO administration, the concentrations of apomorphine in the blood rise slowly, allowing time for the apomorphine to pass through the blood-brain barrier and enter the brain itself, where it suppresses the activity in the brainstem, including the emetic center. Thus, as the concentration gradually rises in the blood to stimulate the CRTZ, it is also rising in the brainstem, where it will depress the emetic center.

    E. False. Ruminatorics stimulate contraction of the rumen. They are not used to relieve bloat.

    F. False. Purgatives are generally more aggressive than cathartics. Both are more aggressive than most laxatives.

    G. True.

    H. True.

APPLICATION QUESTIONS

1. Because phenothiazines are also α-receptor blockers, they can block the vasoconstriction effect of α_1 receptors on

peripheral blood vessels, resulting in a reflex vasodilation and a drop in blood pressure. If an animal is hypovolemic (low blood volume) from dehydration or any cause, the blood pressure is already going to be low. Using acepromazine or any other phenothiazine tranquilizer would only drop that blood pressure further.

2. An anticholinergic drug is one that produces an effect opposite to acetylcholine, the neurotransmitter associated with parasympathetic nervous system responses. Because they block the parasympathetic nervous system, they have a general depressant effect on the GI tract. While blocking the parasympathetic nervous system might decrease some vagal stimulation of the CRTZ and emetic center, it is usually not sufficient to prevent vomiting. However, anticholinergic drugs have been effective in decreasing vomiting associated with inflammation of the colon (irritable bowel syndrome) or vomiting associated with overstimulation of the parasympathetic nervous system. But generally, they are not considered very effective antiemetics.

3. Metoclopramide acts centrally by blocking dopamine receptors in the CRTZ. It acts locally by increasing the lower esophageal tone, relaxing the pyloric exit of the stomach, and increasing the motility of the stomach in the normal direction.

4. Serotonin receptors play an important role in producing vomiting by stimulation of the CRTZ. Because this is also the site where chemotherapeutic agents (cancer-fighting drugs) also stimulate vomiting, serotonin antagonists can be quite effective in blocking vomiting.

5. Hypomotility results in decreased movement, including segmental contractions. The intestinal tract becomes a garden hose through which everything

can slide. Hypermotility can cause diarrhea also, but usually results from acute irritation or burst of motility that is short lasting. Hypermotility is associated with irritated colon, and the resulting straining to pass feces (even when none are present) is called tenesmus.

6. The subsalicylate of Pepto-Bismol (bismuth subsalicylate) is an aspirinlike compound that decreases prostaglandin formation and inflammation in the bowel, which is one of the major stimuli for excessive intestinal secretion of fluids. The bismuth acts as an adsorbent for intestinal toxins and irritants, but it is really the subsalicylate that affects the diarrhea more.

7. While there is the possibility that an animal with intestinal disease might be having some small bowel hemorrhage, there is a greater probability that what the owner is seeing is the change in stool color from the bismuth (turns the stool a dark color).

8. While bismuth subsalicylate can be given to cats, it has to be done very carefully because the subsalicylate can be absorbed into the body and cats are not very effective metabolizers of salicylate (aspirinlike) drugs. Therefore, do not use a dog dose of this compound in cats.

9. In some cases the kaolin-pectin combination can decrease absorption of orally administered drugs by adsorbing the drug and preventing the drug from reaching the wall of the intestine. Better to give the other drugs 2 hours before or 3 hours after the kaolin-pectin compound.

10. The use of oil-based laxatives for chronic constipation, hairballs, etc. can result in a decrease in absorption of fat-soluble vitamins A, D, E, and K.

11. NSAIDs block prostaglandin formation as a means to reduce

inflammation. Unfortunately many of these antiinflammatories also block prostaglandins that help stimulate mucus production, normal perfusion, and healing of the stomach, all of which increase the risk for ulcer formation.

12. Nonsystemic or local antacids simply neutralize the acid produced in the stomach at that point of time, and when the neutralized stomach contents have moved into the duodenum, receptors there tell the stomach to produce even more acid to compensate for the alkaline contents coming into the duodenum. Unfortunately, when the additional acid is produced, the neutralizing local antacid has moved from the stomach into the intestine.

13. Ruminatorics stimulate the rumen. Antibloat medications cause froth associated with bloat to turn into a large bubble that can be eructated. Neostigmine is a parasympathetic-like drug, so it will stimulate the rumen as a ruminatoric. DSS is an antibloat medication.

14. Tylosin can causes severe diarrhea in horses.

15. Livestock producers often use oral electrolyte solutions because it is impractical to hook up IV lines to calves or other young livestock with scours. In small animals, significant dehydration should be corrected with IV administered fluids. The oral electrolyte solutions can follow IV therapy after the animal has begun to stabilize.

16. Lipase enzyme is very difficult to keep in an active form because of its easy breakdown in the acidic environment of the stomach, the need for a specific pH for it to work, and the proper temperature. Several other factors also play a role in getting the lipase to work properly.

For this reason, fats still are not very well digested and used by the body, resulting in stools that often still have a greasy appearance to them and an animal that may not readily regain its weight.

Chapter 5

REVIEW QUESTIONS

1. SA node

2. AV node

3. sodium (Na^+)

4. β_1

5. α_1

6. β_1

7. PR interval (end of P wave to beginning of large R wave in QRS complex)

8. muscarinic and nicotinic

9. norepinephrine, epinephrine (catecholamines)

10. ectopic focus

11. lidocaine

12. β-blocker antiarrhythmics like atenolol and propranolol

13. digoxin

14. mexiletine

15. dobutamine (catecholamine)

16. furosemide

17. spironolactone

18. enalapril

19. aspirin

20. nitroglycerin

21. atropine

22. A. False. QRS is the ventricles depolarizing. The P wave is atria depolarizing.

B. True.

C. True.

D. True.

E. True.

F. False. Positive inotropic drugs increase the force of contraction. Negative inotropic drugs decrease the force of contraction. A positive inotropic drug would increase the heart rate, and a negative inotropic drug would decrease the heart rate.

G. False. The left ventricle, being the larger of the two ventricles, pumps the blood to the rest of the body. The smaller right ventricle pumps the blood the relatively short distance to the lungs and then back to the left atrium.

H. False. Stopping the β blockers suddenly can put the animal at great risk for an increase in arrhythmias and possibly death. When the β blocker drugs are used, the catecholamine neurotransmitters (epinephrine and norepinephrine) cannot reach the β_1 receptors on the heart. In response to this, over time the heart cells begin to sprout new β_1 receptors, allowing the heart muscle to regain its responsiveness to the catecholamines and prompting an increase in β-blocker dose. This is the process of upregulation and it refers to the increase in number of new receptors to the β-adrenergic agonists. If all of the β-blocker drug molecules are allowed to disappear by stopping the β-blocking drug, then all the original β_1 receptors as well as the new upregulated β_1 receptors are available to respond to the catecholamine neurotransmitters. This means in response to a mild release of norepinephrine with excitement or exercise, the heart muscle is going to respond with greater force of contraction and the conduction system is going to conduct the depolarization wave quicker. An ectopic focus could also fire more readily, giving rise to arrhythmias. β_1 blocker antiarrhythmic drugs should be tapered off over time and never stopped "cold turkey."

I. False. Tablets typically have a lower bioavailability than liquids. Digoxin tablets have a 60% bioavailability and the elixir typically has around a 75% bioavailability. Thus, if 2 mg of elixir are administered we are getting 75% of that, or 1.50 mg (0.75 × 2 mg = 1.50 mg) of digoxin, actually into systemic circulation. Because the tablets are absorbed to a lesser degree (only 60% bioavailability compared with 75% for the elixir) then only 1.20 mg of a 2-mg tablet dose (0.60 × 2 mg = 1.20 mg) is going to reach the systemic circulation. To give enough tablet dose to equal the 1.50 mg absorbed after 2 mg of elixir, we would have to give more of the tablet form of the drug. In other words, the dose of the tablet would have to be more than the dose of the elixir to achieve 1.50 mg of drug actually reaching systemic circulation. The actual amount needed for the equivalent tablet dose is shown below:

Dose tablet × 0.60 = Dose elixir × 0.75

Dose tablet × 0.60 = 2 mg elixir dose × 0.75

Dose tablet × 0.60 = 1.50 mg (amount of drug that is absorbed into systemic circulation)

Dose tablet = 1.50 mg/0.60 = 2.50 mg

Dose tablet = 2.50-mg tablet dose needed to achieve the same systemic concentration of drug as the 2.0-mg elixir.

J. True. The origin of the problem is above the ventricles in the atria, and the heart rate is increased.

K. True. The dominance of the parasympathetic effect of digoxin on the SA and AV nodes slows the overall rate of contraction as well as increases the delay of the impulse passing through the AV node.

L. True.

M. True.

N. False. Angiotensin II is the body's most potent vasoconstrictor. It is released as a result of a drop in arterial blood pressure and thus it causes vasoconstriction at the point where the arteries dump blood into the capillaries, essentially squeezing the terminal opening of the arteries. The arterial blood pressure increases in response to the vasoconstriction in the same way that squeezing one end of a rubber tube while blowing into the opposite end would cause air pressure to increase inside the rubber tube.

O. True.

P. True.

Q. True.

R. False. β_2 receptors on the bronchioles cause bronchodilation when stimulated. β-blocker (antagonist) drugs that block β_2 receptors will block this bronchodilating effect and allow the bronchoconstricting effect from parasympathetic (acetylcholine) stimulation or histamine stimulation to dominate. The net effect is the potential for bronchoconstriction.

23. Sedatives or tranquilizers are often given to animals with aerophagia ("eating air," or gasping for breath) to relieve the fear that comes with struggling to breathe. By reducing the fear, the sympathetic nervous system stimulation on the heart is reduced, slowing it down but also allowing the heart to beat more efficiently with fewer beats and reducing the work of the heart.

Reducing the work on the heart means less need for oxygen. Reducing the fear also reduces other muscle movement (pacing, panting, anxious behavior) and therefore also reduces the need for more oxygen.

24. Digoxin. Digoxin slows conduction through the AV node, thus reducing the number of impulses that reach the ventricles and thus reducing the ventricular heart rate. Digoxin slows the SA node, but the SA node is not in control anyway in animals with atrial fibrillation. Thus digoxin does not really reduce the atrial fibrillation, it only reduces the ventricular rate.

25. Kidney.

APPLICATION QUESTIONS

1. A catheter threaded from the jugular vein would enter the anterior vena cava and then the right atrium. A femoral artery catheter threaded against the blood flow would work its way back up the dorsal aorta to the aortic arch and eventually enter the left ventricle.

2. SA node, atria, AV node, bundle branches, Purkinje fibers, apex of the ventricles.

3. The P wave represents atrial depolarization. The large QRS complex (small Q wave + very large R wave + small S wave) represents ventricular depolarization. When the depolarization wave is passing through the AV node, the line is flat, indicating minimal electrical activity. The end of the P wave to the beginning of the QRS complex is called the PR interval and indicates when the AV node is conducting the impulse from the atria to the ventricles.

4. Depolarization occurs when sodium ions move into the cell. Repolarization occurs when potassium ions move out of the cell.

5. Sympathetic nervous system effects (fight or flight).

6. Muscarinic and nicotinic cholinergic receptors. Muscarinic receptors are associated with parasympathetic nervous system effects, and nicotinic receptors are associated with sympathetic nervous system effects (plus voluntary muscle contraction). Muscarinic effects would cause the heart rate to decrease, pupils to constrict, and GI function to increase. Nicotinic effects would cause an increased heart rate, pupillary dilation, and decreased GI function as a result of stimulating part of the sympathetic nervous system neurons. Even though acetylcholine neurotransmitter is associated with parasympathetic nervous system effects, acetylcholine stimulates nicotinic receptors in the sympathetic nervous system that in turn release norepinephrine, which gives us the classic sympathetic nervous system signs.

7. A. Supraventricular tachycardia

   B. Supraventricular bradycardia

   C. Ventricular tachycardia

8. A paroxysm of PVCs is a series of PVCs in a row. Ventricular flutter is when the PVCs continue for an extended period. In both of these cases the wave of depolarization is organized even if it starts from an abnormal location and causes the QRS complex to look bizarre. In ventricular fibrillation the wave of depolarization is totally disorganized and the ventricles contract as a disconnected series of seemingly random contractions in different areas of the ventricles. The net effect is no effective pumping of blood. The ventricle appears to look like a bag of worms because of the disorganized contractions.

9. AV block is the slowing or blocking of the impulse passing through the AV node.

In first-degree AV block the impulse is only slowed as it passes through and the PR interval on the ECG is prolonged. In second-degree AV block the impulse is slowed so much it dies out and fails to make it to the ventricles. This is seen on the ECG as a P wave (atrial depolarization) without a corresponding QRS complex (ventricular depolarization). Because these AV blocks are often caused by overstimulation of the AV node by the parasympathetic nervous system, using the cholinergic antagonist atropine (which competes against acetylcholine for cholinergic receptors) blocks the parasympathetic stimulation and reverses the AV block.

10. Lidocaine at lower doses of toxicity inhibits some excitatory neurons, producing sedation and ataxia. As the concentration of the lidocaine toxicity increases, inhibitory neurons begin to be depressed, allowing remaining excitatory neurons to fire more readily. This can result in tremors or seizures (the inhibitory neurons are disinhibited in their neuronal activity).

11. Local anesthesia lidocaine has epinephrine in it to reduce absorption of the lidocaine (keep it at the site of injection). Lidocaine used for antiarrhythmias does not have epinephrine in it. In fact, giving epinephrine to an animal with arrhythmias can increase the severity of the arrhythmias. Hence the need to clearly distinguish the two different types of lidocaine.

12. Quinidine displaces digoxin from its binding sites in muscle, increasing digoxin concentrations in plasma and increasing the possibility of digoxin toxicosis. When quinidine and digoxin are used together, the digoxin dose should be halved to prevent digoxin toxicosis.

13. Sustained-release medications are often formulated so the tablet dissolves very

predictably from the outside inward at a controlled rate. If you break the tablet, this exposes the more readily dissolved drug inside of the tablet, negating the sustained-release effect.

14. β-blocking drugs (β$_1$ antagonists) decrease sympathetic stimulation on the heart, which allows the parasympathetic stimulation on the heart to dominate. Because parasympathetic stimulation slows impulses traveling through the AV node, this can result in a prolonged PR interval, which is first-degree AV block. The high sympathetic nervous system tone generated by the body may be essential for stimulating the weakened heart to maintain adequate cardiac output. Reducing sympathetic tone by blocking the β$_1$ receptors in the heart may reduce contractility, resulting in insufficient pumping of blood.

15. When β-blocker drugs occupy the β$_1$ receptors on the heart muscle and prevent them from being stimulated, the body responds by increasing the number of receptors on the heart muscle and, in turn, increases the sensitivity of the heart muscle to stimulation. This increased sensitivity allows the heart muscle to begin to respond to the epinephrine/norepinephrine again seemingly causing a decreased effectiveness of the β-blocker drug. This increased number of receptors is called up-regulation. The opposite occurs with β$_1$ receptor stimulating drugs (β agonists) like dobutamine or epinephrine. With excessive stimulation of beta receptors the body begins to remove receptors, making the heart muscle less sensitive to the effects of the catecholamines like epinephrine, norepinephrine, or dobutamine. This is called downregulation.

16. Propranolol blocks β$_1$ receptors in the heart and is used to combat arrhythmias. However, it may also block the bronchodilating effect of the β$_2$ receptors in the airways, resulting in bronchoconstriction by blocking the bronchodilating effects of the sympathetic nervous system.

17. Catecholamines include the group of compounds that stimulate catecholamine receptors (α and β receptors) to produce sympathetic nervous system–type effects. These include (among others) epinephrine, norepinephrine, dopamine, and dobutamine (dobutamine is a drug very similar to dopamine). Although they produce an increase in the rate and force of contraction, downregulation of the number of catecholamine receptors on the heart muscle makes them only effective for a short period. Also, all the catecholamines must be delivered by injection, which makes it impractical for long-term use. The half-life of these catecholamines is very short, so their effect lasts only minutes, which would require multiple doses.

18. Digoxin increases the parasympathetic stimulation of the heart. In so doing, it slows the SA node rate (slows heart rate) and slows conduction through the AV node (AV block). Although first- and second-degree AV block can occur because of parasympathetic stimulation, third-degree AV block (total disconnect between the atria and ventricles; no impulses are getting through the AV node) is typically only because of a physical disruption of the conduction pathway through the heart.

19. Digoxin is eliminated by the kidneys. Thus compromised renal function means that the digoxin cannot leave the body as quickly and is prone to accumulate in the body, producing toxicity. Hypokalemia (low potassium in the blood) has been shown to contribute to digoxin toxicity.

20. The parasympathetic effect of digoxin on the SA node would show a slower overall heart rate, and the parasympathetic effect on the AV node would show a prolonged PR interval (first-degree AV block) or an occasional P wave (atrial depolarization) without a QRS complex (ventricular depolarization), which is second-degree AV block.

21. Dosing digoxin on the basis of milligrams of digoxin per meter squared of body surface area, as opposed to milligrams per pound or kilogram, is more accurate for dosing very small dogs and large-breed dogs.

22. Set up an algebraic equation: dose in tablet × 0.6 = dose in elixir × 0.75. 0.2 mg × 0.6 = × mg elixir dose × 0.75. This equals 0.16 mg of elixir.

23. When a heart begins to fail, the arterial blood pressure decreases. This signals the body to increase arterial blood pressure by vasoconstriction plus increased force and rate of contraction of the heart. Unfortunately, by causing vasoconstriction between the end of the arterial system and the beginning of the capillary system, this increases the resistance to blood flow from arteries to capillaries. It takes greater force to push the blood through the collectively narrower openings. In a heart that is already weakened, this increased workload can cause the heart to eventually fail even further.

24. Renin is released from the kidney when renal perfusion decreases from arterial blood pressure decreases, such as occurs with a weakened heart. Renin quickly converts inactive angiotensinogen to angiotensin I. Angiotensin I is, in turn, converted by ACE to angiotensin II. Angiotensin II is a potent vasoconstrictor. Angiotensin II also stimulates release of aldosterone, which increases sodium resorption from the kidneys, with water following the sodium back into the body. The increased retention of sodium and water increases the blood volume and helps restore arterial blood pressure. Although both actions return blood pressure toward normal, they also increase the workload of the heart.

25. Vasodilators will tend to cause a drop in arterial blood pressure (hypotension), resulting in the animal appearing weak, lethargic, or staggering after rising.

26. Always wear latex gloves when applying nitroglycerin because topical formulations of the drug are easily absorbed through the skin of the person applying the nitroglycerin cream or ointment.

27. Enalapril blocks formation of angiotensin II, a potent vasoconstrictor normally produced in response to falling blood pressure associated with congestive heart failure. In normal animals, little of angiotensin II is produced, and so enalapril does not have anything to block.

28. Loop diuretics such as furosemide work best in most veterinary patients. Furosemide prevents reabsorption of sodium from the renal tubules back into the body. This means that more sodium remains in the urine, more water remains in the urine because of the osmotic effect of the sodium, and a greater volume of urine is produced (diuresis). Although furosemide blocks sodium reabsorption from the renal tubules in the loop of Henle, when the sodium in the renal tubule flows further downstream to the distal convoluted tubule, the body exchanges the sodium for potassium (sodium is taken out of the urine and potassium is put into the urine). Thus the use of furosemide can potentially result in hypokalemia.

29. Furosemide is a loop diuretic because it blocks sodium reabsorption in the segment of the renal tubule called the loop of Henle. Because furosemide works on the loop of Henle where most of the sodium is reabsorbed, blocking sodium at this point produces a much greater diuretic effect than thiazide or spironolactone diuretics that work farther downstream in the renal tubules where there is less sodium reabsorption to be blocked.

30. Mannitol is a sugar compound that is excreted into the renal tubules and osmotically holds water within the renal tubules, creating diuresis. Unfortunately, when it circulates in the blood it also osmotically pulls water from the tissues and has the capacity to dehydrate tissues. This is why mannitol is used to reduce cerebral edema (brain edema) caused by swelling from head trauma. However, this overall body dehydration effect is no advantage in an animal with congestive heart failure and thus mannitol is not used as a diuretic in those cases.

31. Spironolactone works by inhibiting aldosterone. Aldosterone normally causes sodium to be taken up (reabsorbed) from the distal convoluted tubule. Because this occurs in the distal convoluted tubule, the sodium/potassium exchange does not occur as it does with furosemide; thus sodium is excreted and potassium is not.

32. Aspirin decreases clumping of platelets and thus reduces the risk of clots. In cats with hypertrophic cardiomyopathy, the heart wall thickens and clots can form thrombi in blood vessels, especially those in the rear legs. Aspirin use reduces that risk, but the dose used in cats is smaller and the dosage interval is longer than in dogs because cats do not metabolize aspirin well.

33. In congestive heart failure, pulmonary edema can occur from the backup of blood in the lungs caused by the failing heart. Pulmonary edema can reduce the ability to get oxygen to the blood and the animal can feel as if it is not getting enough air. This stimulates a fear response that causes the sympathetic nervous system to stimulate the heart to work harder. In congestive heart failure the heart cannot work any harder because it is weak and diseased. Therefore using sedatives or tranquilizers to reduce the anxiety reduces the fear, reduces the stimulation on the heart, and actually allows the heart to beat slower but with greater efficiency, actually improving the animal's ability to oxygenate its body tissues.

Chapter 6

REVIEW QUESTIONS

1. nebulization or aerosol therapy

2. mucociliary apparatus

3. cor pulmonale

4. antitussive

5. expectorant (a mucolytic breaks apart the mucus)

6. β_2

7. dyspnea

8. metered-dose inhaler

9. guaifenesin

10. butorphanol

11. aminophylline (theophylline is the active ingredient)

12. glucocorticoids, corticosteroids

13. acetylcysteine

14. antihistamine

15. hydrocodone (codeine is less potent)

16. diuretic

17. dextromethorphan

18. guaifenesin

19. acetylcysteine

20. theophylline

21. albuterol, terbutaline

22. A. True.

B. False. Dyspnea is difficult breathing. Rapid breathing is tachypnea.

C. True.

D. False. Drying out the mucus makes it more sticky and harder for the cilia to move.

E. False. Hydrocodone is much more potent. Dextromethorphan is the OTC antitussive and does not work very well in veterinary patients.

F. True.

G. True. They stimulate catecholamine α_1 receptors to cause vasoconstriction and typically have some ability to stimulate β_1 receptors to cause an increased heart rate.

H. False. Antihistamines only work before the histamine is released. Antihistamines are competitive antagonists for histamine at the H_1 receptor. If bronchoconstriction has occurred, the H_1 receptor has most likely already been stimulated by histamine and other chemical mediators that stimulate bronchoconstriction. A direct bronchodilator such as a β_2 agonist drug is needed.

I. True.

J. False. It is an OTC drug requiring no prescription. Some OTC decongestants that contain pseudoephedrine are now more tightly regulated because of their use in manufacturing methamphetamine.

K. False. Nebulization, or aerosol therapy, is the delivery of drug in a mist that is inhaled.

L. True.

M. True.

N. True.

O. True.

P. True.

Q. True.

R. True.

S. True.

23. sympathetic nervous system

24. α_1

25. they stimulate the central nervous system

26. acetylcholine

27. histamine

28. productive cough

29. expectorant (expectorate means "to spit")

APPLICATION QUESTIONS

1. The larynx is very sensitive to stimulation and causes gagging, violent coughing, and spastic closing of the vocal folds of the larynx (laryngospasm) when stimulated. This prevents larger particles from entering the trachea. The bronchi and trachea have cough receptors that stimulate a deeper sounding cough but not as gagging of a cough as the larynx, although the upper trachea can also produce a harsh-type coughing reflex. Cough receptors are not found in the terminal bronchioles or alveoli for the simple reason that the cough mechanism

would be of little value so deep in the respiratory tree. The only way a cough helps is if a sufficient volume of air is able to get behind (deeper into the respiratory tree) the material to be coughed up so that pressure can be built up and then forcefully released, expelling the material with the cough. You cannot get behind the alveoli and there is very little air deeper in the respiratory tree to get behind the bronchioles. Bronchioles can constrict only because they are small enough for smooth muscle rings to squeeze and collapse the small-diameter airway. The alveoli have macrophages (scavenger white blood cells) that enter the airway within the alveolus and attempt to "eat" foreign particles that have entered that far. Unfortunately this is often an inefficient removal and materials in the alveoli may remain there for years or for the rest of the patient's life.

2. Once the animal is rehydrated the nature of the cough may change to a productive cough in which secretions are being brought up. It may also be that once the animal is rehydrated, the mucociliary apparatus is able to work better and the cough may loosen up.

3. Locally acting antitussives act by providing a soothing effect on the throat and respiratory mucosa as they dissolve in the mouth. Unfortunately veterinary patients do not leave them in their mouths long enough to do any good.

4. Drying out the mucus in the respiratory tree results in cilia being unable to move the mucus layer very effectively. Expectorants cause an increase in watery secretions that help dilute the mucus and make it more liquid. Mucolytics such as acetylcysteine chemically break apart the mucus so it is less sticky or stringy. Acetylcysteine breaks the disulfide (S—S)

bonds that contribute to this stickiness, thus making it easier for the mucociliary apparatus to move the mucus out.

5. Most decongestants have drugs that stimulate the sympathetic nervous system receptors to cause vasoconstriction. They also stimulate other sympathetic receptors, and therefore we would expect to see more excited behavior (pacing, panting), increased heart rate, increased force of contraction of the heart, and dilated pupils.

6. Stimulating β_2 receptors causes bronchodilation. Blocking β_2 receptors would allow parasympathetic effects (acetylcholine) or other bronchoconstrictive effects (e.g., histamine stimulation) to dominate. Propranolol is a β_1-blocking (antagonist) antiarrhythmic agent that can also antagonize β_2 receptors, potentially allowing bronchoconstrictive effects to dominate.

7. Epinephrine stimulates many sympathetic nervous system receptors, including β_1 (increased heart rate), α_1 (vasoconstriction), and β_2 (bronchodilation). Therefore it is very nonspecific in its effects compared to albuterol or terbutaline, which primarily target β_2 receptors.

8. Aminophylline is composed of theophylline and a salt. Theophylline is the active ingredient. Both aminophylline and theophylline as well as theobromine (in chocolate) are grouped together as methylxanthines.

9. Clinical signs of respiratory disease will lessen much sooner than the actual underlying bacteria disappear. Stopping treatment too early will result in an increased risk of antibiotic resistance.

10. Nebulization delivers the drug by a mist directly to the surface of the respiratory airways where the airborne bacteria

landed and established an infection. The problem is that animals do not breathe the mist deeply into their lungs like human beings can be instructed to do by taking deep breaths. Also, some compounds can stimulate the reflex that results in bronchoconstriction (the mist is a foreign substance). Use of the MDI has improved the amount of drug delivered to dogs and cats. The MDI avoids spraying the drug directly into the mouth or airway and instead allows the mist to be sprayed into a closed container where it mixes with air and is then breathed in by the animal.

11. Corticosteroids reduce inflammation and in the process they relieve bronchoconstriction, decrease the cough associated with cough receptors stimulated by inflammation, and improve the integrity of the capillaries, reducing formation of edema from injury or inflammation. Corticosteroids also suppress part of the body's immune response; therefore corticosteroids must be used cautiously so as not to allow the pathogen (especially fungal agents) to proliferate to a greater degree. If, however, the inflammation itself is more life threatening than the underlying organism that may have set off the inflammation in the first place, then corticosteroids are indicated to help the animal survive long enough for the pathogen to be killed by other medications.

12. Diuretics can be used to reduce pulmonary edema. Because diuretics dehydrate the tissues by increasing the excretion of water (diuresis), this can result in the mucociliary apparatus becoming dryer and therefore less effective in its removal of particles that it has trapped.

13. Oxygen is a very dry gas; therefore it can dry out the mucous membranes and the mucus in the mucociliary apparatus.

Chapter 7

REVIEW QUESTIONS

1. β cells

2. Secondary hypothyroidism. Hypothyroidism caused by diseases of the thyroid is primary hypothyroidism, and hypothyroidism from a problem with the hypothalamus and lack of TRH is tertiary hypothyroidism.

3. estrus (the noun), not estrous (the adjective)

4. Drugs are exogenous compounds, meaning that they are from outside of the body.

5. follicular phase

6. luteal phase

7. goiter

8. myometrium

9. gluconeogenesis

10. carcinogenic

11. They are oral medications used to lower blood glucose in diabetic animals and people.

12. glycogenolysis

13. prostaglandin

14. TSH

15. estrogen

16. progesterone directly, estrogen by increasing the sensitivity of the uterus to progesterone

17. FSH

18. dinoprost tromethamine, cloprostenol, or fenprostalene (the prostaglandins)

19. diethylstilbestrol (DES)

20. dinoprost tromethamine (Lutalyse)

21. progesterone

22. LH

23. levothyroxine (T$_4$, tetraiodothyronine, thyroxine)

24. TSH and TRH because of the excessive amounts of T$_3$ and T$_4$ generated by the cancerous thyroid gland.

25. NPH insulin

26. regular or crystalline insulin

27. progesterone

28. estrogen

29. oxytocin

30. altrenogest (progestins, progestogens)

31. glipizide; sulfonylurea compound

32. progesterone compounds

33. TSH from the pituitary

34. T$_3$ (triiodothyronine)

35. T$_4$ (tetraiodothyronine, thyroxine)

36. GnRH

37. FSH

38. LH

39. oxytocin

40. ACTH

41. methimazole

42. ^{131}I

43. propranolol

44. megestrol acetate

45. altrenogest

46. estrogens (ECG, DES)

47. Ultralente, PZI insulin

48. dinoprost tromethamine (prostaglandin F$_{2\alpha}$)

49. dinoprost tromethamine

50. A. True. Insulin moves glucose from the blood into the cells.

    B. False. Human beings are much more sensitive to thyrotoxicosis than dogs.

    C. True.

APPLICATION QUESTIONS

1. Hormone B has the effect on the body. Hormone A simply tells gland B that the body needs more of its hormone. Thus when there is sufficient hormone B, the concentration of hormone B will inhibit gland A production of hormone A, which in turn stops stimulating gland B to produce hormone because the body has enough of hormone B.

2. In primary hypothyroidism there is a problem with the thyroid gland's ability to produce T$_3$ and T$_4$. Thus T$_3$/T$_4$ levels should be lower than normal. Because T$_3$/T$_4$ levels are lower than normal, there is not as much negative feedback from T$_4$ on the hypothalamus and pituitary. Without the negative feedback, the hypothalamus releases TRH, which in turn releases TSH, which is intended to stimulate the thyroid to produce more T$_3$/T$_4$ and to bring concentrations of these thyroid gland hormones up to their normal levels. Because the thyroid is incapable of responding, the T$_3$/T$_4$ levels stay low. In secondary hypothyroidism the thyroid is functionally fine but the pituitary gland is not producing sufficient TSH to stimulate the thyroid gland. Thus T$_3$/T$_4$ levels are low because the thyroid gland is not being stimulated. In secondary hypothyroidism T$_3$/T$_4$ levels would be low, as would be TSH levels. In tertiary hypothyroidism the hypothalamus is not producing TRH and therefore TSH levels

from the pituitary would be low and so would levels of T_3/T_4 from the thyroid gland.

3. Because the thyroid hormones control the basal metabolic rate of tissues in the body, hypothyroidism is going to reflect a slower metabolism. The skin changes in texture and thickness, the hair growth is retarded and the hair coat is thin, calories are not burned up as quickly so the animals often get fatter, and they tend to seek warmth because they are not generating as much body heat. They may be lethargic and have other clinical signs that relate to a slower metabolism (slower heart rate, mental dullness, etc.). Cats rarely become hypothyroid from natural disease. Cats are much more prone to hyperthyroidism caused by cancer of the thyroid gland. Hyperthyroid cats tend to be active, thin, tachycardic (fast heart rate), and good eaters, but have bouts of diarrhea.

4. Different body tissues have different needs for thyroid hormone. Because of that, enzymes at the tissue sites convert T_4 to the active T_3 form as needed. Using the T_4 form of medication (levothyroxine) allows the body to convert T_4 to the T_3 form in the amount needed by local tissues. If T_3 is used, dosing would have to take place according to the tissue that needs the most T_3, which means other tissues would receive more T_3 than they needed. The combination drugs of T_3/T_4 are geared towards the ideal T_3/T_4 ratio in human beings, which is quite different from the ratio in dogs. Plus the product is much more expensive than the veterinary T_4 products. For these reasons, combination T_3/T_4 products are rarely used in veterinary medicine.

5. The increase in T_3/T_4 with supplementation will cause increased gluconeogenesis (conversion of protein's amino acids to glucose), which increases blood glucose. Thus an increase in insulin dose may be required to compensate. T_3/T_4 increase the actions of catecholamines (epinephrine, norepinephrine) and thus they would increase the stimulation on the heart to beat faster and stronger. If a cardiovascular patient had arrhythmias, this increased stimulation could increase the severity of these arrhythmias.

6. Surgical removal of the cancerous portion of the thyroid, ^{131}I to kill the tumor, or control production of excessive T_3/T_4 with methimazole. Surgical removal is complete (except accessory tumors not associated with the thyroid might be missed) but it requires anesthesia and there is the risk of the parathyroid glands also being removed, resulting in poor regulation of body calcium. [131]I is effective and targets even accessory locations of the tumor, but it requires a special facility to handle radiation and a more prolonged hospital stay. Methimazole must be given daily and does not kill the tumor causing the problem. Methimazole has some potentially serious side effects that may discourage its use. Propranolol is a β blocker (see Chapter 5). By blocking the β receptors on the heart this drug normally slows the heart rate and decreases arrhythmias. Hyperthyroid cats usually exhibit tachycardia that can make them a poorer anesthetic risk if they are going to have the thyroid tumor removed. By using propranolol, or other $β_1$-blocking drugs, the veterinarian can slow the heart rate and stabilize the electrical activity of the heart.

7. Cats more often have NIDDM than dogs. Sometimes oral hypoglycemic agents such as glipizide can be used in cats with NIDDM. IDDM must be treated with injectable insulin. In NIDDM the hyperglycemia is caused by either

resistance of the insulin receptors to the effect of insulin (such as occurs in overweight human beings) or insufficient (but not absence of) insulin being produced by the β cells in the pancreas. Drugs such as glipizide can increase the amount of insulin produced by β cells and hence help the body better regulate the blood sugar. In IDDM, there are not enough functional β cells left to produce the needed insulin; therefore the insulin must be provided by injection.

8. Cats require the longer acting insulin. PZI insulin is preferred.

9. Insulin concentration is measured in units. A unit is a measure of the biologic activity of the insulin (as opposed to the mass of insulin, as measured by milligrams, grams, etc.). Because insulin in a bottle is measured by units, the syringes used for insulin are marked in units instead of cubic centimeters or milliliters. A bottle of insulin that is listed as a U-40 has 40 U per mL. U-40 bottles need to be used with U-40 syringes so the proper amount of insulin is removed from the bottle. The same applies to U-100 and U-500 designations. Because the insulin is in suspension and not in solution, the bottle has to be carefully inverted several times to mix it. The insulin molecule itself is somewhat fragile and can be broken by physical agitation (vigorous shaking).

10. Cats. If there are enough functional β cells in the pancreas left to be stimulated, this drug may work. Insulin cannot be given by mouth because it is a protein and would be readily damaged by stomach acid or digested by protein-digesting enzymes (proteases).

11. If Mr. Smith is injecting the insulin into fat tissue, which generally has a poor blood supply, the insulin may remain at the site of injection and be very poorly absorbed, essentially resulting in no insulin being delivered to the body. While the painless spot on Spot is easier for Mr. Smith, it might be detrimental to Spot's health. Clients need to understand that they should not deviate much from the injection sites and methods that you or the veterinarian has shown them. It is not a bad idea to have an owner of a poorly regulated animal demonstrate his or her technique for you on the pet so you can see exactly where and how they are injecting the insulin into the animal.

12. Estrus = noun = state of being in heat. Estrous = adjective used to describe a noun = type of cycle, as in the estrous cycle. Mucus is the noun, mucous (as with mucous membranes) is an adjective. The suffix -ous refers to an adjective.

13. DES is a potential carcinogen and using it in any animal that potentially could be used for food is illegal.

14. Dopamine agonists decrease the hormone prolactin. Prolactin normally helps maintain the function of the CL. The CL is producing progesterone, which is maintaining pregnancy. By inhibiting the CL function, progesterone is decreased and pregnancy is terminated.

15. Dexamethasone is a glucocorticoid (corticosteroid) drug. Corticosteroids may induce abortion in mares by mimicking the elevated levels of natural cortisol that occur at the beginning of parturition.

16. In the past, estrogens were used in large doses to prevent implantation of fertilized ova. Because of the high risk for potentially fatal side effects and better alternatives, estrogen can no longer be recommended in any form for preventing conception after mismating. Estrogens can no longer be recommended for

benign prostatic hyperplasia in intact male dogs. Likewise, the use of estrogens as a supplement to castration in male dogs with perianal adenomas and perianal adenocarcinomas has decreased significantly.

Chapter 8

REVIEW QUESTIONS

1. analgesics
2. sedative (a narcotic produces more profound sleep; narcosis)
3. tranquilizer
4. anesthetic
5. visceral pain
6. somatic pain
7. transduction
8. hyperalgesia
9. wind-up
10. opiates
11. opioids
12. euphoria
13. dysphoria
14. partial agonist/partial antagonist
15. mixed agonist/antagonist
16. neuroleptanalgesic
17. α_2
18. hypoproteinemic
19. compound A
20. thiopental
21. xylazine, detomidine, medetomidine
22. yohimbine, tolazoline, atipamezole
23. methohexital
24. sevoflurane
25. acepromazine
26. nitrous oxide
27. diazepam or other benzodiazepine tranquilizers
28. pentobarbital
29. halothane
30. ketamine, tiletamine
31. propofol
32. opioids
33. ketamine, tiletamine (dissociatives)
34. acepromazine
35. butorphanol
36. fentanyl
37. theobromine
38. doxapram
39. A. True.

   B. True.

   C. True.

   D. False. Opioids depress the brainstem, where the respiratory center is located. This is the reason why opioids are used for cough suppression.
40. Cattle: 10× more sensitive than equine patients.

APPLICATION QUESTIONS

1. Many sedatives do not have analgesic (pain-killing) activity. While the animal appears to be resting comfortably, as soon as you begin to move the animal, it will respond (biting, moving, vocalizing) because the sedative did nothing to

reduce the perception of pain. This is a potentially dangerous situation because the animal appears to be without pain, but is merely in a state of feeling relaxed and sleepy. A local anesthetic is not going to cover all the areas that need to be anesthetized. A general anesthetic would decrease all perception, including perception of pain for the entire body. However, a general anesthetic by itself would allow wind-up to occur in the spinal cord, and there is more of a risk of using a general anesthetic than some of the other drugs. An analgesic at doses high enough to suppress visceral pain would probably be the best choice.

2. The difference between the various barbiturate drugs is primarily their duration of activity. Thiopental is considered to be ultrashort in its duration, whereas pentobarbital is classified as a short-acting drug. Phenobarbital has a much longer duration of activity and is classified as a long-acting drug. Thiopental is the thiobarbiturate, and pentobarbital and phenobarbital are oxybarbiturates. Thiobarbiturates penetrate the blood-brain barrier better than oxybarbiturates, and because of their short duration, they are more suited for intubation with an endotracheal tube than the oxybarbiturates.

3. The reason an animal quickly becomes anesthetized with thiobarbiturates is that this drug distributes to the well-perfused tissues first (muscle, lungs, liver, kidney, and brain) but distributes much more slowly to the poorer perfused tissues such as fat. Thus, when the animal receives a bolus IV dose, it goes to sleep quickly. However, as the drug in the blood continues to distribute to the fat, the concentration in the blood decreases. When the blood concentration of barbiturate decreases below the brain concentration,

barbiturate starts to move out of the brain and into the blood following the concentration gradient for the drug. As the concentration of barbiturate decreases in the brain, the animal wakes up. Because this distribution to fat occurs over the first few minutes after the drug is given, the animal can be expected to become more and more alert over those few minutes. If the animal is "light" enough to need a second dose, the second dose needs to be smaller than the first because the drug will not be able to distribute into the fat tissue as well because the drug from the first dose has already established some concentrations within the fat (and other tissues). Thus recovery from distribution of the drug from brain to blood to fat (redistribution) will not occur as quickly.

4. Cats have a reduced ability to metabolize barbiturates. For the fat versus lean dog, it is important to remember that the initial IV bolus dose is going to go primarily to the well-perfused tissues such as the brain, and only after several minutes will the drug distribute to the fat. Therefore, in a 30-kg dog who has a large amount of fat making up his 30-kg body weight, more of the drug is going to go to the brain than in the lean dog, which has less fat. In other words, the initial dose of barbiturate should be calculated for the lean animal inside of the fat animal. That 30-kg fat dog may only need a dose equivalent for a 25-kg animal.

5. Distribution of barbiturates into fat is limited by perfusion. So is movement of the drug out of fat. Thus if the fat has become saturated with barbiturate through repeated doses being given, it will take a longer time for the fat to come back out and be eliminated/metabolized by the body. Therefore, the obese animal will take longer to recover than the lean animal.

6. Repeated exposure to barbiturates by the liver results in stimulation of the MFO system of enzymes that break down barbiturates. The liver becomes more efficient in removing the drug and thus concentrations drop more rapidly. Because the drug is broken down quicker, the dose has to be increased to produce the same effect for the same amount of time.

7. Animals often have a transient period of apnea that reflects high concentrations of barbiturate distributed to the brain after the initial bolus. This effect is seen especially with thiopental because of its high lipid solubility and easy distribution into the CNS. Fortunately, within a few minutes the initial dose of barbiturate redistributes to fat and less perfused tissues, lowering the concentration in the blood and brain, lessening CNS depression, and allowing spontaneous breathing to resume.

8. Thiopental is very irritating to tissues. Extravascular injection can result in swelling and sloughing of tissue. If thiopental is given perivascularly (around the vasculature), then the area can be infiltrated with saline or saline plus lidocaine.

9. Bigeminy, the appearance of a normal QRS wave followed by an abnormal QRS wave, is very common with many injectable anesthetic agents. Generally they spontaneously disappear within a few minutes without any significant compromise of cardiac function. If ventricular arrhythmias become severe the veterinarian can administer lidocaine IV.

10. Propofol is not a barbiturate, but is an injectable anesthetic agent that can be used for short diagnostic procedures. It has minimal analgesic activity, and therefore would not be a good choice for painful procedures such as manipulating fracture sites for radiographs. It is usually injected as an IV bolus, but does not cause tissue necrosis as thiobarbiturates do if they leak out perivascularly.

11. Propofol is dissolved in a liquid that contains protein and other substances that could support bacterial growth. Therefore it is meant to be used as a single dose and the remainder discarded.

12. Telazol is composed of a combination of dissociative anesthetic, tiletamine, plus a benzodiazepine tranquilizer, zolazepam. Ketamine is a dissociative anesthetic similar to tiletamine, whereas diazepam (Valium) is a benzodiazepine tranquilizer like zolazepam.

13. Ketamine and tiletamine do not have very good visceral analgesia. In addition, these dissociatives have poor muscle relaxation (muscle tone is often increased), making it difficult to manipulate large muscle masses (e.g., retraction of abdominal muscles, manipulation of large limb muscles).

14. The cat's eyes remain open and the corneas can dry out unless protected by a lubricant or other moisturizing agent.

15. Ketamine is very similar to phencyclidine, which is a street abuse drug. For that reason, veterinary hospitals have been broken into and bottles of ketamine stolen.

16. Speed of induction of anesthesia and recovery are fastest for sevoflurane, second fastest for isoflurane, and then halothane.

17. MAC = minimum alveolar concentration of anesthetic gas needed to produce anesthesia. Thus the lower the MAC, the lower the concentration of gas required for anesthesia, and hence the less amount of anesthetic gas needed. There is quicker onset of activity with the lower MAC gas (all else being equal).

18. Halothane sensitizes the heart (makes it more susceptible) to arrhythmias caused by epinephrine (released in frightened, excited, or nervous animals). Giving a tranquilizer before anesthesia induction will reduce the fear (fight or flight) response and hence reduce the amount of epinephrine released. This is not a problem with isoflurane or sevoflurane.

19. Malignant hyperthermia, a very high elevation in body temperature, has been associated with veterinary patients on halothane anesthesia. Its cause is not well understood and the ability to determine which patients are at risk is even less understood. Aggressive treatment with cooling the body (cold water enemas, chilled IV fluids, ice packs in the groin area, etc.) may help if given before the body temperature gets too high.

20. Halothane causes the brain vasculature to dilate, resulting in increased cranial pressure. This plus traumatic swelling could produce marked cerebral edema resulting in death of the nervous tissue in the brain.

21. Tranquilizers generally are not considered to be analgesics. Thus, while an animal appears more relaxed, it may still feel the same intensity of pain if it has only been given a tranquilizer like acepromazine. Xylazine and detomidine both have some analgesic effect in addition to their sedative effect.

22. Acepromazine blocks receptors on the CRTZ and thus blocks some of the stimulus on the CRTZ that would in turn trigger vomiting.

23. Acepromazine has a weak antihistamine effect that helps reduce vomiting from car sickness but also interferes with skin testing for allergies by blocking the histamine response to injected allergens (allergy-producing substances).

24. Benzodiazepine tranquilizers work by enhancing the effect of an inhibitory neurotransmitter called GABA. Thus, the CNS becomes more inhibited and the animal becomes more calm.

25. Benzodiazepines have neither analgesic effect nor blocking effect on the CRTZ. They do, however, provide muscle relaxation.

26. Because of the risk of hepatic (liver) failure after the administration of diazepam in cats, this drug is no longer recommended for appetite stimulation.

27. The analgesia appears to wear off before the sedation, meaning the sedated animal is capable of responding to pain after the analgesia begins to wear off. When a dose has been given and the analgesic effect has been achieved, giving additional doses does not increase the sedation as much as it just prolongs the duration of the drug. Thus, if a deeper level of analgesia is needed, a different drug would be required.

28. Xylazine sometimes produces a sudden onset of abdominal distension from increased gas in the stomach (bloat). This is especially true in deep-chested large-breed dogs and can result in bloat and possibly gastric dilatation/volvulus in which the stomach twists on itself, shutting off its blood supply. Gastric dilatation and volvulus are potentially life-threatening conditions.

29. When the α_2-agonist drug (xylazine, detomidine, medetomidine) is given, it will also stimulate α_1 receptors on the precapillary arterioles (small blood vessels going into the capillaries), where it will cause vasoconstriction. This vasoconstriction causes an increase in arterial blood pressure (heart pumps blood into the arteries but blood flow

out of the arteries into the capillaries is restricted). In response to the increased arterial blood pressure the baroreceptor stimulates the vagus nerve to slow the heart rate and bring the blood pressure down. Thus many animals on these drugs show a slower heart rate but near-normal blood pressure.

30. μ Receptors are found in the brain and spinal cord and produce strong analgesia. κ Receptors produce a milder degree of analgesia than the μ receptors. κ Receptors may be involved with the dysphoria effect. δ Receptors have some analgesia but are not thought to play a critical role in animals.

31. An opioid agonist stimulates an opioid receptor. An antagonist occupies the receptor but has no intrinsic activity (does not stimulate it); thus it blocks the agonist's receptor site. A partial agonist has some degree of intrinsic activity when combined with a receptor (it generates some cellular change) but not as much a change as some of the stronger agonists. Thus it is said to be a partial agonist. A partial agonist is often called a partial agonist/partial antagonist because if it occupies a receptor site instead of a stronger agonist, the partial agonist appears to reverse some of the effects of the stronger agonist drug. But because the partial agonist has some activity of its own on the receptor, the reversal is not complete. Thus this partial agonist is also a partial antagonist against some of the stronger agonist drugs. A mixed agonist means that the drug has effect on more than one type of opioid receptor.

32. Opioids tend to enhance the reactivity of the patient to sound.

33. Opioid drugs tend to cause dog and human pupils to constrict. In cats it causes dilation.

34. Hydromorphone and fentanyl can change the setting in the hypothalamus for body temperature, making the body's set point for temperature below normal. The result of this effect is that the body tries to lose heat to bring the body temperature down to the new set point. Panting is one mechanism by which the dog loses heat. Because panting is shallow breathing, there is not efficient oxygen/carbon dioxide exchange at the alveolus. Thus even though the animal appears to be breathing rapidly, the animal may still be accumulating carbon dioxide and not getting sufficient oxygen.

35. Bradycardia (slow heart rate) from opioids involves the parasympathetic nervous system. Therefore atropine, which blocks acetylcholine receptors in the parasympathetic nervous system, can help reverse the bradycardia and bring the heart rate back up closer to normal.

36. The ceiling effect, which is seen with several drugs, means that once the drug achieves a certain level of analgesic or other effect, adding additional drug does not increase the effect but only prolongs the existing maximal effect. The dose administered has hit the ceiling of its effect and can go no higher.

37. Because it is a highly sought-after abuse narcotic.

38. Butorphanol and buprenorphine are partial agonists/partial antagonists. Therefore although they reverse the stronger agonist effects, they provide some agonist effect of their own. Thus the animal still has some analgesia with butorphanol or buprenorphine.

39. To disinhibit is to inhibit an inhibitor. Essentially, a disinhibitor takes the brake off the CNS and allows excitatory neurotransmitters to dominate,

thus creating greater stimulation of the nervous system.

40. The LD_{50} for theobromine in dogs as listed in the text is 250 to 500 mg of theobromine per kilogram of body weight. This dog is 65 pounds (29.5 kg; make sure to convert from pounds to kilograms). Thus the LD_{50} for this particular dog would be 7500 to 15,000 mg of theobromine. LD_{50} means the dose that would be fatal to half of the animals to which it was given. The dose at which toxicity, without death, occurs is lower than this. The lowest dose at which toxicity may occur is 90 mg/kg, so for this dog 2700 mg of theobromine may cause signs of toxicity. A typical chocolate candy bar has 2 to 3 ounces of milk chocolate, which translates to about 120 to 180 mg of theobromine. If we assume most candy bars are approximately 3 oz (although they are steadily shrinking), then 180 mg of theobromine is well below the toxic dose for this size of animal. A much smaller dog getting into the same amount or getting into 3 ounces of baking chocolate might have a greater risk for toxicosis.

Chapter 9

REVIEW QUESTIONS

1. anticonvulsant
2. convulsions
3. epilepsy
4. grain
5. idiopathic epilepsy
6. status epilepticus
7. drug-induced hepatopathy
8. ictus
9. polydipsia
10. partial seizure
11. induced
12. polyphagia
13. generalized seizures
14. preictal phase or aura
15. limbic system
16. antidepressants
17. anxiolytic
18. γ-aminobutyric acid
19. phenobarbital
20. selective serotonin reuptake inhibitor; antidepressant
21. potassium bromide
22. primidone
23. diazepam
24. phenothiazine tranquilizers (acepromazine, etc.)
25. clomipramine
26. phenytoin
27. selegiline (deprenyl)
28. A. False. Phenobarbital induces its own metabolism; thus the rate at which the drug is converted to a less active form is sped up. The concentrations of phenobarbital drop quicker with induced metabolism, thus more drug would have to be given to compensate. The dose would need to be increased, not decreased.

    B. True. They metabolize phenobarbital slower than dogs who need a smaller mg per pound dose.

    C. False. This is a normal side effect of phenobarbital with many dogs.

D. False. PO administered diazepam is largely removed by the liver before it gets a chance to reach systemic circulation (first-pass effect); therefore the PO route of administration is not very effective compared with the IV route of administration.

E. False. Potassium bromide has a very long half-life of 21 to 24 days. Thus the time to reach steady state for potassium bromide is approximately 3 to 4 months (steady state = five times the half life).

F. True. Phenothiazine tranquilizers may remove learned behaviors that control aggression, allowing the natural aggressive behavior to show itself.

G. True.

H. False. Decreased dopamine is associated with senility-like syndrome in dogs; therefore drugs that increase the amount or effect of dopamine tend to reverse some of the signs associated with this syndrome.

I. True.

J. True. Behavior modification is a complex process for which drugs may help but typically are not the sole component of successful modification.

APPLICATION QUESTIONS

1. Status epilepticus, the active state of seizing, is often controlled with diazepam (Valium) administered as an IV bolus. However, although diazepam works quickly, it is also metabolized very quickly. Where the drug, disease, or chemical causing the seizure activity is likely to produce seizures for some time, either administration of diazepam by IV infusion, or IV infusion or repeated IV bolus of one of the barbiturates (phenobarbital or pentobarbital) can be used.

2. Diazepam works quickly to control seizure activity when it is administered IV. However, it is much less effective when given PO because diazepam has a very short half-life and the majority of the drug is removed by the liver before it has the opportunity to reach the systemic circulation (first-pass effect). Phenobarbital has a much longer half-life, has minimal first-pass effect, and can be conveniently given only once or twice a day.

3. Primidone metabolizes to phenobarbital plus a couple of other compounds that have weak anticonvulsant activity. But because the phenobarbital component of primidone metabolism is really what is doing the anticonvulsant activity, why not just use phenobarbital to begin with? The other problem with primidone is that there is an increased risk of drug-induced hepatopathy, a potentially fatal condition in which the liver ceases to function.

4. Generally, 250 mg of primidone is roughly equivalent to 60 mg of phenobarbital. Thus, 500 mg primidone = 120 mg of phenobarbital.

5. 1 grain = 60 mg and this dog is supposed to get ½ grain every 12 hours. Thus this dog needs 30 mg every 12 hours. Because the tablets are 15-mg tablets, this dog gets 2 of the 15-mg tablets every 12 hours.

6. Phenobarbital can have a idiosyncratic reaction that results in the animal becoming anxious and excitable. For animals having this reaction, the phenobarbital typically needs to be discontinued and an alternate anticonvulsant drug used.

7. This is classic for the tolerance a patient develops to phenobarbital. While it is possible that the underlying pathology (disease) is progressing, making it harder for the phenobarbital to control the seizures, a more likely reason for the seizures

is that the concentrations of phenobarbital are dropping. As the drug induces its own metabolism, the liver removes the drug at a faster rate. This means that the dose of drug will be changed from an active to inactive form more rapidly and the concentrations overall of active drug will drop. Once concentrations drop low enough, the seizure activity will resume. The veterinarian in this case would submit blood to determine the plasma (blood) concentrations of phenobarbital and increase the dose to get the concentrations back into the normal therapeutic range. For a review of metabolic induction, see Chapter 3.

8. It never hurts to ask if you suspect something is not quite right. In this case, an increase in serum alkaline phosphatase and alkaline phosphatase from the liver are normal when an animal is on phenobarbital, especially after therapy is initiated. As long as the other liver enzymes are not markedly elevated, it is unlikely that this represents a diseased state of the liver. In drug-induced hepatopathy all the liver enzymes are markedly increased, and there is often severe icterus (jaundice).

9. Potassium bromide has a very long half-life (approximately 3 weeks). This also means that it takes a long time for the drug to achieve its final steady-state concentration (time to achieve steady state equals five times the half-life). While the drug will begin to achieve some significant concentrations in a few days, it will take months for the drug to achieve steady-state concentrations. Thus how much of an effect this new dose of potassium bromide will have won't be known until after several weeks of therapy. Potassium bromide has a narrow therapeutic index, meaning the concentrations at which beneficial effects occur are very close to the concentrations at which toxic side effects occur. Because

loading doses are large doses of the drug, and accurately predicting what concentrations of drug will be achieved with a loading dose is impossible because of variables in the animal's physiology, giving a loading dose of KBr is considered risky. If too much drug is given, the long half-life means that the animal will be toxic for a very long time.

10. Vomiting from KBr can be reduced by dividing the daily dose into two or three daily doses (e.g., 60 mg daily dose = 30 mg b.i.d. = 20 mg t.i.d.). A liquid formulation instead of a solid formulation may reduce vomiting, as may feeding some foods with the oral administration of KBr.

11. Increased dopamine appears to contribute to abnormal behaviors by stimulation of the limbic system. Thus dopamine agonists might appear to be more likely to cause abnormal emotional behaviors. However, dopamine antagonists such as phenothiazines may also have side effects from suppression of learned behaviors.

12. Both TCAs and phenothiazine tranquilizers lower the threshold needed for seizure activity to occur. Thus seizures may increase in frequency or duration from these drugs, allowing seizures to start with less stimulation.

13. GABA is an inhibitory neurotransmitter. Thus anything that enhances GABA neurotransmitter or increases the effect of the GABA receptor will cause inhibition of parts of the CNS and hence tranquilization. A drug that blocks destruction of GABA would prolong GABA's effect and thus produce tranquilization. A drug that binds GABA receptor but doesn't stimulate it (no intrinsic activity) will act as a GABA antagonist and would cause disinhibition (allow stimulation) of the CNS. Benzodiazepine tranquilizers act by increasing stimulation of GABA receptors.

Chapter 10

REVIEW QUESTIONS

1. minimum inhibitory concentration (MIC)
2. thrombocytopenia
3. pathogens
4. spectrum of activity
5. bactericidal
6. residue
7. β-lactam ring
8. hypersensitivity
9. chelate
10. nephrotoxicosis
11. crystalluria
12. dermatophyte
13. myelosuppression
14. DNA gyrase
15. Fanconi's syndrome
16. bacteriostatic
17. leukopenia
18. sensitive
19. superinfection, suprainfection
20. ototoxic
21. keratoconjunctivitis sicca
22. culture and sensitivity
23. anaerobic
24. pyogenic
25. antibiotic
26. cross resistance
27. β-lactamase
28. resistant
29. aerobic
30. aminoglycosides
31. doxycycline and minocycline
32. sulfonamides
33. amoxicillin, ampicillin
34. enrofloxacin
35. cloxacillin, dicloxacillin, oxacillin
36. tetracycline or oxytetracycline
37. penicillins
38. amphotericin B
39. tetracycline and oxytetracycline
40. procaine
41. chloramphenicol
42. cephalosporins
43. aminoglycosides
44. quinolones
45. carbenicillin, ticarcillin, piperacillin
46. tetracycline and oxytetracycline
47. aminoglycosides: amikacin, gentamicin, neomycin, kanamycin, tobramycin, and netilmicin
48. quinolones – enrofloxacin (Baytril)
49. penicillins and cephalosporins
50. sulfasalazine (Azulfidine)
51. quinolones – enrofloxacin (Baytril)
52. sulfonamides
53. tetracyclines
54. aminoglycosides
55. griseofulvin
56. neomycin

57. tetracycline and oxytetracycline

58. penicillins and cephalosporins

59. doxycycline

60. trimethoprim and ormetoprim

61. benzathine

62. sulfonamides

63. penicillin G

64. clindamycin (Antirobe)

65. erythromycin

66. tilmicosin (Micotil)

67. metronidazole (Flagyl)

68. florfenicol (Nuflor)

69. bacitracin

70. clavulanic acid or sulbactam

71. imidazoles: ketoconazole, itraconazole, fluconazole, miconazole, clotrimazole

72. penicillins

73. A. False. Although cloxacillin is effective against β-lactamase–producing bacteria, its overall spectrum of activity is actually narrower than the aminopenicillins such as ampicillin and amoxicillin.

    B. False. Cross reactivity between all members of penicillin is too strong. A similar reaction is likely to occur with all members of the penicillin group.

    C. True.

    D. False. The key to safety with aminogly-cosides is allowing enough time between doses for the drug concentration to drop well below the therapeutic range. Giving the drug in small doses frequently does not allow concentrations to get as high as a single dose once daily, and it doesn't allow for enough time between doses for the trough concentration (lowest

concentration) to get very low before the next dose is given. Once daily doses of aminoglycosides have largely replaced the t.i.d. and even b.i.d. dosing of the drug.

E. False. Aminoglycosides are ionized at body pH; therefore they are not lipophilic and do not readily penetrate cellular membranes like the blood-brain barrier or prostate barrier.

F. True. This is why renal disease or poorly functioning kidneys result in a greater risk for aminoglycoside toxicosis.

G. False. Casts and protein reflect inflammation and injury to the renal tubules. BUN and creatinine do not begin to rise until at least 75% of the kidney function or renal tubule function has been eliminated.

H. False. The magnesium in antacids, kaolin, or bismuth in Pepto Bismol will chelate with the orally administered tetracycline.

I. True. Systemic sulfonamides are absorbed into the body; orally administered enteric sulfonamides stay in the GI tract.

J. True.

K. False. Ultramicrosized is smaller and therefore better absorbed than the microsized formulation. Because of that, you would have to use a smaller dose when switching from the microsized to the smaller ultramicrosized.

APPLICATION QUESTIONS

1. Penicillins, aminoglycosides, cephalosporins, and many other antibiotics are ionized (charged) molecules at body pH. Therefore they are hydrophilic and unable to pass through

a cellular barrier such as the blood-brain barrier or the barrier between the blood supply to the globe of the eye and the globe itself. In those cases the drug can not distribute to these sites with any significant concentration.

2. Some reactions with penicillin injections show up as skin rashes, swelling of the face, swelling of the lymph nodes, and fever. The veterinarian would want to check to see if the signs were related to the dental work and tooth extraction; and, if not, start treatment for an allergic drug reaction.

3. Bacteriostatic antimicrobials only inhibit the growth and replication of the bacteria. They largely rely on the body's immune system to help out and kill off the bacteria. If the immune system is compromised by disease, then the veterinarian needs to limit the use of antimicrobials to those that are bactericidal and will kill the bacteria outright.

4. Enrofloxacin works at a site in bacterial nucleic acids that is not found in mammalian cells. Specifically, enrofloxacin works on an enzyme (DNA gyrase) and disrupts its function. Without DNA gyrase, the bacterial DNA becomes unable to replicate. Gyrases in the mammals are very different in structure from bacterial DNA gyrases; thus enrofloxacin will not bind with the mammalian gyrase and affect mammalian cells.

5. Penicillins must have bacteria dividing to disrupt formation of cell walls in the newly formed bacteria. Bacterial colonies that are static and not dividing will not be affected by the penicillins. Many of the sulfas are bacteriostatic. Thus using these drugs together would inhibit bacterial replication and essentially render the penicillin useless. If this was a potentiated sulfonamide drug, that combination

would more likely be bactericidal. Still, there would be no need to use the potentiated sulfa with the penicillin because either one of the drugs alone (properly dosed) would kill the bacteria.

6. Both drugs are actively excreted into the urinary tract. Thus they achieve concentrations in the urine that far exceed concentrations elsewhere in the body. In a way, the body is delivering high concentrations of antibiotic directly to where the infection is located.

Chapter 11

REVIEW QUESTIONS

1. antiseptics

2. sanitizers

3. disinfectants

4. sporicidal

5. nosocomial infection

6. protozoacidal

7. biofilm

8. virucidal

9. sterilizers

10. cytotoxic

11. Naked virus. Enveloped viruses are easier to kill by disrupting the lipid envelope.

12. fungicidal

13. scrub

14. tincture

15. bactericidal

16. chlorhexidine

17. phenols

18. iodine

19. chlorine

20. quaternary ammonium compound

21. alcohol

22. iodine

23. chlorine

24. glutaraldehyde

25. A. False. Color-fast bleaches have no chlorine despite the "bleach" designation. Color-fast bleaches tend to be peroxide-based compounds (like hydrogen peroxide).

    B. False. Static agents only inhibit the pathogen or microorganism without actually killing it. To kill it requires the action of the immune system. Inanimate objects like a surgery table do not have an immune system, thus the disease-causing agents would not be killed. Disinfectants need to be microbicidal.

    C. True.

    D. False. Organic material, such as dirt, secretions, feces, and blood, often reacts with many antiseptic or disinfectants and reduces their effectiveness. Thus it is much better to scrub a site with a soap or soap/antiseptic combination to reduce the amount of organic material present prior to applying the antiseptic agent itself. This is why at least three cleanings of a surgical site with a surgical scrub compound are recommended.

    E. True. It takes several seconds or even a few minutes for the alcohol to produce a bactericidal effect. In addition, if there is dirt or organic debris at the site, most of the alcohol may be inactivated.

    F. True for the use of phenols to control gram-positive bacteria (less effective against gram-negatives). But, because the phenol residue can irritate the animal's skin with prolonged contact, the bird perch or reptile cage would have to be thoroughly rinsed of any phenol to avoid dermal irritation or ulceration.

    G. False. These two terms are often confused because they both have "hex" and "chloro" in their names. Hexachlorophene is a phenol and has a history of neurotoxicity. Chlorhexidine is a biguanide and is widely and safely used in veterinary medicine as a disinfectant and antiseptic.

    H. True. The longer acting effect of iodophors is from the slow release of iodine over time. This is less irritating, lasts longer, but will not achieve as high of a concentration of iodine as the same amount of free iodine compounds because the iodophor stretches out its release of iodine over a longer period.

APPLICATION QUESTIONS

1. Cytotoxic means the compound is toxic to cells. And the cells to which it is toxic are typically the animal's own cells. Many disinfectants can be cytotoxic at certain levels. It is therefore important to avoid use of disinfectants as antiseptics and to make sure the appropriate concentration of antiseptic is used on tissue.

2. Parvovirus is a naked virus and hence is less susceptible to antiseptics and disinfectants such as alcohol, iodine, or chlorhexidine. If any fecal material containing parvovirus were left on the thermometer, the presence of alcohol would not inactivate the virus. Potentially the virus could be introduced rectally into the next animal on which the thermometer is used.

3. Chlorines need time in contact with the parvovirus to inactivate it. A single swipe or short contact is not sufficient.

However, in the case of a metal surface, chlorine is very corrosive and can cause pitting of the metal surfaces with prolonged exposure. So the chlorine has to be left on for 3 minutes (approximately) to kill the virus but needs to be thoroughly rinsed after that to reduce corrosion.

4. The residue is likely not of high enough concentration to eliminate the virus. Second, and more importantly in this case, the residue can be very irritating to the skin. Thus the standing animal will get irritated foot pads and the recumbent animal will get skin irritation from the part of the body in contact with the chlorine residue. The chlorine needs to be thoroughly rinsed off after its application to any surface.

5. No. Peroxides are not virucidal.

6. Some of the compounds, like chlorhexidine, are precipitated and may be partially inactivated by the minerals found in "hard water" such as found in tap water.

7. Chlorhexidine and quaternary ammonium compounds may be inactivated by soaps and detergents.

8. Chlorhexidine binds to skin, oral mucous membranes, and teeth and has residual activity for several hours.

Chapter 12

REVIEW QUESTIONS

1. GABA

2. proglottids

3. nicotinic receptors

4. coccidiostats

5. mydriasis

6. antitrematodal

7. vermifuge

8. delayed neurotoxicity

9. muscarinic receptors

10. endectocides

11. acetylcholine

12. anthelmintic

13. P-glycoprotein

14. antinematodal

15. glutamate

16. emboli

17. adulticide

18. antiprotozoal

19. ectoparasites

20. hemoptysis

21. ovicidal

22. acetylcholinesterase

23. pruritus

24. anticestodal, cestocides, or taeniacides

25. microfilaricide

26. selective toxicity

27. A. imidacloprid

B. lufenuron

C. melarsomine

D. selamectin

E. milbemycin oxime

F. ivermectin

G. milbemycin oxime + lufenuron

H. fenbendazole

I. pyrantel

J. praziquantel

K. fipronil

L. nitenpyram

28. pyrethrins

29. macrolides (avermectins and milbemycins)

30. amitraz

31. ivermectin

32. piperazine

33. selamectin

34. amprolium

35. melarsomine

36. macrolides (avermectins and milbemycins)

37. organophosphates and carbamates

38. moxidectin (Cydectin in cattle, Quest in horses)

39. thiabendazole

40. ponazuril

41. ivermectin

42. fenbendazole

43. pyrantel

44. organophosphate

45. praziquantel

46. ivermectin

47. milbemycin oxime

48. imidacloprid

49. lufenuron

50. diethylcarbamazine (DEC)

51. milbemycin

52. metronidazole

53. doramectin

54. organophosphates and carbamates

55. piperonyl butoxide

56. fipronil

57. atropine

58. nitenpyram

59. pyriproxyfen

60. DEET (diethyltoluamide)

61. A. False. Microfilaria are not capable of developing into adult heartworms until they are picked up by the mosquito and molt within the mosquito. The infective larvae injected into another animal by the mosquito migrate through tissue and spend a relatively small amount of time in the blood. Also, because there are very few migrating infective larvae in the body, the chances of the infective larvae being in the blood and being taken up in a transfusion are very, very slim.

B. False. Cats with adult heartworms are not treated with adulticides, as the risk of fatal emboli and lung inflammatory reactions is too great. Thus the adult heartworms are allowed to die naturally one at a time and any inflammatory reaction is treated with corticosteroids or other medications.

C. False. Lacrimation (tear production).

D. False. It is an inhibitory neurotransmitter. Stimulation of the glutamate receptor inhibits the nervous system, and blocking glutamate's effect allows domination of excitatory neurotransmitters.

E. True.

62. collie

APPLICATION QUESTIONS

1. Atropine is always the first drug of choice. Atropine will block the muscarinic acetylcholine receptors and

reverse the SLUDDE signs. This reduces the respiratory secretions and helps bronchodilate the airways, thus reducing dyspnea. Glycopyrrolate is also a drug that acts similar to atropine and is used as a preanesthetic agent like atropine. However, glycopyrrolate does not penetrate the blood-brain barrier as readily and therefore will not produce a significant reversal of OP toxicosis signs in the brain compared with atropine. The other drug used is 2-PAM. This drug does not block the acetylcholine receptor like atropine but actually pulls the organophosphate molecule away from the acetylcholinesterase enzyme molecule to allow the acetylcholinesterase to begin working again.

2. Praziquantel (Droncit) is given to eliminate tapeworms. Because it breaks down the tapeworm's ability to protect itself against intestinal enzymes, the worm is digested and does not appear in the stool.

3. While the dead adult heartworms are breaking down, large chunks of these worms may float down the bloodstream from the heart and lodge in the lungs, where they can cause pulmonary emboli and severe inflammation that can potentially kill the dog. If the dog exercises or gets really excited and the heart beats more rapidly and forcefully, there is a greater chance of a large chunk of worm breaking off and causing this severe reaction. While this is more likely to occur during the first 2 weeks after adulticide therapy, these reactions can occur up to 4 to 6 weeks after adulticide therapy.

4. Diethylcarbamazine was known to produce a potentially severe reaction in approximately 20% of dogs that had adult heartworms. This type of reaction is not seen with the macrolide heartworm preventatives. There may be a reaction ranging from diarrhea to even a mild shocklike syndrome in heartworm-positive dogs put on once-a-month heartworm preventatives; however, these reactions are rare.

5. Although pyrethrins and pyrethroids have selective toxicity and are quite safe in mammals when properly used, fish unfortunately readily absorb pyrethrins and do not have the enzymes to break these products down very efficiently. Therefore all the fish (and perhaps the amphibians) may be at risk from exposure to the fogger. It might be better to use a directed premise spray on problem areas instead of using a fogger.

6. Amitraz has been reported to cause illness and even death if ingested by pets or children. Often flea and tick collars have excess length that needs to be trimmed off to properly fit the collar to the pet. The soft, chewable material of the collar makes it attractive to teething children or chewing pets. It is extremely important that these trimmed parts are disposed of in a way that prevents children or other pets from having access to them.

7. Amitraz inhibits the enzyme MAO. Certain behavior modification drugs are also MAOIs. Thus the combined MAO inhibiting effects of both drugs could have significant side effects (CNS stimulation, hyperactivity, behavioral disturbances, etc.). The use of TCAs and SSRIs should also be avoided when amitraz is being used.

8. All these compounds only prevent the immature stages of fleas from progressing. They are not effective in killing the already existing population of adult fleas. Thus the owner needs to use a flea adulticide drug along with these products to provide immediate relief from the biting of the adult fleas living on the pet.

Chapter 13

REVIEW QUESTIONS

1. glucocorticoids

2. thromboxanes

3. alopecia

4. humoral immunity

5. renal papillary necrosis

6. leukotrienes

7. autoimmune reactions

8. neutrophilia

9. catabolic effects

10. B-lymphocytes

11. cortex

12. Cushing's syndrome

13. cyclooxygenase

14. eicosanoids

15. eosinopenia

16. Addison's disease

17. glycogenesis

18. corticotropin-releasing factor

19. monocytopenia

20. atrophy

21. hyperadrenocorticism

22. hypoadrenocorticism

23. iatrogenic

24. aldosterone

25. lipoxygenase

26. mineralocorticoids

27. gluconeogenesis

28. lymphopenia

29. propionic acid

30. cell-mediated immunity

31. prostaglandins

32. arachidonic acid pathway

33. T-lymphocytes

34. ACTH (adrenocorticotropic hormone)

35. tepoxalin

36. hyaluronic acid

37. triamcinolone

38. phenylbutazone

39. carprofen (Rimadyl)

40. prednisolone, methylprednisolone, triamcinolone

41. DMSO

42. hydrocortisone

43. etodolac (EtoGesic), deracoxib (Deramaxx), and meloxicam (Metacam)

44. dexamethasone

45. aspirin

46. ibuprofen, ketoprofen, naproxen

47. flunixin meglumine

48. PSGAGs

49. prednisone

50. glucosamine and chondroitin sulfate

51. acetaminophen

52. A. False. Acetate, diacetate, pivalate, or valerate extensions on drugs such as dexamethasone identify it as suspension formulation. Although an aqueous solution drug can be given IV, a suspension must never be given IV.

B. False. B-lymphocyte responses are not suppressed by normal doses of glucocorticoids. B-lymphocytes are responsible for producing antibodies.

C. False. Less blood protein means less protein for the NSAIDs to bind to in the blood. Thus more of the NSAID molecules are available in the free form to distribute to the tissues. If anything, the dose would have to be decreased to compensate for a greater percentage of the drug being able to get to the target tissues.

D. False. Kidney (renal papillary necrosis) and GI tract (ulcerations). Although the liver is listed as a target organ for some COX-2 selective toxicities, these are fairly rare incidences.

E. False. NSAIDs are not true analgesics in that they do not reduce the perception of pain at the brain level to any great degree. An opioid analgesic is needed for this type of procedure.

53. A. No. That would be a mineralocorticoid effect.

B. Yes.

C. Yes.

D. Yes. This is why fungal diseases and other pathogens normally killed or suppressed by cell-mediated immunity can get worse when on glucocorticoid drugs.

E. Yes. Decreased fibroblasts decrease the amount of scar tissue laid down.

F. No. It affects primarily T-lymphocyte activity and cell-mediated immunity; much less so for antibody formation.

G. Lymphocytosis is an increased number of lymphocytes. Glucocorticoids cause lymphopenia.

H. No. Glucocorticoids cause eosinopenia and monocytopenia.

I. Yes.

J. Yes.

54. Prostaglandins increase mucus production, increase sodium bicarbonate secretion, and increase the rate at which GI epithelial cells turn over and the GI tract wall repairs itself; thus NSAIDs that block these prostaglandins will decrease mucus and bicarbonate secretion and slow healing of the GI tract wall. This is what predisposes the GI tract to ulcers when nonselective COX inhibiting NSAIDs are used.

APPLICATION QUESTIONS

1. Glucocorticoids increase gluconeogenesis (increased amino acid conversion to glucose), which can increase the amount of glucose in the blood. In diabetics, there is a decreased amount of insulin hormone present, and without insulin glucose cannot move from the blood into the cells (with the exception of nervous system cells). Thus more glucose in the blood from glucocorticoid drugs could increase the blood glucose in a diabetic animal. This increase may not necessarily be clinically significant with short-term use of intermediate-acting glucocorticoids.

2. The tumor is producing glucocorticoids regardless of whether the adrenal gland is being stimulated to do so. Thus the adrenal gland is expected to produce massive amounts of cortisol. Because the cortisol levels are so high, there is a significant amount of negative feedback on the hypothalamus and pituitary to stop secretions of CRF and ACTH. Thus CRF and ACTH levels would be very low. This condition is either hyperadrenocorticism or Cushing's syndrome.

3. This is hyperadrenocorticism caused by administration of the dexamethasone.

The administration of drug results in cortisol-like effects and thus the clinical signs of iatrogenic Cushing's are seen. This condition would be called iatrogenic hyperadrenocorticism because it is caused by the physician or the medication and not by a tumor on the adrenal gland. Like natural cortisol, dexamethasone also suppresses the activity of the pituitary and hypothalamus. Therefore, CRF and ACTH would both be decreased below normal. Although this animal is showing signs of iatrogenic Cushing's, dexamethasone should not be stopped immediately because the animal may be thrown into a state of hypoadrenocorticism because of atrophy of the adrenal gland. The atrophy of the adrenal gland is caused by ACTH release being suppressed by the dexamethasone and thus blocking any ACTH stimulation of the adrenal gland. Without stimulation, the adrenal gland atrophies. If dexamethasone is stopped immediately, the levels of dexamethasone would decrease but the atrophied adrenal gland would not be able to respond to the increased need for natural cortisol to take its place. The net effect would be below-normal levels of glucocorticoids. This is Addison's disease or hypoadrenocorticism. Instead of stopping the dexamethasone immediately, the dose of dexamethasone needs to be tapered off over 2 to 3 weeks until the animal is weaned completely off the drug.

4. A COX-2 inhibitor is more selective for decreasing the production of inflammatory prostaglandins than a drug such as aspirin that suppresses both COX-2 and COX-1 enzymes. The COX-1 enzyme produces prostaglandins that are required for normal functions such as maintaining local blood flow (kidneys) or for maintaining the normal health of the stomach and intestinal wall. Because aspirin blocks both COX-1 (enzyme that produces helpful eicosanoids) and COX-2 (enzyme that produces prostaglandins that are associated with inflammation), the aspirin may compromise the health of the GI tract and increase the risk for ulcer formation. Although they are more expensive, selective COX-2 inhibitors tend to be safer at normal doses than aspirin because they block inflammatory prostaglandin formation while still allowing the healthy prostaglandins to be formed by COX-1 enzymes.

5. The use of NSAIDs or other analgesics before surgery is to decrease the amount of pain signals being sent up the spinal cord to the brain from the pain receptors around the site of the surgical procedure and bone manipulation. When many pain signals are sent up the spinal cord, the neurons in the spinal cord change and over time will more readily send pain signals to the brain with less stimulation from the pain receptors. This is the process called windup and it contributes significantly to the pain felt after the surgical procedure. By using NSAIDs (the aspirinlike compound) to decrease inflammation, decrease pain receptors depolarizing, and decrease the wind-up process, the perception of pain by the brain after surgery can be significantly reduced.

6. DMSO can penetrate the skin and also carry toxins or other chemicals into the skin with it. Always wear good-quality gloves when applying this compound topically.

7. This client needs to understand that aspirin is not Tylenol, which is not ibuprofen, which is not Aleve, and so forth. This is a common misperception by the public. The only safe one of these

drugs for use in the cat is aspirin. Aspirin has to be used at a lower dose than for dogs because of the slow metabolism of cats, but it can still be safely used at the "baby" aspirin dose every 2 days. Acetaminophen, on the other hand, is converted by the cat liver into a toxic substance. Unfortunately, the cat's liver does not have much of the necessary compound available to convert the toxic substance into a nontoxic substance. Thus cats can die from accumulation of the toxic metabolite of acetaminophen.

8. Typically the acetaminophen metabolite causes changes in the red blood cells that result in hemolysis and changes in the hemoglobin so that the mucous membranes appear chocolate-colored. The urine also turns black because of the hemolysis of the red blood cells and excretion of the methemoglobin. The face of a cat with acetaminophen toxicosis will often swell. Treatment is acetylcysteine, which provides the materials the liver needs to convert the toxic metabolite to a nontoxic metabolite.

Index